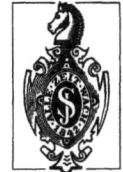

Modern Neurosurgery 1

Edited by M. Brock

With 158 Figures and 95 Tables

Springer-Verlag
Berlin Heidelberg GmbH 1982

Prof. Dr. Mario Brock
Abteilung für Neurochirurgie
Neurochirurgische/Neurologische Klinik und Poliklinik
Universitätsklinikum Steglitz, Freie Universität Berlin
Hindenburgdamm 30, D-1000 Berlin 45

ISBN 978-3-662-08803-6   ISBN 978-3-662-08801-2 (eBook)
DOI 10.1007/978-3-662-08801-2

© Springer-Verlag Berlin Heidelberg 1982
Originally published by Springer-Verlag Berlin Heidelberg New York in 1982

2122/3140-543210

Preface

More than 800 papers were presented by neurosurgeons from 66 countries during the 7th International Congress of Neurological Surgery, held in Munich on 12–18 July 1981. With the present scope and problems of neurosurgery as its theme, the congress achieved its aims in making possible the exchange and dissemination of new knowledge and ideas and in facilitating personal contact between neurosurgeons from all parts of the world. Of such importance are the regional differences within our branch of science that we should spare no effort in acquainting ourselves with those neurosurgical problems which lie beyond the boundaries of our local horizons.

From the vast number of papers the editor has selected those whose high scientific standard merits greater exposure than that given by the conference itself. I should like to thank the editor for his work and Springer-Verlag for their involvement in our discipline. It is to be hoped that this book will find a worldwide audience, in accordance with the intentions of the World Federation of Neurosurgical Societies.

Prof. Dr. K.-A. Bushe
President of the Congress

Editor's Preface

This is the first volume of a new series which aims to provide an overview of the state of the art of neurosurgery every four years. It will contain papers covering various fields of our specialty, selected from among those presented at each International Congress of Neurological Surgery.

Modern Neurosurgery is meant to be more than just a book of proceedings: We hope that it will become a reference volume. Rather than being a mere chronicle, it should enable future generations to evaluate the progress of neurosurgery.

With full approval of the Executive and the Administrative Councils of the World Federation of Neurosurgical Societies (WFNS), another important function of *Modern Neurosurgery* has become possible: to introduce our specialty as practiced nowadays to medical students in selected countries. For this purpose the WFNS is donating copies of this volume to 200 libraries of medical schools in selected countries in all continents. We hope that this new practice will become a tradition in the future.

I wish to express my appreciation to all authors for their cooperation and especially to Charles Langmaid, who has been responsible for the hard task of language editing. The technological support provided by Springer-Verlag has contributed significantly to the quality and speed of publication.

The WFNS hopes that *Modern Neurosurgery* fulfils its ambitious goals and expectations.

Prof. Dr. Mario Brock
Editor of Congress Publications

Contents

Chemotherapy of Brain Tumours

Surgery of the Pituitary Region

Surgery of Ventricular Tumours

Spinal Cord

Reconstructive Vascular Surgery

Vasospasm

Aneurysm Surgery

Functional Neurosurgery

List of Senior Authors

Áfra, D.: National Institute of Neurosurgery, Amerikai út 57, H-1145 Budapest, Hungary

Antunes, J.L.: Department of Neurological Surgery, College of Physicians and Surgeons of Colombia University, 710 West 168th Street, New York, NY 10032, USA

Brandt, L.: Department of Neurosurgery, University Hospital, University of Lund, S-221 85 Lund, Sweden

Chehrazi, B.: Section of Neurosurgery, Department of Surgery, Yale University, School of Medicine, 333 Cedar Street, New Haven, CT 06510, USA

Costal, M.: Instituto de Enfermedades Nerviosas, San Lorenzo 139, 4000 – S.M. De Tucman, Argentina

Dean, D.F.: Department of Neurological Surgery, College of Medicine, University of South Alabama, 2451 Fillingim Street, Mobile, AL 36617, USA

Deruty, R.: Hôpital Neurologique, Hospices Civils de Lyon, 59, Boulevard Pinel Lyon 3^e, B.P. Lyon Montchat, F-69394 Lyon Cedex 3, France

Fornari, M.: Divisione di Neurochirurgia, Istituto Neurologico "C. Besta", Via Celoria 11, I-20133 Milano, Italy

Friedrich, H.: Abteilung für Neurochirurgie, Medizinische Hochschule Hannover, Karl-Wiechert-Allee 9, D-3000 Hannover 61, Germany

Frowein, R.A.: Neurochirurgische Universitätsklinik, Joseph-Stelzmann-Strasse 9, D-5000 Köln 41, Germany

Fujita, Y.: Department of Neurosurgery, Kurashiki Central Hospital, Miwa 1–1, Kurashiki-City, Okayama 710, Japan

Grisoli, F.: Service de Neurochirurgie, C.H.U. Timone, 264, Rue Saint-Pierre, F-13385 Marseille Cedex 4, France

Guarnaschelli, J.J.: Department of Neurological Surgery, University of Louisville, School of Medicine, 568 Medical Towers South, Floyd & Gray Streets, Louisville, KY 40202, USA

Hashi, K.: Department of Neurosurgery, Kitano Hospital, 13—3 Kamiyama-cho, Kita-Ku, Osaka 530, Japan

Hatanaka, H.: Department of Neurosurgery, Teikyo University Hospital, 2—11—1 Kaga, Itabashi-ku, Tokyo 173, Japan

Higuchi, H.: Iwate Central Hospital, 1—1 Honcho Dori, Morioka 020, Japan

Ito, Z.: Department of Surgical Neurology, Research Institute for Brain and Blood Vessels, 6—10, Senshu-kubota-machi, Akita 010, Japan

Kadoya, S.: Department of Neurosurgery, Kanazawa Medical University, Uchinada-cho, Kahoku-gun, Ishikawa-ken 920—02, Japan

Kassell, N.F.: Department of Surgery, The University of Iowa Hospitals and Clinics, Iowa City, IA 52243, USA

Koos, W.Th.: Neurochirurgische Universitätsklinik, Alserstrasse 4, A-1097 Wien, Austria

Kuramoto, S.: Department of Neurosurgery, Kurume University Hospital, 67 Asahi-machi, Kurume 830, Japan

Kuroiwa, T.: Department of Neurosurgery, Tokyo Medical and Dental University, 1—5—45, Yushima, Bunkyo-ku, Tokyo, Japan

Lassen, N.A.: Department of Clinical Physiology, Bispebjerg Hospital, DK-2400 Copenhagen N.V., Denmark

Laws, E.R., Jr.: Department of Neurosurgery, Mayo Medical School, Mayo Clinic, 200 First Street SW, Rochester, MN 55905, USA

Lifson, A.: Institute for Low Back Care, 2727 Chicago Avenue, Minneapolis, MN 55407, USA

Lin, D.-K.: Neurosurgery Department, Affiliated Hospital, Nantung Medical College, Nantung, Jiangsu Province, People's Republic of China

Lobato, R.D.: Servicio de Neurocirurgia, Ciudad Sanitaria "1⁰ de Octubre", Carretera Andalucia KM. 5,400, Madrid, Spain

Masuzawa, H.: Department of Neurosurgery, The Kanto Teishin Hospital, 5-Chome, Higashigotanda 5—9—22, Shinagawa-ku, Tokyo 141, Japan

Nadjmi, M.: Abteilung für Neuroradiologie in der Kopfklinik der Universität Würzburg, Josef-Schneider-Strasse 11, D-8700 Würzburg, Germany

Nashold, B.S.: Division of Neurosurgery, Duke Medical Center, Durham, NC 27710, USA

Newcombe, R.L.G.: Department of Neurosurgery, Royal Canberra Hospital, Acton, A.C.T., 2601, Australia

Nugent, G.R.: Department of Neurosurgery, School of Medicine, Medical Center, West Virginia University, Morgantown, WV 26506, USA

Nukui, H.: Department of Neurosurgery, Gunma University, School of Medicine, 3–39–22, Showa-machi, Maebashi, Gunma 371, Japan

Olteanu-Nerbe, V.: Abteilung für Neurochirurgie, Klinikum Grosshadern, Universität München, Marchioninistrasse 15, D-8000 München 70, Germany

Philippon, J.: Service de Neurochirurgie, Hôpital de la Salpétrière, Boulevard de l'Hôpital, F-75634 Paris Cedex 13, France

Plotkin, R.: 3 Wycombe Medical Mews, 25 Bruce Street, Hillbrow 2001, Johannisburg, South Africa

Price, D.J.: Pinderfields Hospital, Aberford Road, GB-Wakefield WFI 4DG, Great Britain

Rand, R.W.: Department of Surgery/Neurosurgery, UCLA School of Medicine, Los Angeles, CA 90024, USA

Ray, Ch.D.: Department of Neurosurgery, The Low Back Clinic, Sister Kenny Institute, University of Minnesota, 2727, Chicago Avenue, Minneapolis, MN 55407, USA

Richardson, D.E.: Department of Neurological Surgery, Tulane University, School of Medicine, 1430 Tulane Avenue, New Orleans, LA 70112, USA

Rosenblum, M.L.: Brain Tumor Research Center of the Department of Neurological Surgery, School of Medicine, 786 HSE, University of California, 350 Parnassus Avenue, San Francisco, CA 94134, USA

Saito, I.: Fuji Noken, 270–12, Sugita, Fujinomiya, Shizuoka 418, Japan

Salar, G.: Istituto di Neurochirurgia, Universita, Ospedale Civile di Padova, Unita Sanitaria Local N. 21, Via Giustiniani 5, I-35100 Padova, Italy

Salem, F.A.: 39, Speak Close, Pinders Heath, GB-Wakefield WFI 4TG, Great Britain

Sambasivan, M.: Medical College, Trivandrum, 695011 Kerala, India

Shigeno, T.: Abteilung für Neurochirurgie, Neurochirurgische/Neurologische Klinik und Poliklinik, Universitätsklinikum Steglitz, Freie Universität Berlin, Hindenburgdamm 30, D-1000 Berlin 45, Germany

Sukoff, M.H.: Neurological Surgery, Western Medical Center, (Santa Ana-Tustin Comm.), 801 North Tustin Avenue, Suite 406, Santa Ana, CA 92705, USA

Symon, L.: Gough Cooper Department of Neurological Surgery, Institute of Neurology, Queen Square, GB-London WC1N 3BG, Great Britain

Teasdale, G.: Department of Neurosurgery, Institute of Neurological Sciences, The Southern General Hospital, University of Glasgow, GB-Glasgow G51 4TF, Great Britain

Teramoto, A.: Department of Neurosurgery, Faculty of Medicine, University of Tokyo & University of Tokyo Hospital, 7–3–1 Hongo, Bunkyo-ku, Tokyo 113, Japan

van Veelen, C.W.M.: Department of Neurosurgery, State University Hospital, Catharijnesingel 101, NL-3500 CG Utrecht, The Netherlands

Vlahovitch, B.: Service de Neurochirurgie, Centre Gui de Chauliac, F-34000 Montpellier, France

Weizsäcker, M.:Neuropathologisches Institut, Universität Düsseldorf, Moorenstrasse 5, D-4000 Düsseldorf 1, Germany

Winn, H.R.: Department of Neurosurgery, School of Medicine, University of Virginia, Charlottesville, VA 22908, USA

Yamamoto, I.: Department of Neurosurgery, Nagoya University, School of Medicine, 65 Tsuruma-cho, Schowa-ku, Nagoya 466, Japan

TECHNICAL DEVELOPMENTS

^{68}Ga-EDTA Positron Emission Tomography in Cases with Brain Tumour

H. Nukui, L.Y. Yamamoto, Ch. Thompson, and W. Feindel

Introduction

Since the first report by Moore in 1948, external counting with radioactive materials for localization of various intracranial lesions has proved a useful screening test. The technique is simple to perform, noninvasive, repeatable at short intervals and has high diagnostic accuracy. Gamma-ray emitting radionuclides have usually been used to locate intracranial lesions, but since 1951 positron emitting radionuclides have also been employed. With recent refinements of both hardware and analytical method, the system for transaxial reconstruction tomography using the positron annihilation coincidence detecting principle has been further developed to take advantage of depth-independent and depth-equal responses by back-to-back emission of 511 KeV gamma rays.

At the Montreal Neurological Institute, positron emission tomography using ^{77}Kr and ^{68}Ga-EDTA has been performed since 1975. In particular, this technique has proved most useful for prognostic evaluation and understanding of basic pathology of intracranial lesions (9, 10). In addition, it is a useful screening test for detection of intracranial tumours.

In this report, results of positron emission tomography using ^{68}Ga-EDTA (^{68}Ga PET) in intracranial tumours are compared with those of radionuclide cerebral image study with ^{99m}Tc-pertechnetate (^{99m}Tc study) and X-ray transmission tomography (X-ray CT) with or without intravenous infusion of contrast medium. Also discussed in this report are special methods such as coronal section static study and tumour uptake kinetic study of ^{68}Ga PET, recently refined in our institute to diagnose intracranial lesions with greater exactitude.

Methods

^{68}Ga PET was performed with Positome II and III in the Montreal Neurological Institute. Positome II had 64 bismuth germanate scintillation detector in a ring of 43 cm in diameter. Positome III, by which three slices of tomographic images can be obtained simultaneously, has 2 ring of the same detector system. The characteristics of Positome III are shown in Table 1. ^{68}Ga-EDTA was eluted from the commercially available ^{68}Ge-^{68}Ga generator. After rapid injection of 1 to 3 mci of ^{68}Ga-EDTA into the anticubital vein, transit time study and immediate horizontal static study at the same level were performed.

Table 1. Characteristics of positome III

No. of detectors: 64 x 2	Efficiency:
Detector type: Trapezoidal bismuth germanate	Outer slice: 110,000 (c/sec) (μci/ml)
No. of slices: 3	Center slice: 200,000 (c/sec) / (μci/ml)
Slice width:	Energy discrimination: 350 – 650 KeV
Outer slice: $21^{\pm}1$ mm	Coincidence resolving time: 13nsec
Center slice: $24^{\pm}5$ mm	Spatial resolution (20 cm field)
	Normal (FWHM): 15 mm
	With 5 point precession: 8 mm

Transit time was calculated by analysis of the down slope rate of radioactivity per 0.5 x 0.5 cm^2 cross-section of the head. Serial 7 tomographic horizontal image study at every 0.5 to 1.5 cm interval was performed by moving the bed, more than 15 minutes after the injection. Recently, the coronal section study was carried out simultaneously with the horizontal study: in selected cases a tumour uptake kinetic study was also performed. In the latter test, static studies at the same level of the brain were performed at 5 minutes intervals for 60 minutes after the injection of ^{68}Ga-EDTA. Sequential changes of isotope accumulation in the lesion, corrected by the time decay of the isotope, were presented in the graphic mode.

^{99m}Tc study was performed in the anterior view using a scintillation camera with the computer, following the intravenous bolus injection of ^{99m}Tc-pertechnetate in doses ranging from 15 to 18 mCi. The sequential cerebral image study was carried out immediately following the injection, and again 1 to 3 hours later.

X-ray CT was performed using EMI 1005 with or without intravenous infusion of a contrast medium.

Cases

Studies were carried out in 16 brain tumour cases. Of these studies 13 were performed as the pre-operative screening test on patients with seizures (6 cases), progressively increased neurological deficits (6 cases), and blackout episodes (1 case). In 3 patients the tests were done as part of the postoperative followup study.

The pathological diagnosis in all 16 cases was confirmed by histological examinations obtained during surgery. Of the tumours 7 were meningioma, 5 gliomas (3 glioblastomas, 1 astrocytoma, (Grade 2) and 1 oligodendroglioma), 3 metastatic tumours, and 1 was a lipoma.

Results

Results of the studies involving detection and localization of brain tumours are summarized in Table 2.

^{68}Ga static study revealed significant focal uptake in all cases except the 1 lipoma. All cases showed focal uptake: abnormal accumulation of the isotope was clearly seen in the later study than in the immediate one.

^{99m}Tc static study also showed abnormal focal uptake in 14 out of 16 cases. X-ray CT with and without infusion revealed abnormal findings in all 16 cases.

In seven cases with meningioma, ^{68}Ga study revealed very clearly a significant focal uptake which was homogeneous and round or oval-shaped (Fig. 1). ^{99m}Tc study showed round-shaped focal uptake in six cases, and no focal uptake in one case with parasellar meningioma. X-ray CT without intravenous infusion of contrast medium showed: an area of slightly higher than normal density, with or without asymmetry of the CSF spaces in four cases, a large calcified mass with mild shift of the midline structure in one case, hyperostosis with asymmetry of the cistern in one case, and the enlargement of the lateral and third ventricles only in one case. In three out of seven cases, changes in brain density associated with the tumour itself or concomitant displacement and deformity of the CSF spaces was very slight; accordingly, detection of the lesions was relatively difficult by X-ray CT. X-ray CT with infusion of 100 ml of 60% Hypaque clearly showed a well-circumscribed high density area in all seven cases.

In five cases with glioma, ^{68}Ga static PET revealed significant focal uptake. In two cases with glioblastoma, local uptake was "doughnut" shaped, in the other three cases it was irregular in outline. The abnormal uptake was better defined in cases with glioblastomas than in cases with benign gliomas, and in the later study than in immediate one (Fig. 2).

Table 2. Results of static studies in 16 cases with brain tumour

	Meningioma	Glioma	Metastasis	Lipoma	Total
^{68}Ga PET	7/7[a]	5/5	3/3	0/1	15/16
^{99m}Tc study	6/7	5/5	3/3	0/1	14/16
X-ray CT	7/7	5/5	2/2	1/1	15/15

[a] Positive/total cases

^{99m}Tc static study showed "doughnut" shaped focal uptake in one case with glioblastoma and irregular-shaped focal uptake in the four other cases.

X-ray CT without infusion, performed in four cases, revealed an irregular-shaped high density area in one case with glioblastoma, a hypodense area with a slight shift of the lateral ventricle in one case with glioblastoma, a large calcified mass in a case with oligodendroglioma, and a low density area only in one case with a benign astrocytoma. X-ray CT with infusion, carried out in all five cases, showed a high density area in four cases with glioblastoma and oligodendroglioma, and a patchy, ill-defined high density area surrounded by a low density zone in one case with benign astrocytoma.

In three cases with metastatic tumours, in which the primary lesions were oat-cell carcinoma, hypernephroma, and of unknown origin, ^{68}Ga static PET showed significant focal uptake that was homogeneous and of irregular shape in all three cases. ^{99m}Tc static study revealed abnormal focal uptake in all three cases. X-ray CT without infusion revealed in one case a high density area, markedly enhanced by infusion of contrast medium, combined with a large low density zone, and in one case a large low density area only, in which a patchy, ill-defined zone of increased density was disclosed after injection of contrast medium.

In one case with intracranial lipoma, ^{68}Ga PET and ^{99m}Tc study showed no significant abnormal findings, but X-ray CT without infusion revealed multiple well-circumscribed low density areas.

3

Positome III was recently used in some cases for a coronal section study of ^{68}Ga PET and tumour uptake kinetic sutdy. Those tests gave precise information regarding characteristics of uptake patterns in the lesions and the possibility of predicting tumour pathology.

The results of haemodynamic studies are summarized in Table 3. In 13 cases ^{68}Ga dynamic PET revealed reduction of cerebral perfusion at the tumour site and/or at areas remote from the tumour, in one case with metastatic tumour the test showed an increase of perfusion at the tumour site and reduction of perfusion at areas remote from the tumour. In two cases the study revealed normal cerebral perfusion with meningioma and lipoma. Haemodynamic changes shown by ^{68}Ga PET correlated with X-ray CT results and neurological findings. Haemodynamic changes were more extensive in cases with brain oedema and cerebral atrophy as revealed by X-ray CT, and in cases with neurological deficits than in cases without these findings (Table 4).

Table 3. Results in dynamic study in 16 cases with brain tumour

	Normal	Abnormal	Total
^{68}Ga PET	2	14	16
^{99m}Tc study	4	12	16

Table 4. Results of ^{68}Ga dynamic study and X-ray CT in 14 cases with brain tumour

	X-ray CT			
	Enlargement of CSF cavity	Perifocal LDA	Enlargement of CSF cavity + LDA	Total
^{68}Ga Dynamic Study				
Normal	1	0	0	1
Abnormal	2	4	7	13
Localized	2	1	0	3
Diffuse	0	3	7	10
Total	3	4	7	14

LDA = low density area

^{99m}Tc dynamic study revealed abnormal findings in 12 out of 16 cases. In six out of the seven with meningioma cases, ^{68}Ga study showed marked reduction of cerebral perfusion at the tumour site and normal perfusion in one case with a small parasagittal meningioma in which the dynamic study was carried out below the tumour level. Reduction of perfusion was disclosed at the tumour site only in two cases, and at areas remote from as well as at the tumour site in four cases. In one case with marked mental retardation and gait disturbance, diffuse reduction of the perfusion in both cerebral hemispheres was particularly noticeable (Fig. 3).

^{99m}Tc dynamic study revealed early progressive increased radioactivity in the same area as focal uptake shown in the static study as well as reduction of perfusion in the affected cerebral hemisphere in three cases, reduction of the perfusion in only one case, and no significant abnormal findings in three cases.

In five cases with gliomas, ^{68}Ga dynamic PET showed marked reduction of cerebral perfusion at the tumour site and areas remote from the tumour in four cases with glioblastoma and recurrent oligodendroglioma, and only at the tumour site in one case with a benign astrocytoma. ^{99m}Tc dynamic study also revealed in all five cases reduction of the perfusion in the large portion of the affected cerebral hemisphere and progressive increased radioactivity at the tumour site in one case with glioblastoma.

In three cases with metastatic brain tumour, ^{68}Ga dynamic study showed marked reduction of perfusion at the tumour site as well as in areas remote from the tumour site and reduced perfusion at areas remote from the tumour in one case.

^{99m}Tc dynamic study showed reduction of cerebral perfusion in the affected cerebral hemisphere in all three cases.

In one case with lipoma, two studies showed no significant abnormal findings.

Discussion

Recently reported PET studies concerning regional cerebral haemodynamics and metabolism have increased our understanding of the physiochemical function of the normal brain and pathophysiology of various disease (1, 3, 6-8). However, there have been few reports about positron emission tomography capacity for detecting and localizing brain tumours (2, 4, 5).

PET with Positome II and III, using ^{68}Ga-EDTA, was performed in 16 cases with brain tumour. The results of ^{68}Ga PET were compared with findings of ^{99m}Tc study and X-ray CT.

The three techniques were of roughly equal accuracy in detecting tumours, at least in cases of meningioma, glioma and metastatic tumours. But ^{68}Ga PET often showed clearer and more precise localization and haemodynamic information than ^{99m}Tc study as previously reported, particularly when a combination of horizontal and coronal section studies of ^{68}Ga PET was used.

Furthermore, ^{68}Ga PET frequently showed the lesions more clearly than X-ray CT without intravenous infusion of contrast medium, in cases with meningioma, benign glioma and metastatic tumours. The former revealed the lesion itself as a focal uptake of ^{68}Ga-EDTA: the latter often showed only indirect evidence of the tumour, such as displacement of intracranial structures such as CSF cavities, or associated brain oedema. In comparing ^{68}Ga PET to X-ray CT with intravenous infusion of contrast medium, there was no noticeable difference in diagnostic accuracy for detecting meningioma, glioma and metastatsis. However, X-ray CT with the infusion was superior in localizing the lesion as compared with ^{68}Ga PET, because it gave more accurate information regarding the anatomical relationship between the tumour and the neighbouring intracranial structures than did ^{68}Ga-EDTA PET. Furthermore, it is easier to predict tumour pathology with X-ray CT. By interpreting the degree of accompanying brain oedema and changes in the density of the lesion before and after intravenous infusion of contrast medium it is possible to make a differential diagnosis of brain tumour. Nevertheless, haemodynamic and kinetic studies with brain tumour by PET provide quantitative information about local permeability in the lesion as well as haemodynamic changes in the tumour and surrounding brain tissue which are vital for effective treatment.

One major disadvantage of X-ray CT with intravenous infusion of contrast medium is the contrast medium itself. There is a small but definite risk of reaction, sometimes with severe results. This reaction to contrast medium was seen in one case of oligoden-droglioma in this series. In contrast, there is believed to be no risk of reaction to ^{68}Ga-EDTA.

One other disadvantage of X-ray CT with contrast enhancement is the radiation dose to intracranial structure, which is large in comparison to ^{68}Ga PET. The radiation dose after intravenous injection of ^{68}Ga-EDTA has been calculated as 0.02–0.03 rads/mCi for the whole body and 0.2 rads/mCi for the kidney (9). If 3 mCi of ^{68}Ga-EDTA were used in ^{68}Ga PET, the radiation dose would be under 0.06 rads for the whole body and 0.6 rads for the kidney. On the other hand, radiation dosage to the patient's head by widely used X-ray CT, ranges from 4 to 20 rads/study. This means that the radiation dose doubles in tests with and without intravenous infusion of contrast medium.

Another advantage in ^{68}Ga PET is its freedom from artifacts caused by the presence of metallic surgical plates, clips and shunt valves etc, which often render interpretation difficult in X-ray CT.

To understanding the pathophysiological aspects of brain tumours additional infor-mation about haemodynamic changes can be obtained by combining ^{68}Ga dynamic PET with static studies. This information does not indicate quantitative regional cerebral blood flow values as do values obtained by ^{77}Kr PET (9, 10). Because ^{68}Ga-EDTA is a non-diffusible indicator, semiquantitative values of transit time are obtained by analysis of the rate of the down slope curve in every 0.5 x 0.5 cm^2 of the cross section of the head. This value is not quantitative, however, because the volume of the vascular bed of the brain, less than 5% of total brain tissue, changes easily under different conditions. Furthermore, abnormal and undetected conditions of cerebral perfusion caused by abnormal vascular pattern in the brain tumour may exist and the information about this condition cannot be known exactly.

According to these results, ^{68}Ga static PET, a non-invasive technique, is a very useful test for detecting and locating brain tumours. The dynamic study adds further informa-tion to understanding of the pathophysiological aspects of brain tumours. X-ray CT, however, remains superior for depicting anatomical detail and demonstrat ɜ cystic tumours which may be difficult to detect in ^{68}Ga PET. Therefore, a combination of these two studies would increase both the diagnostic accuracy and our understanding of the pathophysiology of brain tumours. Accordingly, both haemodynamic and me-tabolic studies will be planned for extensive cases of brain tumour using Positome III. Such studies will clarify the exact pathophysiological aspects of brain tumours, and may contribute valuable and objective information for evaluating various methods of treat-ment.

Conclusion

^{68}Ga PET was performed in cases with brain tumour. In almost all cases this study showed a significant focal uptake in static study, and haemodynamic changes in dynamic study. Compared to ^{99m}Tc study and X-ray CT, the ^{68}Ga diagnostic rate for detecting brain tumour was almost equal at least in cases with meningioma, glioma and metastatic tumour. However, detection and localization of brain tumour was both easier and clearer in ^{68}Ga PET than in ^{99m}Tc study and X-ray CT without contrast enhancement.

Concerning ^{68}Ga dynamic PET, semiquantitative values obtained by this method correlated well with findings of X-ray CT, and were thought to be more precise and detailed than findings by ^{99m}Tc dynamic study.

In conclusion, ^{68}Ga PET is a useful diagnostic method in cases with brain tumour without any attendant complications. Furthermore, the combination of PET and X-ray CT appears to be outstandingly effective not only for detecting the lesion, but also for understanding its pathophysiological aspects.

References

1. Comer, D., Zarifian, E., Verhas, M., Soussaline, F., Maziere, M., Berger, G., Loo, H., Cuche, C., Kellershohn, C., Deniker, P.: Brain distribution and kinetics of ^{11}C-chlorpromazine in schizophrenics: positron emission tomography. Psychiat. Research *1*, 23-29 (1979)
2. Ericson, K., Bergström, M., Eriksson, L.: Positron emission tomography in the evaluation of subdural hematomas. J. Comput. Assist. Tomogr. *4*, 737-745 (1980)
3. Farckowiak, R.S.J., Lenzi, G-L., Jones, T., Heather, J.D.: Quantitative measurement of regional cerebral blood flow and oxygen metabolism in man using ^{15}O and positron emission tomography: Theory, procedure and normal values. J. Comput. Assist. Tomogr. *4*, 727-736 (1980)
4. Hatter, R.S., Lim, C.B., Swann, S.J., Kaufman, L., Perez-Mendez, V., Chu, D., Huberty, J.P., Price, D.C., Wilson, C.B.: Cerebral imaging using ^{68}Ga-DTPA and U.C.S.F. multiwire proportional chamber positron camera. IEEE Trans. Nucl. Sci. NS-23, 523-527 (1976)
5. Hoop, B., Hnatowich, D.J., Brownell, G.L., Jones, T., McKusick, K.A., Ojemann, R.G., Panker, J.A., Subramanyan, R., Taveras, J.M.: Techniques for positron scintigraphy of the brain. J. Nucl. Med. *17*, 473-479 (1976)
6. Kuhl, D.E., Engel, J., Phelps, M.E., Selin, C.: Epileptic pattern of local cerebral metabolism and perfusion in humans determined by emission computed tomography of ^{18}FDG and ^{13}NH$_3$. Ann. Neurol. *8*, 348-360 (1980)
7. Phelps, M.E., Kuhl, D.E., Mazziotta, J.C.: Metabolic mapping of the brain's response to visual stimulation: Studies in humans. Science *211*, 1445-1448 (1981)
8. Reivich, M., Kuhl, D., Wolf, A., Greenberg, J., Phelps, M., Ido, T., Casella, V., Fowler, J., Hoffman, E., Alani, A., Som, P., Sokoloff, L.: The ^{18}F-fluorodeoxyglucose method for the measurement of local cerebral glucose utilization in man, Circ. Res. *44*, 127-137 (1979)
9. Yamamoto, Y.L., Thompson, C.J., Meyer, E., Robertson, J.S., Feindel, W.: Dynamic positron emission tomography for study of cerebral hemodynamics in a cross section of the head using positron-emitting ^{68}Ga-EDTA and ^{77}Kr. J. Comput. Assist. Tomogr. *1*, 43-56 (1977)
10. Yamamoto, Y.L., Meyer, E., Thompson, C.J., Feindel, W.H.: ^{77}Kr clearance technique for measurement of regional cerebral blood flow by positron emission tomography. In: Positron and single-photon emission tomography. Kuhl, D.E. (ed.), Chap. 10. New York: G & T Management Inc. (1980)

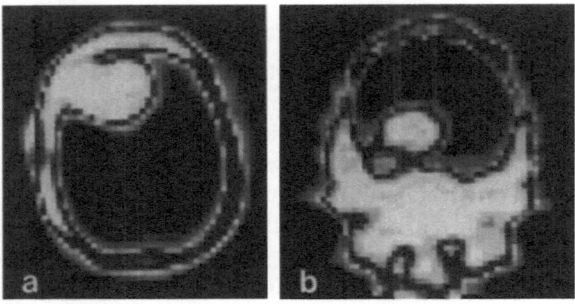

Fig. 1 a,b. 49-year-old female, convexity meningioma. Horizontal (**a**) and coronal (**b**) section ^{68}Ga static PET, showing a significant, homogeneous and oval-shaped focal uptake in the left frontal region

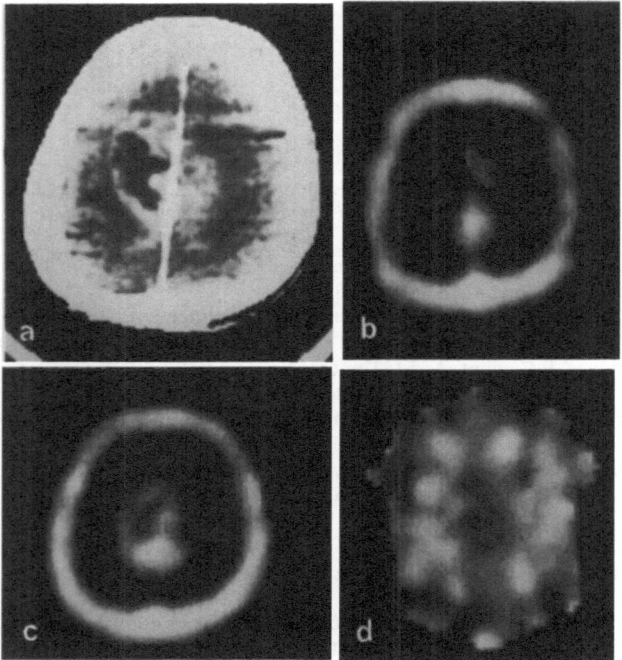

Fig. 2 a-d. 59-year-old male, glioblastoma. X-ray CT with infusion (**a**), showing an irregular-shaped, non-homogeneous enhanced area in the midline, parietal region of both cerebral hemispheres. ^{68}Ga static PET immediately after the injection of ^{68}Ga-EDTA (**b**), showing a significant focal uptake in the midline, parietal region. ^{68}Ga static PET two hours after the injection (**c**), showing an irregular-shaped focal uptake with doughnut-shaped focal uptake in the same place as shown by X-ray CT. ^{68}Ga dynamic PET (**d**), showing markedly slower perfusion rate at the tumour site as well as areas remote from the tumour

Fig. 3 a-e. 58-year-old female, right sphenoid ridge meningioma. X-ray CT without infusion (**a**, *above*) showing the enlargement of lateral and third ventricles, but no areas of abnormal density. X-ray CT with infusion (**b**, *below*) showing a large enhanced area in the middle fossa, extending along the right lateral ventricle

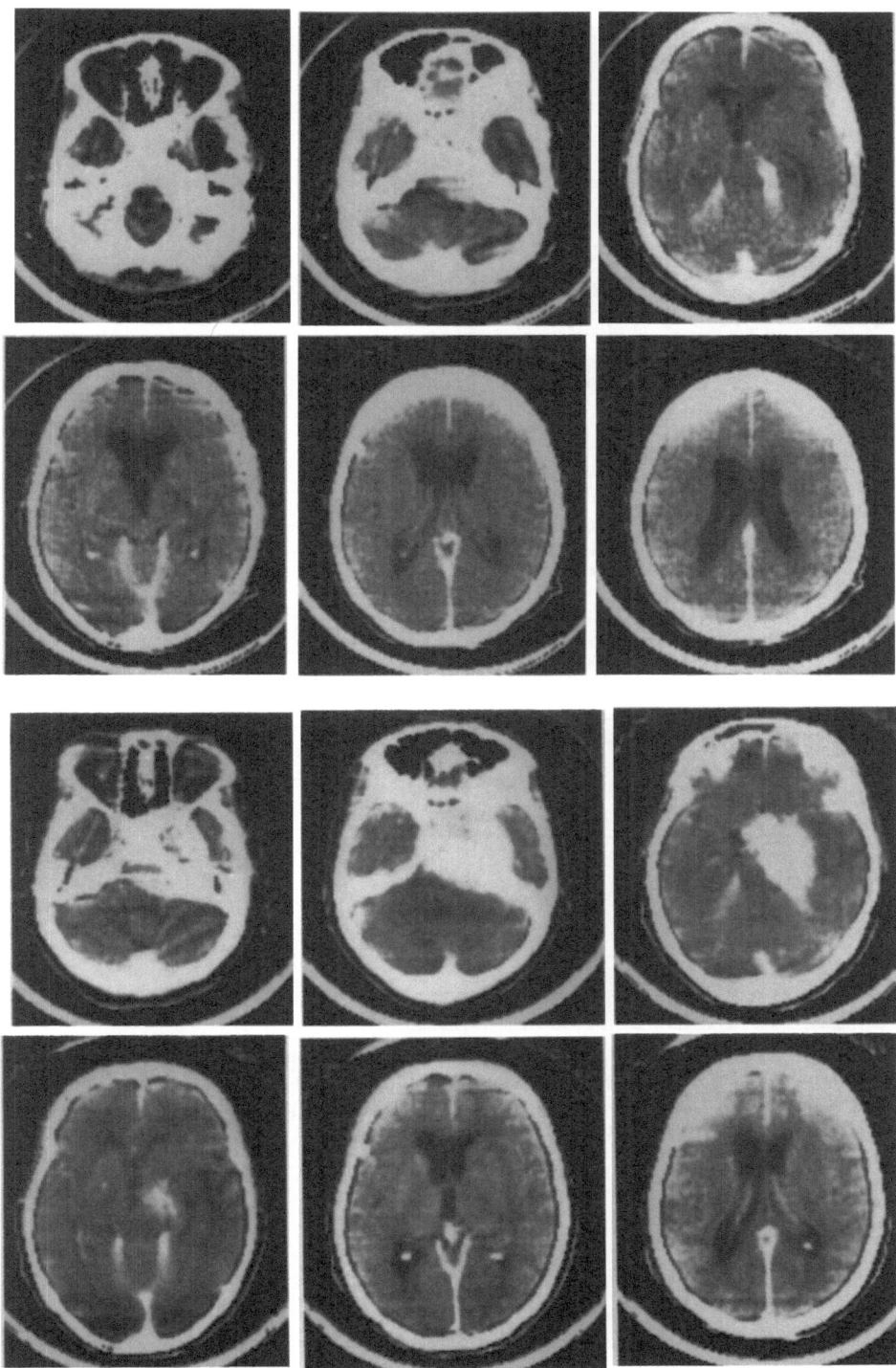

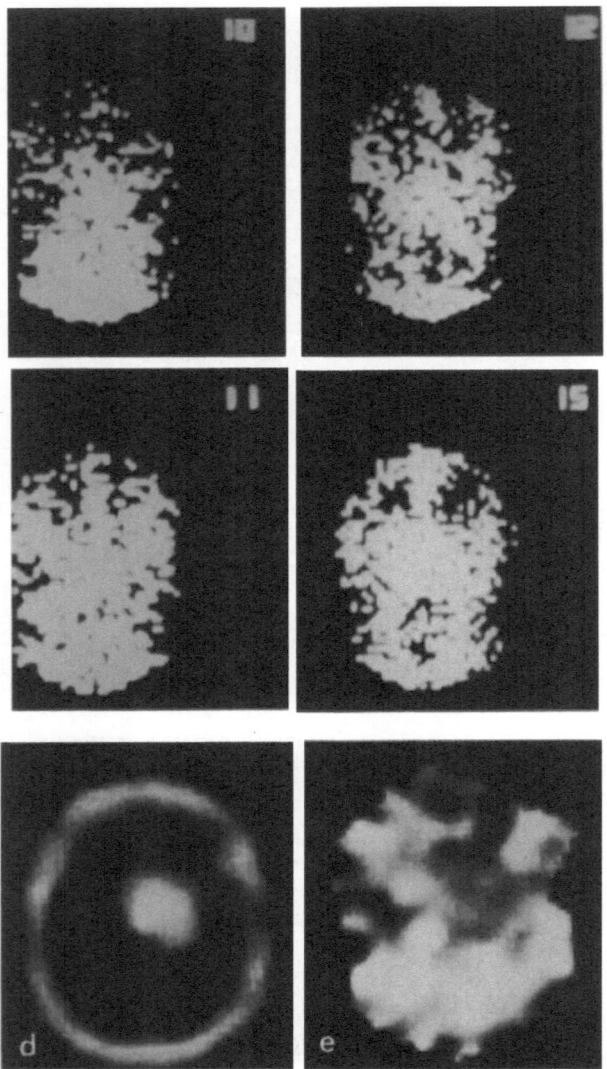

Fig. 3 a-e. ^{99m}Tc dynamic study (**c**, *above*), showing no abnormal findings. ^{68}Ga static PET
(**d**), showing a significant, homogeneous and round-shaped focal uptake in the same place as
shown by X-ray CT. ^{68}Ga dynamic PET (**e**), showing markedly slower perfusion rate at the
tumour site as well as in areas remote from the tumour

Angiotomosynthesis

M. Nadjmi

The principle of classical tomography is based on motion which causes the conditions of blurring. Existing tomographic procedures differ in minor ways mainly because movement of the x-ray tube and the film may be linear, circular, elliptical, spiral and hypocycloidal (1).

Tomosynthesis is a new tomographic method, the results of which can be compared with those of the tomographic procedure which we all are familiar with. However, the main difference from classical tomography is that:

1. all the information necessary for the tomography of an object is obtained with only one exposure;
2. neither the x-ray tubes, nor the film, nor the patient are moved during this process.

By means of this procedure the time of the actual investigation which is relatively long in classical tomography, is reduced to seconds (2, 3).

Principle of Tomosynthesis

Tomosynthesis is a codes-aperture imaging system in two stages, recording and reconstructing. In the first step, the three-dimensional object is imaged by an array of x-ray tubes, resulting in a coded image. This coded image is then processed in the second step to reconstruct arbitrary layers of the object. Initially, the decoding was performed using holography. Later a decoding unit using only lenses was constructed, because this technique is better suited for a hospital environment. The coding-decoding procedure is shown in Fig. 1. Imagine an object which, for the sake of simplicity, consists of only two layers, a disk and a square. We image this object with three immovable x-ray tubes (P) simultaneously and produce an image on which three squares and three disks can be seen. Because of the distance between the disk and the square in the object, the distances from the shadows of the squares and the shadows of the disks to the middle of the film are different. With this procedure the actual tomography of this object is theoretically completed. We call this the recording step, and in a second procedure we try to decode this x-ray image. This second procedure, whereby the presence of the patient is not longer required, is known as the decoding or reconstruction step. If we stay with our simple example of the disk and the square, the decoding step proceeds as follows:

The coded image is projected onto a lens matrix with the same number of lenses as x-ray tubes and in the same position.

© Springer-Verlag Berlin · Heidelberg 1982

The shadows which result with the lenses now contain nine disks and nine squares, whereby each time three disks or three squares are superimposed in the centre of the picture, thus forming a more intense image. This is the precisely adjusted tomography of the disk or the square. All other disks and squares are unclear and therefore artifacts.

In this example the layer chosen is three times more intense than the artifacts. When more tubes are used, the resolution is better.

Figure 2 demonstrates the coding and reconstruction procedure on another example with four x-ray tubes. We see the tubes, the object, the coded picture, the lens matrix and finally the tomograms of the object.

The prototype of the equipment in the Department of Neuroradiology in Würzburg — made by Philips, Hamburg — contains 24 x-ray tubes that can be exposed simultaneously. Our main goal with the tomosynthesis was to exploit the advantages of this method in cerebral angiography to a maximum. A special cassette was developed with which we could carry out the serial angiotomography. We call this angiotomosynthesis.

Since the investigation is a selective angiographic examination, the indication should be performed after the regular angiography. This is why we combined the equipment of angiotomosynthesis with that of cerebral angiography.

Figure 3 shows the results of angiotomosyhtesis in connexion with the diagnosis of cerebral aneurysms in different locations.

Conclusions

With previously known conventional tomographic methods either a multisection cassette or a tomographic procedure is necessary for showing each object layer. With tomosynthesis all the information necessary for the tomography of an object is obtained in one procedure without moving the x-ray tube, the film or the object. In practice there are two essential advantages as compared with conventional tomography:
1. The investigation process is reduced to a few seconds and the x-ray load to an individual tube which plays an important part in conventional tomography is reduced.
2. Tomosynthesis can be used in practice wherever tomography particularly is necessary. An interesting application is for tomography of cerebral and spinal angiography which can be carried out in combination with the usual serial angiography.

References

1. Nadjmi, M.: Atlas der zerebralen Gefäße im Angiotomogramm. Stuttgart: Thieme 1977
2. Nadjmi, M., H. Weiss, E. Klotz, R. Linde: Flashing tomosynthesis – A new tomographic method. Neuroradiology 19, 113-117 (1980)
3. Nadjmi, M., H. Weiss, E. Klotz, R. Linde: Kurzzeit-Tomosynthese – klinische Erfahrungen. Röntgenpraxis 34, 247-252 (1981)

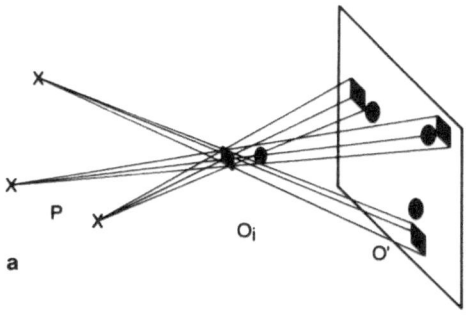

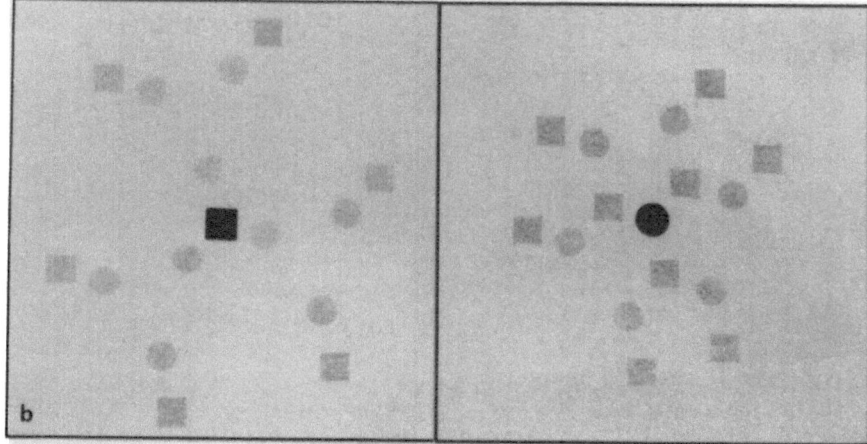

Fig. 1 a,b. Tomosynthesis. **a** Stage of recording, **b** Stage of reconstruction

Fig. 2. Principle of tomosynthesis

X-ray tubes

Object

Coded
picture

Lens matrix

Tomograms

Fig. 3 a ▽

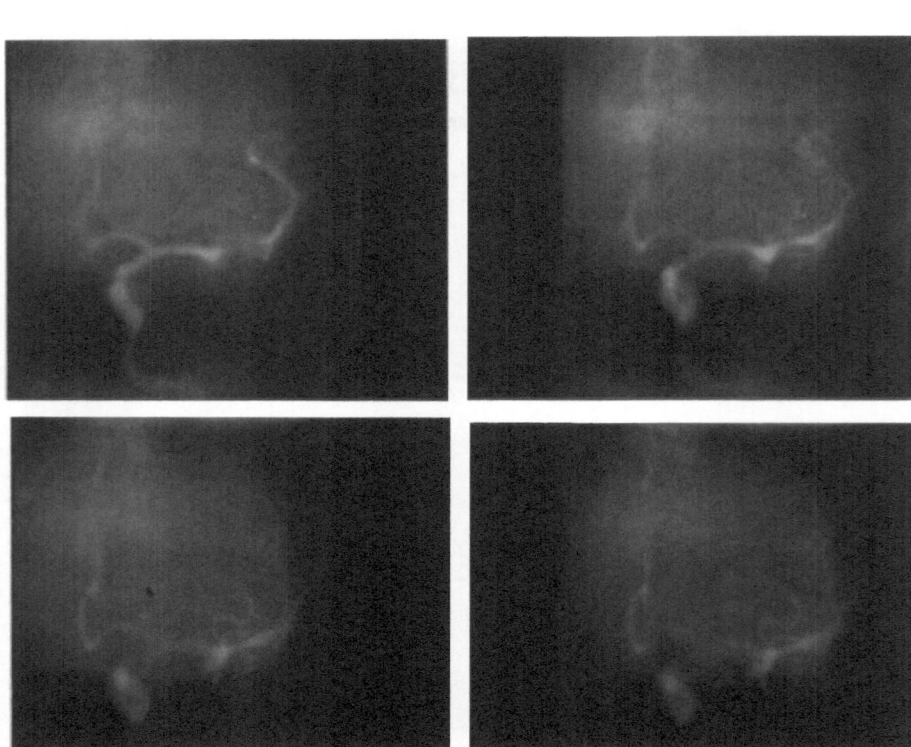

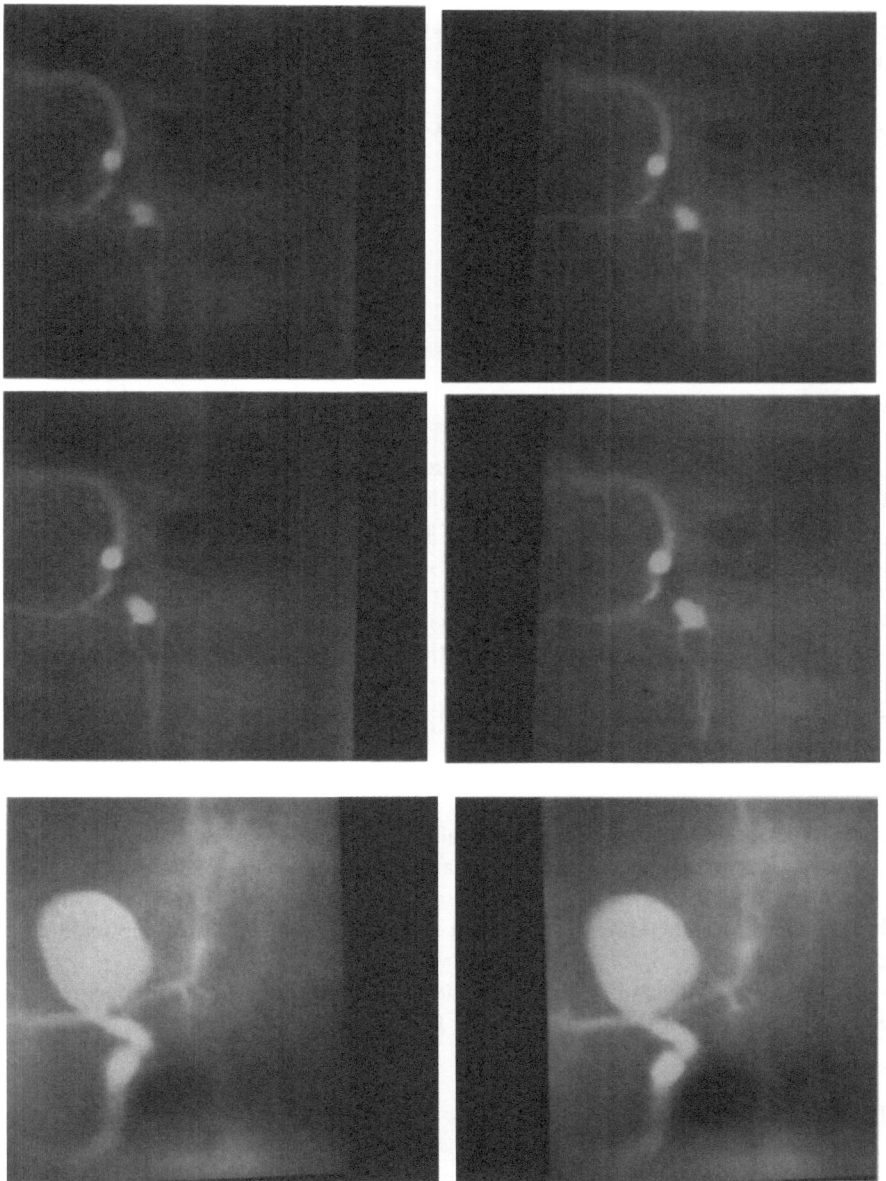

Fig. 3 a-c. Angiotomosynthesis of cerebral aneurysms. **a** Small aneurysm of the trifurcation of the middle cerebral artery (see p. 14), **b** Aneurysm of the anterior communicating artery (*above*), **c** Huge aneurysm of the middle cerebral artery and the bifurcation of the internal carotid artery *(below)*

Age and Other Complicating Factors in Neurosurgical Operations in the Sitting Position

R.A. Frowein, W. Köning, and G.C. Loeschcke

Clinical Material

Our report is based on 203 patients who were operated in the sitting position during the last 4 1/2 years for tumours, vascular malformations, hemorrhages etc. The lesions were situated in the occipital, tentorial, pineal, cerebello-pontine, cerebellar and cervical regions.

In Fig. 1 each of the 203 patients is shown in relation to the most important features of his course. In 111 of these patients the course was uneventful or only slight alterations in the blood pressure occurred when the patient was brought into a sitting position or during the extirpation of the tumour.

In less than half of the cases factors which might have been expected to exercise a negative influence on the course were present. These factors were: elevated intracranial pressure before the operation in only nine cases (in most patients with hydrocephalus a pre-operative external or internal CSF drainage was carried out); air embolism in nine cases; operations and anaesthesia of especially long duration (more than 5 1/2 hours) in 26 cases; haemorrhage or brain swelling after the operation in 21 cases; and a long period of postoperative disturbance of consciousness in 27 cases. In the discussion which follows we have, for the sake of convenience, labelled these factors "complicating factors".

There were 29 deaths among the 203 patients, that is 14%; 26 of them occurred after courses in which one or more complicating factors played a role.

Influence of Multiple Complicating Factors

The only single complicating factor which proved decisive for the outcome was arterial haemorrhage. Apart from this, we invariably found that several factors were responsible for a poor postoperative state or a lethal course. For instance, a 53-year-old woman had a meningeoma in the internal falco-tentorial angle in the pineal region, with hydrocephalus (40/80). At the start of the operation during the skin incision, the Doppler ultrasound monitoring indicated air in the heart and 100 ml of air were withdrawn from the right atrium (Fig. 2). The blood pressure then remained steady. The operation on the deep-seated tumour in the pineal region lasted 6 1/2 hours. After the operation the patient remained in a state of clouded consciousness and died of a secondary lung complication four weeks later.

16   Modern Neurosurgery 1. Edited by M. Brock
© Springer-Verlag Berlin · Heidelberg 1982

Thus at least five complicating factors were operative in this case and it is not possible to point to any one of them as the immediate cause of death. Nevertheless further analysis of the various factors is necessary, especially because of the growing number of tumours which are diagnosed in these locations, particularly in older patients. By examining the data relating to our 203 patients we hope to identify the circumstances under which complications are likely to arise.

Air Embolism

A doppler monitoring system (7) has been used in all 80 operations performed during the past two years (Fig. 3). Air aspiration into the vascular system was detected in eight cases and suspected in one case, i.e., in about 11% of the operations [Hunter (1) 8% in 37 cases; Marshall (2) 15% in 34 cases; Michenfelder et al. (3) 4.1% in 751 cases; Albin et al. (4) 25% in 180 cases]. These cases occurred in operations in all locations and in all age groups.

During the anaesthesia the usual monitoring, end-expired CO_2 and intra-arterial blood pressure measurements were carried out (3, 5).

Attention was paid to:
a) sufficient infusion of colloidal solutions so that before the patient was brought into the sitting position the central venous pressure had reached high normal values of 10-12 mm H_2O;
b) precise placement of the tip of the central venous catheter in the right atrium by means of the ECG, so that in case of air embolism, air could be promptly aspirated;
c) application of the Doppler ultrasonic device on the anterior surface of the chest at the level of the right atrium; a test for correct positioning was carried out by intravenous injection of carbon dioxide and by producing turbulence by injecting sodium chloride solution into the central venous catheter;
d) controlled respiration with PEEP.

When air embolism occurred, the following measures were undertaken: aspiration of intracardiac air; ventilation with pure oxygen; increase of PEEP; compression of the jugular veins to increase the venous pressure; placing of the patient in a more horizontal position; occlusion of a possible leak (6).

Because of the speed with which the anaesthetist was able to deal with circulatory disturbances, we do not believe that air embolisms were decisive in these cases. The two lethal cases were the patient with the meningioma in the pineal region mentioned above and a child with a recurrence of a cerebellar astrocytoma involving the brain system.

Lengthy Operations

Because of servere neurological and psychological defects in four cases, after operations of unusually long duration, we asked ourselves whether lengthy operations in the sitting position, especially in older patients, resulted in a poorer prognosis than shorter operations in the same position.

In one of the four cases, that of a 53-year-old man (13/79), the operation on a supra-tentorial and infratentorial meningioma took six hours. The operation on a large cere-bello-pontine meningioma in a 55-year-old patient (24/79) lasted 9 1/2 hours, the anaesthetic 11 hours.

Anaesthesia and operations in the sitting position of more than 5 1/2 hours were carried out in 26 cases. Figure 4 shows the outcome in relation to the length of the operation and to the age of the patient.

There were four cases of severe postoperative defects: the two already mentioned, a man with an acoustic neurinoma, and a child operated on for a ponto-cerebellar tumour. The two lethal results occurred after operations of less than six hours. Five of these six cases were more than 50 years of age. In the majority of the younger patients a lengthy operation had no negative effects on the course. Thus, age seems to be an important factor.

Analysis of the Progress in Relation to Tumour Location and Age of the Patient

Finally we analysed the relation between age and the immediate postoperative course for each of the principal tumour sites.

Thirty-two tumours, angiomas and haemorrhages were operated in the *occipital, ten-torial and pineal regions* (Fig. 5). The progress of 18 was normal. Of the remaining 14 with pre-operative elevated intracranial pressure, air embolism, lengthy anaesthesia and operation, intraoperative bleeding and/or long postoperative periods of disturbances of consciousness, 11 achieved full recovery, one was postoperatively defective and two died. These last three patients belonged to the group of eight who were over 50 years of age.

Sixty-one patients had meningiomas or acoustic neuromas, as well as some rare tu-mours in the *cerebello-pontine angle* (Fig. 6). Most of them were, as was to be expected, between the ages of 40 and 60. Deaths and poor postoperative states occurred in pa-tients with intra-operative circulatory problems, difficult and lengthy operations on very large tumours and intraoperative haemorrhages; but the largest number of such cases occurred in patients over 53 years of age. Nevertheless five patients over 50 achieved a complete recovery in spite of long-lasting disturbances of consciousness.

In the group of *cerebellar* gliomas the mean age of the patients was 29 years (Fig. 7). Small children operated in the sitting position had an uneventful course. The percent-age of postoperative disturbances increases with age, especially in cases of cerebellar space-occupying lesions other than gliomas and in patients over 50 years of age (Fig. 8).

There were no deaths among the 14 patients with cervical lesions operated on in the sitting position.

Our experience of patients over 60 years is too limited to allow us to judge whether the frequency of deaths or serious defects increases still further in this age group.

However, the individual case does not necessarily correspond to the statistical expec-tation. Thus a 59-year-old patient with a very large meningioma in the cerebello-pontine angle made a full recovery (45/80).

To summarize our results, in all locations age is the one complicating factor which appears to influence the statistical outcome of operations in the sitting position.

References

1. Hunter, A.R.: Air embolism in the sitting position. Anaesthesia *17*, 467-472 (1962)
2. Marshall, B.M.: Air embolus in neurosurgical anaesthesia: its diagnosis and treatment. Can. Anaes. Soc. J. *12*, 55-261 (1965)
3. Michenfelder, J.D., J.T. Martin, B.M. Altenburg, Rehder, K.: Air embolism during neurosurgery. JAMA *208*, 1353-58 (1969)
4. Albin, M.S., Babinski, M., Maroon, J.C., Jannetta, P.J.: Anaesthetic management of posterior fossa surgery in the sitting position. Acta anaesth. scand. *20*, 117-128 (1976)
5. Smith, W.H., Harp, J.R.: Anaesthesia for neurosurgery in the sitting position. In: Surgery of the posterior fossa. New York: Raven Press 1979
6. Star, E.G., Sehhati, Th.: Diagnose und Therapie von Luftembolien bei neurochirurgischen Operationen. Anästhesiologie u. Intensivmedizin *11*, 306-309 (1980)
7. Gildenberg, Ph. L., O'Brien, R.P., Britt, W.J., Prost, E.A.M.: The efficacy of doppler monitoring for the detection of venous air embolism. J Neurosurgery *54*, 75-78 (1981)

Location	Tumour	Complicating factors						
		Uneventful	Circulatory disturbance	Elevated ICP	Air embolism	Lengthy operation	Haemorrhage Brain swelling	Postop. dist. of consc.
Occipital	Meningioma	OOO	O			O	O	O
	Metastasis	O			O			
	Glioma	O	OO					
	Angioma	OO	O			O		
	Haematoma	O 8	4		O 2	2	1	1	18
Tentorial, Pineal		OOOOO 5	O 1		O● 2	OOOO 4	O● 2	14
Cerebello-pontine angle	Meningioma	OO	OOO		O	OOOO	O●	
	Acoustic Neur.	(symbols)	(symbols)●		O	(symbols)OO●	●●●	(symbols)OOOO
	Others	O 15	OOO 17		2	O 16	5	6	61
Cerebellar	Meningioma		O					
	Glioma	(symbols)●	(symbols)●	OO●●●	O●	OO	O●●●●●	(symbols)●●
	Angioblastoma	OOO	OO	OO			O●	O
	Metastasis	OOOOO	O				●●	O
	Angioma	O		O			O●	OO
	Others	(symbols) 31	OOO 18	● 9	2	● 3	● 13	O 20	96
Cervical	Neuroma	OOOOO			O			
	Metastasis							
	Glioma	OOO 8	OOOO 4		1	O	1	14
		66 ↑	1 ⊹ 42 ↑	2 ⊹ 5 ↑	4 ⊹ 7 ↑	2 ⊹ 24 ↑	2 ⊹ 6 ↑	15 ⊹ 24 ↑	3 ⊹ 203

●= fatalities , O= survivors

Fig. 1. Most important features in the progress of 203 patients operated on in the sitting position

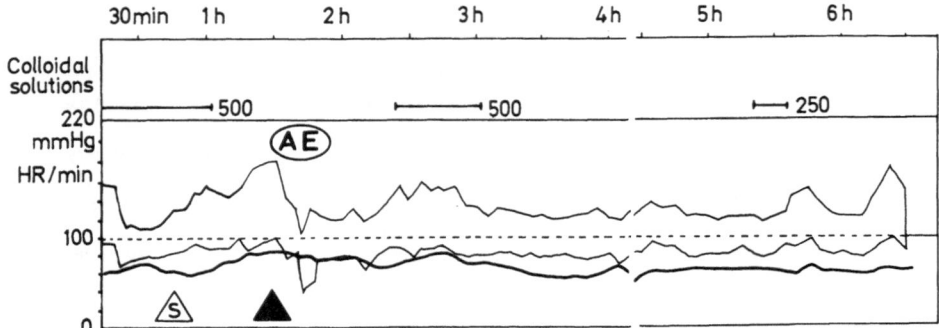

Fig. 2. Anaesthetic record of the operation on a meningioma in the pineal region (K., M. 53 years , female). Anaesthesia was carried out with flunitrazepam, fentanyl, nitrous oxide and halothane; intravenous infusions consisted of crystalline and colloidal solutions and banked blood. *HR*, heart rate; *S*, sitting position; ▲ start of operation; *AE*, air embolism

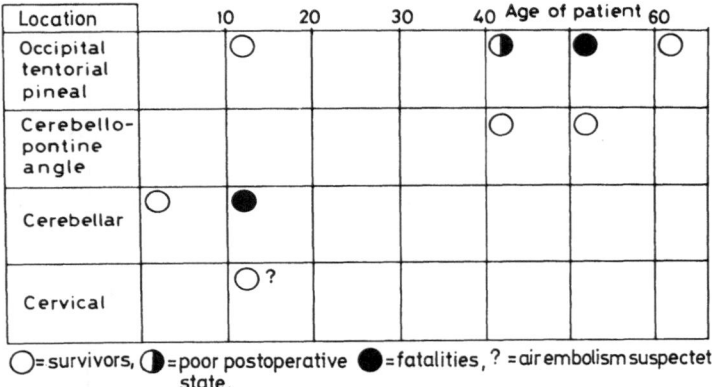

◯= survivors, ◖=poor postoperative state, ●=fatalities, ? =air embolism suspectet

Fig. 3. Operations in the sitting position: air embolism

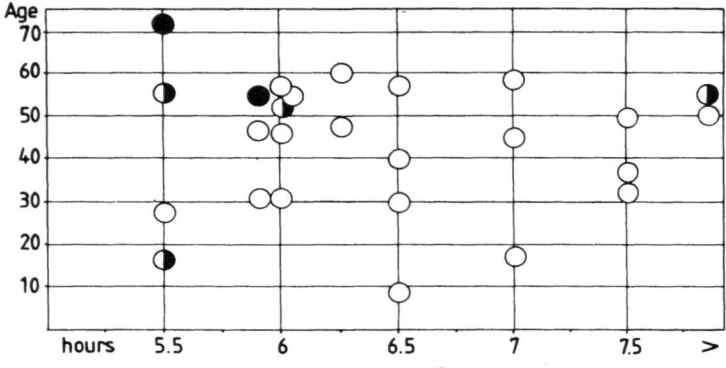

● = fatalities, ◖ = poor postoperative state, ◯= survivors

Fig. 4. Lengthy operations in the sitting position: age of patients in relation to duration of anaesthesia and operation

20

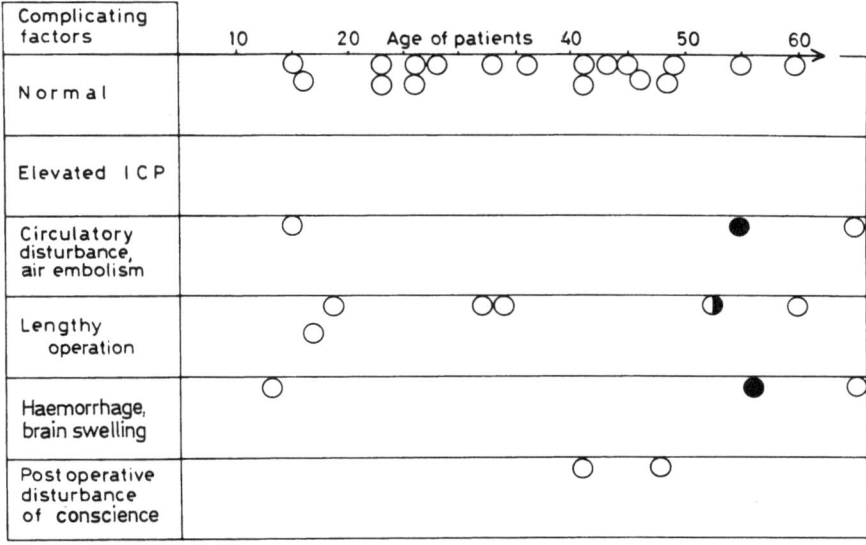

● = fatalities, ◑ = poor postoperative state, ○ = survivors

Fig. 5. Progress of operations in the occipital, tentorial and pineal regions in relation to the age of patient

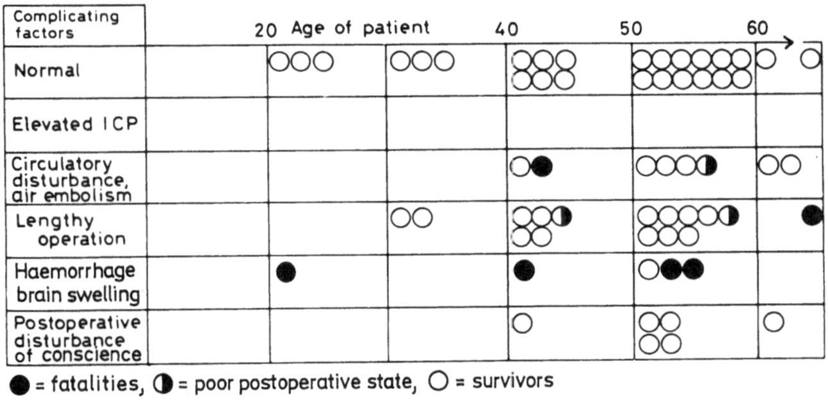

Complicating factors		20 Age of patient		40	50	60	
Normal		○○○	○○○	○○○ ○○○	○○○○○○○○ ○○○○○○○○	○	○
Elevated ICP							
Circulatory disturbance, air embolism				○●	○○○○◑	○○	
Lengthy operation			○○	○○○ ◑ ○○	○○○○○◑ ○○○		●
Haemorrhage brain swelling		●		●	○●●		
Postoperative disturbance of conscience				○	○○ ○○	○	

● = fatalities, ◑ = poor postoperative state, ○ = survivors

Fig. 6. Operations in the cerebello-pontine angle

21

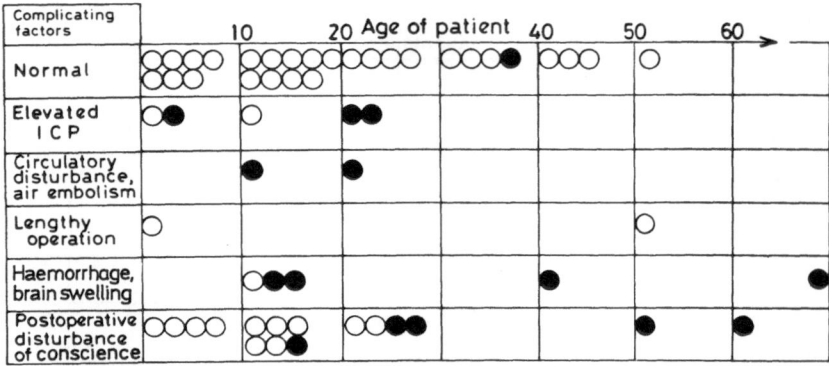

● = fatalities, ○ = survivors

Fig. 7. Cerebellar tumours: gliomas

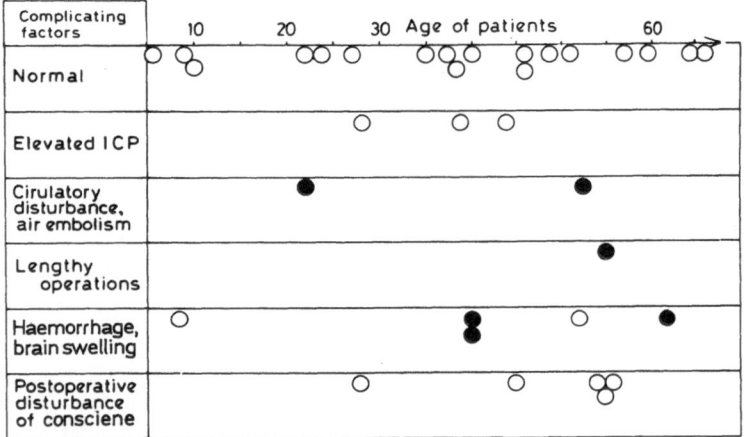

● = fatalities, ○ = survivors

Fig. 8. Cerebellar tumours: other space-occupying lesions

CO₂-Micro-Laser-Neurosurgery – Clinical and Laboratory Experiences

T. Kuroiwa, T. Fujimoto, and Y. Inaba

The CO_2 laser has been expected to be quite useful in future of neurosurgery, because of its potential ability of bloodless and precise operation without direct touch. Stellar (11, 12) was the first who used a CO_2 laser in a neurosurgical field and Heppner (6, 7), Ascher (1), Takizawa (13, 14), Kamikawa et al. (10) are advancing CO_2 laser surgery. However, many problems still remain unsolved for its indication and safety as well as the development of the laser unit. We have had experience of the combined use of operating microscope and CO_2 laser since 1978 in both the fundamental experimental study (4, 5) and in operating on clinical cases (8, 9). Still we feel micro-laser-neurosurgery is just at the beginning and the accumulation of basic knowledge is urgently needed. We have used the CO_2 surgical laser unit Model 400 and Model 450 (since 1980) (Coherent Company, USA). This has a flexible arm using mirrors, micromanipulator and a control system for power (0-30W) and time (interrupted and continuous). The size of the focus is 2.0 mm (through microscope) and 0.4 mm (hand piece) in diameter.

Clinical Cases

We have operated on 40 cases of brain tumour including one case of AVM. The summary of these cases is shown in Table 1. The power used was from 5 to 20W and the exposure time was interrupted or continuous depending on the situation. For removal of a tumour, we coagulated with defocused laser then excavated the inside of the tumour in order to reduce its volume using focused laser and conventional techniques. At the present time we are quite anxious to use laser at the borderline between the tumour and surrounding tissue especially if important vital organs are involved, according to our data (4, 5). In such an area, we have used conventional microsurgical technique. Tumours were removed successfully and we did not have any accident or trouble using the CO_2 laser. It was quite useful to reduce haemorrhage and lessen retraction.

Experimental Studies

To see the effect of the CO_2 laser on living brain tissue under various conditions, the following studies were performed using Japanese white rabbits (2.8-4.2 kg, both sexes) under general anaesthesia with 50 mg/kg of pentobarbital. The CO_2 laser was exposed

Table 1. Microneurosurgery combined with CO_2 laser

Glioblastoma		8
Other gliomas		7
Meningioma		12
Neurinoma		6
Acoustic	4	
Trigeminal	2	
Cavernous angioma		2
Craniopharyngioma		1
Osteochondroma		1
Reticulum cell sarcoma		1
A V M		2
Total		40

Age range: 4-75 years/o– January 1978–August 1980

through the surgical microscope in all cases. For histological examination, the removed brain was fixed with 10% neutral paraformaldehyde. After fixation the tissues were embedded in paraffin and tissue sections were stained with haematoxylin and eosin.

Experiment 1

Skull openings were made in the parietal region of 20 animals. After opening the dura mater, the brain surface was irradiated with laser beam under various combinations of power and exposure time. Immediately after the irradiation, the brains were prepared for histological examination. The thickness of the damaged brain tissue composed of three layers, charred, necrotic and oedematous layers, was measured.

Experiment 2 (1)

To assess the damage to brain tissue at a late phase after laser irradiation, 15 animals were used in this experiment. The brain surface was irradiated through the skull opening with the laser beam at 15W for 3 s. Animals were killed at intervals, immediately and then 5 h, 24 h, 1W and 2Ws after the irradiation. Except for the immediate case, 1.0 ml/kg of 2% Evans-blue was injected intravenously one hour before being killed. After observing the extravasation of Evans-blue, the brains were prepared for histological examination.

Experiment 2 (2)

This experiment was performed to investigate the pathomechanism of "late effect", namely spreading brain tissue damage after CO_2 laser irradiation. Twenty animals were used and laser beam of 15W was irradiated on the exposed brain surface for three seconds as in Experiment 2 (1). In ten animals, immediately after the irradiation, 1.0 ml/kg of carbon black solution was injected into the heart percutaneously then the animals were decapitated. The remaining ten animals were kept alive for 24 h after the laser beam irradiation. After injection of carbon black, the animals were decapitated. The removed brains were inspected and then prepared for histological examination.

Experiment 3

The effect of hypertension on the brain tissue damage after the irradiation was examined using 12 animals. Under general anaesthesia, the right femoral artery was exposed and a polyethylene catheter was inserted for continuous blood pressure monitoring and re-peated injection of norepinephrine. Hypertension higher than 200 mm Hg was induced just before the laser beam irradiation and this level was maintained for 5 h. After the various time intervals, namely, immediately after the exposure, 5 h, 24 h, 1W and 2Ws after the exposure, the animals were killed. 1.0 ml/kg of Evans-blue was injected one hour before they were killed except in the immediate case. The removed brains were examined and prepared for histological examination.

Results

Experiment 1

The area of thermal damage consisted of three layers, as mentioned before, in the area surrounding the central vapourized tissue defect. The thickness of the thermal damaged area is shown in Table 2. The longer the exposure time, the thicker the tissue damage. On the other hand, the thickness was slightly increased but did not correspond with the strength of the laser beam. The size of the tissue defect "crater" increased depending on both the exposure time and the strength of the laser beam.

Experiment 2 (1)

Immediately after the exposure, brain damage was limited, but 5 h or 24 h after the irradiation, the damaged area was much more extensive and prominent extravasation of Evans-blue was seen (Fig. 1). In the case of 1W and 2Ws after the exposure, the thickness was similar to that after 24 h, although extravasation of Evans-blue was now no longer apparent.

Table 2. The average extent and the standard deviation of the thermal damage (μ) for the different situations

Power output (w)	Exposure times (s)					
	0.1	0.2	0.5	1,0	3.0	5.0
5			108 ± 12		277 ± 25	
10			213 ± 18		356 ± 42	
15	56 ± 8	203 ± 15	296 ± 31	308 ± 26	386 ± 19	463 ± 36
27			302 ± 23		400 ± 37	

Experiment 2 (2)

Immediately after the irradiation (Fig. 2), a bright halo was recognized surrounding the central tissue defect. Microscopically, capillaries were obscured and carbon black was not recognized in the necrotic layer. Oedematous changes were also not clear. In the oedematous layer, no carbon black was recognized although capillaries were dilated. On the other hand, 24 h after the irradiation, tissue damage was significant (Fig. 3). In the necrotic layer, no significant changes were seen compared to the immediate case, but in the oedematous layer, significant changes were observed. The thickness of this layer progressed and haemorrhages were seen prominently in this layer in all cases. Oedematous changes and neuronal changes were quite remarkable. Carbon black was scattered here and there.

Experiment 3

Under hypertensive condition, the thickness of brain damage and extravasation was greater than under normotensive condition (Fig. 4). Extravasation was not seen in the one week or two weeks cases after the irradiation.

Discussion

The CO_2 laser combined with the surgical-microscope has been expected to be quite a powerful tool in the neurosurgical field. In the near future we should be able to do more precise operations with less bleeding and retraction through a more restricted access. But that "the thermal damage following CO_2 laser irradiation is quite limited" seems to be stressed too much. Even if the damaged area seems to be quite limited immediately after the irradiation, it might extend considerably at a later stage. We already reported this phenomenon as "late effect", and we found that the microcirculatory disturbance which occurs in the early phase and late changes depends mainly on haemorrhage and extension of brain oedema. Hypertension will also accentuate the thermal damage. These mean the effect of the laser beam on the living brain may well be affected by multiple factors and it might not correspond directly with the result got from isolated brain or other organs. These things must be very important when we want to do a precise operation using the laser in an area especially close to an important structure. At the present time, we should use CO_2 laser only for excavation of the tumour and the dissection between the tumour and surrounding tissue should be done not by CO_2 laser but by conventional microneurosurgical technique. Many problems still remain unsolved for its indications and safety as well as the development of the machine. We need a more precise and exact power controlling system as well as the smaller focus. Moreover we need complete changeability of the laser beam direction together with that of the operating microscope during operation. If these requirement for CO_2 laser unit could be satisfied and various basic experimental studies could be accumulated in future, CO_2 laser would be used regularly and routinely not only for the purpose of tumour tissue removal but also for dissection close to the brain tissue, nerve fibres and blood vessels. For the progression of "micro-laser-neurosurgery", the combination of CO_2 laser and Nd:YAG laser, which seems more suitable for coagulation (2, 3) should be investigated.

Conclusion

We have used the CO_2 laser combined with the surgical microscope in 40 cases of brain tumour since 1978. Simultaneously we examined brain tissue damage caused by laser using rabbits. We found extension of tissue damage at a late phase ("late effect") and significant increase of tissue damage under hypertension. The CO_2 surgical laser is quite useful but we should know about the possible damage to brain tissue under certain condition because it could be afffected by multiple factors.

References

1. Ascher, P.W., Oberbauer, R., Holzer, P., Knoetgen, I.: Vorteile und Möglichkeiten des CO_2-Laser's in der Neurochirurgie. Wien. Med. Wschr. *127*, 260 (1977)
2. Beck, O.J., Wilske, J., Schönberger, J.L., Gorisch, W.: Tissue changes following application of lasers to the rabbit brain. Neurosurg. Rev. *1*, 31-36 (1979)
3. Beck, O.J.: The use of the Nd-YAG and the CO_2 Laser in neurosurgery. Neurosurg. Rev. *3*, 261-266 (1980)
4. Fujimoto, T., Inaba, Y., Kuroiwa, T., Fujiwara, K.: Basic experimental study for CO_2-Laser Microsurgery – Especially about the late effect of CO_2–Laser beam. Laser surgery *3* (2), 166-175 (1979)
5. Fujimoto, T., Inaba, Y., Kuroiwa, T.: Fundamental study for CO_2-micro-laser-surgery. J. of Japan Association of Medical Laser *1* (1), 279-286 (1980)
6. Heppner, F., Ascher, P.W.: Über den Einsatz des Laserstrahls in der Neurochirurgie. Act. Medicotechm. *24*, 424 (1976)
7. Heppner, F., Ascher, P.W.: Operationen an Hirn und Rückenmark mit dem Sharplan 791 CO_2-Laser. Acta Chir. Austriaca *9*, 32-34 (1977)
8. Inaba, Y., Fujimoto, T., Fujiwara, K., Nishimoto, K.: CO_2-surgical laser combined with microneurosurgery – clinical and experimental study. Neurologia med. chir. 18 (Suppl.) 123 (1978)
9. Inaba, Y., Fujimoto, T., Kuroiwa, T., Fujiwara, K.: CO_2-laser microsurgery of brain tumors. Laser surgery *3* (2), 119-127 (1979)

10. Kamikawa, K., Ikeda, T., Hayakawa, T., Onishi, T.: Application of laser surgical unit in neurosurgery. Surgical Therapy *35* (6), 626-636 (1976)
11. Stellar, S.: Effects of laser energy on brain and nerve tissue. Abst. 1st Ann. Biomed., Laser Conf., Boston 1965
12. Stellar, S.: Laser studies on nervous system tissue, neoplasms and related biological systems. Proc. Rudolf Virchow Med. Coc. (New York) Suppl. *26*, 416 (1968)
13. Takizawa, T.: Comparison between the laser surgical unit and the electrosurgical unit. Neurologia. Med. Chir. *17* (1), 95-105 (1977)
14. Takizawa, T.: Laser surgery of brain tumors. Advances in Neurological Sciences *22* (1), 101 (1978)

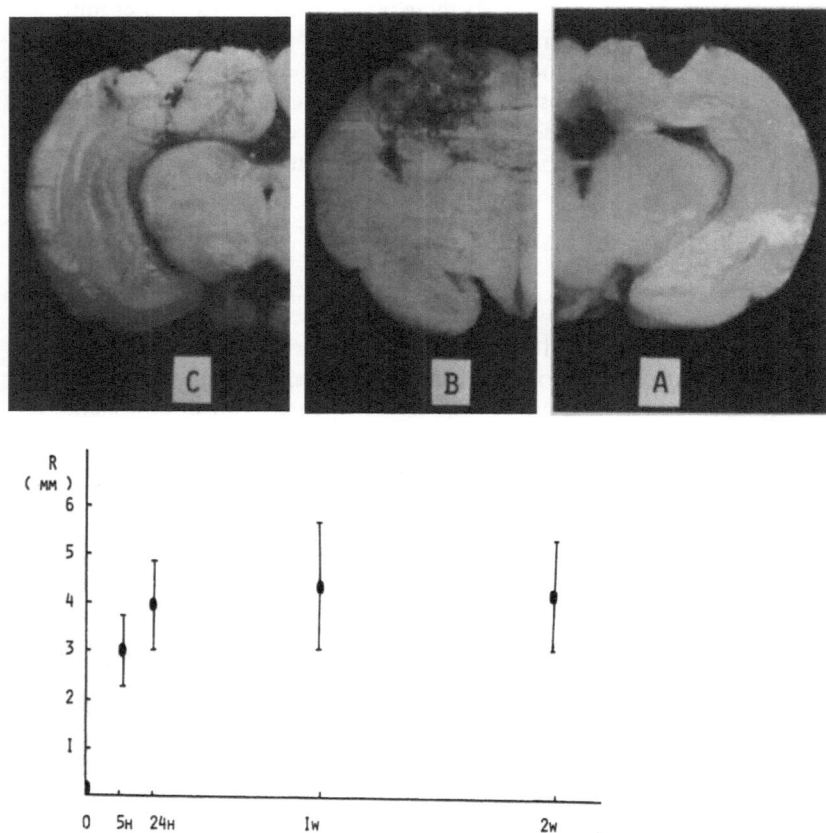

Fig. 1. Coronal section of the brain immediately after (*A*), 24 h (*B*) and 1W (*C*) after the CO_2 irradiation (15W, 3 s) (*above*). The average extent and standard deviation (mm) of the tissue damage at various time interval after laser-irradiation (n=6) (*below*). Output power is 15W and exposure time is 3 s

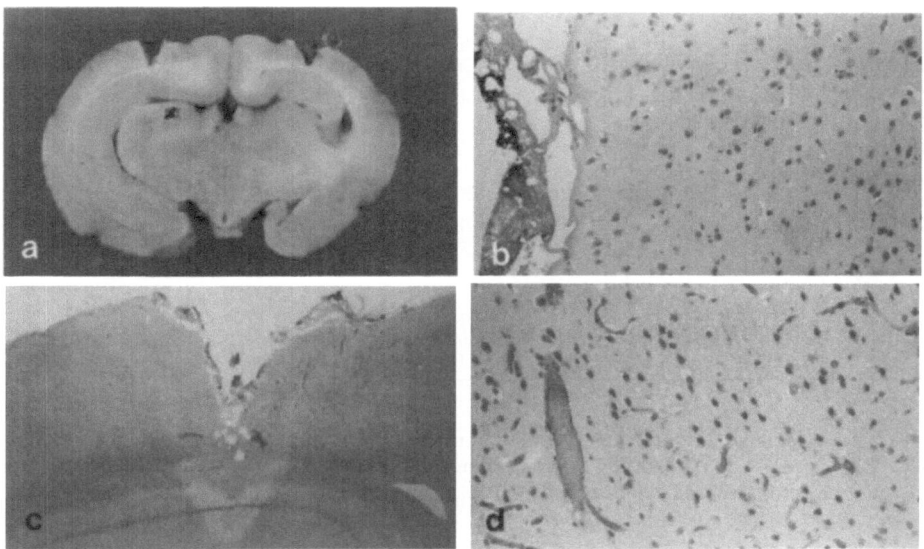

Fig. 2 a-d. Coronal section of a brain removed immediately after laser-irradiation and carbon-black injection (15W, 3 s) (**a**). Light micrograph of the irradiated brain cortex (x 66). Three layers of tissue damage surrounding vaporized tissue defect are seen (**b**). Tissue changes in charred and necrotic layer (**c**) and oedematous layer (x 66) (**d**)

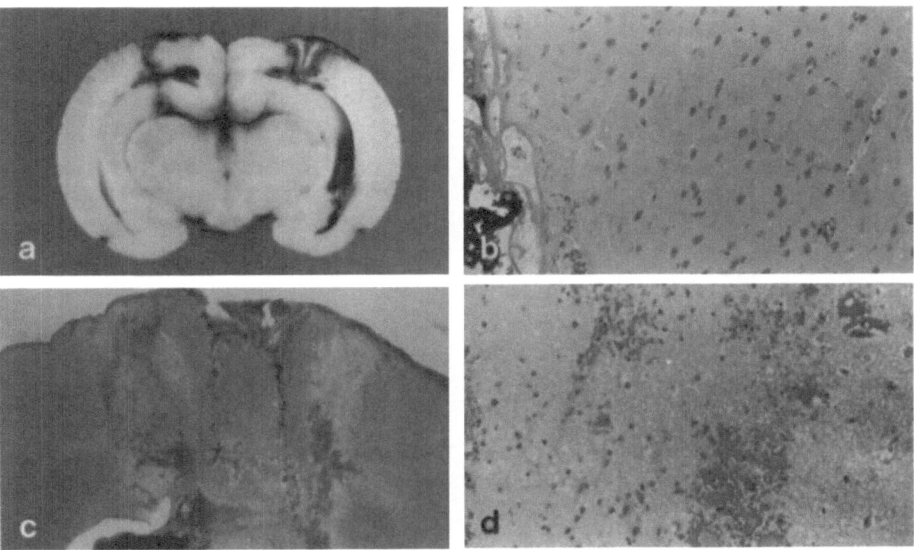

Fig. 3 a-d. Coronal section of a brain removed 24 h after laser-irradiation (15W, 3 s). Carbon black was injected just before the animal was killed (**a**). Light micrograph of the irradiated brain cortex (x 66) (**b**). The charred and necrotic layer (**c**) and oedematous layer (x 66) (**d**)

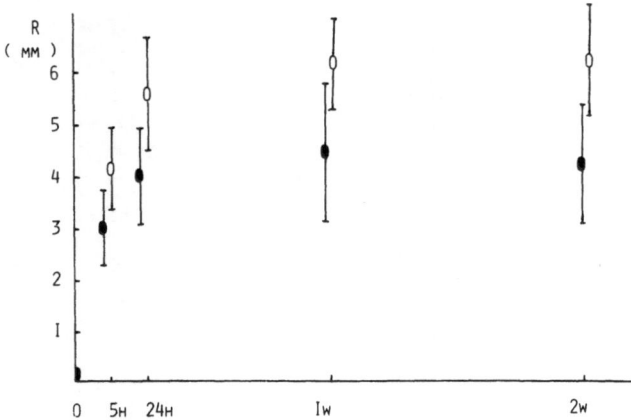

Fig. 4. The average extent and the standard deviation (mm) of the brain tissue damage under normotensive (●) or hypertensive (o) condition at various time intervals after the CO_2-laser irradiation (n=6). Output power is 15W and exposure time is 3s

Decompression in Lumbar Stenosis – New Techniques for Decompression in Lumbar Spinal Stenosis "Guided" by High Resolution CT Scans

Ch. D. Ray and K.B. Heithoff

Abstract

Central and lateral stenosis of the lumbar neural canal are a relatively less common cause of chronic pain in the lumbar region and lower limbs. Accurate anatomical diagnosis has been difficult until the advent of high resolution computerized tomographic scanning. Appropriate decompression surgery can then be focussed or "guided" by the scans as well by the clinical syndrome. Good to exellent clinical results have been seen in as many as 75% of the cases, depending upon the technique chosen. Good results are seen even in cases with very long standing pain and disorder.

Introduction

Syndromes of compression of the cauda equina and lumbar nerve roots by bony changes in the lumbar spine have been known for many years (1, 6). Because of the great difficulty in establishing a diagnosis, however, no more than "rare" cases were thought to exist. More recently attention has been called to both developmental and acquired (traumatic) stenosis and their associated clinical syndromes which often resemble vascular claudication (17, 18).

Since its inception, our department has been devoted to the use of specialized, principally implantable neurostimulation equipment for the control of chronic pain syndromes. In 1976 we began specifically to study failed back surgery cases who had implanted devices for chronic low back and radiating leg pain, where the pain proved greater than that which could be treated by the stimulation. We began to use intermediate–resolution and then when it became available high-resolution CT scanning to establish an anatomical diagnosis, to study the pathology involved, and also to guide the development of new surgical techniques (2, 4, 5, 7, 8, 16).

Entrapment

The entrapment of neural structures typically produces pain and reduction in function of the structures innervated. An entrapped nerve will undergo gradual, usually reversible changes. With the loss of space around a nerve root where it leaves the spinal canal, there will be a decrease in the fat and loose connective tissue. With further compression axons will slowly alter their conduction, principally due to a change in axonal transport, both centripetal and centrifugal (12). Further, there will be vascular compression and accumulation of tissue fluid, producing oedema of the root and perhaps of the ganglion. A cyclic entrapment ensues, often precipitated by small events.

Anatomy of Stenosis

Central stenosis is well known and generally produces bilateral pain, weakness and disturbances of bladder control, etc. Of greater interest, however, is the lateral stenosis syndrome. There may be a considerable overlap with other lumbar problems, notably the ruptured disc or the mechanical low back syndrome. However, the lateral stenosis syndrome more commonly consists of chronic sensitivity of the sciatic nerve in the pelvic notch, and neurogenic claudication (3, 9, 10, 13, 14, 19). Stenosis in the fibro-osseous foramen may arise from hypertrophy of the pedicle, enlargement of the superior articular facet, osseous changes in the posterior structures around the disc space, or hypertrophy of lateral ligaments embracing the foramen. Spurs and displacement (as with spondylolisthesis) may be a factor.

Medial hypertrophy with a narrowed "lateral recess" may produce subarticular stenosis (3). Here the nerve root is caught in a tight "pulley" around which it must pass before passing into the lateral foramen. Further, a very slight bulging of a rather superiorly placed disc may easily compress this tethered root. At the Sl level, the subarticular portion is particularly prone to stenotic entrapment.

Methods of Decompression

The important elements in an appropriate approach to decompression are based on careful analysis of the high resolution CT scan. (High resolution means the ability to visualize nerve, connective tissue, ligament, fat and blood vessels as well as bone and joint.) There are other important considerations as well, e.g., the decompression must be adequate not only for the present but for the future; in case further collapse occurs, for example, there must be space for the root. Potential regrowth of bone should be anticipated by generous decompression and, wherever possible, the leaving of cortical bone or protective membrane adjacent to nerve tissue. Consideration must also be given to the possibility of instability. If on the CT scan one can see that there is a considerable amount of ligamentous hypertrophy and ossification all around the disc space, even on the anterior aspect, it is far less likely that stability will be affected by a radical removal of posterior structures. As a general rule, however, if posterior structures (including facets) are removed, the simultaneous removal of the disc renders the spine quite likely to slip unless some form of fusion (preferably interbody fusion) is performed.

One must also try to avoid the creation of new problems such as excessive fibrosis or direct injury to roots. The utilization of free fat grafts taken from the white fat deposits of the superior buttock and the gathering of globules of white intramuscular fat during the surgical approach can be used to isolate the nerve and dura, thus helping to reduce postoperative scarring and fibrosis (2, 9, 11). The location of and quantity of the fat stores available during the decompression can be estimated from the scan itself. Further, the patient who continues to show irreversible and disagreeable leg pain in the future may respond to the use of an implanted neurostimulation device placed higher in the spinal extradural space.

Surgical Techniques

Three "types" of approach have been utilized. The transverse "wedge" technique is a transection of the pars interarticularis bilaterally (preceded by a denuding of the facet capsules and total detachment of the ligaments between laminae and spinous processes). One first visualizes the posterior dura and nerves, then makes medial-to-lateral bites utilizing a bone punch to remove as much of the pars interarticularis as possible. Straight osteotomes are used to cut out a triangular wedge just inferior to where the pars is attached to the pedicle. This is done on both sides. Then with a simple levering action from an elevator placed inside the facet space, the neural arch is removed *en bloc* (see Fig. 1). After having removed the arch, cuts in the overhanging superior facets and pedicles are easily made to permit total decompression of the roots (Fig. 2). This approach is remarkably atraumatic providing the posterior structures had been cleansed of as much ligamentous attachment as possible. The location of the pedicle and foramen should be determined by a nerve probe passed through the foramen prior to cutting the wedge. One should not cut too high into the pedicle. A second wedge may be cut out of the remaining pedicle so that its medial and inferior cortical surfaces may be displaced upwards and laterally thus relieving the root from subarticular stenosis or relative tethering. One often sees a swollen ganglion and vessels (which almost instantly dilate) as the offending structures are removed (see Fig. 2).

The lateral "wedge" is a decompressive canal cut out of the pars interarticularis leaving the ligaments intact. This is somewhat more difficult to do and the results are not as good, probably because of residual stenosis. Lateral "wedging" at S-1 is the method of choice, however, in decompressing subarticular stenosis at this site.

Bilateral cuts in the laminae which are made parallel to the long axis of the spine may be used for removing the more central parts of the neural arch to relieve central stenosis and the medial subarticular entrapment. In Fig. 1 this is shown on one side only but the other side must also be cut to remove the medial lamina and spinous process. Wedge techniques should be reserved for adults beyond the age when their spine is hypermobile. Otherwise, there may be a slippage (although to date we have only seen one); such instability may require subsequent or intraoperative fusion.

Results

Up to the present 63 "wedge" procedures have been performed. In Table 1, the surgical results of the three approaches are given. Although the lateral "wedge" was used first, results with this method are not as good as with the others. In general, I would recommend, as does Rosomoff, that the more radical removal is more likely to yield good

Table 1. Surgical results, new lumbar decompressions for stenosis: A. Transverse "wedge" procedure. B. Lateral "wedge" — laminoforaminotomy. C. Parallel "wedge" procedure

No. of PTS ::	M/F	AVG age (years)	Average Duration of pain (years)	Surgical levels decompressed 1 2 3 4				Average follow-up (months)	Results [a] nil	min	mod	ex
A. 44	27/17	35.9	14.5	22	14	7	1	7.7	4	6	20	10
B. 15	11/4	46.0	6.5	7	6	1	1	10.2	1	6	3	4
C. 4	3/1	40.5	10.9	3	1	0'	0	5,1	0	1	1	2

A. Transverse "wedge" procedure results: 75% moderate to excellent
B. Lateral "wedge" laminoforaminotomy: 50% moderate to excellent
C. Parallel "wedge" procedure results: 75% moderate to excellent

[a] Results do not include non-pain (weakness) or immediate post-operative cases

results (15). Two cases included in the transverse approach did not have pain in the presence of lateral stenosis but had weakness. The decompression was performed in hope of restoring motor function but so far, little improvement has been seen.

On the other hand, alterations in neurogenic claudication, chronic pain and disability has often been quite dramatic, even in cases where pain has been present for many years.

In conclusion, the diagnosis of spinal stenosis should be made principally on the basis of the clinical syndrome (extent of pain and disability) together with a high resolution CT scan..There should be a generous exposure utilizing the large MacElroy retractor, a clean posterior dissection before cutting the wedge, good haemostasis, good exploration of the entire nerve root (out to the transverse process), and the placement of generous fat grafts. Bleeding is controlled by bipolar coagulation and no other haemostatic agents (such as oxidized cellulose or gelatin foam) should be used, as they contribute to fibrosis. If necessary, the posterior aspect of the vertebral body and its disc margins or prominent osteophytes should be removed either with small osteotomes or by the air drill.

Although follow-up in months has been short, to date there have been no cases showing a relapse in their improvement. In some, it may take a year or more for the improvement to reach a point of relative comfort. More often, however, patients are remarkably comfortable after the massive procedure probably due in part to a partial denervation of the posterior sensory branches serving facets, ligaments and wound areas.

References

1. Brodsky, A.E.: Low back pain syndromes due to spinal stenosis and posterior cauda equina compression. Bull. Hosp. Joint. Dis. *30*, 66-79 (1969)
2. Burton, C.V., Heithoff, K.B., Kirkaldy-Willis, W., Ray, C.D.: Computed tomograpic scanning and the lumbar spine. Part II: Clinical considerations. Spine *4*, 356-363
3. Ciric, I., Mikhael, M.A., Tarkington, J.A., Vick, N.A.: The lateral recess syndrome. A variant of spinal stenosis. J. Neurosurg. *53*, 433-443 (1980)

4. Epstein, J.A., Epstein, B.S., Rosenthal, A.D., Carras, R., Lavine, L.S.: Sciatica caused by nerve root entrapment in the lateral recess: The superior facet syndrome. J. Neurosurg. *36*, 484-489 (1972)
5. Glenn, W.V., Rhodes, M.L., Altschuler, E.M., Wiltse, L.L., Kostanek, C., Kuo, Y.M.: Multiplanar display computerized body tomography. Applications in the lumbar spine. Spine *4*, 282-352 (1979)
6. Gill, G.C., Manning, J.G., White, H.L.: Surgical treatment of spondylolisthesis without spine fusion; excision of loose lamina with decompression of nerve roots. J. Bone Joint, Surg. *37*, 493-520 (1955)
7. Jacobson, R.E., Gargano, F.P., Rosomoff, H.: Transerve axial tomography of the spine. Part II. The stenotic spinal canal. J Neurosurg *42*, 412-419 (1975)
8. Kestler, O.C.: Overgrowth (hypertrophy) of lumbosacral grafts, causing a complete block. Bull Hosp. Joint Dis. *27*, 51-57 (1966)
9. Kirkaldy-Willis, W.H., McIvor, G.W.D.: Symposium: Spinal stenosis. Clin Orthop *115*, 1-144 (1796)
10. Kirkaldy-Willis, W.H., Wedge, J.H., Yong-Hing, K., Reilly, J.: Pathology and pathogenesis of lumbar spondylosis and stenosis. Spine *3*, 319-328 (1978)
11. Langenskold, A., Kiviluoto, O.: Free fat transplants in the prevention of epidural scar formation after lumbar disk surgery. A preliminary report. Clin. Orthop. *115*, 92-95 (1976)
12. Mayfield, F.H., True, C.W.: Chronic injuries of peripheral nerves by entrapment. In: Neurological Surgery. Youmans, J. (ed), pp. 1141-1161. Philadelphia: Saunders 1973
13. Nelson, M.A.: Lumbar spinal stenosis. J. Bone Joint Surg. *55*, 596-512 (1973)
14. Robertson, G.H., Llewellyn, H.T., Taveras, J.M.: The narrow lumbar spinal canal syndrome. Neurosurg *107*, 89-97 (1973)
15. Rosomoff, H.: Neural arch resection for lumbar spinal stenosis. Clin. Orthop. *154*, 83-89 (1980)
16. Sheldon, J.J., Russin, L.A., Gargano, F.P.: Lumbar spinal stenosis; radiographic diagnosis with special reference to transverse axial tomography. Clin. Orthop. *115*, 53-67 (1976)
17. Verbiest, H.: A radicular syndrome from developmental narrowing of the lumbar vertebral canal. J. Bone Joint Surg. *36*, 230-237 (1954)
18. Verbiest, H.: The significance and principles of computerized axial tomography in idiopathic developmental stenosis of the bony lumbar vertebral canal. Spine *4*, 369-378 (1979)
19. Wiltse, L.L., Kirkaldy-Willis, W.H., McIvor, G.W.D.: The treatment of spinal stenosis. Clin. Orthop. *115*, 83-91 (1976)

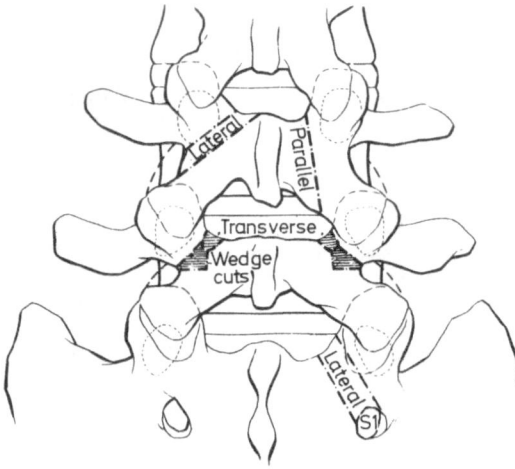

Fig. 1. Composite drawing of "wedge" procedures for lumbar spinal stenosis. Transverse wedge begins with removal of medial portions of the pars interarticularis. A triangular wedge is then cut in the pars using sharp osteotomes. A nerve probe passed through the foramen determines the location of the pedicle relative to the pars. The facet capsule and all interlaminar and interspinous ligaments are removed. The entire neural arch is then broken upward while pulling on a towel clip attached to the base of the spinous process. The parallel wedge utilizes two cuts on both sides of the lamina (only the right-sided cut shown). The lateral wedge is a deep canal cut in the lamina with sharp osteotomes; again, a probe is used to determine the location of the root and pedicle before and while cutting. ©Ch.D. Ray, 1982

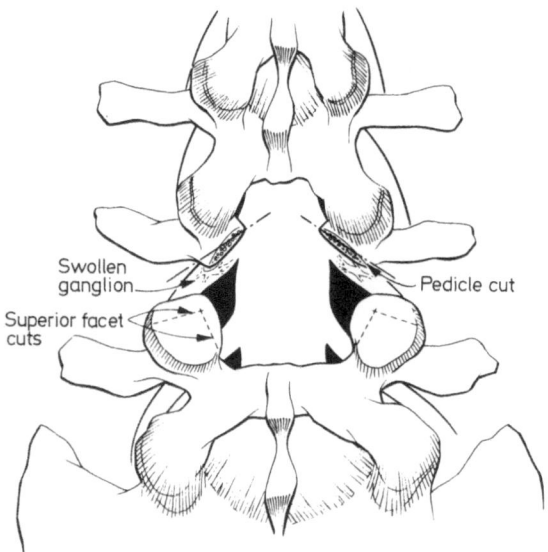

Fig. 2. Exposure after the neural arch of L-4 has been removed. Additional pedicle and superior facet cuts are now easily done to achieve good decompression. Swollen ganglia with dilated surface vessels are shown immediately after removal of the compressive bone. ©Ch.D. Ray, 1982

Intraoperative Use of Sector Scanning Ultrasonography in Neurosurgery

H. Masuzawa, H. Kamitani, J. Sato, and F. Sakai

Introduction

Intraoperative A-mode ultrasound imaging of the brain has been described (1-3, 5, 8, 11-13, 15, 16, 18, 19). B-mode dural echoencephalography using a contact compound method has also been reported (7, 17, 19), but this could not be applied directly to the brain surface because it might cause cortical bruising (19). Recent advances in computerized tomography apparently lessened the enthusiasm for the use of ultrasonography in neurosurgery. Interest in intraoperative ultrasonography has now been renewed because of technologically advanced ultrasound equipment (4, 6, 9, 10, 14). We have found that intraoperative use of ultrasonography proves to be easy, safe and valuable, especially in obtaining precise topographic localization of subcortical lesions, as well as in puncturing ventricles and cysts.

Material and Approach

Since November 1979, ultrasound examination was carried out during neurosurgical operations in 50 cases using an electronic sector scanning ultrasonograph[1] with a 2.4 MHz sector scanning probe. Details of the lesions found are listed in Table 1. A 3.0 MHz sector scanning probe was also tried. The probe and the connecting cord were sterilized pre-operatively by formalin gas for not less than twelve hours. The probe, moistened with normal saline, was gently pressed against the dura mater or saline-wetted brain surface (Fig. 1). In two cases it was also placed over a burr-hole. The space between the dura mater and the probe tip was filled with water or moistened cottonoid. In three cases it was placed directly into an intracerebral operative cavity. In nine cases needle puncture of the ventricles or needling of the tumour was carried out. For such cases we used a needle guide which had been specially designed. The contribution of the ultrasound examination to the operative procedure in each case was assessed (Table 1).

---

[1] Sonolayergraph SSH-10A, manufactured by Toshiba Corporation, Uchisaiwai-cho, Chiyoda-ku, Tokyo 100, Japan

Table 1. Summary of 50 intracranial lesions studied by intra-operative sector scanning ultrasonography

Diagnosis	No. of cases	US[a] positive	US contributary
Metastasis	11 (9)[b]	10 (9)	9 (9)
Glioma	7 (3)	7 (3)	4 (2)
Meningioma	3	3	3
Pituitary adenoma	2	1	0
Other tumours	4	3	0
Subarachnoid haemorrhage	13	0	2
Intracerebral haematoma	6 (5)	6 (5)	4 (4)
Miscellaneous	4	1	0
Total	50 (17)	31 (17)	22 (15)

[a] US= ultrasonography

[b] Numerals in parenthesis indicate the number of cases with subcortical lesions

Result

The ultrasonograph offers fan-shaped (78°), real-time, grey-scale cathode ray tube (CRT) images at a rate of 30 frames per second, which can be photographed by polaroid films (Figs. 2-4) or by 16mm movie films. The wide visible field is accounted for not only by the fan-shaped scanning field but also by the easy manipulation or angulation of the relatively small scanning probe.

Ventricles, falx or tentorium and the inner surface of the skull were consistently visualized and these served as identifiable landmarks. In three cases, ventricular tapping was successfully performed under ultrasonic guidance, in two manually and in the other by using the needle guide device. The trial use of a 3.0 MHz probe in nine cases gave images of generally better resolution than the ordinary 2.4 MHz probe (Fig. 4).

Among 46 cases of supratentorial craniotomy there were ten cases of metastatic tumours or fourteen metastatic nodules. Eleven nodules were subcortical. One of the latter, 5 mm in diameter, was not clearly shown. The rest, all 8mm or larger in diameter, were clearly shown (Figs. 2, 3). The images were valuable in selecting the corticotomy site and in dissecting out the nodule. Two nodules were transcortically needled under ultrasonic monitoring (Fig. 3) and dissection was successfully performed along the needle. In another two cases, the cystic component of the tumour was located and was easily punctured under ultrasonic monitoring (Fig. 1). Images of the needles were more easily identified on the CRT or in the 16mm movie than in polaroid films (Fig. 3) because in the two former instances, manual motion of the needle could be observed and served for identification.

Six supratentorially approached gliomas were all echogenic, although they were either high dense or low dense in the pre-operative enhanced computerized tomography. In one of them, needle biopsy was successfully performed under ultrasonic monitoring.

Six intracerebral haematomas were all detected and evacuated. Three of them were fresh haematomas and all were echogenic. Another three were relatively old haematomas, 9, 17, and 35 days old, respectively. They were shown as cysts transparent to ultrasound, although two were still high dense and the oldest was iso-dense in computerized tomography.

Meningiomas were clearly shown with sharp margins. Intracavitary introduction of the ultrasound probe during subcapsular removal of the tumour served to outline the remaining tumour mass.

Two small skull base tumours, a 3 mm suprasellar pituitary adenoma and a 5 mm adenoid cystic carcinoma of the foramen ovale, escaped ultrasound detection, probably because of their size and location. A large pituitary adenoma, a suprasellar germinoma, and a glioma in the pineal region were visualized but their images contributed little to the operation. They were all easily found, without resort to the ultrasound, by a routine approach through the subarachnoidal space. A chronic subdural haematoma was seen ultrasonically, but this did not influence the surgical approach. It was found, however, that placing the ultrasound probe over a comparatively smaller burr-hole could yield ultrasound images of fair quality.

There were four infratentorial tumours approached suboccipitally. They were clearly visualized but, again, this made little difference to the surgical approach.

Therefore, intra-operative ultrasound contributed to the operation in 44% of all the neurosurgical cases examined as shown in Table 1, or in 88% of 17 supratentorial subcortical lesions. We have not so far observed any cerebral cortical injruy due to manipulation of the probe. There has been no case of meningitis or other infectious lesion after these examinations.

Discussion

Since the advent of computerized tomography, neurosurgical operations on small subcortical lesions have generally increased. These lesions require precise topographic localization so that they can be biopsied or removed with a minimum of operative insult to cortical and surrounding brain tissues.

Linear scanning ultrasonography was tried once by the authors during operation (6, 10). However, it proved unsatisfactory because of poor contact between the probe and the brain and also because of the relatively narrow scanning field.

Recently, the usefulness of intra-operative sector scanning ultrasound examinations was reported (4, 6, 9, 10, 14). Rubin et al. (14), applied a mechanical sector scanning probe to the dura mater (dural echoencephalography). We (6, 9, 10) used electronic sector scanning ultrasonography and applied the probe to both the dura mater and the brain cortex (to the arachnoid membrane, correctly speaking). This gives a precise topographic orientation of the lesion relative to the operative field and, especially, to the various cortical landmarks. Tomographic planes can be chosen with manual control of the probe by the operator himself. Corticotomy, biopsy or removal of the lesion can be correctly performed. Under ultrasonic guidance puncture of the ventricles or of cysts can also be performed with confidence.

The manipulatory motion of the puncture needles can be actually observed as long as the needle is in alignment with the ultrasonic beams. Our needle guiding device was useful in maintaining such alignment. Future progress in technology would make it possible to perform stereotactic biopsy under ultrasonic monitoring (1). Ultrasonography through a burr-hole might be a promising technique both in ventricular punctures and in stereotactic needle biopsies.

There were occasional discrepancies between the computerized tomographic density and the echogenicity of a lesion. This is understandable because the echogenicity is based on reflection of ultrasound waves or differences in tissue density rather than the density itself. A glioma of low density in computerized tomography was as echogenic as gliomas of high density. Contrary to a previous concept (7), relatively old intracerebral haematomas were ultrasonically transparent even though they were still coagulated and of high density in pre-operative computerized tomography.

Ultrasonography in our posterior fossa tumours made no particular contribution, but this does not exclude its possible value in posterior fossa operations.

It should be mentioned that all the cases reported here were pre-operatively examined by computerized tomography. Intra-operative ultrasonography cannot replace preoperative computerized tomography but rather supplements it in the operating theatre where the latter cannot readily be performed.

Conclusion

Electronic sector scanning ultrasonography was performed, during operation, through the dura mater and through the brain cortex in 50 cases of craniotomy. Topographic identication of the subcortical lesions, ventricles or cysts was easily obtained relative to the operative field. Needle biopsies and needle punctures were confidently performed under ultrasonic monitoring or guidance. A needle guiding device was designed. Intracavitary introduction of the ultrasound probe served to outline the residual tumour. A 3.0 MHz probe gave images of better resolution than the ordinary 2.4 MHz probe.

References

1. Backlund, E., Levander, B., Greitz, T.: Stereotactic exploration of brain tumours by ultrasound. Acta Radiol. [Diagn.] (Stockh.) *16*, 117-122 (1975)
2. Ch'en, K.P., P'an, Y.H.: Intracerebral ultrasonic exploration. Chinese Med. J. *83*, 506-510 (1964)
3. Dyck, P., Kurze, T., Barrows, H.S.: Intra-operative ultrasonic encephalography of cerebral mass lesions. Bull. Los Angeles Neurol. Soc. *31*, 114-124 (1966)
4. Enzmann, D., Britt, R.H., Lyons, B., Buxton, T.L., Wilson, D.A.: Experimental study of high-resolution ultrasound imaging of hemorrhage, bone fragments, and foreign bodies in head trauma. J. Neurosurg. *54*, 304-309 (1981)
5. Glasauer, F.E., Schlagenhauff, E.: The use of intraoperative echoencephalography. Neurology (NY) *20*, 1103-1107 (1970)
6. Kamitani, H., Inoya, H., Sato, J., Masuzawa, H., Sakai, F., Hachiya, J.: Ultrasonography in neurosurgery. Teishin Igaku *32*, 580 (1980)
7. Kanaya, H., Saiki, I., Furukawa, K.: Ultrasonography in cerebrovascular diseases. Rinsho To Kenkyu *51*, 975-980 (1974)

8. Kanaya, H., Yamasaki, H., Saiki, I., Furukawa, K.: The use of echoencephalography to differentiate intracerebral hemorrhage and brain softening. J. Neurosurg. *28*, 539-543 (1968)

9. Masuzawa, H.: Intraoperative ultrasonography of the brain. Jpn. J.Med.Ultrasonics *7*, 277-279 (1980)

10. Masuzawa, H., Kamitani, H., Sato, J., Inoya, H., Hachiya, J., Sakai, F.: Intraoperative application of sector scanning electronic ultrasound in neurosurgery. Neurol. Med. Chir. (Tokyo) *31*, 277-285 (1981)

11. Mitsuno, T., Kanaya, H., Shirakata, S., Ohsawa, K., Ishikawa, Y.: Surgical treatment of hypertensive intracerebral hemorrhage. J. Neurosurg. *24*, 70-76 (1966)

12. Müller, H.R., Lévy, A.: A simple method of twodimensional intra-operative sonencephalography, employing the A-scan technique. Europ. Neurol. *1*, 31-40 (1968)

13. Nakajima, K., Taguma, N., Tsutsumi, Y.: Angiosteomatous hamartoma. Report of a case. No To Shinkei *24*, 1509-1513 (1972)

14. Rubin, J.M., Mirfakhraee, M., Duda, E.E., Dohrmann, G.J., Brown, F.: Intraoperative ultrasound examination of the brain. Radiology *137*, 831-832 (1980)

15. Sugar, O., Uematsu, S.: The use of ultrasound in the diagnosis of intracranial lesions. Surg. Clin. North Am. *44*, 55-64 (1964)

16. Tanaka, K., Ito, K., Wagai, T.: The localization of brain tumors by ultrasonic techniques. A clinical review of 111 cases. J. Neurosurg. *23*, 135-147 (1965)

17. Ueda, S.: Ultrasonic tomography of intracranial tumors by dural contact compound scan. Medical Ultrasonics *6*, 9-23 (1968)

18. Walker, A.E., Uematsu, S.: Dural echoencephalography. J. Neurosurg. *25*, 634-637 (1966)

19. Wood, J.H., Parver, M., Doppman, J.L., Ommaya, A.K.: Experimental intraoperative localization of retained intracerebral bone fragments using transdural ultrasound. J. Neurosurg. *46*, 65-71 (1977)

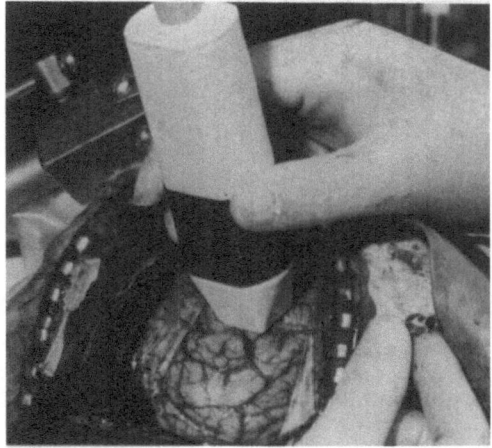

Fig. 1. Intra-operative application of an electronic sector scanning probe during right occipital craniotomy in a 57-year-old woman with a breast cancer metastasis. The probe is pressed against the brain surface moistened with saline solution. A needle is inserted manually to evacuate an intra-tumoural cyst under ultrasonic monitoring

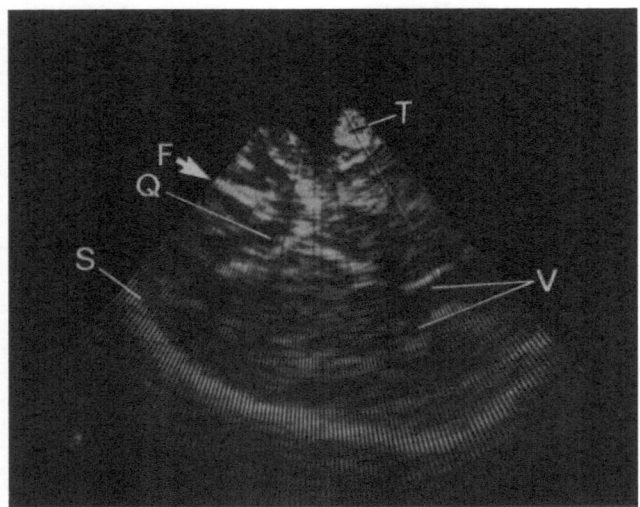

Fig. 2. Transaxial sector scan using a 2.4 MHz probe through a left parietal craniotomy during operation. The dotted line along the right margin indicates 1 cm intervals. A well-circumscribed metastatic nodule 1.5 cm in diameter (*T*) is clearly displayed slightly cephalad and 1.5 cm from the brain surface. Included are the falx (*F*), ventricles (*V*), quadrigeminal cistern (*Q*) and the inner surface of the skull (*S*)

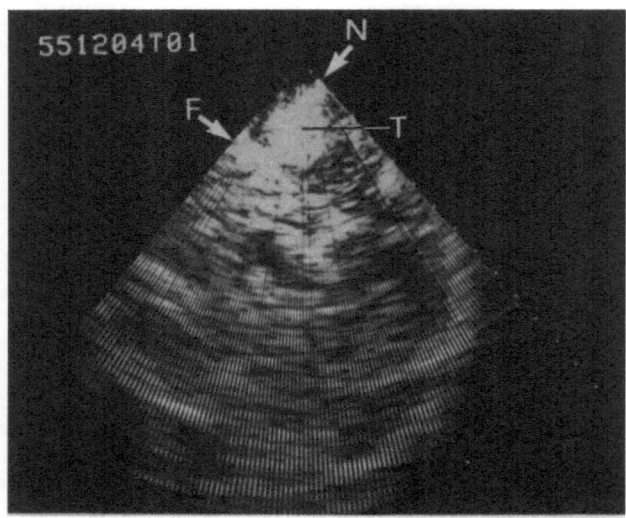

Fig. 3. Transaxial sector scan through a left occipital craniotomy in a 50-year-old woman with pulmonary cancer. A highly echogenic metastatic tumour 2 cm in diameter (*T*) is seen adjacent to the falx (*F*). Exploratory needling (*N*) through the cortex is being performed

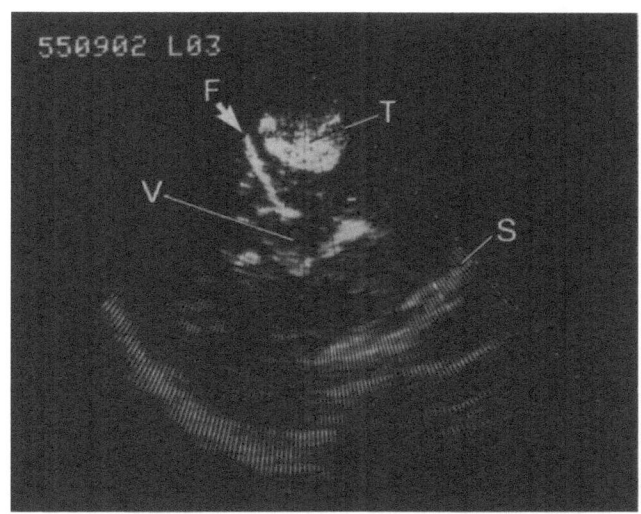

Fig. 4. Transcoronal¡sector scan using a 3.0MHz probe through a left parietal craniotomy, exposing a high convexity meningioma in a 56-year-old woman. This section shows the tumour with a sharp margin (*T*) adjacent to, but separate from the falx (*F*). The distorted bodies of the lateral ventricles (*V*) are depicted and also the skull base (*S*)

Monitoring of Head Injuries

F.A. Salem and D.J. Price

Recognition leading to early surgical evacuation of post-traumatic intracranial haematomas in patients transferred to the care of the neurosurgeons has improved considerably over the last decade. This significant advance in management has been almost entirely attributed to the use of the CT scanner and some reduction both in mortality and morbidity has been reported (2).

Unfortunately, this technological advance has only exerted a small influence on the total strategy. In many countries, it is rightly considered that neurosurgical facilities should be centralized to provide an economic well-structured service for a population of between one and three million. Apart from the combination of a very high density city population with very rapid transit facilities directly to a neurosurgical centre, most patients with head injuries are first seen in the local district hospital.

If emergency services are developed to a sophisticated degree, a direct admission policy even for urban and rural areas can be considered (1). Such emergency services can, however, only be provided by ambulance staff highly trained in emergency intubation, intravenous fluid replacement and all other resuscitative procedures necessary for treating patients with multiple injuries during transit. It is unlikely that this concept would be financially viable or widely accepted, and most countries will continue with a secondary referral policy.

The selection of patients for secondary referral usually proves to be the most difficult decision in the whole strategy of management and only those who are working in emergency departments fully recognize these difficulties. The first decision involves the greatest number of patients and is concerned with the option as to whether to telephone the neurosurgeon or not. The second decision is a little simpler, involving a shared responsibility over the telephone with the neurosurgeon. A subjective correlation of the individual patient's risk of developing a complication with the cost and time of transfer, level of expertise at the referring hospital and the availability of beds at the neurosurgical centre is used.

When CT scanning became available, it was thought that the problems of deciding about possible surgical intervention would be solved. We therefore decided to review the options for selection for an initial CT scan and these are listed as follows:

1. Carrying out serial CT scans on all patients admitted using the scanner installed in the district hospital.
2. Reserve CT scanning at the district hospital for patients with a skull fracture and/or impairment of consciousness on admission or those with localising neurological signs.

3. Transfer to a neurosurgical centre all head injuries requiring admission, for neurological monitoring and CT scanning if necessary.
4. Transfer to a neurosurgical centre only those patients with skull fracture and/or impairment of consciousness or neurological signs.
5. Only transfer patients to a neurosurgical centre if they are in coma or if there has been any evidence of neurological deterioration.

The selection of an optimum option needs a clear understanding of both head injury statistics and financial resources. A detailed retrospective survey of all patients with head injuries who were seen in emergency departments in Scottish hospitals during two periods in summer and winter provided very useful information (7). Based on these data, an estimated 19,000 head injuries per million population would be seen in emergency departments in Britain each year (Fig. 1). Of these many are unnecessarily admitted for observation (3) but 785 will have been admitted for good clinical reasons, such as altered consciousness on arrival, localising neurological signs or a fractured skull.

With these statistics in mind and considering an average district hospital serving a 200,000 suburban and rural population with its neurosurgical unit a few miles away serving a population of 2 million, none of the five options are viable.

For the first two options, the selection of the seven patients a year with a haematoma out of 876 patients admitted or 157 with a skull fracture or altered consciousness would not justify the installation and running costs of the CT scanner with a reliable 24-h radiographic and radiological service at a district hospital. The third and fourth options would involve transfer to the neurosurgical centre of 8,760 and 1,570 patients respectively. These numbers are well in excess of the 400 non-head injured neurosurgical admissions per million population in Britain and centres would need considerable expansion.

The fifth option is probably that most commonly applied. In this entire group approximately 60% have haematomas.

Patients First Seen in Coma

There seems no question that every patient in coma after a head injury should be intensively monitored and treated by a specialist team. A recent report concerning head injuries admitted in coma (defined by the absence of recognisable speech, obedience to commands or eye-opening to pain) confirmed the high incidence of intracranial haematoma, intracranial hypertension and hypoxia (5).

Quite apart from the haematoma risk, the high incidence of the other complications makes transfer to a neurosurgical unit for CT scanning, ICP monitoring and possible operation mandatory.

Patients with Neurological Deterioration

If criteria for transfer are based on this traditional advice, delays are inevitable. Mendelow (4) has clearly shown the alarming correlation between delay from the onset of deterioration in conscious level to surgical evacuation of a haematoma and quality of outcome. Undoubtedly, some of this delay can be overcome by the use of coma scales designed for detection of deterioration. If, however, scales such as the Glasgow Coma Scale are used for this particular purpose, their lack of sensitivity causes unnecessary delays due to failure of the nursing staff to be alerted to an impending significant fall in conscious level. Of those patients with significant 4 or 5 point falls in conscious level on a sensitive scale in a neurosurgical ward, 60% are not detected as showing deterioration on the Glasgow Coma Scale (6).

Disadvantages of CT Scanning

The ideal patient for CT scanning is alert and fully cooperative. The patients who are the subject of most concern are unforunately restless and confused. As most haematomas develop at any time during the first 24 hours of injury, a single initial CT scan is of limited value in excluding the possibility of a haematoma developing. Serial CT scanning of patients with some impairment of consciousness requires anaesthesia or sedation and hence this diagnostic test becomes very impractical.

Selection of One Predictive Indicator

As we were disillusioned with the practical use of CT scanning for the large group of patients who are neither fully conscious nor in coma, we examined the case records of 500 patients admitted to the neurosurgical department. Table 1 lists the clinical, radiological and ultrasound data collected. Before embarking on a full Bayesian Analysis using all the data to define the risk of a haematoma developing, we selected one single factor which proved to be the most powerful predictive indicator in the largest proportion of patients.

Table 1

1. Conscious level	initial & trend
2. Pupil signs	initial & trend
3. Motor signs	initial & trend
4. Headache	whether present
5. Seizures	whether present
6. Fracture vault	whether present
7. Fracture base	whether present
8. Midline shift	mm shift
9. Outcome	disability grading
10. Haematoma	type, size and means of diagnosis

The Need to Improve Selection for the Transfer

None of the five options for transfer already considered proved satisfactory and we found that no single clinical feature could indicate a haematoma risk level between 10% and 40% on the risk scale (Fig. 2). Patients with a fractured skull have an approximately 10% risk of developing a haematoma and those in coma have approximately a 40% risk. Transfer of all patients with a 40% or more risk involves only 90 patients per million per year, but lowering that threshold risk level to 10% or more, increases that number to 360. Twenty per cent might well be considered a reasonable compromise provided a predictive indicator can be found to influence the risk level to either well below or well above that arbitrary management threshold.

Measurement of Midline Shift by Computerised Ultrasound

The reliability of a single reading of midline shift by conventional A-mode ultrasound is entirely dependent on the expertise of the operator. It was for this reason that most neurosurgeons abandoned this diagnostic aid.

The introduction of computerized equipment with digital display and filtration of the extraneous echos has much improved the accuracy. With minimal training, a radiographer or nurse can learn the technique and obtain consistently reliable results. A series of at least 30 readings is taken within a few minutes and statistical analysis can be carried out by manual histogram to obtain a median or by a programmable calculator to produce a mean and a standard deviation. The equipment is portable and it can be used with irritable and restless patients. It is relatively inexpensive, takes less time than a CT-scan and the ease of serial estimations every few hours provides a very useful adjunct to clinical monitoring.

Evaluation of Ultrasound as a Predictive Indicator for Posttraumatic Intracranial Haematoma

Ultrasound data from 400 consecutive patients admitted to the neurosurgical unit with head injuries were analysed by the computer for the median, mean and standard deviation and merged with the operative, CT-scan and autopsy data. The data from five of the patients were inadequate for technical reasons. Of the remaining 395 patients 168 (42.5%) had a significant haematoma. Figure 3 shows how the mean midline shift influences the percentage chance of having a haematoma. If the mean value was less than 1.0 and the median was also zero, there was a 10% chance of haematoma development. This risk is no more than that associated with a skull fracture. We found that the patients within this group had either frontal haematomas which had developed slowly or they were in coma with bilateral haematomas. Those in coma qualified for a CT-scan for clinical reasons alone.

It could be suggested that as the risk of a haematoma developing in this selected group of patients exceeded 20%, they could all have a CT-scan. Over one third of this group would have required anaesthesia to prevent unacceptable movement artefacts caused by restlessness, and such inconvenience is not readily accepted by anaesthetists.

When these statistics are applied to patients admitted to a district hospital with impaired consciousness or a fractured skull, the advantages of ultrasound become dramatically apparent. To take an example, a patient with a vault fracture has a risk of 10% of developing a haematoma (Fig. 4). If there is no midline shift on the ultrasound, this is reduced to 1.5%, whilst if there is a 4 mm shift, the risk is increased to 85%. This single investigation influences the calculated risk by a factor of over 50 in this example.

The data base has now been transfered to a pocket computer and the percentage risk can be obtained by typing in only three numbers.

Conclusion

Neurosurgeons have a responsibility for guiding their colleagues in primary care hospitals in the selection of patients for transfer to the central neurosurgical unit. If beds in the neurosurgical department are limited, transfers may have to be limited to those with a risk of developing a haematoma of 20% or over. If an arbitrary level is chosen well below that, too many patients are transferred unnecessarily and if this threshold is much higher, waiting for patients to deteriorate may cause an unacceptable morbidity and mortality.

Computerised ultrasound measurement of midline shift has proved to be the most useful single factor in helping to bridge the gap between the 10% and the 40% risk levels.

We are now planning to incorporate the information obtained from ultrasound with the clinical data and apply Bayesian Analyses. Within the next few months, pocket computers capable of such complex analyses will be available for use as a guide to management in the emergency department or at the patient's bedside.

References

1. Bowers, S.A., Marshall, L.F.: Outcome in 200 consecutive cases of severe head injury treated in San Diego County: a prospective analysis. Neurosurgery 6, 237-242 (1980)
2. Cordobés, F., Lobato, R.D., Rivas, J.J., Munoz, M.J., Chillón, O., Portillo, J.M., Lamas, E.: Observations on 82 patients with extradural haematoma. J. Neurosurg. 54, 179-186 (1981)
3. Galbraith, S., Smith, J.: Acute traumatic intracranial haematoma without skull fracture. Lancet 1, 501-503 (1976)
4. Mendelow, A.D., Karmi, M.Z., Paul, K.S., Fuller, G.A.G., Gillingham, F.J.: Extradural haematoma: effect of delayed treatment. Br. Med. J. 1, 1240-1242 (1979)
5. Miller, J.D., Butterworth, J.F., Gudeman, S.K., Faulkner, J.E., Choi, S.C., Selhorst, J.B., Harbison, J.W., Lutz, H., Young, H.F., Becker, D.P.: Further experience in the management of severe head injury. J. Neurosurg. 54, 289-299 (1981)
6. Price, D.J., Marsden, A.K.: A practical coma scale for monitoring head injuries. In: Progressive care of the acutely ill and injured. Wilson, D.H., Marsden, A.K. (eds.). New York: John Wiley & Sons Inc. (in press)
7. Strang, I., MacMillan, R., Jennett, B.: Head injuries in accident and emergency departments at Scottish hospitals. Injury 10, 154-159 (1979)

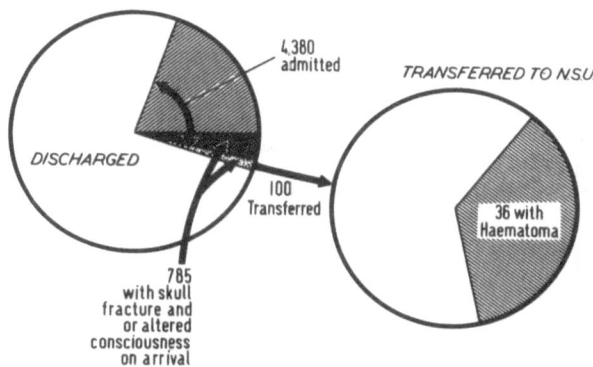

Fig. 1. Of 19,000 patients seen in hospital after head injury per million population per year, 4,380 are admitted. If beds in a neurosurgical unit (NSU) are limited, only 100 may be transferred and selection is of the utmost importance

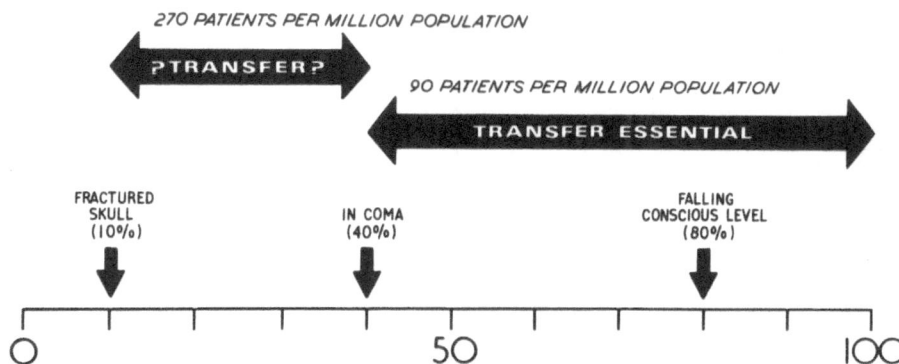

Fig. 2. Percentage risk of patients developing a haematoma related to number of patients per million population per year

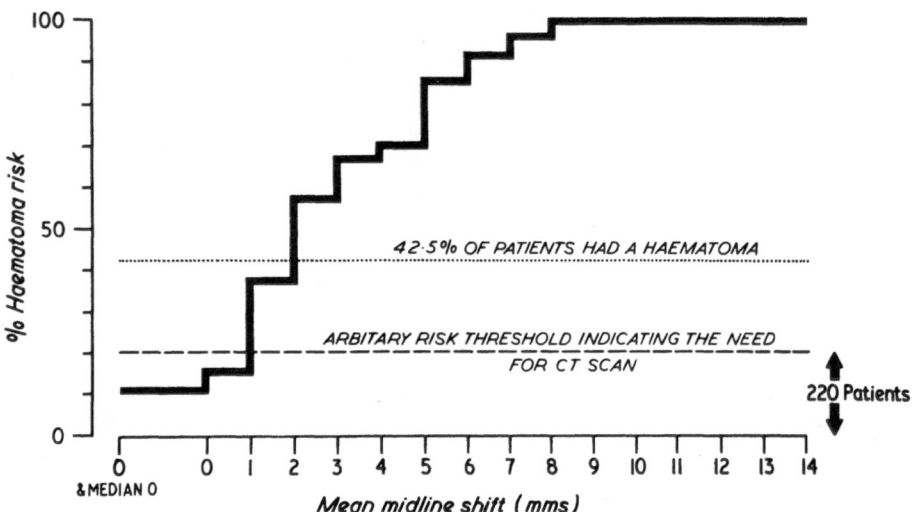

Fig. 3. Correlation of haematoma risk related to mean ultrasound midline shift in 394 patients admitted to a neurosurgical unit

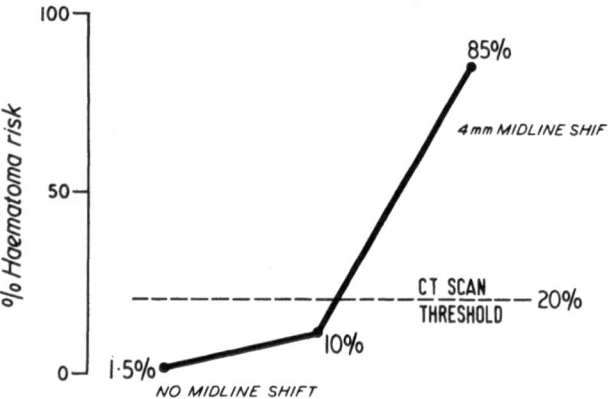

Fig. 4. Without knowledge of midline shift, a conscious patient seen in an emergency department with a fractured skull has a 10% haematoma risk.
This figure is modified by the presence or absence of midline shift

Long-Term Analysis of Cerebrospinal Fluid Dynamics in Pseudotumour Cerebri

R.D. Lobato, M.J. Muñoz, J.J. Rivas, J.M. Portillo, F. Cordobes, and E. Lamas

Introduction

Pseudotumour cerebri (PC) may have variable causes and run different courses (1–3). Most often it occurs as a self-limiting benign disease without apparent oetiology but in many cases it follows a chronic course threatening the patient's visual function. Since the occurrence of both remissions and relapses in cases of PC is usually established on clinical grounds without determining the changes in CSF pressure, the outcome of this entity is not well known at the present time (3).

The aim of this work was to analyse the changes in CSF dynamics occurring in a series of patients with idiopathic PC. Apart from determining the spontaneous variations in the CSF pressure throughout the course of the illness we tried to clarify the effects on the CSF dynamics of available medical and surgical treatment.

Material and Methods

The 32 patients included in this series presented symptoms and signs of intracranial hypertension and had definitively raised CSF pressure with normal neuroradiological studies and CSF analysis. Fluorescein angiography was performed in 18 cases, cerebral angiography in 27, EEG in 22 and isotope cisternography in 6. All patients had plain and enhanced CT scans. On the first admission and before any treatment was initiated we made continuous CSF pressure measurements over periods ranging from 12 hours to 7 days; pressure recordings were made by the lumbar route in 14 patients and intracranially in 18 more patients (either intraventricular or epidural). Apart from being displayed on a chart recorder, the pressure signal was stored by using a semi-automatic analyser, into 20 predetermined proportional pressure classes (5 mm Hg each) at time intervals of 1 sec. Once the pressure profile and the pressure histograms had been determined under basal conditions the effect of the different measures upon the pressure regime was analysed. Firstly we drained CSF until the pressure was reduced to normal level; then the AYALA index ($\frac{\Delta V}{\Delta P}$) was determined and by measuring the time taken for the pressure to return to predrainage levels the rate of CSF formation was roughly estimated. We then assessed the effect of the administration of dexamethasone (8–32 mg/day) or acetazolamide (Diamox) (500 to 3000 mg/day) on the pressure profile and on the pressure histograms. Once the best type of treatment had been determined

Table 1. CSF pressure in a series of 32 patients with Pseudotumour cerebri. Cases 1–13 form group I; cases 14–27 form group II; group III is formed by cases 28–30 and group IV by cases 31 and 32

Case No.	Age Sex	Site of pressure measurement Initial controls	Mean CSF pressure ± S.E.M. (mmHg) [a]	Total reduction in pressure with Acetazolamide dexamethasone (%)	Total time (years)	Follow-up Course Treatment-Cure-Recurrences (time) (C) (R)
1	39 f	L L	15 ± 2.1	73 69	1.5	3 weeks-C-1.5 years
2	12 f	L L	14.1 ± 3.9	– 52	1.6	2 weeks-C-1.6 years
3	38 f	IC L	25.6 ± 3.2	– 84	1.5	1 month-C-1.5 years
4	29 f	IC L	24 ± 4.1	58 –	1.7	3 months-C-1.7 years
5	27 f	IC O	21.5 ± 4.2	72 –	1.4	2 months-C-1.4 years
6	12 m	IC L	28 ± 6.1	72 76	3.1	1.5 months-C-3 years
7	23 f	IC L	32.1 ± 7	62 62	2.5	1 month-C-1.5 years-R-1 month-C-11 months
8	42 f	L O	19 ± 1.6	– 68	5	2 weeks-C-5 years
9	29 f	IC O	57 ± 8.5	92 96	2.3	2 months-C-2.3 years
10	38 f	IC L	36 ± 6.2	70 70	1	1 month-C-0.9 years
11	12 m	IC L	22.1 ± 3.2	54 –	2	3 months-C-1.8 years
12	28 f	L O	19.6 ± 2.1	72 68	1.9	1 week-C-4 months-R-1 month-C-1.5 years

13	24		L						
		f	L		22 ± 4.6	68	50	1.2	3 months-C-1 year
14	37		L						
		m		O	17 ± 5.1	26	—	2.3	3 months-C- 1 year-R-1.5 months-C-1.5 years
15	33		IC						
		f		O	22.6 ± 3.1	45	71	2.1	6 months-C-6 months-R-7 months-C-6 months
16	51		IC						
		m		O	27 ± 6.2	46	50	2.1	5 months-C-7 months-R-1 month-C-1.6
17	43		IC						
		f		O	14.5 ± 3.1	14	22	2	6 months-C-3 months-R-3 months-C-1 year
18	57		IC						
		f		O	28 ± 3.1	31	57	2.4	3 weeks-C-1.5 years-R-2 weeks-C-8 months
19	43		IC						
		m		O	20.1 ± 3.1	42	43	1.2	1.2 years-treatment tapered off
20	44		L						
		f		O	32 ± 6.3	30	35	4.3	1 month-C-8 months-R-1 month-C-1 year-R-2 months-C-1 month-R-2 months-C-2 years-R-7 months-C-6 months
21	46		L						
		f		O	17.1 ± 5.2	40	40	1.8	6 months-C-1 year-R-1 month-C-1 month
22	32		L						
		f		O	24 ± 6.2	45	36	2.3	2.3 years-treatment continues
23	52		IC						
		m		L	22.5 ± 1.2	50	—	3.9	3 months-C-2 years-R-2 months-C-1.6 years
24	43		L						
		m		O	52.8 ± 10.1	66	58	1.4	1.2 year-C-3 months
25	44		IC						
		m		O	31.7 ± 5.7	66	33	3	2 years-C-1 year
26	30		IC						
		m		O	21.6 ± 2.3	None	7	1.1	3 days-Shunt-C-Sr-C-Sr-C-So-1

Table 1 *(continued)*

Case No.	Age Sex	Site of pressure measurement Initial controls	Mean CSF pressure ± S.E.M. (mmHg) [a]	Total reduction in pressure with Acetazolamide dexamethasone (%)	Total time (years)	Follow-up (time) Course Treatment-Cure-Recurrences (C) (R)
27	31 f	L L	34 ± 7.2	36 34	1.2	1.2 years-treatment continues
28	32 f	L O	31 ± 7.1	18 11	2	7 months-treatment tapered off
29	18 f	L L	35 ± 2.1	13 18	1.2	1.2 years-treatment continues
30	30 f	L L	22.2 ± 4.1	11 8	1	8 months-treatment tapered off
31	36 f	IC L	64 ± 16.6	None None	2	6 days-Shunt-3 months-Sr-2 months-So-6 months-R-2 months-C-5 months-R-2 months-C-3 months
32	46 m	IC O	40 ± 10.1	– None	2.6	3 days-DC-4 days-shunt-1 month-Sr-5 months-C-So-2.2 years-R-1 month-C-1 month

Abbreviations: *L* lumbar; *IC* intracranial; *O* Ommaya reservoir; *So* Shunt obstruction; *Sr* Shunt revision; *C* cure; *R* recurrence; *f* femal; *m* male; *DC* decompressive craniectomy

[a] Mean pressure values and the standard error of the mean were calculated from the pressure histograms

patients were discharged and were followed for periods ranging from one (minimum) to five (maximum) years after the initial diagnosis (Table 1).

During this time we performed 382 continuous recordings of CSF pressure in order to relate the patient's clinical progress to both the spontaneous and the drug-induced changes in pressure. Control recordings were performed at lumbar level in cases presenting a short benign course, but in patients with threatened vision or a chronic course they were achieved by means of an OMMAYA reservoir implanted in the right frontal horn. In this way we could not only evaluate the effectiveness of the medical treatment but also determine the influence on CSF dynamics of permanent CSF shunting, decompressive craniectomy, menstruation, pregnancy and tapering off dexamethasone and Diamox.

Results

The age and the sex of the patients are shown in Table 1. Cases have been separated into four groups on the basis of their different clinical course. In the 13 patients who form group I the illness was short-lasting and had a benign course; these patients were not prone to present recurrences. Patients in group II had a chronic course and needed medical treatment over a long period. Group III includes three patients in whom the clinical response to medical treatment was fairly good despite the fact that CSF pressure did not change significantly. Finally, group IV consists of two patients presenting severe intracranial hypertension in whom permanent CSF shunting was the only way to control the raised pressure.

Group I. There were 11 young women and two boys (mean age= 27.1 ± 2.8 years). None had a known disease or was taking drugs. One patient had been diagnosed as PC in another hospital five years before and was given a short-term course of steroids. Present histories were short (two months on average). All patients complained of headaches and blurring or transient obscurations of vision. Two had diplopia. All women except one were obese and also one of the boys. Mild papilloedema was present in 11 cases the remainder two presenting haemorrhages and exudates. Fluorescein angiography was abnormal in the eight cases in which it was performed. Visual acuity was 10/10 in seven cases, 8/10 in three cases, and 5/10 in three more cases. Visual field examination showed enlarged blind spots and slight concentric reduction in most patients. One patient had homonymous hemianopia. EEG, CT scans and cerebral angiography were normal. The clearance of the isotope from over the brain convexity was abnormally delayed in the four patients in whom cisternography was performed. CSF pressure recordings were abnormal in all cases (Fig. 1A and Table 1). Infrequent typical or atypical A waves and B-wave activity were observed in three and nine cases respectively. Three patients had a sustained high pressure. All patients experienced a significant reduction in pressure within the first hours of receiving steroids or Diamox (Table 1). Although these two agents induced a similar quantitative decrease in pressure, the first provoked a more marked stabilisation that the second, (Fig. 1, 2). In fact, despite reducing basal pressure by 58 to 92% Diamox did not suppress A and B waves in most cases. Medical treatment could be tapered off in less than 1–2 months in most cases (Fig. 3A and Table 1). From the clinical point of view a more or less complete remission of the symptoms occurred in all cases within the first days of treatment. Clinical improvement coincided with pressure decrease except in three cases in which a return to normal pressure took a further three weeks. Only two patients in this group had a late and short-lasting recurrence of the syndrome. Three patients who became pregnant several months after discharge presented a moderate increase in CSF pressure which was unaccompanied by clinical manifestations and faded off with delivery.

Group II. Males and females were equally represented in this group (Table 1). They were older than patients in group I (mean age = 43.2 ± 2.3 years) but had a similar clinical presentation. All had headaches and blurring of vision or transient amblyopia. Four complained of decreased vision and two had diplopia. Bilateral papilloedema was present in all instances and fluorescein angiography was abnormal in the eight cases in which it was performed. As a rule visual acuity was more affected than in group I being 8/10 in eight cases, 5/10 in two cases, 10/10 in one case and 1/10 or less in two more cases (cases 24 and 26). These last two patients had been treated with sporadic short-term courses of steroids over the past two years in another department and came to us almost blind, showing intense optic atrophy and chronic papilloedema. As in group I, enlarged blind spot and concentric reduction of the visual fields were commonly found. One patient had homonymous hemianopia and another a quadrantic defect. EEG, cerebral angiography and CT scans were normal. Isotope cisternography was performed in two patients and was abnormal. Mean CSF pressure was abnormally raised in all patients (Table 1). True A waves, which occurred in five patients, were not associated with headaches or increases in systemic blood pressure in spite of the fact that in one case mean pressure at the peak of the A wave was 82 mm Hg. Most patients showed B waves of high amplitude superimposed on the base line of the pressure recording. Apart from one patient who did not respond at all, both Diamox and steroids were effective in lowering CSF pressure in all cases. However, the response was quantitatively less marked than in group I. In fact, total reductions oscillated from 7 to 66%, pressure remaining above normal limits in seven patients despite high drug dosage. Apart from being more refractory, the patients required treatment over considerably long periods of time before the first remission occurred (Fig. 3B, Table 1). In two cases the first spontaneous remission, i.e. the maintence of normal pressure without treatment, did not occur until 12 or more months after initial diagnosis had elapsed and in three more patients it has still not occurred 15, 16 and 28 months after the initial diagnosis. Once clinical improvement was achieved we always tried to reduce drug dosage to a minimum. Using this policy we realized that routine sequential pressure measurement was the only way to detect acute outbursts of high pressure which were unaccompanied by headaches. Another feature shared by patients in this group was the tendency to develop recurrences. Remarkably enough, pressure rises with recurrences tend to present always at the same level in a given patient, and in three patients Diamox and steroids were considerably less efficient in lowering pressure with a recurrence than at the first treatment. As shown in Table 1 there was one patient (case 26) in whom a CSF shunt had to be used because visual acuity was dramatically impaired and there was no response to steroids. In spite of the relatively modest reductions in CSF pressure, all patients in this Group experienced a marked or even complete clinical improvement with medical treatment. However, in many

56

cases regression of the symptoms was incomplete. For instance the optic fundi did not return completely to normal in many patients, discrete blurring persisting despite the fact that improvement of the visual function was total and that CSF pressure was kept within normal limits for long periods of time. Conversely in another two patients showing complete clinical remission and good venous pulsation in the optic discs, CSF pressure remained above normal.

Group III. These three obese young women showed similar clinicoradiological findings to patients in groups I and II (Table 1). The distinctive feature in these patients is that both Diamox and steroids although inducing a marked clinical improvement were ineffective in lowering CSF pressure (Fig. 4A). For remission of symptoms to be maintained patients had to take Diamox over long periods of time. As with patients in group II we assessed the need for treatment at a given moment by tapering off the drug and checking the changes occurring in the clinical status and the CSF pressure; provided that a spontaneous remission had not occurred the recurrence of the symptoms was very clear whereas the related changes in CSF dynamics were hardly discernable. Nevertheless when comparing pressure recordings obtained with and without treatment we observed that although steroids did not significantly decrease mean CSF pressure they blunted the pressure peaks (B and atypical A waves). Two patients in this group are clinically cured at the present time and show spontaneous venous pulsation in the optic disc despite the fact that mean CSF pressure without treatment is 18 and 23 mm Hg respectively.

Group IV. There were two patients in this series in whom medical treatment failed to modify either the clinical status or the CSF pressure level. They presented short histories (10 and 25 days) consisting of violent headaches and frequent transient amblyopic attacks followed by severe impairment of visual acuity. Both had intense papilloedema with haemorrhages and exudates. Although the CT scan was normal, cerebral angiography disclosed slowing of the circulation and defective filling of the dural sinuses. Mean CSF pressure was extremely high and could be decreased only be establishing an external CSF drainage (Figs. 1B and 4B). Interestingly enough, both Diamox and steroids were effective in decreasing CSF formation because the amount of drained fluid was reduced by more than 50%. However, pressure was unchanged so that we had to implant a permanent CSF shunt in these cases. In one of these patients we performed a decompressive craniectomy before implanting the shunt and although some stabilization of pressure occurred, mean pressure was not significantly modified (Fig. 1B). In these two patients clinical improvement was dramatic after shunting, but a residual optic atrophy and moderate impairment of visual acuity occurred. Shunts became definitively obstructed at the time that patients presented a spontaneous regression of the syndrome. Both patients have had a short-lasting recurrence but the intensity of the symptoms and the pressure rise were much less marked than initially so that they could be successfully managed with Diamox (Fig. 4B).

In the study of CSF dynamics there were certain findings that were common to patients in all four groups. The Ayala index was increased in all cases in which it was estimated (mean value = 1.02 ± 0.21; n= 22). We also found a distended subarachnoid spaces over the brain convexity when we implanted the Ommaya reservoirs and the ventricular catheters or performed the decompressive craniectomy. Moreover, 19 patients had CSF protein levels of 0.10 mg% or less. All these findings suggest the existence of increased CSF volume in our patients. The constant infusion test, performed with a 0.76 ml/min infusion rate, was abnormal in nine instances and normal in two more. When CSF pressure returned to normal by means of draining variable amounts of fluid, it returned to the predrainage levels within one hour in most patients. This time was shorter when the initial pressure was higher, being very short in cases 31 and 32. The rate of CSF formation was estimated by dividing the amount of extracted fluid in ml by the time required for pressure to return to predrainage levels in minutes. It varied between 0.18 and 0.38 ml/min (mean= 0.25 ± 0.01 ml/min; n= 22).

Discussion

The course of the illness and the effectiveness of treatment in patients with PC have been evaluated by resorting to serial visual field examinations and assessing the blurring of the optic discs. Since many patients so managed continue to develop serious visual loss or even blindness, the need for more reliable criteria of evaluating the outcome becomes apparent (2, 3).

After carrying out a close survey of the visual function and the CSF pressure changes occurring in our series of patients we feel that long-term pressure monitoring is mandatory for the correct management of chronic cases. Apart from its practical value, serial pressure measurements help to clarify the poorly understood physiopathology of PC and to outline its natural history. As has been shown here the outcome may be quite different in cases presenting identical symptoms and signs. For reasons as yet unknown the illness follows a chronic course in many patients who seem prone to de-) velop recurrences, whereas in other cases remission occurs promptly and recurrences are exceptional. The response to medical treatment is also different and whereas there are some patients who show a rapid improvement with steroids or acetazolamide, others are more or less refractory. Moreover we observed discrepancies between the degree of clinical improvement and the spontaneous or the drug-induced changes in pressure in our patients. In fact, many patients showed marked clinical improvement with only a moderate or minimum decrease in pressure. Forty per cent reductions in pressure may be sufficient while waiting for a spontaneous remission, with the certainty that vision will not deteriorate in the meantime. Since many patients improve without showing significant changes in CSF pressure and clinical improvement is the ultimate goal of treatment, it may be argued that CSF pressure monitoring is superfluous. However, serial pressure measurements represent the only reliable mean for detecting the occurrence of clinically silent outbursts of high pressure which may be followed by visual deterioration. The unfortunate outcome in patients No. 24 and 26 who received sporadic steroid treatment for two years in another department, clearly illustrate the need for frequent pressure controls in cases with a chronic course.

Although we treated all patients in group I, we wonder whether most of them would have achieved a favourable outcome without any treatment. It is uncertain whether witholding treatment in these benign cases represents a risk for evolving into chronicity. However, since the final outcome cannot be predicted on the basis of the clinical presentation or the initial changes in CSF dynamics we feel that treatment is indicated in all patients. According to our experience acetazolamide rather that steroids must be tried first. These two drugs may act by reducing CSF formation rate and steroids also by decreasing the outflow resistance to CSF drainage (3, 4). The number of cases in which clinical improvement cannot be achieved with medical treatment is small. Only in three patients were the above mentioned drugs ineffective in lowering CSF pressure so that they had to be submitted to CSF shunting. Since both steroids and Diamox were seen to decrease CSF formation a physio-pathological mechanism other than, or concurrent with CSF malabsorption had to be involved in these cases; two of these patients showed definite defects in cerebral venous drainage and the occurrence of venous engorgement could explain the failure of the medical treatment in them. It was the negative response to treatment and not the level of pressure which set up the indication for CSF shunting in patients with severe impairment of vision. The high pressure level in case 24 could be successfully controlled with Diamox and shunting was not needed in spite of the advanced optic atrophy.

In our experience repeated lumbar puncture (1−2 per day) as well as decompressive craniectomy are worthless in the management of patients with PC and should be abandoned. Finally our observations support the findings of other authors (3−5), suggesting that CSF formation rate is normal or slightly decreased in patients with PC whereas CSF absorption is diminished.

References

1. Boddie, H.G., Banna, M., Bradley, W.G.: Benign intracranial hypertension: A survey of the clinical and radiological features and long-term prognosis. Brain *97*, 313−326 (1974)
2. Gucer, G., Viernstein, L.: Long-term intracranial pressure recording in the management of pseudotumor cerebri. J. Neurosurg. *49*, 256−263 (1978)
3. Johnston, I., Paterson, A.: Benign intracranial hypertension. I. Diagnosis and prognosis. II. CSF pressure and circulation. Brain, *97*, 289−312 (1978)
4. Man, J.D., Johnson, R.N., Butler, A.B., Bass, N.H.: Impairment of cerebrospinal fluid circulatory dynamics in pseudotumor cerebri and responses to steroid treatment. Neurology *29*, 550 (1979) (Abstract)
5. Sklar, F.H., Beyer, Ch.W., Ramannthan, M., Cooper, P.R., Clark, W.K.: Cerebrospinal fluid dynamics in patients with Pseudotumor cerebri. Neurosurgery *5*, 208−214 (1979)

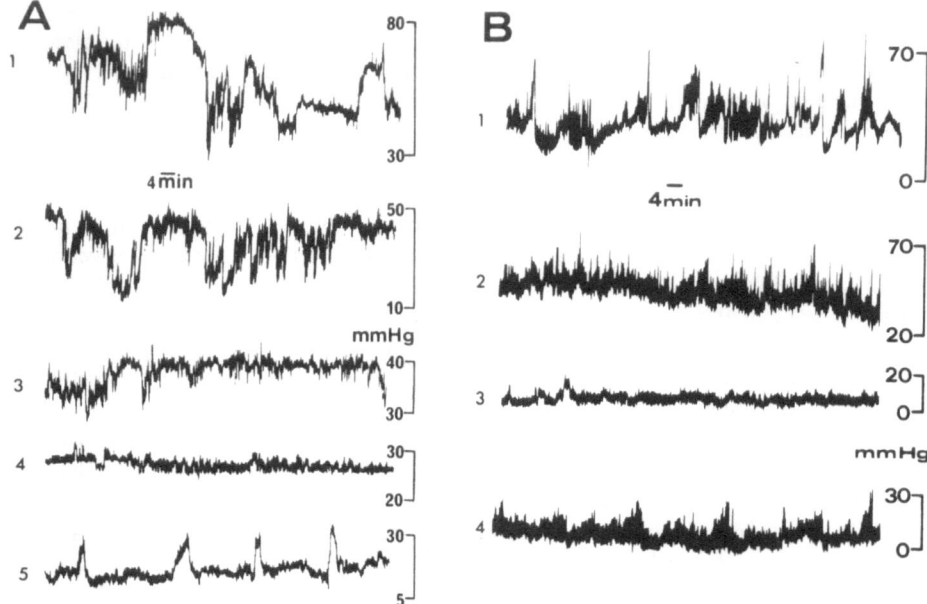

Fig. 1. A Intraventricular pressure recordings in case 9. Recording No. 1 is a basal one and No. 2 and 3 were obtained three and five days respectively after treatment with acetazolamide (2000 mg/day). Recording No. 4 was made when dexamethasone (16 mg/day) had been administered for five days; stabilization of pressure is greater than with acetazolamide although pressure is still above normal. Recording No. 5 was obtained six days after both acetazolamide (1500 mg/day) and dexamethasone (16 mg/day) had been given; mean pressure was normal at this time but small plateau waves were recorded. **B** Intracranial epidural pressure recording (Ladd fibre optic sensor) in case 32. No. 1 is a basal recording and No. 2 was obtained immediately after decompressive craniectomy had been performed; No. 3 was made after free external CSF drainage had been established. Recording No. 4 correspond to a post-shunting control

60

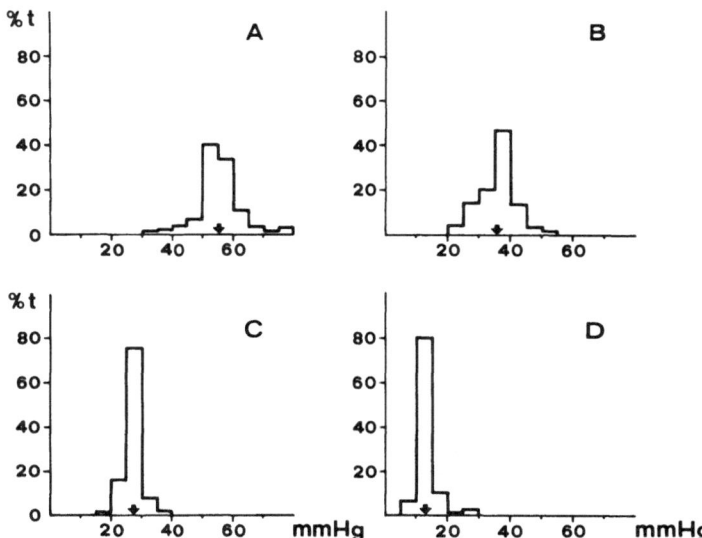

Fig. 2 A–C. Pressure-frequency histograms in case 9. **A** is the histogram obtained under basal conditions. **B, C** and **D** are histograms obtained after treatment with acetazolamide (2000 mg/day), dexamethasone (16 mg/day) and both acetazolamide (1500 mg/day) and dexamethasone (16 mg/day) respectively

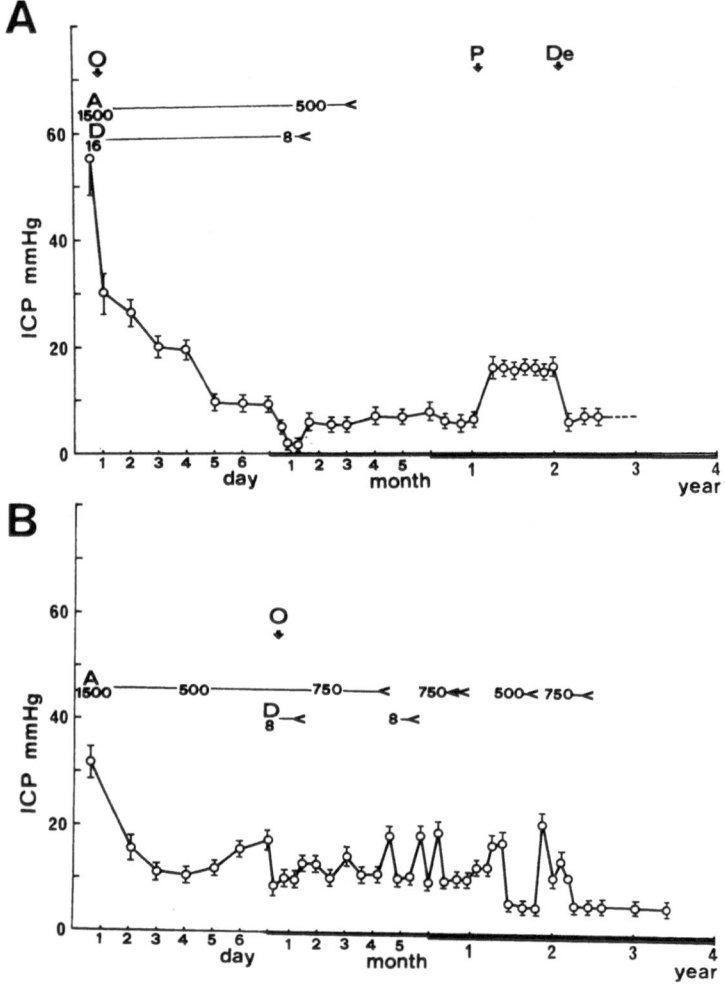

Fig. 3. A Long-term intracranial pressure (ICP) plotted daily and monthly from the first admission to May, 1981, in case 9. Acetazolamide (*A*) and dexamethasone (*D*) could be tapered off in a few months. Pregnancy (*P*) caused a slight increase in pressure which was well tolerated and subsided with delivery (*De*). Because of the severe intracranial hypertension seen at admission an Ommaya reservoir (*O*) was implanted. Each point represents the mean CSF pressure $\pm$ standard error of the mean Figures under drug abbreviations (*A, D*) indicate the total dose per day. **B** Plotting of the ICP changes in case 25. Despite treatment pressure remains above normal and rebounds were frequent. Treatment could not be tapered off until two years after first admission

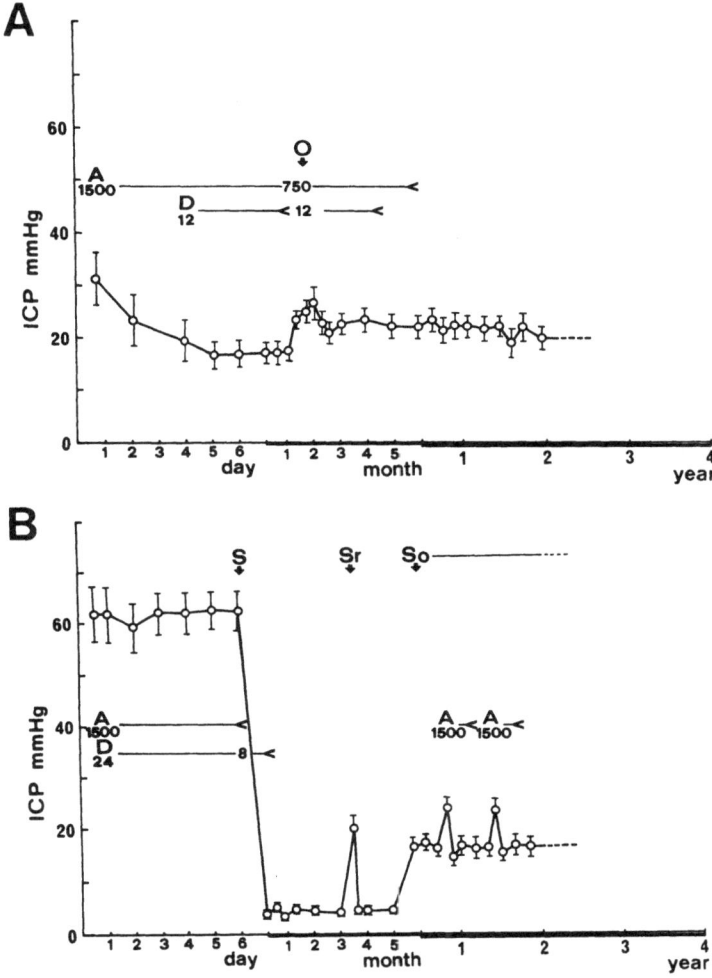

Fig. 4. A Plotting of the ICP changes in case 28. Treatment reduced pressure by less than 20%. Nevertheless clinical improvement was almost complete and treatment cbuld be tapered off seven months after first admission. This patient shows spontaneous venous pulsation in the optic discs with a CSF pressure of 18–20 mm Hg. Symbols are the same as in Fig. 3. **B** Plotting of the ICP pressure changes in case 31. Both acetazolamide and dexamethasone were ineffective in lowering CSF pressure, so a CSF shunt (S) was placed. Shunt obstruction 3 months later caused a pressure rebound which subsided after shunt revision (Sr). Pressure set around 17 mm Hg at the time that the shunt was definitively obstructed (So). In the last years there were two recurrences and raised pressure was controlled with acetazolamide

Analysis of Intracranial Pressure in Neonates and Infants

S. Kuramoto, T. Shirouzu, T. Hayashi, E. Honda, T. Shojima, S. Anegawa, Y. Ohshima, O. Nakashima, and T. Hashimoto

Introduction

Extensive studies have been undertaken to develop methods for the noninvasive, continuous measurement of intracranial pressure (ICP) via the anterior fontanelle. Wealthall and Smallwood (4) reported on an instrument which is based on the applanation principle, the Hewlet-Packard APT-16 transducer. However, the size and weight severely limits continuous, accurate ICP monitoring. We have developed a miniature transducer to overcome this problem, and we present data demonstrating its successful application.

Method and Materials

With our applanation transducer, we measured ICP via the anterior fontanelle. In order to fix the transducer to the fontanelle, the guide ring is first fixed to the scalp at three points with an adhesive agent (methyl cyanoacrylate) and then, the transducer is connected to the guide ring by the flanged springs. The footplate and the pressure-sensoring plunger is located in the central portion of the transducer (Fig. 1). The plunger transmits the pressure directly to the paper strain gauge.

The ICP was measured in normal neonates with no intracranial lesions within a week of their birth. Daily changes in ICP were recorded in 17 cases. We also followed the time pattern of ICP changes by measuring ICP in 32 normal infants. In neonates and infants with intracranial lesions, measurements were carried out six times in six cases of asphyxia or dyspnoea, 15 times in 12 cases of intracranial haemorrhage and 22 times in 14 cases of hydrocephalus. All measurements were performed on infants in the supine position during natural sleep and recording time was 3–12 hours.

Results

ICP in normal neonates ranged from 40–140 mm H_2O with an average value 84.7 (SD: 34) mm H_2O. The amplitude of the ICP pulse wave was approximately 10 mm H_2O. Characteristically, the ICP of normal neonates showed fluctuations of 15–30 minutes duration. ICP recordings during non-REM and REM sleep were similar. Premature and full-term neonates with hyperbilirubinaemia produced almost the same ICP recording as that of normal full term neonates.

Table 1. ICP value

	No. of case	No. of measurement	Non-REM		REM	
			Baseline pressure	Amplitude	Baseline pressure	Amplitude
Control group			mm H$_2$O	mm H$_2$O	mm H$_2$O	mm H$_2$O
Neonates	17	64	84.7(SD:34.0)	10.5(SD:4.3)		
Infants	32	32	89.3(SD:12.9)	y=0.236, x=12.1 [a]	135.7(SD:24.5)	
Abnormal group						
Asphyxia or dyspnoea	6	6	158.3(SD:67.7)	69.2(SD:98.8)		
Intracranial haemorrhage	12	17	165.8(SD:105.9)	28.8(SD:32.3)		
Hydrocephalus	14	22	208.3(SD:42.3)	25.0(SD:24.6)	216.0(SD:49.5)	96(SD:118.3)

[a] y= amplitude, X= month old of infants

In normal infants, baseline pressures during non-REM sleep ranged from 80 — 120 mm H$_2$O. With age, baseline pressures remained the same, but the amplitude of the pulse wave tendend to increase (y= 0.235x+12.3; y: amplitude, mm H$_2$O; x: month old). However, ICP during REM sleep behaved differently. During the first two and half months of life ICP during non-REM and REM sleep is the same. After that period, baseline pressures in addition to amplitude of pulse wave (pressure wave) were noted to increase during REM sleep. Pressure waves of more than 250 mm H$_2$O noted during the same period (Fig. 2).

ICP in patients with intracranial haemorrhage (6 subarachnoid haemorrhages, 3 intraventricular haemorrhages and 3 subdural haematomas) did not show any characteristic findings according to the site of haemorrhage.

It varied greatly according to the amount of haemorrhage, and in moderate haemorrhage, there were slight increases in baseline pressure during non-REM sleep and marked increases during REM sleep. In massive haemorrhages, REM sleep was not observed, presumably owing to disturbances of consciousness and marked increases in the baseline pressure were noted (Fig. 3). In cases in which intracranial haematomas were removed, the ICP improved after operation.

In three neonates with asphyxia, the ICP was 80–120 mm H$_2$O, that is, within normal range; slight apnoeic attacks did not effect ICP. These cases survived. However, a fourth, more severe case with an ICP of 200 mm H$_2$O, died. In two one month old patients with dyspnea, ICP rose to 200–250 mm H$_2$O and increased further during episodes of apnoea; ICP was reduced to normal range with hyperventilation or controlled respiration.

In hydrocephalic infants, the baseline pressure in the non-REM sleep was elevated to 208.3 (SD:42.5) mm H$_2$O. Although the ICP was within the normal range in two of these cases, marked elevations of pressure were observed during REM sleep in all patients.

Shunting operations were performed in ten of these cases. After the operation the ventricular size was not reduced in two cases. These cases, whose preoperative baseline pressures were 180–260 mm H_2O and whose amplitudes of 5–25 mm H_2O were low, showed poor results. However, in cases of ICP with a high amplitude, even though the preoperative baseline pressure was almost the same as above, the ventricular size was reduced and clinical results were good after the operation (Fig. 4).

Discussion

Methods for the non-invasive, continuous ICP monitoring include the fibre optic (3) and Wealthall's applanation transducers. With the former, although it is capable of estimating the mean pressure, it is impossible to analyse the ICP wave which is indispensable for analysis of the ICP. In the latter, the weight and size of the Hewlett-Packard APT-16 transducer make it unsuitable for prolonged monitoring. In contrast, our transducer is well-suited for prolonged, continuous monitoring. However, the size of the fontanelle remains a limitation, as it is impossible to measure ICP when the open fontanelle is less than 2 cm in diameter.

This is the first description of ICP measurements in neonates during non-REM and REM sleep. Cooper (1) stated that the ICP rose during sleep, especially during REM sleep and that the amplitude also increased in intracranial lesions. We observed the ICP in normal infants and neonates during non-REM and REM sleep and found similar results during REM sleep. During the period of two and half months after birth, fluctuations in ICP during REM sleep were not observed. This seems to depends upon the physical characteristics of the skull in this period. Therefore REM sleep, increases in cerebral blood flow or a slight haemorrhage lead to increases in the intracranial volume but do not seem to exert any influence on ICP. However, marked increases in the intracranial volume seem to cause changes in ICP during REM sleep first, which then leads to elevations in the baseline pressure. As the skull of the infant becomes hard with age, the intracranial compliance lowers. Consequently, at two and half months of age elevation in ICP as well as increase in amplitude are observed during REM sleep. The pressure volume relationship was generally observed in the skull (2). When the ICP rises, the amplitude is increased; however, in the case of advanced hydrocephalus, the amplitude was low in spite of a high baseline pressure. In such a case, the paper-like brain mantle and reduced cerebral blood flow is suggested. From the unfavorable prognosis of the cerebral function after shunting operation, it may be assumed that irreversible changes occur in the brain mantle and cerebral blood vessels.

Summary

1. With our newly-developed applanation transducer, the ICP was measured non-invasively and continuously via the fontanelle in neonates and infants.
2. In normal neonates, ICP ranged from 40–140 mm H_2O with average of 84.7 mm H_2O with slow fluctuations. The amplitude was small and measured approximately 10 mm H_2O.

3. In normal infants, ICP varied little with increasing age, except that amplitude increased. Pressure waves of more than 250 mm H_2O during REM sleep were noted after 2 1/2 months of age.
4. The skull of neonates has a high compliance and ICP does not necessarily reflect changes in intracranial volume.
5. Most of the hydrocephalic patients showed high ICP, but, in some cases ICP was normal and abnormality was detected only during REM sleep.

References

1. Cooper, R., Hulme, A.: Intracranial pressure and related phenomena during sleep. J. Neurol. Neurosurg. Psychiat. *29*, 564–570 (1966)
2. Miller, J.D., Garibi, J.: Intracranial volume-pressure relationship during continuous monitoring of ventricular fluid pressure. In: Intracranial Pressure. Brock, M., Dietz, H. (eds), pp. 270–274, Berlin, Heidelberg, New York: Springer 1972
3. Vidyasagar, D., Raju, T.N.K.: A simple noninvasive technique of intracranial pressure in the newborn. Pediatrics *59*, 957–961 (1971)
4. Wealthall, S.R., Smallwood, R.: Method of measuring intracranial pressure via the fontanelle without puncture. J. Neurol. Neurosurg. Psychiat. *37*, 88–96 (1974)

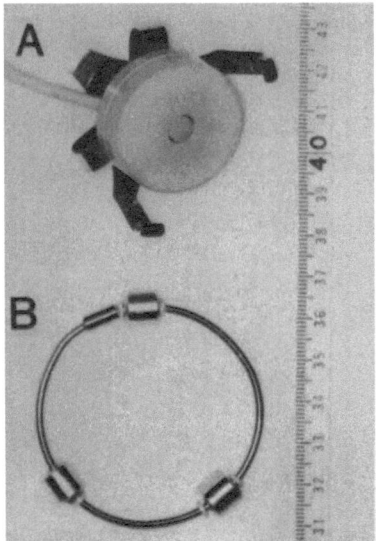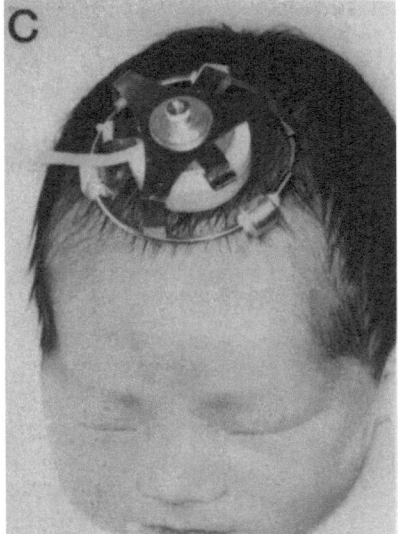

Fig. 1. A Transducer with three flanged spring, **B** guide ring, **C** transducer and guide ring was fixed on fontanelle in neonates

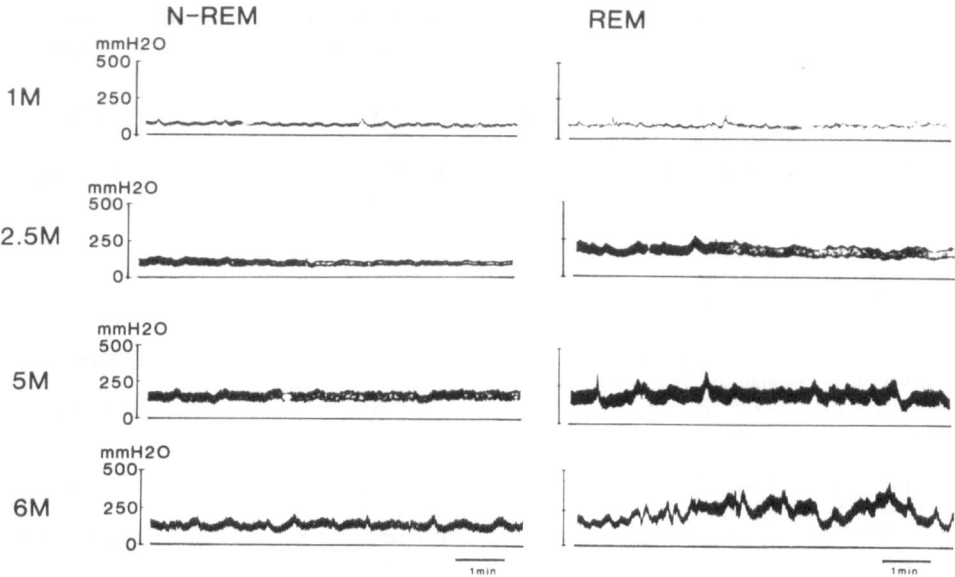

Fig. 2. Changes in ICP recordings in normal infants with age. During non-REM sleep, baseline pressure remained almost the same but the amplitudes were increased with age. ICP and amplitude were elevated in patients older than 2.5 months of age during REM sleep

Non-REM

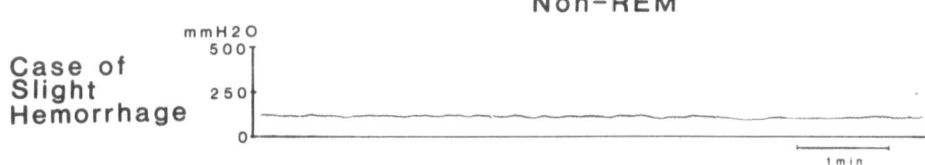

Case of
Slight
Hemorrhage

mmH2O
500
250
0
1 min

Non-REM   REM

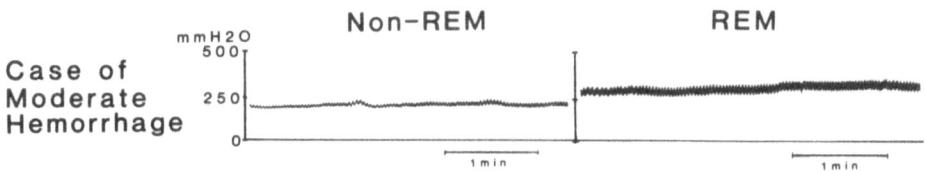

Case of
Moderate
Hemorrhage

mmH2O
500
250
0
1 min   1 min

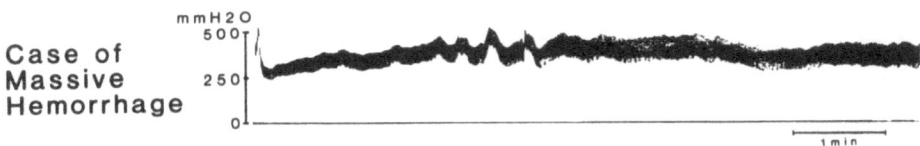

Case of
Massive
Hemorrhage

mmH2O
500
250
0
1 min

Fig. 3. ICP recordings in neonates with intracranial haemorrhages. ICP increased according to degree of haemorrhage

69

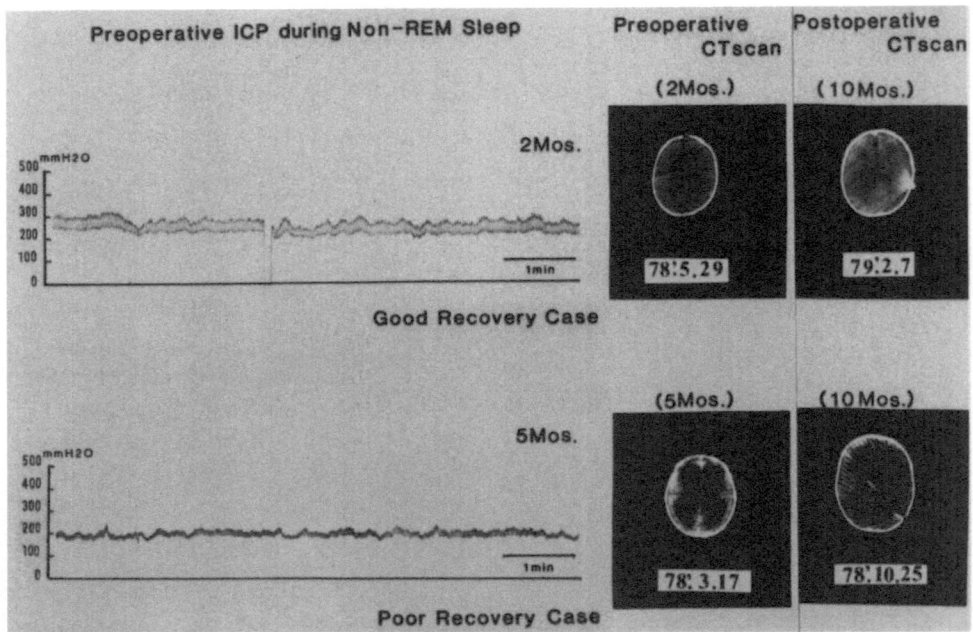

Fig. 4. Preoperative ICP and CT scans in hydrocephalic patients. Preoperative ICP shows comparable pressures for both cases, though the amplitudes were different. In the case of lower amplitude a shunting operation did not produce any reduction in ventricular size

Automated Prophylaxis of Postoperative and Posttraumatic Intracranial Hypertension

D.J. Price and J. Mason

Any serious insult to the brain, whether the result of spontaneous haemorrhage, trauma or surgical manipulation may initiate a potentially preventable progressive process of secondary brain damage. The severity of such a secondary event is determined by its pathogenesis and the length of time it remains unrecognised and untreated. The aetiology of this continuing insult is the result of any combination of the three component factors of cerebral hypoxia, hypoperfusion and mechanical distortion. All three cause a reduction of delivery of oxygen to the vulnerable brain cells and distortion also produces localised compression of the neurones in addition to its influence on vessels.

These basic pathophysiological principles have been widely understood for many years and yet in practice, they are often ignored (3, 4). A high morbidity and mortality in this relatively small but important group of neurosurgical patients then becomes inevitable. If we wish to improve our results in the management of these patients, we need to concentrate our energy and enthusiasm on those patients who become comatose after head injury, subarachnoid haemorrhage or spontaneous intracerebral haemorrhage.

Monitoring

Both the recognition of these three components of secondary brain damage and the monitoring of their treatment demand the ability to measure arterial oxygen levels, intracranial perfusion pressure and lateral shift of midline structures. In practice, continuous rather than intermittent measurement of arterial paO_2 intracranial pressure (ICP) and arterial pressure are more convenient and are less demanding on nursing and medical staff.

Serial measurements of midline shift are easier to obtain using portable computerized ultrasound equipment in the ward than by transferring the patient to a CT scanner every few hours and disrupting the continuity of management and supervision. The reliability of this technique has been assessed recently in a group of 400 patients with head injuries (9).

Reproduceability within 1.0 mm and high levels of reliability for those patients with unilateral haematomas were reported.

On-Line Signal Processing

Continuous monitoring of paO_2, ICP and arterial pressure are familiar techniques in the intensive care environment. Analogue displays either as a wave-form on a screen or as a trend on a pen recorder are usually generated. Both forms of presentation are unfortunately difficult to interpret and in particular, the ICP often proves too unstable to allow accurate visual evaluation of a mean value over a defined period. A comparison of visually assessed mean ICPs from a chart recorder with concurrent computer analysis of the same signal shows alarming discrepancies (1). This inevitably brings into question the advisability of basing clinical decisions on even the most careful observations of conventional chart records when there are large spontaneous fluctuations in the measured signal.

The advent of inexpensive computer technology has revolutionized this situation (5) and in addition, nursing staff need no longer spend so much of their time watching the bedside equipment and they can concentrate on more direct nursing care.

Continuous on-line analysis is particularly applicable to the ICP waveform as it contains useful information concerning cerebral elastance. By sampling at an adequate frequency, the amplitude of the ICP pulse wave can be determined and related to the diastolic ICP to produce a Pulse Wave Index (5). Changes in this index coincide with those in the elastance constant and when using drugs which influence the intracranial interstitial fluid volume, the selection of an optimum dose requires an estimate of the defining ing constants of the current pressure-volume relationship.

Treatment of Intracranial Hypertension

In those patients in coma after head injury or spontaneous intracranial haemorrhage, brain tissue pressure is far from uniform and we have found considerable pressure gradients between interstitial pressure within contusions and the ventricular pressure, during the first two days after head injury. Pressure gradients also develop along the vascular tree due to a narrowing of the larger vessels following subarachnoid haemorrhage, and are seen in both the macrocirculation and microcirculation after head injury. The combination of low mean capillary pressures and high surrounding interstitial pressures in the vicinity of contusions produces severe reduction in local perfusion pressure and jeopardizes the viability of the major portion of tissue which has usually escaped the primary impact injury (7, 8).

The prevention of severe secondary brain damage due to low-perfusion ischaemia is an essential feature of early intensive management. It is normal custom to reduce the ICP as measured in the subdural space or ventricle to less than 25 mmHg and to maintain a perfusion pressure in excess of 70 mmHg. The apparent "overtreatment" is necessary to offset the early interstitial pressure gradients, to provide space for their more rapid dissipation and halt further expansion of the pericontusional ischaemic areas.

For those patients with ventricular catheters, CSF drainage remains the treatment of choice for initial management but unfortunately, conventional gravity drainage is difficult to control. When elastance is high and ventricles are small, aspiration of 1 ml may produce a dramatic fall in pressure. If the outflow is too rapid the ventricles collapse down on to the catheter causing the choroid plexus to block the tip.

As the majority of patients are adequately controlled by CSF drainage and Mannitol infusion, we chose to apply closed-loop methods to these methods initially, reserving the other two drugs (Table 1) for manual administration if necessary.

Principles of Medical Application of Closed-Loop Techniques

Computerised closed-loop therapeutic techniques have only enjoyed limited success in very few intensive care situations. One reason for this failure to be accepted by the medical profession despite the availability of suitable and relatively inexpensive equipment has been due to the lack of adherence to the following basic principles:
1. Safety alarms at the bedside are essential.
2. Repeated assessment of the current effectiveness of the drug used is necessary for the inclusion of an adaptive element which compensates for variability in the individual patient and between different patients.
3. The controller must have access to the patient data base containing all the other information which might influence the signal.
4. The pharmacokinetics of the drug of choice should be fully understood.
5. If possible, the impulse response of the controlled variable should be determined.
6. Clinicians must be able to select control parameters and maximum infusion rates for each individual patient.

We have already attempted to use these principles for automated control of status epilepticus (6), of arterial pO_2 in patients with head injuries and for ICP control by CSF aspiration. All the principles had to be applied for the control of ICP by intermittent Mannitol bolus infusion.

Closed-Loop Administration of Mannitol

As the ICP pressure volume curve is non-linear, normal mathematical models familiar to control engineers are neither applicable nor safe. We have therefore approached the problem by developing control laws based on clinical, physiological and pharmacological

Table 1

Method	↓ CSF volume	Mode of action ↓ Interstitial fluid volume	↓ CBF	↓ Intracranial blood volume
CSF drainage	★			
I.v. Mannitol		★		★
I.v. Frusemide	★	★		★
I.v. Althesin			★	★

principles and incorporating necessary safety limitations. This concept resembles a fuzzy controller which has already been successfully used for the control of left atrial pressure with automatic infusions of blood (10).

In order to monitor the unpredictable and potentially dangerous patient response to Mannitol, intermittent bolus rather than continuous infusions are used.

Characteristics of the System

1. Safety Alarms

Mannitol is infused using an Imed 929 computer pump, controlled by the ward computer through a serial line interface. If the outflow pressure rises to suggest venous occlusion, if a bubble of air is detected in the line or if hardware faults develop in the pump or at the host computer, a pump alarm sounds and relevant messages are displayed on a screen at the nurses' station. Any such fault causes the pump to revert automatically to manual mode.

2. Monitoring Mannitol Effectiveness

Optimum drug administration whether conventional or automated depends on a continuing learning process related to knowledge of changes in the patient's response to that drug. If the last dose proved relatively ineffective the next dose must be proportionally higher. After each infusion of Mannitol, its effectiveness is determined and expressed as a perventage fall in ICP per ml of Mannitol per kilogram of body weight.

If the effectiveness falls below preset limits the computer informs the medical staff and suggests a check for midline shift. If that is satisfactory, enhancement of Mannitol with Frusemide or a change to a CBF suppressant such as Althesin is considered.

Most patients respond to 20% Mannitol which has a maximum effectiveness between 20 and 30 minutes after a bolus dose (2). Although it is reasonable to base an initial dosage on the patient's estimated weight, it is naive to suggest that subsequent doses should be the same. Not even the seniority of the neurosurgeon seems to have any beneficial influence on the choice of an optimum dose (Fig. 1) and the rather complex task of calculating the volume of each dose is best delegated to a computer.

3. Inclusion Within a Patient Data Base

The control of a single physiological parameter divorced from other clinical information is potentially dangerous. Automated drug therapy should therefore only be considered if the logical algorithm involves access to all relevant data concerning the patient's progress. For Mannitol administration, such essential information includes that concerning procedures which might influence the ICP and the effect of Mannitol istself on fluid and electrolyte balance.

For many years, nurses' charts with partly digital and partly graphic display have been satisfactory. Current shortages in numbers of nurses stimulated us to attempt to replace the charts with a small inexpensive data terminal for input and retrieval and for transmission to the minicomputer data base. It is not acceptable to require nurses to enter data on a chart and then duplicate entries to a computer data base.

This terminal was designed by our nurses in conjunction with ergonomists and acceptibility was only achieved when we were able to prove that this was superior to the charting system in all respects. The latest prototype is proving satisfactory but further adaptions are required. Preliminary studies suggest a reduction in data input times of 50% in comparison with charts.

4. Plasma Clearance

The repeated administration of any drug has to be judged according to its rate of clearance from the plasma. As mannitol is cleared entirely by glomerular filtration, its half-life is related to the glomerular filtration rate. In the absence of renal failure, a constant half-life can be presumed and the proportion of the last dose in circulation at any subsequent time can be calculated. For example, if one hour after a 300 ml infusion had been given and a further plasma concentration to that original level is required, the "top up dose" needed would be 300 minus that volume remaining in circulation (Fig. 2).

5. Clinician Control

During the first 24 hours after injury or operation very aggressive control of ICP below 20 mm Hg. is advisable to dissipate the initial high interstitial cerebral pressure gradients. When these gradients gradually resolve over the next few days, control values may then be relaxed.

We consider that the neurosurgeon should be able to manipulate these control values in order to tailor the treatment regime to the needs of each individual patient. This involves simple access to the program constants through the keyboard at the nurses' station and any of the four following values may be changed:
1. bolus infusion rate,
2. threshold ICP level,
3. target ICP level,
4. maximum plasma concentration.

1. Bolus Infusion Rate. This solves a purely mechanical problem related to the size of the vein used for the infusion. In practice, we have found the need for only two alternatives — one for children and one for adults.

2. Threshold ICP Level. This is the pressure above which treatment should be instituted and is usually within the range of 15—25 mm Hg. As Mannitol only becomes effective some ten minutes after the start of infusion, a calculation is necessary to estimate what the ICP will be at that time. If this forward projection of the current trend exceeds the selected threshold level, treatment proceeds (Fig. 3). In practice, a decision concerning treatment is made at the end of each fifteen minute period.

The "success" of treatment is expressed as the period in each 24 hours during which the pressure is below a defined level 5 mm Hg. above the selected threshold.

3. Target ICP Level. Each Mannitol infusion aims to reduce the ICP to a pressure below the threshold level. This is the target pressure and we chose it within a range of between 3 and 10 mm Hg. below the threshold. The dosage is calculated to achieve that target by the end of 30 minutes and the actual proportional fall achieved during that time is used to update the effectiveness constant.

4. Maximum Plasma Concentration. To avoid electrolyte and fluid inbalance, plasma Mannitol concentration calculated from the clearance equation is not allowed to exceed this level. The relationship between this concentration and serum osmolality is presumed to be linear but this subject is under study at present. When the chosen maximum level is reached a message is displayed at the nurses' station to suggest the possible need for a change to Althesin therapy.

Work in Progress

It is now apparent that the combination of CSF aspiration with carefully controlled Mannitol treatment is sufficient for the majority of patients with intracranial hypertension. Similar principles of closed-loop control are being applied to a CSF aspiration system with automated catheter clearance.

Results

The closed-loop Mannitol administration has now been used on 30 patients. When we compare tracings of patients treated by manual and computer it becomes clear that manually, we have often used too high a dose too late, resulting in poor control (Fig. 4). Despite the considerable improvement in control achieved by the computer system, the total dosage of Mannitol given each 24 hours is no more than when under manual control.

Apart from the availability on display at the nurses' station of trends over a selected time period, graphs are printed summarizing 24 hours of ICP data correlated with dosage of Mannitol given (Fig. 5).

References

1. Driscoll, P.A., Price, D.J., Mason, J.: A comparison of graphical trends on a chart recorder with computer generated displays. Critical Care Medicine 9, 216 (1981)
2. Ferrer, E., Villa, F., Isamat, F.: Mannitol response and histogram analysis in raised ICP. In: Intracranial pressure IV. Shulman, K., Marmarou, A., Miller, J.D., Becker, D.P., Hochwald, G.M., Brock, M. (eds.), pp. 647–649. Berlin, Heidelberg, New York: Springer (1980)

3. Graham, D.I., Adams, J.H., Doyle, D.: Ischaemic brain damage in fatal non-missile head injuries. J. Neurol. Sci. *39*, 213–234 (1978)
4. Pathologists and head injuries. Brit. Med. J. *1*, 1344 (1981)
5. Price, D.J., Dugdale, R.E., Mason, J.: The control of ICP using three asynchronous closed loops. In: Intracranial pressure IV. Shulman, K., Marmarou, A., Miller, J.D., Becker, D.P., Hochwald, G.M., Brock, M. (eds.), pp. 395–399. Berlin, Heidelberg, New York: Springer (1980)
6. Price, D.J.: The efficiency of Sodium Valproate as the only anticonvulsant administered to neuro-surgical patients. In: The place of Sodium Valproate in the treatment of epilepsy. Parsonage, M.J., Caldwell, A.D.S. (eds.), pp. 23–34. London, Toronto, Sydney: Academic Press 1980
7. Price, D.J.: Intracranial pressure monitoring. Brit. J. Clin. Equipment *5*, 92–98 (1980)
8. Price, D.J.: Severe head injuries: In care of the critically ill patient. Tinker, J., Rapin, M. (eds.). Berlin, Heidelberg, New York: Springer (in press)
9. Salem, F.A., Price, D.J.: Monitoring of head injuries. In: Modern Neurosurgery 1. Brock, M. (ed.), pp. 44–50. Berlin, Heidelberg, New York: Springer (1982)
10. Sheppard, L.C., Kouchoukos, N.T., Kurtts, M.A., Kirklin, J.W.: Automated treatment of critically ill patients following operation. Ann. Surg. *168*, 596–604 (1968)

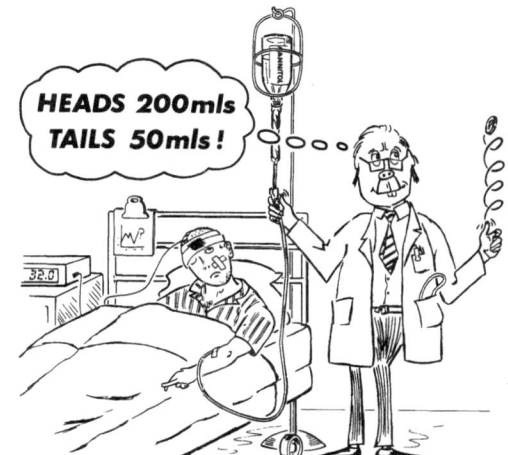

Fig. 1. A method of random selection of an optimum dose of Mannitol. The older the neurosurgeon, the less dispute there is about his "judgment"

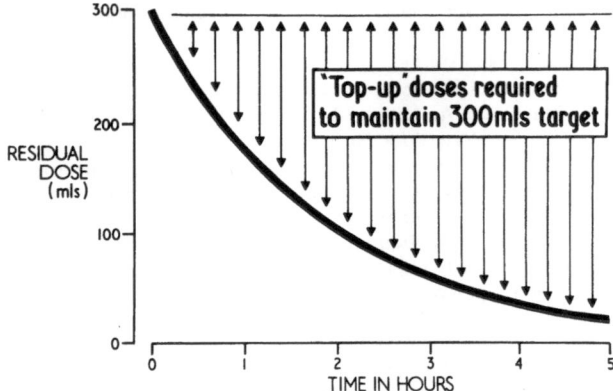

Fig. 2. Plasma clearance of Mannitol following a large 300 ml bolus infusion. The "top up doses" (*arrows*) required to produce the same circulating plasma levels increase as time proceeds

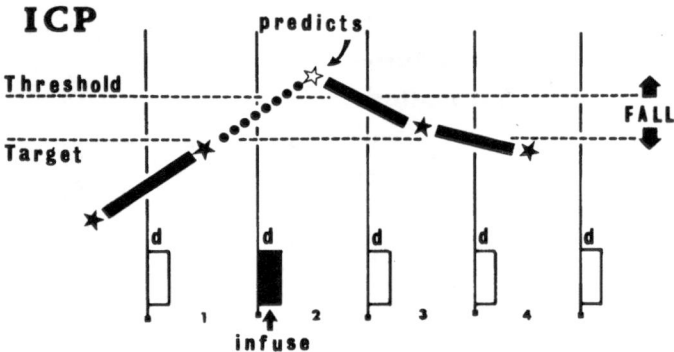

Fig. 3. A graph showing the decision to infuse Mannitol at the second fifteen minute period, based on the projected pressure rising above the selected threshold. The volume of the infusion is related to the proportional reduction required to achieve the target level (d= decision)

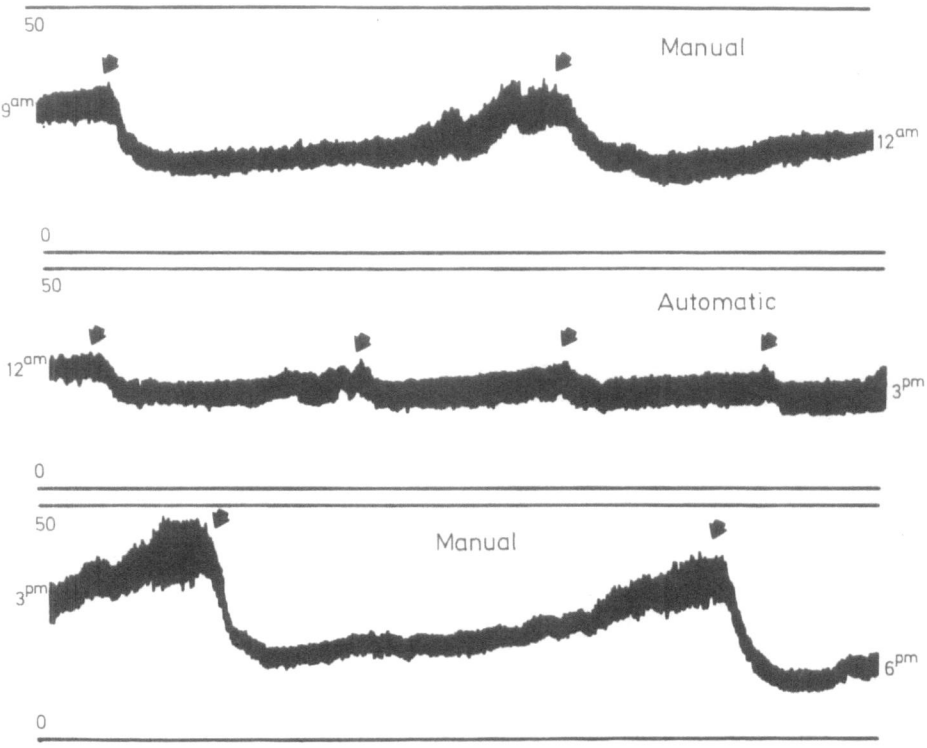

Fig. 4. Three consecutive periods of an ICP recored demonstrating the difference between manual and computer control. This illustrates that despite an attempted rigid regime under manual control, too high a dosage is often given too late (*arrows*)

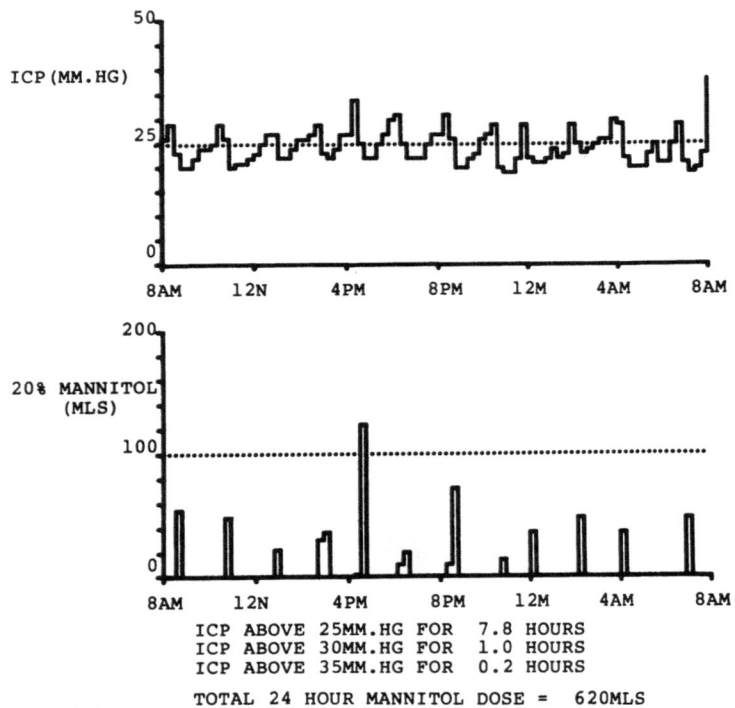

ICP ABOVE 25MM.HG FOR   7.8 HOURS
ICP ABOVE 30MM.HG FOR   1.0 HOURS
ICP ABOVE 35MM.HG FOR   0.2 HOURS

TOTAL 24 HOUR MANNITOL DOSE =   620MLS

Fig. 5. A 24 hour computer plot for the patient records of mean ICP with volumes of Mannitol infused under computer control. This patient had a large acute subdural haematoma removed two days previously and the threshold level had by then been raised to 28 mm Hg and the target level to 22 mm Hg

Penetration of Antimicrobial Drugs into the Cerebrospinal Fluid —
Its Relevance in Postoperative CSF Infections

H. Friedrich, G. Hänsel-Friedrich, H. Dietz, and J. Potel

Introduction

The serum and tissue levels of most antibiotics which are used for the therapy of infections in the central nervous system (CNS) are known. Despite the enormous literature on CNS infections and their treatment, little information is available regarding penetration of the newer antibiotics into the cerebrospinal fluid (CSF).

The relative exclusion of antibiotics from the CSF is generally attributed to the blood-brain and the blood-CSF barrier. Histologically the brain capillary walls and the adjacent layer of glial cells are impermeable to many small molecules but permeable to certain others. All organic compounds have to pass this lipid membrane. Numerous factors regulate entry, distribution and concentration of antibiotics within the CSF. The penetration rate from blood into CSF is not only dependent on lipid solubility, ionisation, protein binding and molecular size but also on cerebral blood flow, and the formation and absorption of CSF. Moreover, active removal of antibiotics from the CSF by mechanisms which transport drugs from the CSF into the blood have been postulated. From the clinical point of view the penetration into the CSF plays an important role in the distribution of an antibiotic within the CSF and brain abscesses. Postoperative CNS infections are life-threatening complications, because their tendency to spontaneous healing is very low. This is due to the lack of defense mechanisms, since the CSF contains only 0.1% of the white blood cells and very few immune globulins.

During recent years we have systematically investigated serum and CSF concentrations of various antimicrobial drugs in patients with and without meningitis. The aim of this study was to establish an optimal regimen of antimicrobial treatment in CSF infections, particularly those which may occur after neurosurgical operations.

Patients and Method

In most neurosurgical operations prophylactic chemotherapy is not indicated (5, 9). In this clinic per-operative short-term chemoprophylaxis is only used in those operations in which a foreign body is implanted into the CSF, i.e. CSF shunts, ventricular drainage systems and stimulators (5, 28). The penetration of several antibiotics into the CSF was investigated by determining serum and CSF levels simultaneously in 68 patients with and without meningitis. The CSF samples were taken from external CSF drainage systems (lumbar or ventricular). In 46 patients without meningitis it was possible to study the penetration of antibiotics into the CSF without violating ethical rules, because in all these cases the CSF drainage system had been inserted for intracranial pressure monitoring or for diagnostic purposes.

Twelve out of 22 patients with meningitis suffered from post-operative shunt sepsis. In these cases the shunt was completely removed and replaced by an external ventricular drainage system. In all patients with meningitis or ventriculitis the diagnosis was confirmed by raised cell count and CSF protein, and by identification of the pathogens. During the investigation the drainage systems were opened only for taking the samples from a three-way tap. All blood samples were taken from a central venous catheter. Blood and CSF samples were collected simultaneously at particular time intervals. The concentrations of most antibiotics were determined biologically by the agar diffusion method of Grave and Randall (11).

The concentrations of Co-trimoxazole were determined by the spectrofluorometric method described by Schwartz et al. (27) (Trimethoprim) and by the absorption-spectrometric technique modified by Rieder (sulfamethoxazole) (22). The analytical technique used for chloramphenicol concentrations was high pressure liquid chromatography as modified by Rosin (23).

Results

The antimicrobial drugs investigated are shown in Table 1. The sulphonamides are known to have an excellent CSF penetration but their antibacterial spectrum is poor. The combination of *trimethoprim (TMP)* and *sulfamethaxazole (SMZ)* interferes with two consecutive steps of the normal bacterial metabolism of folinic acid (1). The synergistic bactericidal effect of the combination has been demonstrated in a wide variety of gram-positive and gram-negative organisms. *Co-trimoxazole* reaches high CSF concentrations irrespective of the degree of meningeal inflammation.

Figure 1 shows continuous TMP and SMZ levels during a 12 hour period in the CSF, while the serum concentrations decrease within 3–4 hours.

Trimethoprim (TMP) (3)

The maximal and minimal CSF concentrations of TMP are shown in the right-hand column of Fig. 1.

The maximum CSF level of 0.7 μg/ml was found two hours after the maximum serum level of 1.75 μg/ml immediately after repeated parenteral administration of 160 mg TMP. The minimum CSF level of 0.32 μg/ml was found 12 hours after administration.

The maximum TMP concentration in the CSF reaches 39.7% of the plasma concentration. The CSF-serum ratio was up to 68.9% after two hours and 109.4% after 12 hours in several patients. These data show that the determination of the CSF-serum ratio is not an adequate method for evaluating the degree of penetration into the CSF, for it is influenced by the sampling time and is dependent on the different rates of decrease in CSF and serum concentrations.

Table 1. Antimicrobial drugs investigated (serum and CSF concentrations determined simultaneously)

Antibiotic	No. of patients	Plasma-CSF-concentrations
I. Combination Trimethoprim Sulfamethoxazole	7	70
II. Chloramphenicol	5	39
III. β-Lactam antibiotics a) Acylureido-penicillin Mezlocillin	17	168
b) Cephalosporins Cephalothin	2	10
Cefazolin	4	25
Cephacetril	6	133
Cefuroxime	5	72
Cefotaxime [a]	4	38
Moxalactam	3	36
IV. Aminoglycosides Gentamicin	9	82
Sisomicin	6	75

[a] With kind permission of PD Dr. med Stolke, Med. Hochschule Hannover

Sulfamethoxazole (3)

The maximum CSF concentration of non protein bound SMZ was 9.5 μg/ml determined 1–3 hours after the maximum serum level of 77 μg/ml.

A ratio of TMP:SMZ of about 1:10 is maintained. In our cases (six patients with normal and one patient with inflammed meninges) the penetration of co-trimoxazole into the CSF was independent of a normal or pathological CSF state. All CSF concentrations found were above the minimal inhibitory concentration (MIC) of co-trimoxazole susceptible pathogens and thus therapeutically effective.

Figure 1 demonstrates the good penetration of TMP and SMZ into the CSF even when the blood-CSF barrier is intact. Consequently TMP alone or the combination co-trimoxazol should be a valuable drug for per-operative chemoprophylaxis in neurosurgery and particularly for the therapy of the postacute state of meningitis (12), since the blood-CSF barrier then becomes tighter again and the CSF concentration of most antibiotics administered during the acute state drops rapidly to ineffective levels.

Chloramphenicol (8)

Chloramphenicol is said to have a good capacity for penetrating the intact blood CSF barrier (14, 15, 24, 29). This antibiotic can cause the rare but irreversible bone marrow aplasia that so justifiably limits its use to a small number of specific infections. Its antibacterial activity is also limited, because chloramphenicol is essentially a bacteriostatic agent.

In 1949 Glatzko et al. described a colorimetric procedure for the determination of chloramphenicol in biological materials (10). With this method CSF concentrations were found between 40% and 100% of the serum concentrations. Windörfer et al. (1981) reported high chloramphenicol levels in the CSF of newborns and babies but noticed "marked variations" of serum and CSF concentrations (30). Using the same method Roy et al. found errors of measurement of up to 40% (24). Kramer et al. (15) determined brain concentrations of chloramphenicol by the agar diffusion method and stated: "The amount of chloramphenicol assayed from the brain was nine times greater than the comparable blood level in a paired sample".

In our study serum and CSF levels of chloramphenicol in five neurosurgical patients with normal meninges were determined with the high pressure liquid chromatography (HPLC) modified by Rosin (23).

Figure 2 shows maximal serum concentrations between 7.45 and 26.14 μg/ml. The maximum CSF levels were about 2.16 μg/ml one hour after injection of 1g of chloramphenicol succinate and decreased to 1.55 μg/ml after two hours.

Compared to the results from the literature we found a much lower concentration of chloramphenicol than expected in the CSF of patients with non-inflamed meninges. Because of its possible side-effects chloramphenicol should not be used for per-operative chemoprophylaxis in neurosurgical operations.

However, it still can be recommended in the postacute stage of meningitis, when most less toxic antibiotics do not reach comparably high CSF levels in slightly inflamed meninges (30). In the acute stage of meningitis therapeutically adequate CSF levels can be achieved even with most betalactam antibiotics.

Mezlocillin (6)

Seventeen neurosurgical patients received 5–15 g Mezlocillin intravenously at eight-hour intervals. Serum and CSF concentrations were determined simultaneously 168 times. In ten patients with intact CSF barrier the maximum CSF level was 0.9 μg/ml three hours after infusion. Of the seven patients with meningitis the maximum CSF concentrations ranged between 10.4 and 32 μg/ml during a period of 2–3 hours (Fig. 3).

The penetration of mezlocillin into the CSF seems to be dependent on the degree of inflammation. Therefore, in the postacute stage of meningitis therapeutically adequate CSF levels cannot be obtained. By additional intraventricular administration of 3x50–100 mg per day, mezlocillin levels can be raised to 50 μg/ml.

According to the MIC of most pathogens these CSF concentrations are in the range of therapeutic efficacy. With these recommended doses no neurotoxic side effects were observed.

In patients with an intact CSF barrier most *cephalosporins* diffuse poorly into the CSF. Even in meningitis the measured concentrations vary over such a wide range, that these drugs have to be rejected in the treatment of meningitis. Mangi et al (19) and Lorber (17) reported a few cases of meningitis occurring during treatment with cephalothin and cefazolin. From the cephalosporins included in our study only the findings with cefuroxime and moxalactam are presented.

Cefuroxime (7)

Five neurosurgical patients, two with normal meninges and three suffering from acute meningitis, received 2g of cefuroxime intravenously every eight hours. In patients without meningitis the CSF concentrations amounted to 0.01–0.09 $\mu g/ml$. With inflamed meninges the hightest CSF concentrations were 3–7.5 $\mu g/ml$ and occurred during the first and second hour after infusion. A progressive decline followed for the next six hours after injection as shown in Fig. 4.

The value of intravenous therapy with cefuroxime is questionable despite these concentrations, because the MIC of cefuroxime against several organisms causing postoperative meningitis often exceeds these levels. In the postacute stage of meningitis the penetration of cefuroxime into the CSF decreases rapidly. However, in patients with cefuroxime susceptible organisms this cephalosporin derivative can be administered in daily doses of at least 100 mg/kg given at six hours intervals.

Moxalactam

This is a new cephalosporin, an oxa-beta-lactam, with a broad spectrum of activity (18). Three patients with meningitis received continuous therapy (2–4 g intravenously every 8 hours) (Fig. 5). Plasma and CSF levels were determined periodically for several days. In all patients peak plasma concentrations of 50–90 $\mu g/ml$ were observed half an hour after intravenous infusion. Peak CSF levels of moxabetalactam ranged from 3.1–9.4 $\mu g/ml$ after the first dose. After repeated administration they rose to 17–30 $\mu g/ml$. Peak levels were obtained 1–2 hours after intravenous administration. In our patients the moxalactam penetration into the CSF seemed to be dependent on the degree of inflammation and the dosage of the antibiotic (13, 16). The mechanism that promotes the diffusion of moxalactam into CSF is unknown. Although moxalactam is hydrophilic and insoluble in organic solvents like the other cephalosporins, its penetration rate into the CSF seems to be higher.

Moxalactam is found to be highly active against certain gram-positive and gram-negative clinical isolates. However, other cephalosporines are superior against staphylococci and pseudomonas (18).

Sisomicin (2)

Sisomicin is an aminoglycoside which closely resembles gentamicin in antimicrobial activity, pharmacology and clinical efficacy. After systemic administration CSF levels of sisomicin and gentamicin are very low in patients with normal meninges (Fig. 6). We measured sisomicin concentrations in the CSF of six patients without meningitis 30 minutes to eight hours after repeated intravenous injections of 80 mg of sisomicin. Concentrations ranging from 0 (in five patients) to 0.4 $\mu g/ml$ were found.

Gentamicin

Gentamicin concentrations were determined in patients with meningitis, and although these levels were higher than those in the patients treated with sisomicin, they were below the detectable limit of 0.1 μg/ml after four hours. These concentrations are therapeutically inadequate. Therefore all our patients with gentamicin susceptible staphylococcus epidermidis or gram-negative meningitis were treated with gentamicin administered both parenterally and intraventricularly. The intraventricular instillation of 5 mg gentamicin every 24 hours resulted in CSF concentrations of 48 μg/ml 30 minutes after administration, 20 μg/ml 2 hours and 2–8 μg/ml 24 hours after administration. Therapeutic CSF levels were maintained for 24 hours after repeated intraventricular instillation. Intrathecal application by repeated lumbar puncture, however, is ineffective (5, 20, 25, 29).

In summary Table 2 demonstrates the penetration rate into the CSF of the antibiotics discussed, related to their maximum serum concentrations, while Table 3 shows the doses of antibiotics recommended for intraventricular administration.

In patients with an *intact blood-CSF barrier* we found no measurable or very low CSF levels of all beta-lactam-antibiotics and of the tested aminoglycosides. Even with chloramphenicol we achieved considerably lower CSF concentrations than expected according to the literature. Only the CSF levels of trimethoprim and sulfamethoxazole showed a satisfactory relation to the plasma concentrations.

All CSF samples were taken from external ventricular or lumbar drainage systems. The site of sampling for concentration assay had little influence on the results. Only in four cases with different protein content of the ventricular and lumbar CSF increased antibiotic levels were determined in the lumbar CSF, despite the CSF pathways being free. This suggests that the CSF concentrations are dependent on the CSF protein content and a somewhat impaired CSF circulation as found in patients with meningitis. On the other hand, in two patients with non-inflamed meninges suffering from acoustic tumours this phenomenon was not observed although there was a marked difference in the protein content of ventricular and lumbar CSF.

Furthermore *hydrocephalus* or severe *head injury* — if there was no contamination of CSF with blood — did not influence the CSF concentrations. With inflamed meninges the CSF levels of most antibiotics increase remarkably, the concentrations being highly dependent upon the degree of meningeal inflammation

Clinical Aspects

In postoperative neurosurgical infections the microorganisms most frequently isolated are Staphylococcus epidermidis and Staphylococcus aureus (Table 4). Since the pathogens involved are often multiresistant it is mandatory to determine the minimal inhibitory concentration, to consider the CSF-patency of the antibiotic in question and the variability of its CSF concentration even in meningitis.

Table 2. Penetration of antibiotics into the CSF of patients with and without meningitis in relation to maximal serum concentrations (poor= below 2%, fair= more than 10%, good= more than 20%)

Antibiotic	CSF − penetration Normal meninges	Meningitis
I. Combination		
Trimethoprim	Good	Good
Sulfamethoxazole	Good	Good
II. Chloramphenicol	Fair	Fair-good
III. β-Lactam antibiotics		
a) Acylureido-penicillin		
Mezlocillin	Poor	Fair-good
b) Cephalosporins		
Cephalothin	Poor	Poor-fair
Cefazolin	Poor	Poor-fair
Cephacetril	Poor	Poor-fair
Cefuroxime	Poor	Poor-fair
Moxalactam	Poor	Fair-good
IV. Aminoglycosides		
Gentamicin	None	Poor-fair
Sisomicin	None	Poor-fair

Table 3. Doses of antibiotics recommended for intraventricular administration

II. Chloramphenicol	25−50 mg
III. β-Lactam antibiotics	
a) Mezlocillin	50−100 mg
b) Cephalosporins	
Cephalothin	25−100 mg
Cefazolin	25−50 mg
Cephacetril	25−100 mg
Cefuroxime	25−50 mg
IV. Aminoglycosides	
Gentamicin	2−8 mg
Sisomicin	2−4 mg

Table 5 shows the antimicrobial drugs investigated and their susceptibility to staphylococcus epidermidis. The susceptibility patterns of Staphylococcus aureus are similar. Although gentamicin has been used extensively in recent years for the treatment of postoperative CSF infections, the incidence of bacterial resistence to this antibiotic has remained low. However, systemic treatment with aminoglycosides alone, is insufficient. Also it must be given by the intraventricular route. Where this is not possible co-trimoxazole may be an good alternative because its efficacy against staphylococci corresponds to that of the aminoglycosides and beside, therapeutically adequate CSF levels of this drug can be achieved even with normal meninges.

Table 4. Micro-organisms involved in 97 postoperative CSF infections

1. 1979 − 6. 1981 (4300 operations)

Organism	No. of patients	No. of positive culturs
Staph. epidermidis alone	64	104
Staph. epidermidis mixed	3	8
Staph. aureus	14	33
Staph. aureus β-haemolytic	1	2
Strep. viridans	4	6
Pseudomonas	3	9
Esch. coli	3	6
Klebsiella pneumonia	2	10
Pneumococci	1	2
Micrococci	1	4
Enterobacter aerogenes	1	16

Table 5. Susceptibility of Staphylococcus epidermidis to the antimicrobial drugs investigated

CSF-infections (1. 79 − 6. 1981) and Staphylococcus epidermidis (64 patients)

Susceptibility (%)	Good	Fair	Non	Not tested
I. Co-Trimoxazol (TMP − SMZ)	68	2	28	2
II. Chloramphenicol	48	−	25	27 [a]
III. β-Lactam antibiotics				
a) Mezlocillin	14	3	9	74 [a]
b) Cephalosporins	53	3	16	28 [a]
c) Pen resistent to penicillinase	60	4	18	18 [a]
IV. Aminoglucoside Gentamicin	73	3	22	2

[a] Because of high resistence

Antibiotic prophylaxis in neurosurgical operations is still under discussion. According to the literature (5, 26) the routine use of antimicrobial prophylaxis does not reduce the infection rate and may even provoke superinfections with resistant pathogens.

Long-term antibiotic prophylaxis in patients with rhinorrhoea does not show any significant effect concerning the development of meningitis.

Two years ago we finished a prospective study on neurosurgical patients undergoing operations of more than six hours duration. There were two groups, one which received per-operative short-term antibiotic prophylaxis with co-trimoxazole and one which did not. Our results from 364 patients demonstrated that the incidence of postoperative infections including meningitis could not be reduced, with the exception of catheter-associated urinary tract infections (9). Antibiotic short-term prophylaxis might be indicated whenever a foreign body is implanted into the CSF space.

In CSF shunts, for instance, the shunt valve with its somewhat stagnant cavity is an ideal culture medium for infectious organisms. Thus, meningitis and ventriculitis are the most frequent causes of mortality and morbidity in shunted patients (25, 28, 29). In a previous study (5) we demonstrated that the well-considered use of a per-operative short-term prophylaxis limits the progression from a transient intra-operative bacteriaemia to an established postoperative shunt infection. Since no complications result from such short-term antibiotic prophylaxis and superinfections as well as changes of the bacterial spectrum are unknown, this method has no disadvantages. Our results correspond to those of other investigations (26, 28). In cases of shunt infection our first treatment consists of intravenous and intra-shunt antibiotic therapy without removal of the shunt system. Only if this procedure fails the infected shunt system is removed, an external ventricular drainage performed and both systemic and intraventricular antibiotics administered according to the resistance test.

Conclusion

Successful control of neurosurgical infections demands appropriate antibiotic concentrations at the site of infection, against the micro-organism involved. Since many antibiotics administered by the systemic route do not reach therapeutically effective CSF levels either with normal meninges or with meningitis, additional intraventricular administration seems to be the only way to avoid disappointing results. This is particularly true for postoperative CSF infections in neurosurgery.

References

1. Daschner, F.: Inhibition of cell wall synthesis by sulfonamides and trimethoprim. Chemotherapy 22, 12–18 (1976)
2. Friedrich, H., Pelz, K., Haensel-Friedrich, G.: Liquorspiegeluntersuchungen zwei neuerer Antibiotika Cefazolin und Sisomicin. Neurochirurgia 20, 123–131 (1977)
3. Friedrich, H., Haensel, G.: Liquorspiegeluntersuchungen einer Trimethoprim-Sulfamethoxazol-Kombination im Ventrikel-liquor bei neurochirurgischen Patienten. Acta Neurochir. 37, 271–280 (1977)
4. Friedrich, H., Pelz, K., Haensel-Friedrich, G.: Lack of penetration of cephacetrile into the cerebrospinal fluid of patients without meningitis. Infection 6, 226–230 (1979)
5. Friedrich, H.: Untersuchungen zur Liquorgängigkeit einiger Chemotherapeutika und zur perioperativen Chemoprophylaxe neurochirurgischer Infektionen. Habilitationsschrift, Medizinische Hochschule Hannover 1980
6. Friedrich, H., Pelz, K., Haensel-Friedrich, G., Isele, E.: Liquorspiegeluntersuchungen von Mezlocillin bei Patienten mit und ohne Meningitis. Inn. Med. 6, 165–172 (1979)
7. Friedrich, H., Haensel-Friedrich, G., Langmaak, H., Daschner, F.D.: Investigations of cefuroxime levels in the cerebrospinal fluid of patients with and without meningitis. Chemotherapy 26, 91–97 (1980)

8. Friedrich, H., Haensel-Friedrich, G.: Liquorgängigkeit von Chloramphenicol – eine kritische Überprüfung. Neurochirurgia *23*, 235–238 (1980)

9. Friedrich, H., Haensel-Friedrich, G., Hüttner, B., Daschner, F.: Perioperative Chemoprophylaxe bei Langzeitoperationen in der Neurochirurgie. Fortschr. Med. (in press)

10. Glatzko, A.J., Loretta, M.W., Wesley, A.D.: Biochemical studies on Chloramphenicol. I. Colorimetric method for the Determination. Arch. Biochem. *23*, 411–418 (1949)

11. Grove, D.C., Randall, W.A.: Assay methods of antibiotics: a laboratory manual. New York: Medical Encyclopedia 1955

12. Hansen, I.B.: The combination trimethoprim-sulphamethoxazole. Antibiot. Chemother. *25*, 217–232 (1978)

13. Kaplan, S.L., Mason, E.O., Garcia, H., Koernland, S.J. et al.: Pharmacokinetics and Cerebrospinal Fluid Penetration of Moxalactam in Children with Bacterial Meningitis. J. Pediatr. *98*, 152–157 (1981)

14. Kelly, R.S., Hunt, A.D., Tashman, S.G.: Studies on the absorption and distribution of chloramphenicol. Pediatrics *8*, 362–367 (1951)

15. Kramer, P.W., Griffith, R.S., Campbell, R.L.: Antibiotic penetration of the brain. J. Neurosurg. *31*, 295–302 (1969)

16. Landesman, S.H., Corado, M.L., Chembin, C.C., Gombert, M., Cleri, D.: Diffusion of a new beta-lactam into cerebrospinal fluid. Am. J. Med. *69*, 92–98 (1980)

17. Lorber, B., Santoro, J., Swenson, R.M.: Listeria meningitis during cefazolin therapy. Ann. Int. Med. *82*, 226–229 (1975)

18. Malottke, R.: Bakteriologische Untersuchungen mit einem neuen halbsynthetischen Oxy-Beta-Lactam Antibiotikum. Infection *8*, 43–45 (1980)

19. Mangi, R.J., Kundargi, R.S., Quintilani, R., Andriole, V.T.: Development of meningitis during cephalothin therapy. Ann. In. Med. *78*, 347–351 (1973)

20. McCracken, G.H., Mize, S.: A controlled study of intrathecal antibiotic therapy in gram negative enteric meningitis of infancy. J. Pediatrics *89*,66–72 (1976)

21. Moellering, R.C., Fisher, B.G.: Relationship of intraventricular gentamicin levels to cure of meningitis. J. Pediatrics *31*, 534–537 (1972)

22. Rieder, J.: Physikalisch – chemische und biologische Untersuchungen an Sulfonamiden. Arzneimitt. Forsch. Drug Research *13*, 81–105 (1963)

23. Rosin, H., Nixdorf, A., Spira, I.: Konzentrationsbestimmung von Antibiotika durch Hochdruck-Flüssigkeits-Chromatographie: Chloramphenicol. Referat Arbeitstagung Deutsche Gesellschaft für Hygiene und Mikrobiologie, Mainz 1978

24. Roy, T.E., Krieger, E., Craig, G., Cohen, D., McNaughton, G.A., Silverthorne, N.: Studies on the absorption of chloramphenicol in normal children in relation to the treatment of meningitis. Antibiot. and Chemother. *1965*, 1044–1050 (1966)

25. Salmon, J.H.: Ventriculitis complicating meningitis. Amer. J. Dis. Child. *124*, 35–40 (1972)

26. Savitz, M.H., Malis, L.J., Meyers, B.R.: Prophylactic antibiotics in neurosurgery. Surg. Neurol. *2*, 95–100 (1974)

27. Schwartz, D.E., Koechlin, B.A., Weinfeld, R.E.: Spectrofluorometric method for the determination of trimethoprim in body fluids. Chemother. *14* (Suppl.) 22–29 (1969)

28. Venes, J.L.: Control of Shunt infection. J. Neurosurg. *45*, 311–314 (1976)

29. Wilson, H.D., Bean, J.R., James, H.E., Pendley, M.M.: Cerebrospinal fluid antibiotic concentrations in ventricular shunt infections. Child's Brain *4*, 74–82 (1978)

30. Windoerfer, A., Bauer, P., Alterthum, K.: Bestimmung von Chloramphenicol in Serum und Liquor bei Neugeborenen und Säuglingen mit bakterieller Meningitis. D.m.W. *106*, 739–743 (1981)

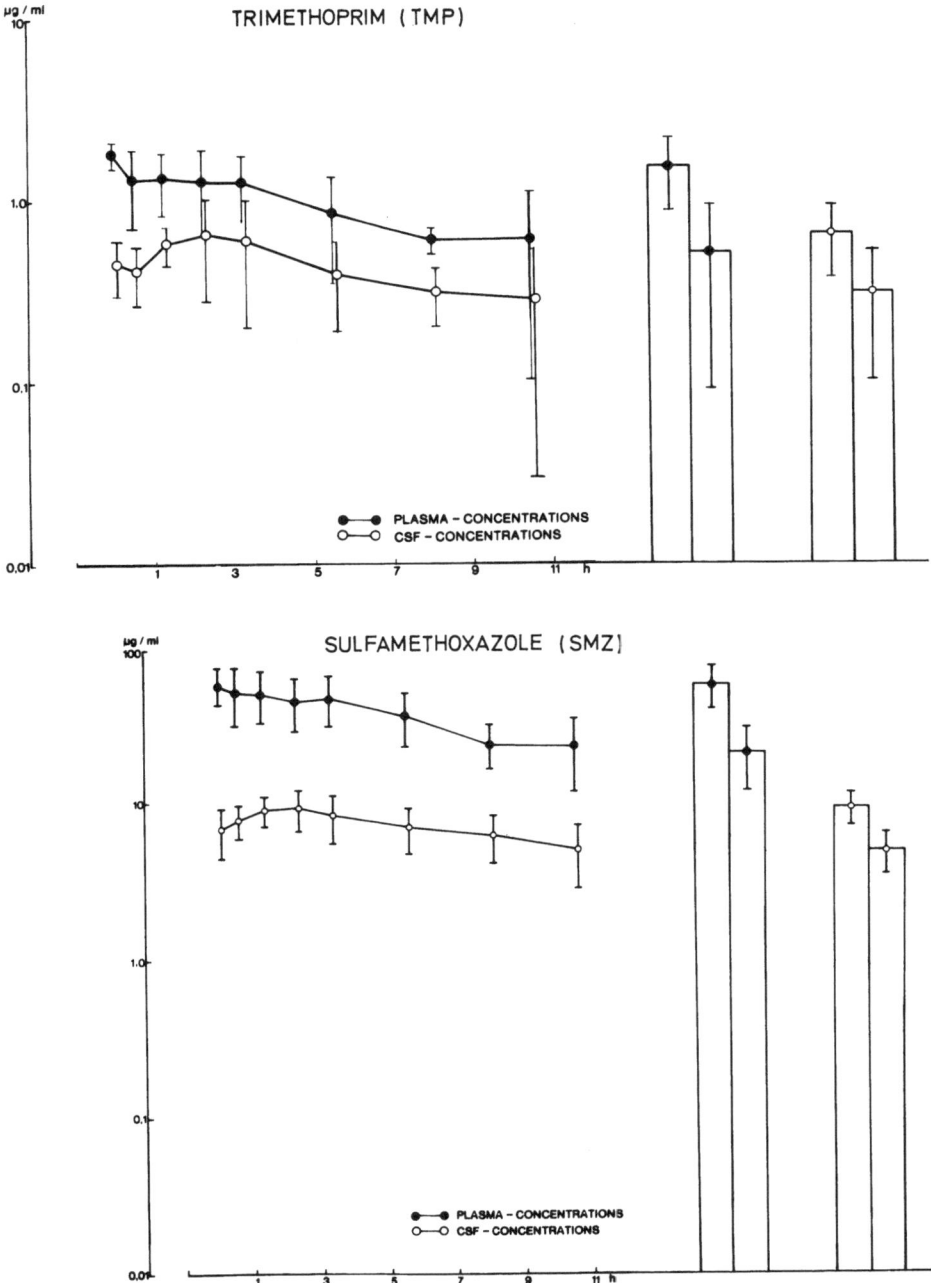

Fig. 1. Trimethoprim and Sulfamethoxazole concentration in plasma and CSF, columns show maximal and minimal concentrations

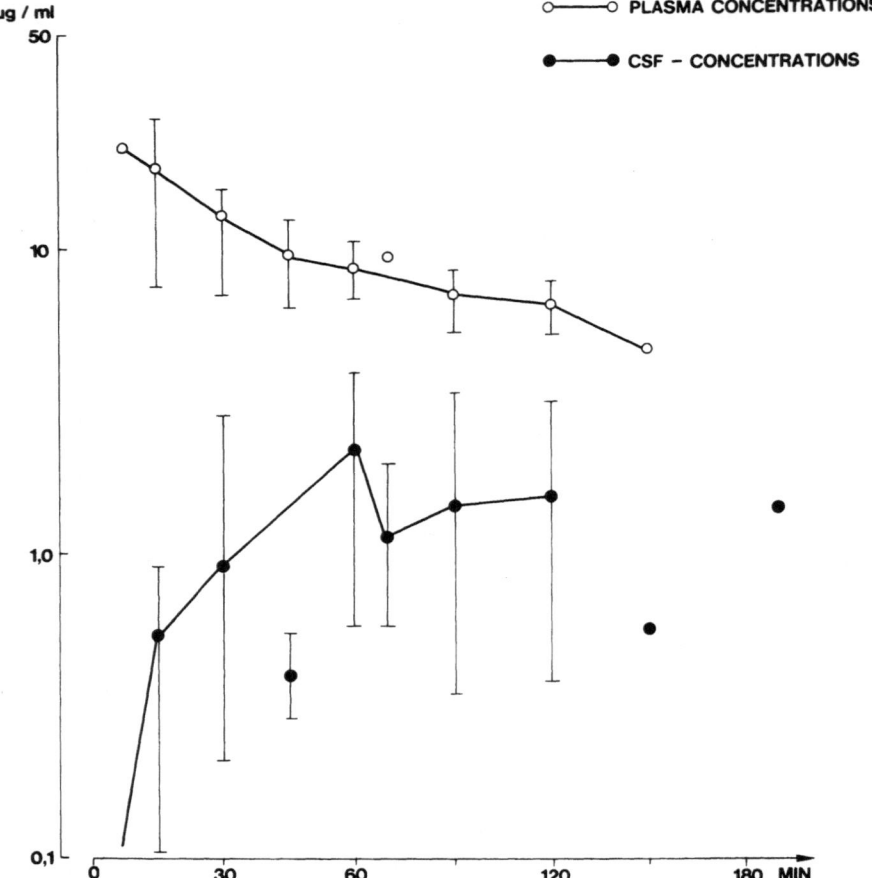

Fig. 2. Chloramphenicol concentrations in patients with non-inflamed meninges (1 g i.v. normal meninges)

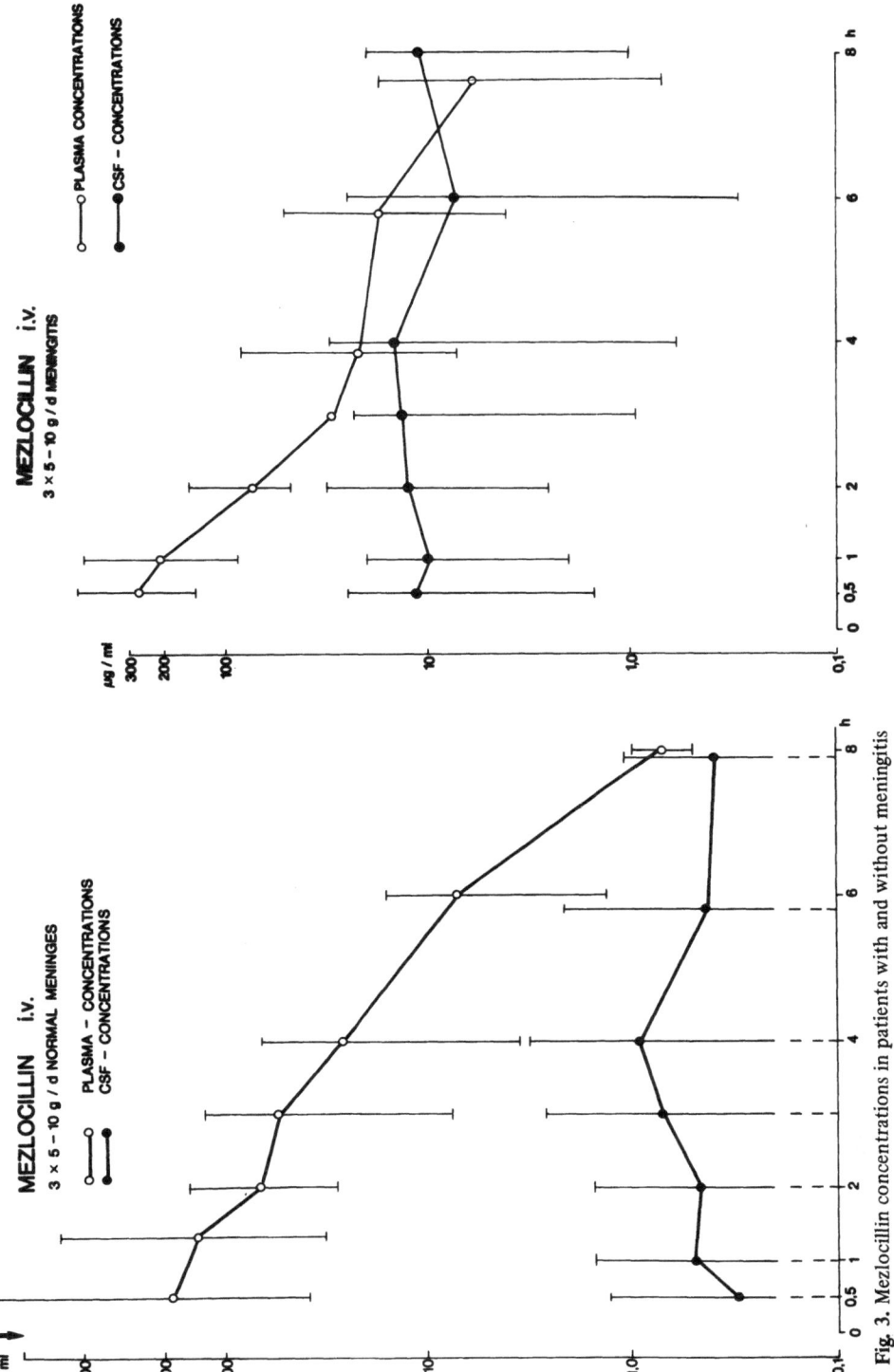

Fig. 3. Mezlocillin concentrations in patients with and without meningitis

93

94

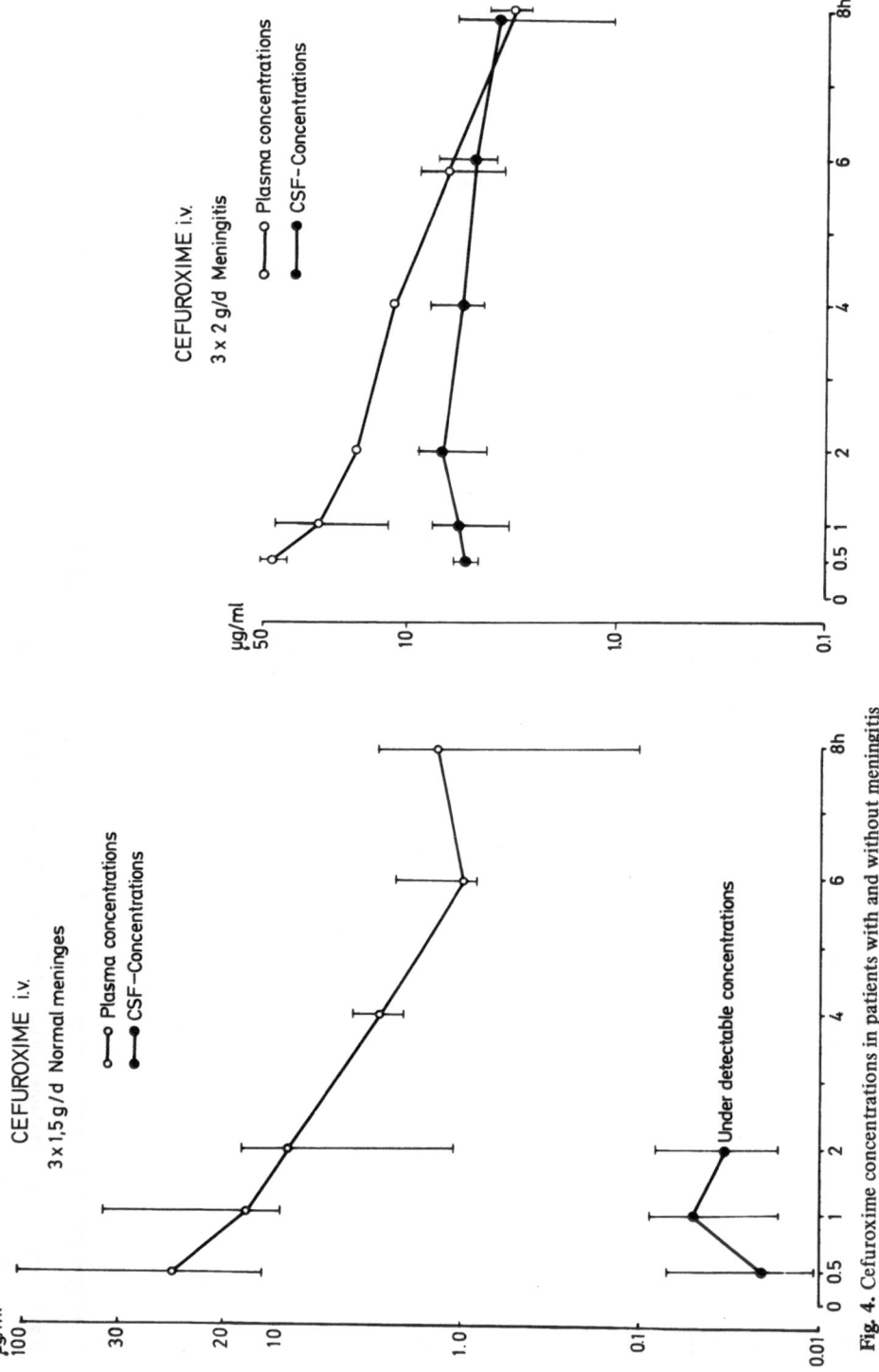

Fig. 4. Cefuroxime concentrations in patients with and without meningitis

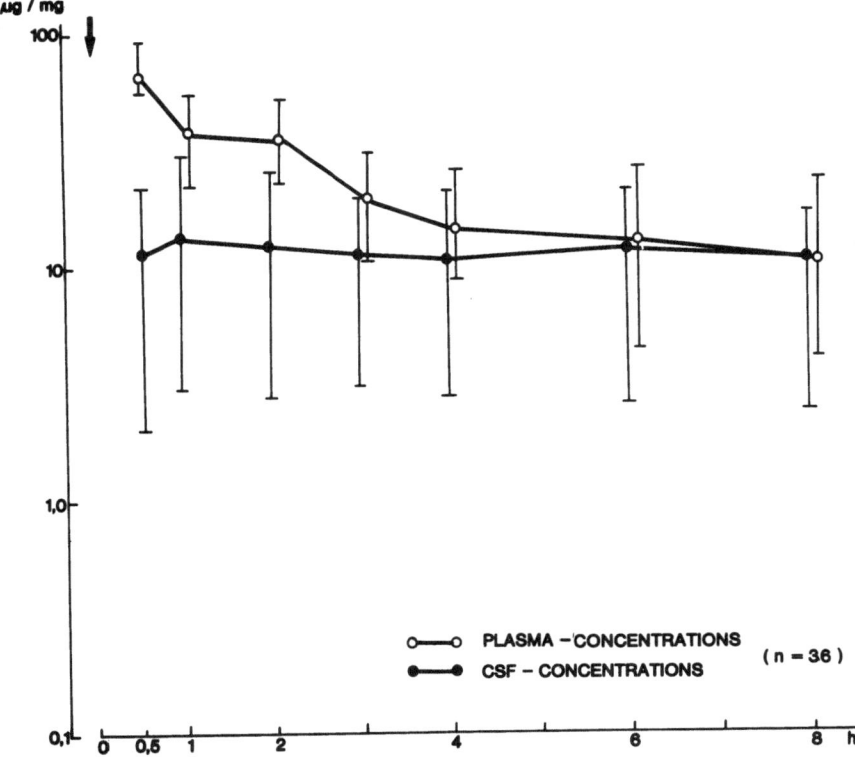

Fig. 5. Moxalactam concentrations in patients with meningitis (3x3 g/d meningitis, three patients)

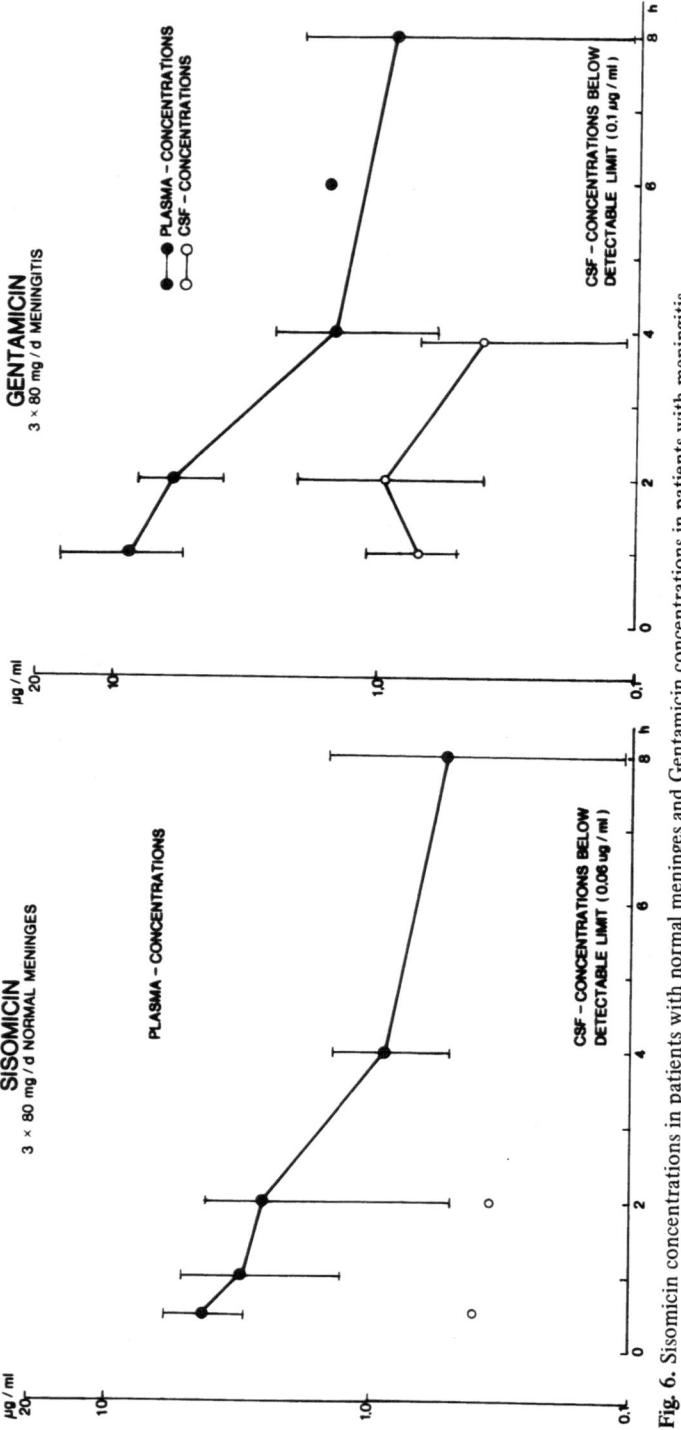

Fig. 6. Sisomicin concentrations in patients with normal meninges and Gentamicin concentrations in patients with meningitis

The Influence of High Dose Barbiturates on Canine Cerebral Blood Flow and Metabolism

N.F. Kassell and P.W. Hitchon

Introduction

In the last few years there has been increased use of barbiturates in very high doses to treat a variety of neurosurgical disorders associated with cerebral ischaemia (12, 17), brain swelling, and intracranial hypertension (21–23, 25, 28). There are two questions that have developed regarding the practical application of this form of treatment. The first relates to techniques for regulating the dose of barbiturates, and the second relates to the role of hyperventilation in patients receiving treatment with high doses of barbiturates.

The purposes of this study were 1. to determine whether the electroencephalogram (EEG) could be used to control the administration of sodium thiopental and 2. to determine whether hypocapnia results in additional cerebral vasoconstriction during the course of high dose barbiturate treatment.

Materials and Methods

Mongrel dogs weighing approximately 15 kg each were used for this study. Anaesthesia was induced with intravenous chloralose (50 mg/kg) and urethane (500 mg/kg), and maintained with a nitrous oxide-oxygen mixture (70%:30%) supplemented with intravenous morphine sulphate. Muscular paralysis was achieved with pancuronium, and ventilation was controlled with a pump respirator. A total of between 2.5 and 5 mg/kg of morphine and 0.1 to 0.3 mg/kg of pancuronium was administered to each dog in divided doses. The animals were hyperventilated and CO_2 added to the inspired gas mixture to maintain the $PaCO_2$ at the desired levels. Oesophageal temperature was measured and maintained at $37.5^{\circ}C$ with a warming blanket.

Cerebral blood flow was determined by the radioactive microsphere technique (5, 11, 19, 20). In each experiment, CBF was measured six times using 15-μm spheres labeled with iodine-125, cerium-145 strontium-85, tin-113, niobium-95, and scandium-46. The microspheres were injected into the left ventricle through a pigtail catheter inserted through the femoral artery and descending aorta. Blood samples were drawn from one femoral and one brachial artery. At the completion of the experiment, the brain was removed and divided into cerebral hemispheres, corpus callosum, brain stem, and cerebellum for determination of blood flow.

End-tidal CO_2, O_2, and nitrous oxide were monitored continuously with a respiratory mass spectrometer. Systemic arterial pressure was measured from a catheter placed in the brachial artery. Central venous pressure was measured from a Swan-Ganz catheter inserted into the pulmonary artery through the femoral vein and descending vena cava. This catheter also served to measure cardiac output utilizing the thermodilution technique. Sagittal sinus pressure was measured from a catheter inserted in the anterior portion of the sagittal sinus and threaded caudally. Heart rate was derived from the electrocardiogram. These physiological data were continuously recorded on an eight-channel strip-chart recorder. Electroencephalograph (EEG) monitoring was performed from leads screwed into the frontal and parietal bones bilaterally and recorded on an eight-channel EEG.

Immediately before each CBF determination, blood was drawn for measurement of arterial blood gases and haematocrit. Oxygen content of the sagittal sinus and systemic arterial blood was also measured.

The cerebral metabolic rate for oxygen ($CMRO_2$) was calculated by multiplying the mean cerebral hemispheric flow by the difference between the systemic arterial and sagittal sinus oxygen content. Cerebral vascular resistance (CVR) was calculated by dividing the systemic arterial pressure minus the sagittal sinus pressure by the total mean hemispheric blood flow. Peripheral vascular resistance was calculated by dividing the systemic arterial pressure by the cardiac index. Cardiac index was estimated by dividing the cardiac output by the animal's body weight.

The data were examined using Analyses of Variance and Student's t-test. Where differences are reported as significant $P < 0.05$ had been established.

Procedure

Two series of experiments were performed and will hereafter be referred to as "EEG" and "CO_2" studies respectively.

1. EEG Study. In nine dogs a control determination of cerebral blood flow was performed following which a slow infusion of sodium thiopentone was started. Cerebral blood flow determinations were repeated when the periods of burst suppression (BS) in the EEG over several minutes averaged 30, 60, 120, and 240 seconds. Arterial PCO_2 was maintained at 40 mm Hg during the course of these experiments.

2. CO_2 Study. In thirteen dogs cerebral blood flow was determined at arterial PCO_2 levels of 20, 30, 40, 50, and 60 torr after administration of sufficient sodium thiopentone to produce EEG burst suppression averaging 30 to 60 seconds. The cerebral metabolic rate of oxygen was determined in seven of these animals.

Results

1. EEG Study

During the course of the experiments no significant variations were noted in arterial PCO_2, PO_2, pH, core temperature, sagittal sinus pressure, or central venous pressure.

The blood sodium thiopental level increased from a control value of 0 to 22 ± 3 μg/ml at 30 seconds BS, to 36 ± 3 at 120 seconds BS, decreasing to 32 ± 4 at 240 seconds BS (Table 1). Mean arterial pressure remained at control levels until 30 seconds BS, and then gradually declined approximately 30% by 240 seconds BS. Administration of sodium thiopentone produced a tachycardia. Heart rate increased approximately 26% at 30 seconds BS, and 56% by 240 seconds BS. Cardiac index decreased by 15% at 30 seconds BS, and by 26% at 240 seconds BS.

Total cerebral blood flow was markedly decreased by the sodium thiopentone. At 30 seconds BS, CBF decreased approximately 45% and by 240 seconds BS the reduction was approximately 57%. The changes in cerebral vascular resistance were of a similar but opposite nature to the changes in cerebral blood flow. Cerebral metabolic rate of oxygen decreased approximately 42% by 30 seconds BS and showed no further significant reduction with increasing levels of burst suppression.

2. CO_2 Study

Following adminstration of sufficient sodium thiopentone to produce 30 to 60 seconds burst suppression in the EEG, there was no significant change in mean arterial pressure, heart rate, cardiac index, or cerebral metabolic rate of oxygen over the range of $PaCO_2$

Table 1. Effect of increasing interval of burst suppression

	Interval of burst suppression (s)				
	0	30	60	120	240
CBF (ml/100g/min)	67 ± 8	37 ± 6	31 ± 5	27 ± 4	28 ± 3
CVR (mmHg/ml/100g/min)	1.6 ± 0.2	3.6 ± 0.5	3.5 ± 0.7	3.7 ± 0.4	2.8 ± 0.2
CMRO$_2$ (mlO$_2$/100g/min)	4.3 ± 0.4	2.5 ± 0.2	2.0 ± 0.3	2.3 ± 0.2	2.7 ± 0.3
MAP mmHg	112 ± 4	111 ± 5	98 ± 7	93 ± 7	78 ± 5
HR (beats/min)	106 ± 11	134 ± 10	145 ± 6	152 ± 10	165 ± 15
CI X 10^2(l/min/kg)	13.0 ± 1.6	11.1 ± 0.9	10.7 ± 1.2	9.8 ± 0.5	9.6 ± 1.2

CBF = total mean cerebral blood flow; CVR = cerebral vascular resistance;
CMRO$_2$ = cerebral metabolic rate of oxygen; MAP = mean arterial pressure;
HR = heart rate; CI = cardiac index

between 20 and 60 torr. Decreasing arterial PCO_2 from 40 to 20 torr resulted in a reduction in total brain blood flow of 19% and an increase in cerebral vascular resistance of 27% (Table 2). However, there were no significant differences in cerebral blood flow or cerebral vascular resistance between arterial PCO_2 of 30 and 20.

Discussion

High dose barbiturate therapy is being used with increasing frequency in neurosurgical patients. Although the value of this form of treatment has not been fully proven, there is strong suggestive evidence that barbiturates are helpful in the management of patients with Reye's syndrome (21, 23), head injuries (22, 25, 28), and in situations where the arterial supply to the brain has been acutely compromised (12, 17). The mechanism(s) whereby high dose barbiturates exert their beneficial actions have not been fully elucidated, but those postulated include: Free radical scavenging (7, 9); decreasing the metabolic demands of the brain to allow it to survive in an environment of decreased substrates (15, 24, 29); and consequently decreased intracranial pressure by decreasing cerebral blood flow and volume. However, in addition to these potentially beneficial actions, barbiturates in high doses are cardiovascular depressants (3, 6, 8, 18) and any decrease in cardiac output or blood pressure resulting from their administration could completely outweigh the useful effects. It appears that there may be a fairly narrow margin between the doses of sodium thiopentone useful for cerebral protection and the cardiovascular depressant doses. Accordingly, it is essential to employ a technique for accurately and reliably regulating the administration of barbiturates in high doses.

There are several methods currently in use. Administration of barbiturates in doses based upon body weight is unreliable because of the variable metabolism of the drug. Measurements of blood levels are helpful, but these are expensive and time-consuming and the relationship between blood level, brain level, and cerebral and cardiovascular depression from barbiturates is unpredictable (2, 4, 27). In contrast, the EEG provides a continuous, readily accessible index of brain activity that can be easily used by medical and paramedical personnel (14). However the use of the EEG for this purpose requires knowledge of the relationship of the EEG to brain metabolism and cerebral and systemic circulatory dynamics.

Table 2. Effect of alterations in $PaCO_2$ during high dose barbiturates

| | $PaCO_2$ (Torr) | | | | |
	20	30	40	50	60
CBF (ml/100 gm/min)	22 ± 1	22 ± 1	27 ± 3	40 ± 15	67 ± 11
CVR	4.0 ± 0.4	3.8 ± 0.6	2.9 ± 0.3	2.3 ± 0.8	1.3 ± 0.1

CBF = total brain mean cerebral blood flow;
CBR = cerebral vascular resistance (mean arterial pressure minus sagittal sinus pressure divided by CBF)

In this study, the administration of sufficient sodium thiopentone to produce burst suppression in the EEG of between 30 and 60 seconds was accompanied by marked reduction in cerebral blood flow. No additional decrement in cerebral blood flow was noted as additional barbiturates were administered to produce burst suppression in excess of 60 seconds. Mean arterial pressure was adequately maintained until burst suppression in excess of 30 to 60 seconds was achieved. There was no correlation between the level of sodium thipentone in the blood, cerebral blood flow, cerebral metabolism, cerebral metabolic rate of oxygen, or mean arterial pressure. This observation confirms the difficulties anticipated in using blood levels as a reliable indicator of the effects of barbiturates on cerebral blood flow and metabolism or cardiovascular function.

Of all the hypothetical beneficial actions of high dose barbiturate therapy, its ability to decrease cerebral blood volume and brain bulk and lower increased intracranial pressure are the most well documented and understood. Hyperventialtion is more commonly used for the same purpose (10, 16, 26). However, in contrast to barbiturates, hypocapnia does not result in decreased cerebral metabolism (1, 13) and accordingly, produces a relatively adverse change in the ratio of cerebral metabolism to blood flow. Hyperventilation is an effective mechanism for controlling intracranial hypertension. However, it is not entirely without risk (30). Since barbiturates result in a significant degree of cerebral vasoconstriction, it is important to determine whether this vasoconstriction is enhanced by hypocapnic levels of arterial PCO_2. In this study, when 30 to 60 seconds of burst suppression in the EEG had been achieved the degree of cerebral vasoconstriction produced by these doses of sodium thiopentone at an arterial PCO_2 of 40 torr was equivalent to that produced by hypocapnia to an arterial PCO_2 of 20 torr in the absence of barbiturates. Minimal additional cerebral vasoconstriction was noted in the animals who received high dose barbiturates when the arterial PCO_2 was reduced from 30 to 20 torr. This would suggest that it is reasonable to maintain arterial PCO_2 at approximately 30 torr during high dose barbiturate therapy.

The above interpretations must be qualified by stating that these studies were performed in dogs with normal central nervous and cardiovascular function and that the results may be different in humans, particularly after trauma to the central nervous system.

References

1. Alexander, S.C., Smith, T.C., Strobel, G., et al.: Cerebral carbohydrate metabolism of man during respiratory and metabolic alkalosis. J. Appl. Physiol. 24, 66–72 (1968)
2. Becker, K.E., Jr.: Plasma levels of thiopental necessary for anaesthesia. Anesthesiology 49, 192–196 (1978)
3. Becker, K.E. Jr., Tonnesen, A.S.: Cardiovascular effects of plasma levels of thiopental necessary for anesthesia. Anesthesiology 49, 197–200 (1978)
4. Brand, L., Mazzia, V.D.B., Van Poznak, A., Burns, J.J., Mark, L.C.: Lack of correlation between electroencephalographic effects and plasma concentrations of thiopentone. Br. J. Anaesth. 33, 92–96 (1961)
5. Buckberg, G.D., Luck, J.C., Payne, D.B., Hoffman, J.I.E., Archie, J.P., Fixler, D.E.: Some sources of error in measuring regional blood flow with radioactive microspheres. J. Appl. Physiol. 31, 598–604 (1971)
6. Chamberlain, J.H., Seed, R.G.F.L., Chung, D.C.W.: Effect of thiopentone on myocardial function. Br. J. Anaesth. 49, 865–870 (1977)

7. Demopoulos, H.B., Flamm, E.S., Seligman, M.L., Jorgensen, E., Ransohoff, J.: Antioxidant effects of barbiturates in model membranes undergoing free radical damage. Acta Neurol Scand (Suppl.) *64*, 152–153 (1977)

8. Etsten, B., Li, T.H.: Hemodynamic changes during thiopental anesthesia in humans: Cardiac output stroke volume, total peripheral resistance and intrathoracic blood volume. J. Clin. Invest. *34*, 500–510 (1955)

9. Flamm, E.S., Demopoulos, H.B., Seligman, M.L., Ransohoff, J.: Possible molecular mechanisms of barbiturate-mediated protection in regional cerebral ischemia. Acta. Neurol. Scand. (Suppl.) *64*, 150–151 (1977)

10. Hayes, G.J., Slocum, H.C.: The achievement of optimal brain relaxation by hyperventilation technics of anesthesia. J. Neurosurg. *19*, 65–79 (1962)

11. Heymann, M.A., Payne, B.D., Hoffman, J.I.E., et al.: Blood flow measurements with radionuclide-labeled particles. Prog. Cardiovasc. Dis. *20*,55–79 (1977)

12. Hoff, J.T., Pitts, L.H., Spetzler, R. et al.: Barbiturates for protection from cerebral ischemia in aneurysm surgery. Acta Neurochir. Scand. (Suppl) *64*, 158–159 (1977)

13. Kety, S.S., Schmidt, C.F.: The effects of altered arterial tensions of carbon dioxide and oxygen on cerebral blood flow and cerebral oxygen consumption of normal young men. J. Clin. Invest. *27*, 484–492 (1948)

14. Kiersey, D.K., Bickford, R.G., Faulconer, A.Jr.: Electroencephalographic patterns produced by thiopental sodium during surgical operations: Description and classification. Br. J. Anaesth. *23*, 141–152 (1951)

15. Lafferty, J.J., Keykhah, M.M., Shapiro, H.M., Van Horn, K., Behar, M.G.: Cerebral hypo-metabolism obtained with deep pentobarbital anesthesia and hypothermia (30°C). Anesthesiology *49*, 159–164 (1978)

16. Langfitt, T.W., Kassell, N.F.: Acute brain swelling in neurosurgical patients. J. Neurosurg. *24*, 975–983 (1966)

17. Lawner, P.M., Simeone, F.A.: Treatment of intraoperative middle cerebral artery occlusion with pentobarbital and extracranial-intracranial bypass. Case report. J. Neurosurg. *51*, 710–712 (1979)

18. Manders, W.T., Vatner, S.F.: Effects of sodium pentobarbital anesthesia on left ventricular function and distribution of cardiac output in dogs with particular reference to the mechanism for tachycardia. Circ. Res. *39*, 512–517 (1976)

19. Marcus, M.L., Heistad, D.D., Ehrhardt, J.C., Abboud, F.M.: Regulation of total and regional spinal cord blood flow. Circ. Res. *41*, 128–134 (1977)

20. Marcus, M.L., Heistad, D.D., Ehrhardt, J.C., Abboud, F.M.: Total and regional cerebral blood flow measurement with 7–, 10–, 15–, 25–, and 50 μm microspheres. J. Appl. Physiol. *40*, 501–507 (1976)

21. Marshall, L.F., Shapiro, H.M., Rauscher, A., Kaufman, N.M.: Pentobarbital therapy for intracranial hypertension in metabolic coma: Reye's syndrome. Crit. Care Med. *6*, 1–5 (1978)

22. Marshall, L.F., Smith, R.W., Shapiro, H.M.: The outcome with aggressive treatment in severe head injuries; Part II. Acute and chronic barbiturate administration in the management of head injury. J. Neurosurg. *50*, 26–30 (1979)

23. Menezes, A., Bell, W.E., Kealey, G.P., Chaves-Carballo, E., Yamada, T.: Experience in management of critical patients with Reye-Johnson syndrome. In: Intracranial Pressure IV. Shulman, K., Marmarou, A., Miller, J.D., Becker, D.P., Hochwald, G.W., Brock, M. (eds.), pp. 553–555. Berlin, Heidelberg, New York: Springer 1980

24. Michenfelder, J.D.: The interdependency of cerebral functional and metabolic effects following massive doses of thiopental in the dog. Anesthesiology *41*, 231–236 (1974)

25. Rockoff, M.A., Marshall, L.F., Shapiro, H.M.: High-dose barbiturate therapy in humans: A clinical review of 60 patients. Ann. Neurol. *6*, 194–199 (1979)

26. Rossanda, M., Collice, M., Porta, M. et al.: Intracranial hypertension in head injury. Clinical significance and relation to respiration. In: Intracranial Pressure II. Lundberg, N., Ponten, U., Brock, M. (eds.), pp. 475–479. Berlin, Heidelberg, New York: Springer 1975

27. Saubermann, A.J., Gallagher, M.L., Hedley-Whyte, J.: Uptake distribution and anesthetic effect of pentobarbital–2–^{14}C after intravenous injection into mice. Anesthesiology *40*, 41–51 (1974)

28. Shapiro, H.M., Wyte, S.R., Loeser, J.: Barbiturate-augmented hypothermia for reduction of persistent intracranial hypertension. J. Neurosurg. *40*, 90–100 (1974)
29. Simeone, F.A., Frazer, G., Lawner, P.: Ischemic brain edema: Comparative effects of barbiturates and hypothermia. Stroke *10*, 8–12 (1979)
30. Sullivan, H.G., Keenan, R.L., Isrow, L. et al.: The critical importance of $PaCO_2$ during intracranial aneurysm surgery. Case report. J. Neurosurg. *52*, 426–430 (1980)

Resistance of Brain Tumours to Chemotherapy: Preliminary Studies of Rat and Human Tumours *

M.L. Rosenblum, D.F. Deen, V.A. Levin, D.V. Dougherty, M.E. Williams, M. Weizsäcker, M. Gerosa, and Ch.B. Wilson

Introduction

There are several possible reasons why malignant brain tumours do not respond to chemotherapy. First, because of impaired drug delivery, chemotherapeutic agents might not reach all tumour cells in cytoxic concentrations. Second, tumour growth kinetics might affect the response to drugs because tumour cells are in an insensitive phase of the cell cycle when the drug is administered (10). Finally, tumour cells may survive therapy because of "inherent" cellular resistance.

We have investigated possible mechanisms of clinical drug resistance in malignant brain tumours using 1,3—bis (2—chloroethyl)—1—nitrosourea (BCNU), a cell cycle nonspecific agent that is the most effective single agent available for the treatment of malignant brain tumours. Drug sensitivity was determined by means of an *in vitro* clonogenic cell assay (8). Investigations on "inherent" cellular resistance were performed in the 9L rat brain tumour model (6).

Materials and Methods

Human Biopsies

A detailed report on the human brain tumour assay has been published (7, 8). Cells were obtained by dissociation of fresh biopsy specimens and, for the studies reported here, were tested after initial dissociation. Cells analysed are probably malignant glial cells because they contain GFAP, a substance that is presumed to be specific for glial cells (1), are recognized by hybridoma-produced monoclonal antibodies that react only with glioma cells (9), and, when cells were injected into nude mice, solid tumours grew (7).

Animal Experiments

The transplantable 9L rat brain tumour was used for these studies (6). The tumour was transplanted into the brains of adult male Fisher 344 rats weighing 150—200 gm (6).

* Supported in part by NCI Grant CA—13525, the Morris Stulsaft Foundation, and a grant from the Deutsche Forschungsgemeinschaft

After tumours had grown to an average weight of 50–70 mg, 27 mg/kg (twice the LD_{10}) of BCNU was administered intraperitoneally. One day after treatment, the rats were killed, tumours were removed, and a single cell suspension was obtained and plated for colony forming efficiency (CFE) (8) and/or grown in culture. Cells that survived *in vivo* treatment were subsequently exposed to a range of BCNU doses *in vitro*. Cells harvested from tumours of untreated rats were used as the control. In other experiments, surviving tumour cells from both treated and untreated rats were treated *in vitro* with equimolar doses of 1–(2–chloroethyl)–3–cyclohexyl–1–nitrosourea (CCNU), 1–(2–chloroethyl) –3–(4–methylcyclohexyl)–1–nitrosourea (MeCCNU), 1–(2–chloroethyl)–3–(2,6– dioxo–3–piperidyl)–1–nitrosourea (PCNU), and spirohydantoin mustard (SHM). A similar *in vitro* experiment was performed with X rays at doses of 500 to 1500 rads.

The transport of nitrosoureas across cell membranes was investigated by measuring the intracellular concentrations of ^{14}C-PCNU added to single cell suspensions of resistant and sensitive cells obtained from exponentially growing cultures.

Results

Human Biopsy Specimens

To date, cells from biopsy specimens of 12 malignant gliomas (glioblastomas) have been analyzed for *in vitro* cell sensitivity to BCNU, and the results have been compared to *in situ* tumour response to nitrosoureas (Table 1). There were two distinct patterns of response to BCNU, First, there was essentially no cell kill *in vitro* for cells from seven specimens and all seven patients were resistant to nitrosoureas clinically (Group I). Second, moderate cell kill was achieved *in vitro* at clinically achievable doses of BCNU for cells from five specimens, with a marked increase in cytotoxicity at higher doses (Group II); three of the five patients with BCNU-sensitive cells were sensitive to nitrosoureas clinically.

Animal Experiments

Cells from tumours treated with BCNU (9L/BCNU) were markedly more resistant to treatment *in vitro* with BCNU than cells from untreated tumours (9L/0) (Fig. 1). The dose-response curve for 9L/0 cells showed an exponential cell kill that exceeding 2 logs, but the dose-response curve of resistant cells (9L/BCNU) showed a maximum of 1 log kill even at very high doses of BCNU. Cells were equally resistant to equimolar doses of CCNU, MeCCNU, and PCNU (Table 2). Cells were partially cross-resistant to the alkylating agent SHM, but were not cross resistant to X rays.

Preliminary studies of nitrosourea transport, in which ^{14}C-PCNU was administered to a single cell suspension of 9L/0 and 9L/BCNU cells, showed a rate of drug influx that was both very rapid and similar for both groups of cells. Thus, for 9L cells, the mechanism of resistance to nitrosoureas is probably not related to altered transport across the cell membrane but to altered biodistribution and/or biotransformation.

Table 1. Correlation between *in vitro* and *in vivo* treatment with BCNU

Specimen No.	*In vitro* treatment (% cell kill)		Clinical response [b]
	Achievable dose [a]	4x achievable dose	
Group I. Resistant cells [c]			
125	0	33	R [d]
127	0	0	R
128	0	10	R
131	14	0	R
134	0	21	R
150	40	14	R
168	0	89	R
Group II. Sensitive cells [c]			
126 [e]	61	99.3	S [d]
167 [e]	85	97	R
159	46	96	R
160	51	--	S
163	45	90	S

[a] Maximum clinically achievable dose at the tumour cell site (8.5 μM) after a single 200 mg/m dose of BCNU (V.A. Levin, personal communication)

[b] Determined from serial computerized tomographic and radionuclide brain scans and neurological evaluations, without knowledge of cell survival results

[c] Sensitive cells = $>$ 40% cell kill; resistant cells = $<$ 40% cell kill; both at maximum clinically achievable doses

[d] S (sensitive) = complete or partial tumour response; R (resistant) = progressive or stable disease

[e] Same patient, before chemotherapy (# 126) and at tumour recurrence after clinical chemotherapy (BCNU) failure (#167)

Discussion

The predictive capability of our clonogenic assay, which is 100% for clinical resistance and 60% for clinical sensitivity, is similar to that of soft agar "stem" cell assays for a variety of tumours (11) and to the oestrogen receptor assay for breast carcinoma (5), the latter of which is considered clinically useful for planning the treatment of patients with malignant mammary neoplasms. The correlation between *in vitro* and *in situ* results implies that the cells disaggregated from a tumour biopsy are representative of the clonogenic cells within the solid tumour, at least with regard to sensitivity to chemotherapeutic agents. Nevertheless, more data are needed to validate our assay.

Table 2. Cell kill for sensitive (9L/0) and resistant (9L/BCNU) cells at equimolar doses of drugs, and for x-irradiation

Treatment	% Cell kill		Log cell cill		Resistance ratio [a]
	Sensitive	Resistant	Sensitive	Resistant	
BCNU					
12 μM	62	45	0.74	0.26	2.85
20 μM	98.9	66	1.96	0.46	4.26
CCNU					
12 μM	90	36	0.98	0.19	5.16
20 μM	99.6	40	2.37	0.22	10.77
MeCCNU					
12 μM	80	34	0.70	0.18	3.89
20 μM	99.5	67	2.32	0.48	4.83
PCNU					
6 μM	47	25	0.27	0.12	2.25
12 μM	NA	42	NA	0.23	- - -
20 μM	NA	62	NA	0.42	- - -
SHM					
12 μM	97	87	1.48	0.89	1.66
20 μM	99.9	98.7	2.85	1.88	1.52
X-rays					
1,000	89	83	0.94	0.77	1.22
1,500	99.2	98.4	2.09	1.79	1.17

[a] Ratio = log kill 9/0% ÷ log kill 9L/BCNU; $\rangle$ 2 = marked cross resistance;
 1.3−2 = mild − moderate cross resistance; $\langle$ 1.3 essentially no cross resistance

Continuous unretarded growth of malignant tumour is the result of the multiplication of clonogenic cells that have the potential for "unlimited" proliferation. In humans tumour resistance to chemotherapy is probably the result of the combined effects of insufficient drug delivery, cell kinetic-imposed insensitivity, and biochemically-mediated resistance. In addition, sensitivity of the tumour may also depend on the participation of host defense mechanisms; clinical resistance may be related to inhibition of the immuno processes by the agent.

Most tumours are presumed to contain various proportions of drug-sensitive and drug-resistant cells. Tumours cells show "intrinsic" and acquired resistance, the latter of which is the result of treatment with various agents. In the former instance, cells appear refractory to treatment from the outset. In the latter instance, resistance might arise by biochemical modification of cells that were initially sensitive to a particular drug. Some of the biochemical and pharmacological mechanisms that accompany the development of resistance include impaired cellular transport, reduced affinity of drug for a target enzyme, metabolic bypass, impaired activation of a pro-drug, increased catabolism, and increased levels of a competing biological substrate (3). The role of each of these "determinants" in the development of resistance to nitrosoureas still needs to be clarified for brain tumours. If drug resistant cells predominate, the tumour will be resistant to therapy, and sampling any region of the tumour will yield predominantly resistant clonogenic cells. When drug sensitive cells predominate, tumour response will occur until the majority of sensitive cells are killed, after which resistant cells will repopulate the tumour.

Our preliminary investigations suggest that in some patients, the clinical failure of chemotherapy may be caused by "inherent" tumour cell resistance in some patients (Group I) and by inadequate drug delivery in others (Group II). Patients whose tumours progressed despite documented *in vitro* cell sensitivity might benefit from being treated with potentially toxic doses of drug, followed by bone marrow rescue (4). The case of Patient No. 126 is illustrative. After subtotal resection of a left frontal glioblastoma multiforme, this 50-year-old woman was treated with BCNU. Cells obtained from a biopsy specimen were sensitive in culture, and she responded clinically. However, her tumour recurred 12 months later and progressed despite further treatment with BCNU. Histological examination of the biopsy specimen from the recurrent tumour showed many areas of necrosis, and cells obtained from the recurrent tumour showed a persistent sensitivity to BCNU.

Because BCNU is the single most effective agent for brain tumour chemotherapy, and because it is a cell cycle nonspecific agent, the mode of action of which is not affected by cell kinetics, results from our animal and cell transport studies suggest that resistance to nitrosoureas in 9L cells is probably the result of biochemical and/or metabolic "determinants".

Conclusion

The presence of cross resistance indicates that various classes of compounds share a common pathway. The complete cross resistance in 9L cells found for five nitrosoureas confirms the clinical impression of cross resistance in patients treated with BCNU and CCNU (2). These results, although preliminary, also suggest that optimum cyclical or sequential delivery of a nitrosourea with another alkylating agent agent such as SHM might produce additive cell kill and improve patient prognosis, if toxicity to normal tissue is not additive.

References

1. Eng, L.F., Rubinstein, L.J.: Contribution of immunohistochemistry to diagnostic problems of human cerebral tumors. J. Histochem. Cytochem. *26*, 513–522 (1978)
2. Fewer, D., Wilson, C.B., Boldrey, E.B., Enot, K.J.: Phase II study of 1-(2-chloroethyl)-3-cyclohexyl-1-nitrosourea (CCNU; NSC-79037) in the treatment of brain tumors. Cancer Chemother. Rep. *56*, 421–427 (1972)
3. Harrap, K.R., Jackson, R.C.: Biochemical mechanisms of resistance to antimetabolites. In: Fundamentals in cancer chemotherapy. Antiobiotic Chemotherapy, Vol. 23, pp. 228–237. Basel: Karger 1978
4. Hochberg, F.H., Parker, L.M., Takvorian, T., Canellos, G.P., Zervas, N.T.: High dose BCNU with autologous bone marrow rescue for recurrent glioblastoma multiforme. J. Neurosurg. *54*, 455–461 (1981)
5. McGuire, W.L., Carbonne, P.P., Sears, M.E., Escher, G.C.: Estrogen receptors in human breast cancer: An overview. In: Estrogen receptors in human breast cancer. McGuire, W.L., Carbonne, P.P., Vollmer, E.P. (eds.), pp. 1–7. New York: Raven Press 1975

6. Rosenblum, M.L., Knebel, K.D., Vasquez, D.A., Wilson, C.B.: Brain tumor therapy: Quantitative analysis using a model system. J. Neurosurg. *46*, 145–154 (1977)
7. Rosenblum, M.L., Vasquez, D.A., Hoshino, T., Wilson, C.B.: Development of a clonogenic cell assay for human brain tumors. Cancer *41*, 2305–2314 (1978)
8. Rosenblum, M.L.: Chemosensitivity testing for human brain tumors. In: Human tumor cloning. Salmon, S.E. (ed.), Chap. 20. (Alan Liss Co., New York), Prog. Clin. Biol. Res. *48*, 223–245 (1980)
9. Schnegg, J.F., Diserens, A.C., Carrel, S., Accolla, R.S., De Tribolet, N.: Human glioma-associated antigens detected by monoclonal antibodies. Cancer Res. *41*, 1209–1213 (1981)
10. Skipper, H.E., Schabel, F.M. Jr., Wilcox, W.S.: Experimental evaluation of potential anticancer agents. XXI. Scheduling of arabinosylcytosine to take advantage of its S-phase specificity against leukemia cells. Cancer Chemother. Rep. *51*, 125–141 (1967)
11. Von Hoff, D.D., Casper, J., Bradley, E., Sandbach, J., Jones, D., Makuch, R.: Association between human tumor colony-forming assay results and response of an individual patient's tumor to chemotherapy. Am. J. Med. *70*, 1027–1032 (1981)

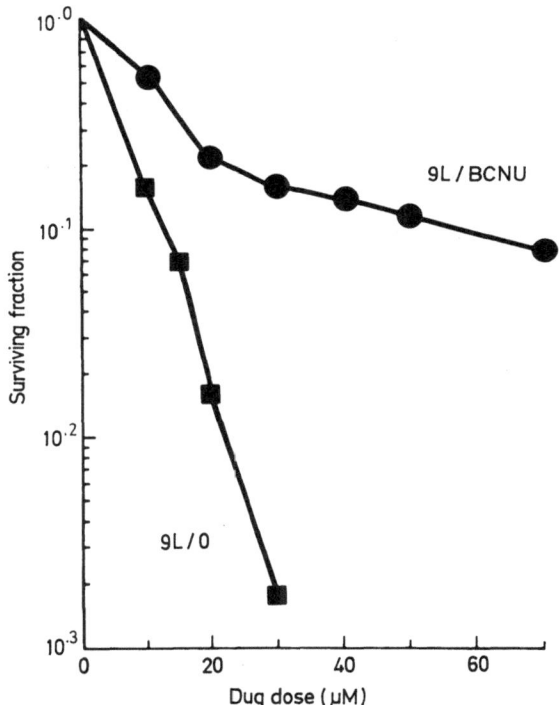

Fig. 1. 9L tumour cells that survived a 2 x LD_{10} dose of BCNU *in vivo* (9L/BCNU), were harvested and exposed to the drug a second time *in vitro*. Cells disaggregated from untreated tumours (9L/0) served as controls. The survival of untreated and previously treated cells was determined by colony formation analysis following graded doses of BCNU *in vitro*. 9L/BCNU cells were markedly more resistant to BCNU than 9L/0 cells

L-α-Alanine Inhibition of Pyruvate Kinase from Tumours of the Human Central Nervous System
A New Aid in the Treatment of Gliomas

C.W.M. van Veelen, H. Verbiest, K.J. Zülch, B. van Ketel, M.J.M. van der Vlist, A.M.C. Vlug, G. Rijksen, and G.E.J. Staal

Introduction

There is ever-increasing literature pointing out that gene expression in tumour cells is different from that in normal cells from which or in which the tumour originates. In general, neoplasia is characterized by misprogramming of protein synthesis (16).

It is now well known that a massive alteration in isozyme composition occurs in cancer tissue as compared to the pattern in normal tissue. These alterations may offer an elegant approach in the study of the genetic basis of neoplasia.

It was first established by Shapira (9) that isozymes present in experimental hepatomas are the predominant or sole form in fetal liver and are absent in adult liver of the host.

Ibsen (5) has collected no fewer than 21 enzymes whose isozyme composition changes in neoplasia of liver from an adult to a fetal form. This developmental gene expression in cancer is not only observed in isozyme shifts in human tumours but also in tumour immunology. Extensive literature exhibits close parallels between immunological and enzymological data (17). A number of fetal tumour-associated proteins have been identified like α-foetoprotein, the angiogenesis factor and plasminogen activators. Also the finding of ectopic hormone production in tumours of respectively endodermal, mesodermal and ectodermal origin suggests an embryonal relationship (17).

Several concepts have been proposed for the understanding of enzyme and isozyme changes in neoplasia (14–16).

The dedifferentiation theory, as proposed by Ibsen (5), deserves particular attention for the explanation of the reappearance of fetal isozymes in neoplasia. The genome responsible for the production of an isozyme during fetal life may be repressed during the development and derepressed in neoplasia (originating from normal adult tissue), due to presence or absence of a repressor molecule. The derepressed genome may code for the neosynthesis of fetal isozymes.

In human developing embryonic brain and gliomas, changes in isozyme composition have been found by Bennet (1) that support this view.

Especially enzymes of glycolysis were studied, particularly hexokinase, phosphofructokinase, pyruvate kinase (1) and lactate dehydrogenase (8). In the present study the isozyme composition of pyruvate kinase was examined, with the aim of investigating the isozyme shift in human intracranial tumours. Pyruvate kinase (ATP: pyruvate phosphotransferase, EC 2.7.1.40) catalyzes the conversion of phospho-enol-pyruvate (PEP) to pyruvate with regeneration of ATP:

$$\text{phospho-enol-pyruvate + ADP} \xrightarrow[K^+]{Mg^+} \text{pyruvate + ATP.}$$

There are at least three mammalian isozymes of pyruvate kinase (PK) each of which is composed of four identical or nearly identical subunits. These isozymes are designated as the liver or L-type, the muscle or M-type and the kidney or K-type (4). The subunit constitution of the isozymes can be designated by a subscript e.g. K_2M_2 to designate a hybrid with 2 subunits of the K-type and 2 subunits of the M-type protomer.

L-type is known to be also present in erythrocytes. K-type is present in spleen, and in many cells of mesodermal origin (4). The three main types of pyruvate kinase not only differ in their kinetic and electrophoretic properties, but also in their sensitivity to the aminoacid alanine. The M-type is not, whereas in contrast the K-type is strongly inhibited by alanine.

An alanine inhibition test was developed to discriminate between M and K type pyruvate kinase. A strong correlationship with the results of scannings of electrophoresis of these isozymes was observed (r= 0.99) (13). The alanine inhibition test can be performed in very short time and thus may be used during a neurosurgical procedure.

Materials and Methods

Patients

One hundred and twelve intracranial space-occupying lesions of various nature were evaluated. The patients age ranged from 1 − 73 years of age. The tumours of children were categorized separately. Histologically normal brain of 5 adults, one newborn and 2 fetuses were examined within 24 hours respectively after death from cardiovascular accidents, fatal cerebellar herniation accompanying Arnold-Chiari malformation and therapeutic abortion. Moreover histologically normal brain specimens could be obtained from cerebellar tissue surrounding large sized neurilemmomas (n= 2) and cortical grey and white matter resected at operations on aneurysms (anterior communicating artery aneurysms, n= 3). Enzymological examination was performed either during operation or at a later stage after storage at $-70^{\circ}C$. Storage appeared to have no influence on the stability of the enzyme.

Enzyme Assays

Investigated were:
a) The electrophoretic pattern of pyruvate kinase.
b) The activity of pyruvate kinase in the absence and presence of 4 mM alanine. The activity of pyruvate kinase in the presence of alanine was expressed as residual activity of the activity in the absence of alanine.

ad a) The extracted enzymes were diluted in the electrophoresis buffer so that the final activity was about 0.5 units/ml. The buffer contained 20 mmol/l Tris-citrate (pH 7.7), 1 mml/l fructose-1,6-diphosphate, 1 mmol/l disodium EDTA and 0.1 mmol/l dithiothreitol. Pyruvate kinase from leucocytes and striated muscle was used as a marker for the electrophoretic mobility of the K_4 and M_4 isozymes, respectively. A sample of 2 μl was applied to cellulose acetate and sub-jected to electrophoresis at 12V/cm for 3 h at 20°C. The staining mixture contained 0.5 mmol/l disodium EDTA, 10 mmol/l glucose, 1.5 mmol/l ADP, 3 mmol/l phospho-enol-pyruvate, 0.2 mmol/l NADP, 10 mmol/l AMP, 100 mmol/l Tris-HCl (pH 8.0), 10 mmol/l $MgCl_2$, 100 mmol/l KCl, 3.5 units hexokinase, and 2 units glucose-6-phosphate dehydrogenase, thiazolyl blue tetra-zolium (1 g/l) and phenazine methosulphate (0.2 g/l). The solution was spread on the cellulose acetate strip and incubated for 10 min at 37°C. The reaction was stopped by the addition of acetic acid solution (5%). The interference of adenylate kinase in this procedure was excluded by running suitable blanks without phospo-enol-pyruvate in the staining mixture. No bands of adenylate kinase could be detected.

ad b) For the alanine inhibition test the assay medium contained in a final volume of 3 ml: 0.1 mol/l Tris-HCl, pH 8.0, 65 mmol/l KCl, 20 mmol/l $MgSO_4$, 0.09 mmol/l NADH, lactate dehydrogenase (27 units), 1 mmol/l phospho-enol-pyruvate, 4 mmol/l alanine and enzyme. The control con-tained no alanine. The mixture was incubated for 5 min at 37°C. The reaction was started by the addition of ADP at a final concentration of 0.2 mmol/l. The 100% value is the activity in the absence of alanine.

Biopsies

Always two adjacent specimens were taken during the operation. The total volume of a twin specimen ranged from 0.5 to 2 cm^3. One piece of the twin specimen was used for the enzymological, the other one for the histological examination. In most cases several twin biopsies were taken from what was estimated to be in or near the centre of the tumour. In some cases also twin biopsies were taken from locations more towards the periphery of the tumour. The "twin" specimen in which the lowest residual activity was found and in which the histological diagnosis concerned the least differentiated part of the tumour was selected for comparative evaluation in respect to classification and grading. Moreover in all individual twin specimens a comparative evaluation of the histo-logical diagnosis tumour or no tumour and the enzymological findings was performed. The histological classification and grading was done according to the World Health Orga-nization Histological Classification of Tumour (18). In gliomas of adults localized in the cerebral hemispheres the results of the afore-mentioned tests were also compared with survival after "total" or "subtotal" resection without adjuvant radiotherapy and/or chemotherapy.

Resection was considered "total" if at macroscopic examination or examination with the magnifying loupe no tumour was left after resection. Resection was considered "sub-total" if after resection of the bulk of the tumour small rests of the tumour were sus-pected to be left in place. For further details see references (11—13).

Results

Figure 1 shows the electropherogram of mixed white and grey matter of two fetuses and a newborn as well as the pattern in white and grey matter of normal adult brain. In fetal brain K_4 isozyme M_4 and the hybrids K_3M and K_2M_2 are present, and at the age of 16 weeks also KM_3. In the newborn only M_4, K_3M and K_4 are present. M_4 is predominant. In adult brain the same pattern is found. However, M_4 is now largely

112

predominant. The isozyme pattern of pyruvate kinase in the various sites in adult brain strongly resembles the pattern in white and grey matter with the exception of the pineal gland in which all five bands were found. In the alanine inhibition test of normal adult white and grey matter residual activities were found between 85 and 93%.

Pyruvate Kinase Isozymes in Neuro-Epithelial Tumours of Adults

Figure 2 shows the electropherogram of a well and a poorly differentiated glioma. With the exception of a medulloblastoma these isozyme patterns appeared to be representative for all neuro-epithelial tumours of adults. A shift in synthesis of M-type towards K-type pyruvate kinase is observed according to loss of differentiation at the histological examination. The electrophoretic findings are confirmed in the alanine inhibition test: when more K-type is present, alanine inhibition is stronger.

Figure 3 shows the correlation between the alanine inhibition of pyruvate kinase expressed as residual activity and the histological classification and grading of 57 neuro-epithelial tumours of adults (12 years and older). Well differentiated tumours are nearly all characterized by relatively high residual activity. In contrast poorly differentiated tumours have low residual activity, with the exception of a medulloblastoma.

There is also a correlation between alanine inhibition of pyruvate kinase and postoperative survival. Figure 4 shows the correlation between the histological grading, the alanine inhibition and the postoperative survival in a series of 45 patients, who had survived the operation and the sequelae possibly related to it. In all these patients the tumours were situated in the cerebral hemispheres. Macroscopically the tumours could be resected either totally or subtotally. In the treatment of three patients operation was followed by non-surgical treatment, i.e. radio- or chemo-therapy. The effect of this treatment has not significantly influenced the correlation between survival after operation and histological grading and alanine inhibition. In 29 tumours a residual activity of 15% or less was found. Only one patient in this group has survived the first 18 months after operation. The group included anaplastic gliomas grade III and IV but also two oligodendrogliomas grade II and one astzocytoma grade II. In 13 tumours a residual activity of 20% or more was found. The patients of this group are all alive to date. Ten patients have now survived 36 months or more. The group included grade I and II astrocytomas and oligodendrogliomas and one glioblastoma. In an intermediate group of four patients a residual activity higher than 15 and less than 20% was found. Two patients in this group died of an anaplastic oligodendroglioma and a glioblastoma after 13 and 20 months respectively. One patient operated on for a glioblastoma is still alive 16 months after operation. One patient operated on for an oligodendroglioma belongs to the longest survivors in the study.

Presence and Absence of Tumour

In earlier reports it was already concluded that in biopsies taken in the periphery of gliomas a positive correlationship exists between presence or absence of tumour in the microscopic examination and alanine inhibition when a residual activity was found less than 70%. In Fig. 5 an illustration of this contention is shown.

Pyruvate Kinase in Gliomas of Children

In this group of patients, age one to eleven years (n = 9) tumours of various degrees of differentiation and classification were examined, including pilocytic astrocytomas, anaplastic glioma, ependymoma and medulloblastoma. All tumours were characterized by low residual activity, from 3 to 18%. No correlation between degree of malignancy and pyruvate kinase activity in the presence of alanine is found.

Non Neuro-Epithelial Tumours

These included haemangioblastoma (n = 1), meningioma (n = 22), chromophobe adenoma (n = 3), craniopharyngioma (n = 1), neurilemmoma (n = 6), fibrosarcoma (n = 1) metastatic tumours (n = 5). Relatively high residual activity of pyruvate kinase was found in the haemangioblastoma, the craniopharyngioma and in the two chromophobe adenomas. Pyruvate kinase from the other tumours within this group shows much less residual activity. Table 1 shows the residual activity of these lesions. No correlations could be detected between degree of malignancy and residual pyruvate kinase activity.

Pyruvate Kinase in Intracranial Lesions of Non-Neoplastic Origin

This group included two cases of long-standing post-traumatic gliosis and scarring, one case of haemorrhagic infarct, leading to death within 24 hours after the onset and two cases of intracerebral haemorrhage with signs of extensive reorganization. One cavernoma and two arteriovenous malformations without haemorrhage were also included in this series. High residual activities equal to those found in normal brain tissue were found in the cases of gliosis and scarring, in the arteriovenous malformation, and in the acute fatal haemorrhage.

Low residual activities equal to those found in gliomas were found in the cavernoma and in the cases of haemorrhage accompanied by regeneration.

Table 1. Residual activity of non-neuro-epithelial tumours and metastatic tumours

	Mean residual activity in %
Meningioma	9 (n = 22)
Chromophobe adenoma	47 (n = 1)
Haemangioblastoma	44 (n = 1)
Craniopharyngioma	37 (n = 1)
Neurilemmoma	8 (n = 6)
Fibrosarcoma	8 (n = 1)
Metastatic tumours	11 (n = 5)

Discussion

As shown in the electropherograms in Fig. 1 human fetal brain of 12 and 16 weeks of age is characterized by the presence of both M and K-type pyruvate kinase and their hybrids. In the brain of a newborn a shift in the synthesis of isozymes is observed. The isozyme synthesis resembles strongly the adult pattern, only its composition is different. In the adult brain the M_4 type is strongly predominant over the K-type. It seems likely that during the development of the human brain the synthesis of K subunits is repressed whereas the reverse is found for the M subunit. It is not certain at what age the adult isozyme composition is obtained. It is however surprising that all childrens gliomas were characterized by low residual activities i.e. predominance of K-subunits of pyruvate kinase, unrespective the degree of differentiation. These findings need further evaluation.

The investigated non-neuroepithelial tumours were all characterized by the predominant occurrence of K_3M and K_4. The same pattern was found in a cavernoma and in cases of long-standing partially organized haemorrhage. In view of the results of examination of isozymes of PK in human tissues of different origin it does appear that the tissue from which or in which non-neuroepithelial tumours originate is already characterized by presence of K-type pyruvate kinase in much greater amounts than in normal adult human brain. Consequently it cannot be surprising that K-type predominates also in lesions of mesodermal origin like cavernoma and re-organization in haemorrhage. There is strong indication that the small amounts of K_3M and K_4 present in normal adult brain are synthesized by non-neuroepithelial elements (10).

The shift of the synthesis of M-type to K-type is shown to correlate well with histological differentiation and growth rate of gliomas of adults. In these tumours a strong relationship appears to exist between the electrophoretic pattern and alanine inhibition on the one hand and histological grading, presence or absence of tumour in the histological examination of paraffin sections and prognosis on the other hand.

The use of enzyme assays for the prognosis of growth rate of tumours is not new. As early as in 1970 Knox et al. (6) were able to show the value of an enzyme assay in the prognosis of growth rate of experimental tumours. Their enzyme assay appeared to have better prognostic significance than pathologic examination. Recently Deshpande et al. (2) showed the value of enzyme assays in the prognosis of human breast cancer.

However, these methods depend on the measurement of total enzyme activities which may vary according to the setting in which the method is applied. Electrophoresis of isozyme patterns of one enzyme as performed by Bennet et al. (1) and Rabow et al. (8) in human gliomas may prove to be more reliable. Such assays however are time-consuming and cannot be used intra-operatively.

For this reason an alanine inhibition test was developed in which the M- and K-type isozymes of pyruvate kinase could be rapidly and reliably discriminated. Because this test can be performed within ten minutes the test can be used for the intra-operative estimation of the degree of growth rate of gliomas and the demarcation of the resection.

Despite the availability of histological examination of frozen sections no certainty exists so far during operation about classification and grading of gliomas. It must await examination of paraffin sections of representative parts of the tumour by the pathologist. From the experience obtained it does appear that besides histological examination of frozen sections, the alanine inhibition test may prove to be a valuable tool in the surgery of gliomas.

115

The reason for the reappearance of K-type pyruvate kinase in gliomas still needs to be elucidated. Gliomas share the predominance of K-type pyruvate kinase with all human and experimental tumours examined to date and with proliferating and fetal cells of various origin (16, 17). Characteristic for most tumour cells is their high rate of glycolysis, i.e. they convert most of the glucose into lactic acid, even in aerobic circumstances, an observation already made by Warburg in 1924. In aerobic glycolysis carbohydrates can be channelled toward nucleic acid synthesis precursors. This can be partly achieved by a blockade on the level of pyruvate kinase. It was shown by Eigenbrodt (3) that the K-type pyruvate kinase may indeed be inactivated by a protein kinase. Such protein kinase might than be linked to the production of proteins, made under the direction of viral genetic material RNA. The recent discovery of protein kinases (7) linked to the presence of cancerous viruses may help in the understanding of the Warburg Effect, in which the isozyme shift of pyruvate kinase does play an important role as it is one of the key enzymes of glycolysis.

Conclusion

More definite conclusions about the applicability of an alanine inhibition test in the treatment of patients suffering from intracranial tumours should be based on results obtained on a larger number of patients than the series presented here.

Nevertheless some preliminary conclusions can be made:
1. In gliomas of adults a shift in the synthesis of isozymes of pyruvate kinase occurs from the M- towards the K-type, according to histological grading and growth rate.
2. The isozyme shift can be rapidly demonstrated with an alanine inhibition test.
3. The alanine inhibition test can be an aid in the intra-operative grading of gliomas of adults and also in the demarcation of the resection of these tumours.
4. Enzymological research not only deserves a place in oncology in general, but there is also strong indication that chemotherapy may be made more effective if it is based on the altered enzyme properties in cancer.

References

1. Bennet, M.J., Timperley, W.R., Taylor, C.B., Hill, A.S.: Isozymes of hexokinase in the developing, normal and neoplastic human brain. Europ. J. Cancer *14*, 189–193 (1978)
2. Deshpande, N., Mitchell, I., Millis, R.: Tumour enzymes and prognosis in human breast cancer. Europ. J. Cancer *17*, 443–448 (1981)
3. Eigenbrodt, E., Glossmann, H.: Glycolysis – one of the keys to cancer? Trends Pharmacol. Sci. *1*, 240–245 (1980)
4. Ibsen, K.H.: Interrelationships and functions of the pyruvate kinase isozymes and their variant forms: a review. Cancer Res. *37*, 341–353 (1977)
5. Ibsen, K.H., Fishman, W.H.: Developmental gene expression in cancer. Biochim. Biophys. Acta Cancer Rev. *560*, 243–280 (1979)
6. Knox, W.E., Linder, M., Friedel, G.H.: A series of transplantable rat mammary tumors with graded differentiation, growth rate and glutaminase content. Cancer Res. *30*, 283–287 (1970)
7. Marx, J.: Tumor viruses and the kinase connection. Science *211*, 1336–1338 (1981)
8. Rabow, L., Kristansson, K.: Changes in lactate dehydrogenase isozyme patterns in patients with tumours of the central nervous system. Acta Neurochir. *36*, 71–81 (1977)

9. Schapira, T.: Isozymes and cancer. Advan. Cancer Res. *18*, 77–153 (1973)
10. Tolle, S.W., Dyson, R.D., Newburgh, R.W., Cardenas, J.M.: Pyruvate kinase isozymes in neurons, glia, neuroblastoma and glioblastoma. J. Neurochem. *27*, 1355–1360 (1976)
11. Van Veelen, C.W.M., Verbiest, H., Vlug, A.M.C., Rijksen, G., Staal, G.E.J.: Isozymes of pyruvate kinase from human brain maningiomas and malignant gliomas. Cancer Res. *38*, 4681–4687 (1978)
12. Van Veelen, C.W.M., Verbiest, H., Zülch, K.J., van Ketel, B.A., van der Vlist, M.J.M., Vlug, A.M.C., Rijksen, G., Staal, G.E.J.: L-α-alanine inhibition of pyruvate kinase from tumors of the human central nervous system. Cancer Res. *39*, 4263–4269 (1979)
13. Van Veelen, C.W.M., Rijksen, G., Vlug, A.M.C., Staal, G.E.J.: Correlation between alanine inhibition of pyruvate kinase and composition of K-M hybrids. Clin. Chim. Acta *110*, 113–120 (1981)
14. Weber, G.: Enzymology of cancer cells. New. Engl. J. Med. *296*, 486–493 (1977)
15. Weinhouse, S.: Metabolism and isozyme alterations in experimental hepatomas. Fed. Proc. *32*, 2162–2167 (1973)
16. Weinhouse, S.: Molecular mechanism of gene regulation. Cancer *36*, 4330–4331 (1976)
17. Weinhouse, S.: New dimensions in the biology of cancer. Cancer *45*, 2975–2980 (1980)
18. Zülch, K.J.: Principles of the new WHO classification of brain tumors. J. Neurosurg. Sci. *22*, 1–5 (1978)

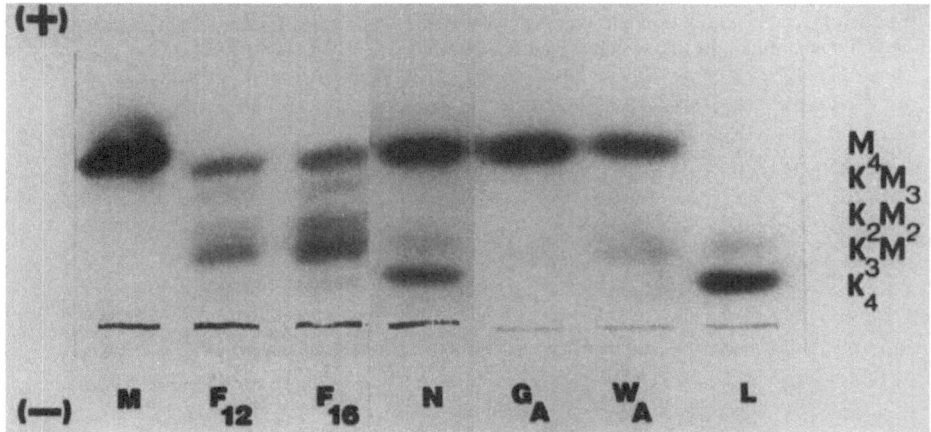

Fig. 1. Electropherogram of pyruvate kinase of (*from left to right*): striated muscle (*M*), whole fetal brain, 12 weeks old (F_{12}) and 16 weeks old (F_{16}), whole brain of a newborn (*N*), cortical grey matter of an adult brain (G_A), white matter of an adult brain (W_A) and leucocytes (*L*)

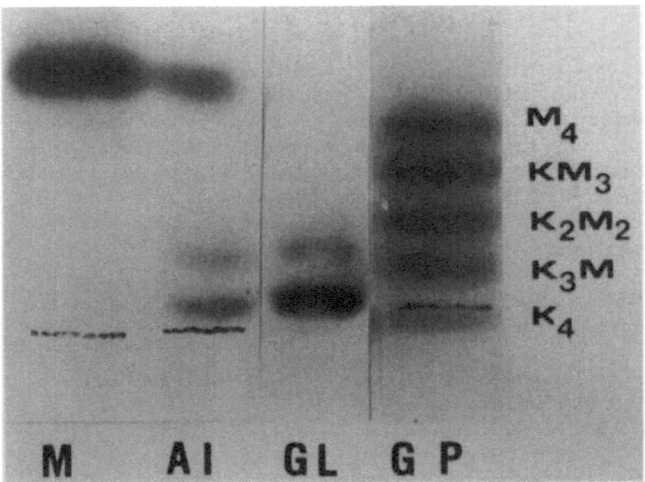

Fig. 2. Electrophoretic pattern of pyruvate kinase of examples of tumors representative for the respective histological classification and grading (AI = astrocytoma grade I; GL = glioblastoma; M = muscle; GP = glandula pinealis, which served as a reference)

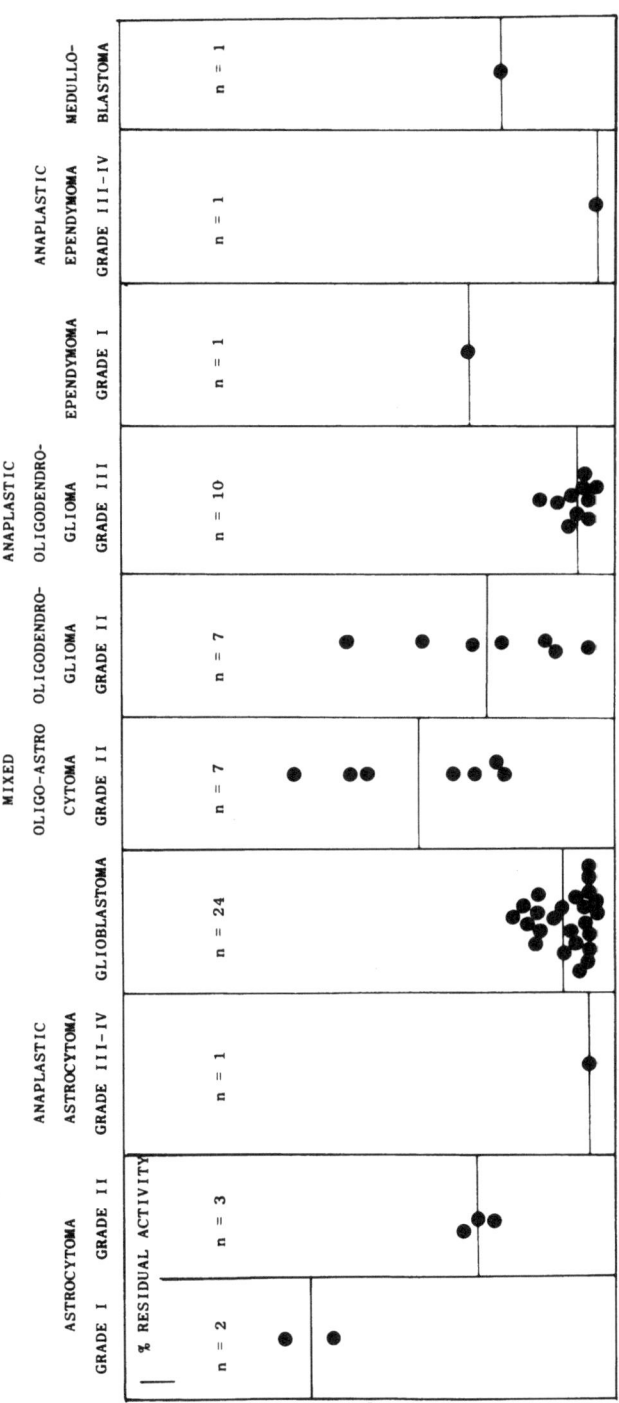

Fig. 3. Correlation between residual activity and histological classification and grading in gliomas

119

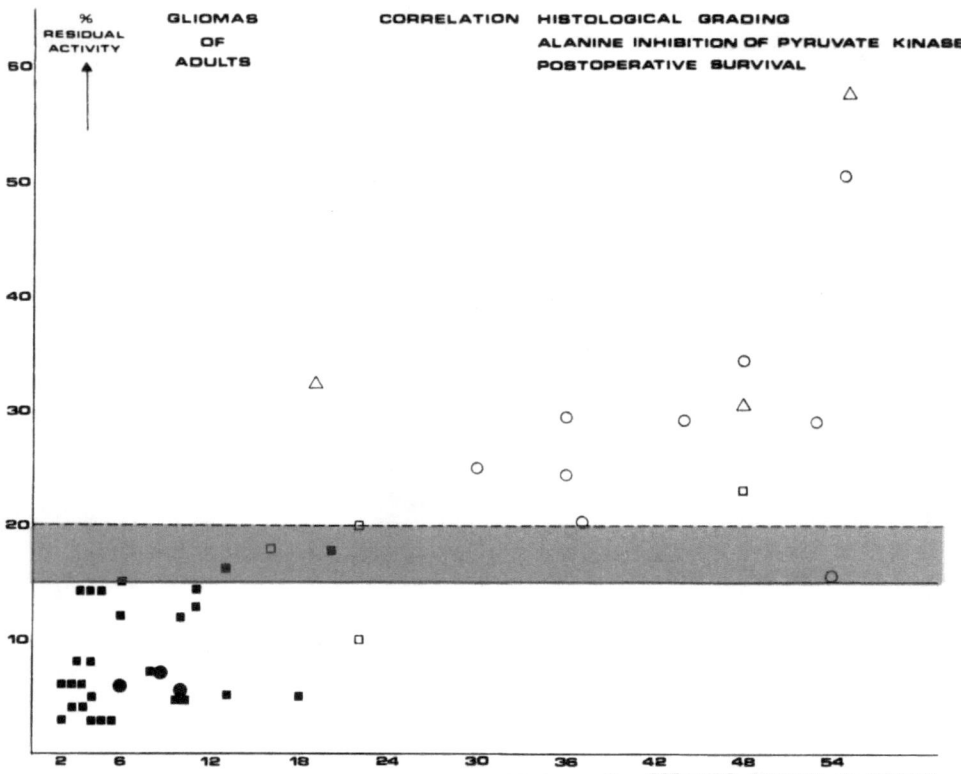

Fig. 4. Residual pyruvate kinase in the presence of alanine and survival after operation in months, of well and poorly differentiated gliomas (n = 45). (△ = astrocytoma grade I; ○ = oligodendroglioma grade II and astrocytoma grade II; □ = poorly differentiated gliomas, glioblastoma, anaplastic oligodendroglioma and anaplastic astrocytoma; open figures = alive; closed figures = dead

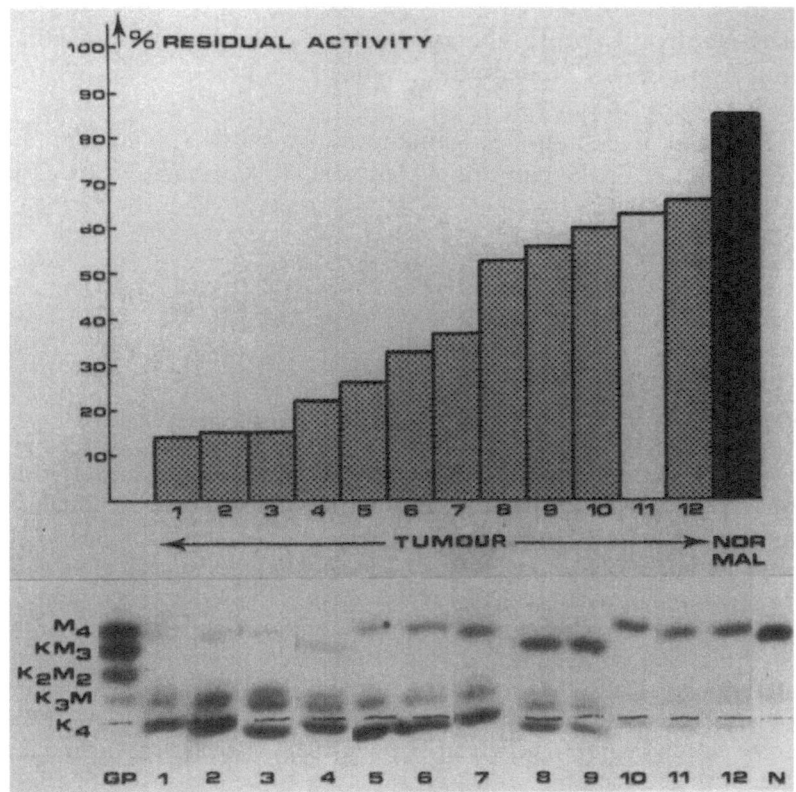

Fig. 5. Residual pyruvate kinase in the presence of alanine of different parts (1–12) of an anaplastic oligodendroglioma, developing into a glioblastoma. The electrophoretic pattern of pyruvate kinase is shown in the photograph (*below*). Glandula pinealis (*GP*) and normal brain tissue (*N*) were used as references. (This figure is presented with kind permission of Cancer Research)

Boron-Neutron Capture Therapy vs. Photon Beam for Malignant Brain Tumours — 12 Years' Experience

H. Hatanaka, K. Amano, S. Kamano, F. Tovaryš, N. Machiyama, T. Matsui, H. Fankhauser, T. Hanamura, T. Nukada, T. Kurihara, N. Ito, and K. Sano

Introduction

Slow neutron capture therapy is intended to irradiate tumor tissue selectively with heavy particles produced by the neutron-capturing reaction of Boron-10, Lithium-6 and certain other nuclides (6, 9, 16, 19, 34). In early trials between 1953 and 1961 p-carboxyphenyl boronic acid or sodium perhydrodecaborate (29, 30), and more recently, since 1968, mercaptoundecahydrododecaborate have been used for brain tumour treatment (8,28). Brain tumours are most suited to this type of therapy, because of the so-called Blood-Brain Barrier phenomenon which allows a discriminative transport of the neutron-capturing isotope into the tumour tissue but not into the surrounding brain matter, yielding a large Tumour/Brain ratio in isotope concentration (1, 4, 20). After the first trial of Boron-Neutron Capture Therapy in Japan in 1968, 44 malignant brain tumours were treated with neutron capture. Thirty-two of the 44 were treated with neutron capture alone, but 12 others were treated only after the failure of preceding conventional radiotherapy with photon. The clinical results were compared with that of 90 patients treated with photon. Most of the photon-treated patients with malignant gliomas underwent adjuvant therapy with chemo- or immuno-therapeutic agents. Tumours with better prognosis with conventional radiotherapy are excluded.

Materials and Methods

Table 1 is the list of the brain tumours included in the present study of radiotherapy. Out of the 308 cases which constitute the series treated by one of the authors (H.H.) up until August 1980, 212 cases were treated with radiation. The material best suited to evaluation of therapeutic effect is high-grade glioma, represented by glioblastoma, as its prognosis is usually extremely poor.

Malignancy Grading. A crucially important pre-requisite to this study is the malignancy grading of each tumour. The histology specimens were examined by two or more pathologists, including Prof. Kurt Jellinger of Vienna, who reclassified them by applying the new grading criteria recommended by WHO (37). The percentage of Grade III–IV glioma in the author's series, as diagnosed by Prof. Jellinger, was 62% — slightly lower than the

Table 1. Radiation-treated brain tumours (Hatanaka, 1963–1964, 1967–1980)

Gliomas	131/133	cases
Supratentorial, grade I–II	30/30	
Supratentorial, grade III–IV	68/68	
Infratentorial, grade I–II	3/5	
Pons-Medulla, grade II–III	21/21	
Optic	5/5	
Medulloblastoma	4/4	
Meningioma	10/31	
Metastases	24/24	
Pituitary adenoma	23/23	
Craniopharyngioma	0/14	
Neurinoma	1/12	
Pinealoma (germinoma)	7/7	
Other pineal tumours	3/3	
Intracranial sarcomas	5/5	
Teratoma	2/4	
Neurofibromatosis	0/4	
Other neoplasms	2/10	
Angioma (AVM)	4/31	
Abscess, granuloma	0/7	
Total	212/308	cases (68%)

66% and 68% of Zülch (36) and Zimmerman's (35) series. This fact suggests that Jellinger's diagnosis of high grade malignancy may be even stricter than that of other prominent brain tumour pathologists.

Patient Selection. All the glioma patients except Grade I cases were radiated either by BNCT or photon. After 1968 when Boron-Neutron Capture Therapy (BNCT) was first applied to a terminally ill recurrent glioblastoma patient, the author H.H. has made it a rule to treat any stage of high-grade glioma by BNCT, however deteriorated the patient's condition might be, except when 1) Boron-10 isotope was not available, 2) the reactor was not in operation, or 3) the operator himself (H.H.) was not available. A patient with a medulla astrocytoma was conveyed to the reactor with his respiration artificially maintained because of respiratory paresis and established tetraplegia (but after BNCT he recovered spontaneous respiration), and a patient in coma was taken to the reactor for a pons-medulla astrocytoma which had recurred after photon therapy (she has by now survived almost 5 years). This steadfast policy of treating any terminal-stage case by BNCT may well render the whole series practically as valid as a randomized study for clinical evaluation, although the present report is not prospective.

Procedures of Treatments

1. Photon (and Chemo-Immunotherapy). After craniotomy and surgical removal of tumours a total of 4000–6000 rad tumour dose was delivered over a period of 4–6 weeks. As a rule, a resection of the brain was avoided. The most common regimen was to give 200 rad per day 20–30 times with either Cobalt-60 or linear accelerator (Lineac). This is approximately equivalent to 1250–1750 ret (Nominal Standard Dose, Ellis). Most of the patients radiated with photon were also treated by adjuvant therapy of chemotherapeutic and/or immunotherapeutic agents (5-fluorouracil, vincristine, cyclophosphamide, bromodeoxyuridine, showdomycin (14), carmustine, bleomycin, autochthonous tumour cells pre-treated with mercaptoundecahydrododecaborate, BCG, and thymosin (18). Only the patients treated with showdomycin underwent a smaller dose photon therapy (1000–1250 ret) because the radiosensitivity effect of showdomycin, which doubles the effect of radiation, had been established. A combined showdomycin-small-dose-radiation effect upon patient survival has been proved not to differ significantly from conventional dose radiotherapy (14), and hence the showdomycin cases are included in the Photon group.

2. Boron-Neutron Capture Therapy. At one or two weeks after a craniotomy for tumour excision or a biopsy, the patient undergoes an intra-arterial infusion of isotonic boron-10 solution on the evening before the scheduled neutron irradiation, and is then conveyed to the reactor where the tumour is apposed to the thermal neutron collimator. Reflection of the scalp is necessary to prevent a boron-10 neutron-capture reaction in the skin that contains a fairly large amount of boron-10. The scalp is shielded against neutron beam to avoid skin necrosis, while the brain matter which holds no boron-10 is exposed. After the neutron irradiation, if the neutron fluence delivered to the tumour bed was satisfactorily large, the tumour undergoes a gradual degeneration, depending on the amount of neutron capture reaction which is in direct proportion to neutron flux and boron-10 concentration. If everything goes well, a patient can go home within 20 days after the first surgical intervention. The infused boron-10 dose is 30–50 mg ^{10}B/kg of body weight. The ^{10}B concentration in tumour attained at the time of neutron irradiation is 13–60 μg/g of tumour, while its concentration in normal brain matter (N) is not measurable. The concentration in blood (B) is usually equal to or less than the concentration in tumour (T). T/B ratio is usually 1–4, greater in children and smaller in the elderly, probably because of the excretion capacity of the individual body. The neutron flux from Musashi Institute of Technology reactor at its medical port is 1.5 x 10^9 n/cm^2/sec. The actual flux can vary depending on the shape of the craniotomy, the patient's head, and on the depth of the tumour bed. The neutron flux delivered to the tumour bed can be improved, in spite of the rapid attenuation of thermal neutron, through the use of certain surgical techniques and multi-directional irradiation (10).

Interim Results

No patient was excluded from statistical evaluation because of inappropriate treatment or discontinuation of the treatment. The whole series corresponds to the so-called valid study group (Table 2).

Table 2. Interim clinical results depending on the types of initial radiotherapy in 1963–64, 1967–1980, out of 308 cases by Hatanaka as of May 31, 1981

Tumour	Initial radiation		Photon	
	Neutron capture		+ Chemo / immuno	+ Neutron capture
Supratentorial glioma, grade III–IV (68 cases)	Mn $>$ 577 $\pm$ 178 days 5/18 alive Karnofsky 73%		Mn $=$ 388 $\pm$ 48 days 0/41 alive Karnofsky 56%	Mn $=$ 531 $\pm$ 124 days 0/9 alive ———
Supratentorial glioma, grade II (30 cases)	Mn $>$ 1176 $\pm$ 107 days 3/5 alive Karnofsky 92%		Mn $>$ 1147 $\pm$ 295 days 5/25 alive Karnofsky 67%	———
Pons-medulla astrocytoma, grade II–IV/ or unverified (21 cases)	Mn $=$ 260 $\pm$ 45 days 0/4 alive Karnofsky 45%		Mn $=$ 245 $\pm$ 66 days 0/16 alive Karnofsky 39%	Mn $>$ 1741 days 1/1 alive Karnofsky 80%
Meningioma (10 cases)	3/3 alive		4/5 alive	0/2 alive
Intracranial sarcomas (5 cases)	1/2 alive Rhabdomyosarcoma 7 years Chondrosarcoma $>$ 3 years		0/3 alive Fibrosarcoma Reticulum cell sarcoma Reticulum cell sarcoma	———

1. Supratentorial Grade III–IV Glioma

(i) By BNCT without preceding photon treatment, an average of 19.2 ± 5.9 months survival was reached at the end of May, 1981, and five patients out of 18 are alive. The longest survival by neutron is a man of 59 with a glioblastoma who has lived nine years after BNCT. (ii) By Photon combined with chemo-immuno-therapy, the mean survival was 12.9 ± 1.6 months. None of the patients lived beyond 4 years. (iii) By BNCT after previous photon therapy, none of the nine patients is now alive, although the survival was 17.7 ± 4.1 months (Table 3). It should be noted that among the 18 patients treated by BNCT without photon, ten patients, who had been operated on from the beginning by one of the authors (H.H.), have done far better than the other eight patients, who had been operated on by other neurosurgeons and then referred for subsequent BNCT. The mean survival for the first ten patients exceeded 26.4 ± 10.1 months as of May 31, 1981, and four of ten are alive, whereas the mean survival for the second eight patients has reached only 10.3 ± 2.4 months and only one of them is alive. This difference may have been caused by various factors such as surgical skill or care to prevent metastases of tumour cells. But a still more important factor may be the difference in the time interval between the first surgical tumour excision and the subsequent neutron bombardment, as the first ten patients were treated, on the average, only two weeks after the surgical excision, while the second eight patients were treated almost six weeks afterwards. This interpretation is probably endorsed by the fact that the patients with tumours smaller than 6 cm in diameter (geometrical average diameter) have lived more than 30.2 months while those with tumours larger than 6 cm have lived only more than 10.5 months. If we limit our analysis to the patients with glioblastomas averaging 5 cm in diameter, their mean survival exceeds four years. This indicates the crucial importance of "Early Detection, and Early Treatment" of a glioblastoma, even in BNCT (Table 4). It is assumed that there is a correlation between the size of the tumour and the survival after BNCT, but the calculated correlation coefficient was -0.41 and a correlation could not be proved at least for dthe moment, probably due to the limited number of cases. The depth of the tumour bed may be important for a good therapeutic result, in view of the unsatisfactory penetration of thermal neutron which attenuates to one half after travelling only 1.7–2.0 cm in the tissue. The correlation coefficient between the depth of the tumour bed and the survival was -0.66, and appears to be more significantly correlated to the survival than is the average diameter of the tumour. If the diameter of the tumour is smaller than 5 cm, although the number of cases is very small (3), the average survival is almost four years for glioblastoma. Two of them are believed to have been cured, judging from radiological and clinical evidence. The third patient died 15 months later because of remote dissemination of the tumour from the anterior genu of the corpus callosum to the IVth ventricle; at autopsy the original tumour site (corpus callosum) did not have viable tumour cells. The reason for the inefficiency in treating a large tumour is accounted for by the fact that the authors have not yet delivered the neutron beam over a large area of the brain. After other neurosurgeons had done a bona fide craniotomy (usually 6–10 cm in diameter), it was quite difficult to enlarge the skin flap and the bone window lest the blood supply to the skin should be disturbed. In two cases we tried a crisscross scalp incision to expose the entire vault and to put the entire vault of the head into the collimator. This procedure necessitates a considerable loss of

Table 3. Supratentorial grade III—IV glioma survival and initial operator (as of May 31, 1980)

Initial operator	Hatanaka	Others
Mean interval (initial excision — neutron capture)	13.8 $\pm$ 2.2 days	46.3 $\pm$ 17.1 days
Mean survival (initial excision — death)	⟩ 26.4 $\pm$ 10.1 months	⟩ 10.3 $\pm$ 2.4 months
Currently alive	4/10	1/8

blood from the scalp and an extra hour to suture when the procedure is over. The bleeding can be minimized when a specially designed head rest is developed to fasten the reflected skin flaps, even if the neurosurgeon may not feel the suturing of such a large skin wound is a nuisance.

A Case Example. A man of 50, M.T. (Fig. 1), presented with mental deterioration, difficulty of speech, and right-sided motor weakness in early 1972, was operated on for a vascular tumour (approximately 6.5 x 5.5 x 4.5 cm on angiograms) in the left posterior frontal lobe. The angiograms were suggestive of a glioblastoma, and the histology also attested to this preoperative diagnosis. On July 22, 1972, the patient was operated on by one of the authors (H.H.) and tumour tissue weighing 20 grams was obtained without removing any brain matter. The tumour residue was seen to be continuous with the corpus callosum. After this partial resection, the patient underwent BNCT on June 29, 1972, and was discharged three weeks later. The only post-operative complication was transient diabetes insipidus caused by BNCT radiation of the pituitary gland that had taken up Boron-10. He was able to resume his occupational activity of farming immediately, and ever since has been active, for nine years (Fig. 3).

2. Supratentorial Grade II Glioma

The mean survival for the photon group is 38.2 $\pm$ 9.8 months and for BNCT 39.2 $\pm$ 3.6 months as of the end of May, 1981. Although superficially the survival does not differ very much for the moment, only 20% (5 out of 25) are alive for the photon group, while 60% (3 of 5) are still alive for the BNCT group. It should be noted that only one half of the Grade II patients treated by photon are in a condition to work, while all the patients treated by BNCT recovered well enough to work. The performance status, as measured by the Karnofsky scale, for the photon group was 67%, and for the BNCT group, was 92%.

127

Table 4. Major reports of mean survivals of anaplastic gliomas

Authors	Gillingham		Walker				Jellinger				Hatanaka		
Year	1975		1978				1979				1981		
Total, No. of cases	238		222				116				68		
Therapy	0	0+R	0	0+C	0+R	0+R+C	0	0+R	0+C	0+R+C	0+N	0+R+C/I	0+R+N
No. of cases	100	138	31	58	51	72	39	31	13	33	18	41	9
Average age	51		57	56	57	57	65	55	58	56	49	45	39
(range)			10-79	28-78	22-78	6-78	30-76	21-67	21-69	27-72	22-70	10-68	29-52
Grade of tumour [a]	3–4		3–4				3.72	3.68	3.68	3.76	3.33	3.39	3.33
Mean survival [b] (month)	5.2	13.8	3.3	4.3	8.4	8.1	5.4	10.6	10.7	13.3	19.2	12.9	17.7
2 year survival	2.0% (3yr)		0%	0%	2.0%	6.9%	0%	3.2%	8.3%	5.6%	30.8%	12.2%	22.2%

0= operation; R= radiation with X-ray, cobalt or lineac; C= chemotherapy; I= immunology; N= neutron capture

[a] Cases by Hatanaka were diagnosed by Jellinger with WHO criteria

[b] As of May 31, 1980. Mean survival for Hatanaka, Gillingham series. Median survival for Walker, Jellinger series

3. Pons-Medulla Grade II–IV Glioma

16 photon-treated cases died with a mean survival of 8.2 ± 2.2 months. Average Karnofsky score was 39%. BNCT group without photon survived an average of 8.7 ± 1.5 months. Karnofsky score was 45%. This sounds as if BNCT did not prove to be significantly more effective than photon, but it is the result of insufficient neutron flux at the tumour bed due to the deep location of the brain stem where there is an inevitable attenuation of neutron flux to 1/16–1/32 of the flux at entry to the brain. This result strongly indicates the need for an epithermal neutron radiation facility which yields a larger neutron flux at the depth of the brain (7). However, one patient who belongs to the BNCT-after-Photon group has been doing well. A 3-year-old child was treated with photon for a Grade III–II astrocytoma and did well for a few months, but then deteriorated and finally fell in coma when BNCT was performed. After a slow recovery, she has been doing well for more than four years and she will have survived five years in August 1981. On CT scan she has no evidence of a mass but the so-called isolated fourth ventricle is apparent. The success of BNCT on this patient is not a combination effect of preceding photon and BNCT, but is probably owing to the shorter distance between the neutron collimator and the tumour bed in the fourth ventricle (rhomboid fossa) in a young child. This patient (R.T.) was the youngest in the BNCT-treated brain stem series. The depth of her tumour was not so great; hence, the neutron flux was larger than in the others.

4. Sarcoma and Other Tumours

A primary intracranial rhabdomyosarcoma, a primary intracranial chondrosarcoma, and three meningiomas were treated by BNCT, and two meningiomas were treated by BNCT after the failure of photon. In addition, five meningiomas were radiated with photon alone. The rhabdomyosarcoma case lived almost seven years. The chondrosarcoma case is alive after four years and is perfectly fit to work.

Discussion

The outlook for brain tumour in general used to be in a pessimistic state. The statistics obtained in the United States indicate that in 1975, 10,700 new brain tumour patients appeared, and almost 80% of them were doomed to die, as 5,000 glioma patients and 3,500 non-glioma patients died in that same year (23). Except for Grade I (WHO) gliomas which take place in the cerebellar hemispheres of infants, only very few glioma patients are cured. In spite of many reports of improved multimodality treatments, the clinical results are far from satisfactory. BCNU or CCNU, which is believed to cross the Blood-Brain Barrier, has been shown ineffective in prolonging the life span (22, 24, 32). If it is combined with radiotherapy, it is believed to prolong survival, but the survival is not much better than that by radiotherapy alone. The results of our Grade III–IV gliomas are compared with the reports from others in Table 4 (13, 32, 33). After histological reclassification, our series will tolerate criticism. It clearly indicates that BNCT is superior to ordinary Photon therapy and probably to the combined modality treatment. Beyond doubt BNCT will yield a much better survival if a randomized clinical trial is attempted, because the presently reported series of Grade III—IV gliomas is mostly an accumulation of cases referred to the author after previous treatment and with clinically proven malignant tumours.

There is no basis on which to compare the present results of BNCT with those obtained by radical surgery (25) on malignant brain tumours, because the author (H.H.) who conducted this series has constantly tried to spare the brain matter and to compare the therapeutic effect with adjuvant therapies other than surgery. It should be remembered that brain stem (pons medulla) tumours are usually not radically removable and that the eventual objective of a radiotherapy is to treat such a surgically untouchable tumour. This objective has not yet been very successfully attained by the presently available BNCT except in one case of ponto-medullary astrocytoma out of five, who has been alive for more than four years (R.T.). But BNCT will be promising in the event that a more effectively penetrating epithermal neutron source reactor becomes available. Although there are fragmentary reports of long survival of brain stem glioma patients, they are uniformly considered to be benign astrocytoma cases (12). The aforementioned case is certainly different from such benign astrocytoma cases because its malignancy had been clinically established through its recurrence after a previous surgical excision and Photon treatment. This case certainly demonstrates the superiority of BNCT to conventional photon therapy.

Fast Neutron (17) and Pi-meson (31) have been tried to treat glioblastoma, but their eventual clinical outcome may not be superior to that of radical surgery, because the extent of such an invasive tumour cannot be precisely determined before radiation even by new means like CT. The results of treatment by such heavy particle radiation have been reported, but they are not superior to photon therapies. Besides short survival, the brain damage that is caused by such heavy particles will be serious unless the radiation is precisely targeted. On the contrary, Boron-10 neutron capture radiation has been proved to be least injurious to the brain matter. Normal dog brains which underwent BNCT regimen could tolerate almost 5000 rad of intravascular $^{10}_{5}B\,(n\alpha)\,^{7}_{3}Li$ reaction (series of dogs that underwent craniotomy, Zamenhof, Brownell, Schoene, Klein and Richardson) (26), and 8000 rad (dogs without craniotomy, Takeuchi and Ushio) (3, 9, 15). Photon-radiation therapy is widely acknowledged to extend the life span, but its radiation hazard cannot be ignored. By radiotherapy with photon and by BNCT, a gram of brain tissue is exposed to an average of 1500 ret and 722 ret, respectively, given an RBE (relative biological effectiveness) of 3.5 for alpha-particle produced by Boron-Neutron capture reaction. The superiority of post-BNCT patients' performance status to that of post-photon patients may be easily accounted for by the difference of radiation exposure of the normal brain.

The clinical trial up to the present is a sort of Phase I—II study, and the patient material tended to be far-advanced cases. If a newly-diagnosed glioblastoma patient is treated without delay by BNCT, one can expect a good result which may well lead to a clinical cure. The use of a more deeply penetrating epithermal neutron will produce an even better therapeutic effect. To attain this aim some physicists [Dr. Fairchild (7) and Prof. An (5)] have been designing an epithermal reactor. Research into some neutron-capturing compounds of Boron-10 or Lithium-6 and the isotope transport across the so-called Blood-Brain Barrier is being conducted, as there is still room to improve the clinical result.

Conclusion

The clinical results on malignant brain tumours by BNCT, BNCT-after-Photon, and Photon were retrospectively compared.

1. Supratentorial grade III–IV gliomas: BNCT conducted after partial excision yielded the best result in length and quality of survival. A mean survival of 20 months will be reached in July, 1981, with 31% patients surviving two years. The longest surviving is a then 50-year-old man with a partially excised glioblastoma who has been perfectly fit to work for the past nine years. All the photon-group patients died before four years with a mean survival of less than 13 months and 12.2% two year survival. BNCT-after-Photon patients had been so destined by the previous photon and subsequent recurrence and all of them died although their life was extended. BNCT patients who had been treated from the onset by the same surgeon (H.H.) without delay have done best with a mean survival of 26 months and 40% still alive.

2. Brain stem (pons-medulla) astrocytomas (grade II–IV): BNCT result was not significantly superior to Photon, due to the insufficient depth dose of thermal neutron. However, a young infant with a smaller distance has lived five years after the initial operation and photon followed by recurrence and subsequent BNCT.

3. The interim results indicate a satisfactory improvement of the future clinical results by introduction of epithermal neutron, by early treatment without delay, and perhaps by discovery of more efficient neutron-capturing isotopes.

References

1. Abe, M., Kitamura, K., Amano, K., Hatanaka, H.: Tissue distribution of ^{10}B compound in ENU-induced tumor-carrying rats and transplanted brain tumor-carrying rats. 39th Annual Meeting of the Japanese Neurosurgical Society, Oct. 16, 1980
2. Aizawa, O., Kanda, K., Nozaki, T., Matsumoto, T.: Remodeling and dosimetry on the neutron irradiation facility of the Musashi Institute of Technology Reactor for Boron Neutron Capture Therapy. Nuclear Technology *48*, 150–163 (1980)
3. Al-Samarrai, S.F., Hatanaka, H., Takeuchi, A.: Electron microscopic study on the response of the normal canine brain to Boron-Neutron Capture Therapy. Gann *66*, 663–672 (1975)
4. Amano, K., Sweet, W.H.: Alpha-autoradiography of ^{10}B compound distribution in tissue by use of superimposition technique. Nippon Acta Radiol. *33*, 267–272 (1973)
5. An, S., Furuhashi, A., Oka, Y., Akiyama, M., Kuga, H., Tanaka, H.: Development studies regarding the construction of epithermal-enriched neutron field for medical purposes at the University of Tokyo Yayoi Fast Reactor. Nuclear Technology *48*, 204–215 (1980)
6. Brownell, G.L., Zamenhof, R.G., Murray, B.W., Wellum, G.R.: Boron Neutron Capture Therapy. In: Therapy in Nuclear Medicine. Spencer, R.P. (ed), pp. 205–222. New York, San Francisco, London: Grune & Stratton 1978
7. Fairchild, R.G.: Development and dosimetry of an 'epithermal' neutron beam for possible use in neutron capture therapy. Physics in Medicine and Biology *10*, 491–503 (1965)
8. Hatanaka, H., Sano, K.: A revised boron-neutron capture therapy for malignant brain tumors. In: Present Limits of Neurosurgery. Fusek, I., Kunc, A. (eds.), pp. 83–85. Prague: Avicenum, Czechoslovak Medical Press 1972
9. Hatanaka, H., Sweet, W.H.: Slow-neutron capture therapy for malignant tumours. Its history and recent development. In: Biomedical Dosimetry. pp. 147–178. Vienna: International Atomic Energy Agency 1975

10. Hatanaka, H., Watanabe, T.: Treatment of brain tumors with slow neutron. Geka-Shinryo (Surgical Diagnosis and Treatment) *12*, 1041–1055 (1970)
11. Hayakawa, Y., Harasawa, S., Nakamoto, A., Amano, K., Hatanaka, H., Egawa, J.: Simultaneous monitoring system of thermal neutron flux for Boron-Neutron Capture Therapy. Radiation Research *75*, 243–251 (1978)
12. Hoffman, H.J., Becker, L., Craven, M.A.: A clinically and pathologically distinct group of benign brain stem gliomas. Neurosurgery *7*, 243–248 (1980)
13. Jellinger, K., Kothbauer, P., Volc, D., Vollmer, R., Weiss, R.: Combination chemotherapy (COMP protocol) and radiotherapy of anaplastic supratentorial gliomas. Acta Neurochirurgica *51*, 1–13 (1979)
14. Kamano, S., Amano, K., Hanamura, T., Fankhauser, H., Hatanaka, H.: Clinical experience of combined therapy of small dose radiation and showdomycin for brain tumors. Brain Nerve *29*, 407–413 (1977)
15. Kitao, K.: A method for calculating the absorbed dose near interface from ^{10}B $(n, \alpha)^7$ Li reaction. Radiation Research *61*, 304–315 (1975)
16. Kruger, P.G.: Some biological effects of nuclear disintegration products on neoplastic tissue. Proc. Nat. Acad. Sci. *26*, 181–192 (1940)
17. Laramore, G.E., Griffin, T.W., Gerdes, A.J., Parker, R.G.: Fast neutron and mixed (neutron/photon) beam teletherapy for grades III and IV astrocytomas. Cancer *42*, 96–103 (1978)
18. Lipson, S.D., Chretien, P.B., Makuch, R., Kenady, D.E., Cohen, M.H.: Thymosin immunotherapy in patients with small cell carcinoma of the lung. Cancer *43*, 863–870 (1979)
19. Locher, G.L.: Biological effects and therapeutic possibilities of neutrons. Am. J. Roentgenol. *36*, 1–13 (1936)
20. Matsuoka, O., Hatanaka, H., Miyamoto, M.: Neutron capture whole body autoradiography of ^{10}B compounds. Acta Pharmacologica et Toxicologica *41* (Suppl. 1), 56–57 (1977)
21. Phillips, T.L., Buschke, F.: Radiation tolerance of the thoracic spinal cord. Am. J. Roentgenol. *105*, 659–664 (1969)
22. Pompili, A., Riccio, A., Jandolo, B., Fontana, M.: CCNU chemotherapy in adult patients with tumors of the basal ganglia and brain stem. J. Neurosurg. *53*, 361–363 (1980)
23. Posner, J.R., Shapiro, W.R.: Brain tumor – Current status of treatment and its complications – Editorial. Arch. Neurol. *32*, 781–784 (1975)
24. Reagan, T.J., Bisel, H.F., Childs, D.S., Jr., Layton, D.D., Rhoton, A.L., Jr., Taylor, W.F.: Controlled study of CCNU and radiation therapy in malignant astrocytoma. J. Neurosurg. *44*, 186–190 (1976)
25. Roth, J.G., Elvidge, A.R.: Glioblastoma multiforme. J. Neurosurg. *17*, 736–750 (1960)
26. Schoene, W.C., Murray, B.W., Rumbaugh, C.L., Shalev, M., Kleinman, G., Zamenhof, R.G., Wellum, G.R., Murphy, J.C., Brownell, G.L.: Morphological assessment of Boron Neutron Capture Therapy (BNCT) effectiveness on experimental brain tumors. 56th Annual Meeting of the American Association of Neuropathologists. June 13–15, 1980. J. Neuropathology Exp. Neurol. *39*, 388–398 (1980)
27. Soloway, A.H.: Boron compounds in cancer therapy. In: Progress in Boron Chemistry, pp. 203–234. New York: Pergamon Press 1964
28. Soloway, A.H., Hatanaka, H., Davis, M.A.: Penetration of brain and brain tumor. VII. Tumor-binding sulfhydryl boron compounds. J. Med. Chemistry *10*, 714–717 (1967)
29. Sweet, W.H., Javid, M.: The possible use of neutron-capturing isotopes such as boron-10 in the treatment of neoplasms. I. Intracranial tumor. J. Neurosurg. *9*, 200–209 (1952)
30. Sweet, W.H., Soloway, A.H., Brownell, G.L.: Boron-Neutron Capture Therapy of gliomas. Acta Radiologica *1*, 114–121 (1963)
31. Takenaka, E.: Negative pion radiation therapy of brain tumor. Neurological Surgery *8*, 1023–1029 (1980)
32. Walker, M.D., Green, S.B., Byar, D.P., Alexander, E., Jr., Batzdorf, U., Brooks, W.H., Hunt, W.E., MacCarty, C.S., Mahaley, M.S., Jr., Mealey, J., Jr., Owens, G., Ransohoff, J., II, Robertson, J.T., Shapiro, W.R., Smith, K.R., Jr., Wilson, C.B., Strike, T.A.: Randomized comparisons of radiotherapy and nitrosoureas for the treatment of malignant glioma after surgery. New Eng. J. Med. *303*, 1323–1329 (1980)

33. Yamashita, J., Gillingham, F.J.: Radiotherapy for glioblastoma. Neurological Surgery *3*, 329–336 (1975)
34. Zahl, P.A., Cooper, F.S., Dunning, J.R.: Some in vivo effects of localized nuclear disintegration products on a transplantable mouse sarcoma. National Academy of Sciences *26*, 589–598 (1940)
35. Zimmerman, H.: Seminar at the 5th International Congress of Neurological Surgeons, 1974
36. Zülch, K.J.: Brain tumors; their biology and pathology. pp. 63. New York: Springer 1965
37. Zülch, K.J.: Principles of the new World Health Organization (WHO) classification of brain tumors. Neuroradiology *19*, 59–66 (1980)

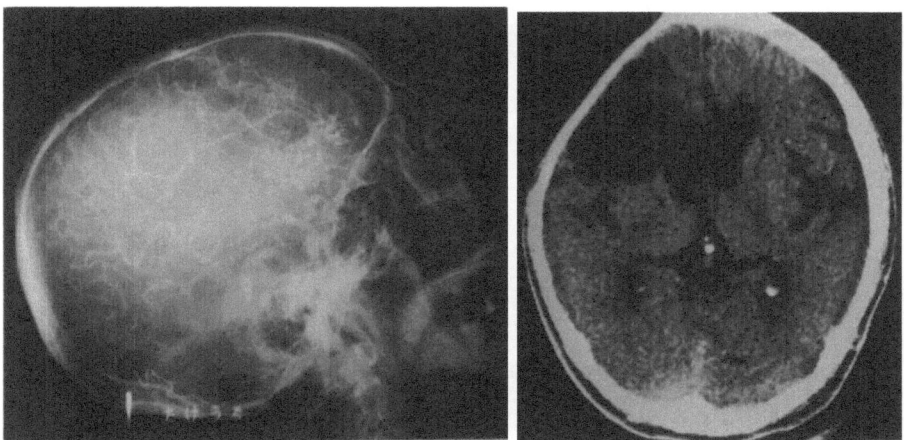

Fig. 1. A 50-year-old right-handed man (MT), treated by BNCT in June, 1972. No clinical sign of recurrence has been observed for the past nine years. *Left:* original angiogram demonstrating a classical glioblastoma tumour circulation in the left posterior frontal lobe. No CT was obtained in 1972. *Right:* CT in January, 1981 demonstrates a large cavity containing normal C.S.F. in the left frontal lobe, which is separated from the left lateral ventricle by a thin membrane. Although not shown here, the CT obtained in 1977 which was his first CT scan in his life and the 1981 CT demonstrate exactly unchanged findings. The latter is his second CT, since his clinical condition does not require a CT follow-up

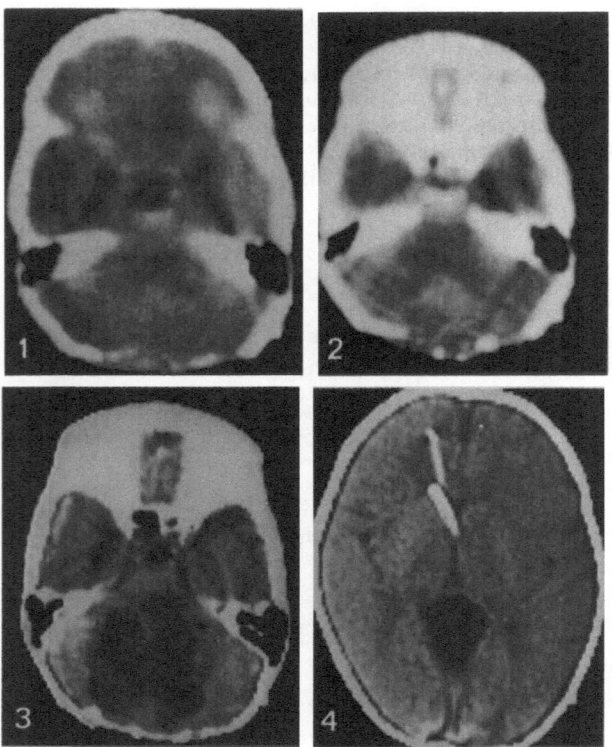

Fig. 2. A 3-year-old female child whose Grade II—III astrocytoma arising from the rhomboid fossa was operated on in August, 1976, and subsequently radiated with 4,000 rad of photon. After a temporary amelioration, the patient gradually deteriorated and fell in coma on March 29. BNCT was carried out on March 30, 1977. After remaining in a vegetative state for a few months, she slowly recovered and even started elementary schooling in April, 1980. She will have survived five years by August, 1981. *From left to right: 1* CT by a primitive apparatus on February 22, 1977. *2* CT by the same apparatus on April 14, 1977. *3* CT by EMI-1010 on March 8, 1979, *4* slice above the level of 3). The last CT taken on March 8, 1979, demonstrates a strikingly dilated 4th ventricle, and the normal size of the lateral ventricles containing two tubes for a ventriculoperitoneostomy and a Torkildsen procedure. The latter procedure had been done for the so-called isolated fourth ventricle which probably resulted from the pre-existing V-P shunt and long standing adhesive and occlusive change in the aqueduct. But the Torkildsen tube slipped off probably due to the growth of the head. Because of the reluctance of the parents no revision of either procedure has been attempted

Fig. 3. Post-radiation change of a large glioblastoma arising at the genu of the corpus callosum. *First line:* Pre-operative. The deepest part of the tumour is apparent just above the olfactory groove. *Second line:* Almost 12 days after the surgical removal of the tumour. Only partial excision was performed but no brain resection. *Third line:* Approximately 12 days after BNCT. The tumour tissue has turned to a low- or iso-density.

These three CT indicate a fairly good response of the tumour, even at the base of the brain. (This patient unfortunately died of constant gastric bleeding which persisted for three months, probably related to the slowly necrotizing process of the extensive tumour tissue)

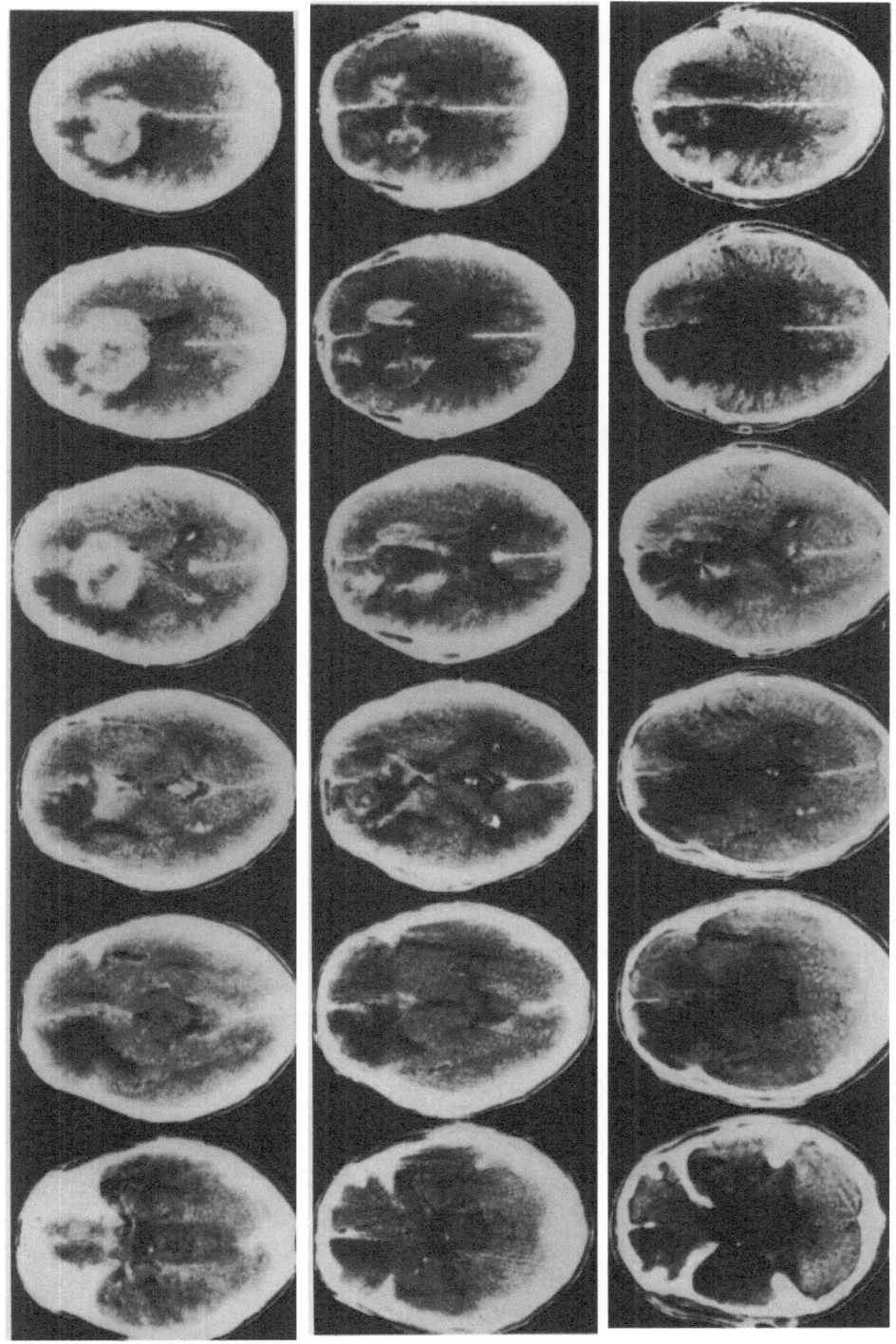

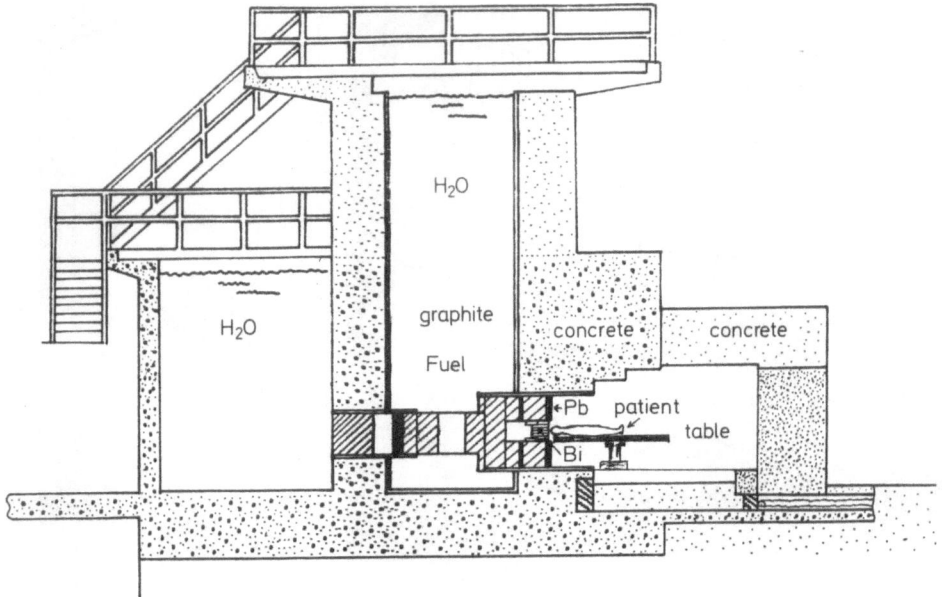

Fig. 4. Cross section of the currently used Musashi Institute of Technology Medical Reactor (100 Kw)

Treatment of Supratentorial Glioma Recurrencies with Re-Operation and Chemotherapy

D. Áfra

For treatment of supratentorial glioma recurrencies there are two main alternatives: either reoperation or conservative treatment, i.e. irradiation and/or chemotherapy. The possibility of repeated surgical intervention seems to be rather limited. According to our earlier experiences a reasonably longer survival-time could be achieved by removal of rather circumscribed located recurrences mostly sited in the poles, with subsequent irradiation (1). Apart from this, surgical evacuation (14) or shunting of cystic recurrences might be mandatory in some cases (2).

Chemotherapy has been widely used in the postoperative period as well as for treatment of recurrences during the last decade. Nitrosoureas, first of all BCNU and CCNU proved to be effective even in the form of monotherapy and they are essential components in the majority of polychemotherapeutic schedules (6, 12, 13, 15, 16, 18). Objective remissions and considerable survival times have been reported in 35—60 % of various recurrences, treated by different drug combinations (7, 8, 11). However, most papers deal with CNS tumours of very different histology and location, and the number of malignant supratentorial gliomas was relatively low.

We are now reporting our experiences obtained in the treatment of recurrent supratentorial gliomas only. In appropriate cases a reoperation had been performed first, and then followed by irradiation and chemotherapy as well. The other group of recurrences was treated by polychemotherapy with two different drug combinations.

Clinical Material and Methods

Since July, 1978 thirty patients with recurrent, supratentorial gliomas have been treated or are still under treatment with one of our protocols. In all cases clinically significant recurrence made some kind of repeated intervention necessary. The time elapsed from primary operation varied between 4 and 78 months, depending mostly on the histology of the tumour. Beside clinical progression, recurrent glioma was verified by angiography, isotope scintigraphy and recently by computed tomography (CT) as well. In all cases a histological diagnosis has been available by biopsy (Table 1).

According to the extension and location of recurrent tumours, reoperation had been performed in ten cases, removing as much of the tumour mass as possible (group 1). The primary histology was glioblastoma in four, low grade astrocytoma in five cases and oligodendroglioma in one patient. Glioblastomas remained unchanged at the second

Table 1. Number of cases according to different treatment schedules and response to therapy

Re-operation + radiotherapy and chemotherapy

	No. of cases	R	NR
Glioblastoma	4	3	1
Malignant glioma	6	6	–
Total	10	9	1

Chemotherapy with CCNU + PCB

	No. of cases	R	S	NR
Glioblastoma	3	2	1	–
Malignant glioma	3	2	1	–

Chemotherapy with BCNU + DBD

Glioblastoma	3	1	–	2
Malignant glioma	11	3	3	5
Total	20	8	5	7

R= responders; S = stable disease; NR= non-responders

histology, but all the other cases have shown malignant transformations up to glioblastoma. Prior to reoperation, only one of the glioblastoma patients was irradiated, but with an insufficient dose (3000 rads). After reoperation all patients have been irradiated with cobalt-60 equipment up to a total amount of 5000–5500 rads. After a six weeks interval we started with chemotherapy. On Day 1 110 mg/m^2 CCNU, on Days 15–29, 60 mg/m^2 Procarbazine (PCB) daily was administered orally. Such courses have been repeated after a rest of one month, up to 18 months or to severe deterioration of the patients. Each patient got 3–10 courses, on the average 6.2.

The second group of patients has been treated by chemotherapy only (group 2). Most patients had earlier been given a complete course of irradiation. The primary histology was glioblastoma in six, high grade astrocytoma in seven, low grade astrocytoma in four and oligodendroglioma in two cases. At the time of recurrence all tumours were classified as malignant, on the basis of the radiological investigations and clinical course.

Six patients have been treated with the same CCNU–PCB combination, as the reoperated recurrences.

In fourteen cases we used a combination of BCNU and Dibromodulcitol (DBD) chemotherapy. On Day 1 BCNU was given intravenously at a dosage of 170–200 mg/m^2 (average 191 mg/m^2). Subsequently DBD was administered beginning on Day 2, later every fifth day, altogether 7– times at a dosage of 200 mg/m^2. Each course took a month. After a rest of 4–6 weeks the course was repeated. Treatment has been continued for 18 months or up to the severe deterioration of the patient. Each patient received 2–9 courses, on the average 5.

138

Before treatment all patients had normal blood and platelet count and laboratory tests for renal and hepatic functions as well as blood sugar. Myelotoxicity and gastrointestinal (GI) toxicity were carefully monitored during the treatment period and dosage was reduced, if necessary. All patients were checked every two months by complete neurological examination. At 2–4 months intervals brain scan, CT and in some cases angiography were performed.

Corticosteroids (Dexamethasone) have not been used routinely during treatment. In some cases we gave Dexamethasone in daily doses of 10–20 mg at the beginning of treatment, but the maintenance dose never exceeded 1.5–3.0 mg/day.

Results

Because of the basically different treatment schedules, the two groups of patients had to be evaluated separately.

In group 1 the neurological symptoms and the degree of improvement were determined by the result of reoperation, in the first place. All subsequent treatments, such as irradiation and chemotherapy could mainly prevent an eventual regrowth. Accordingly, in these cases the survival time alone had to be taken for evaluation. In group 2, response to treatment was determined by the results of periodical neurological examinations and brain scan or CT, as compared to the results of preceding tests. "Response" was defined if improvement in the clinical status,was supported by evaluable regression or, at least, by no change in radiological tests. "Stable disease" meant no basic change at clinical and radiological control examinations. Only patients who were given a minimum of two courses of chemotherapy were evaluated. Those who rapidly deteriorated or died in the interval before the second treatment were classified as non-responders or failures.

Out of four glioblastoma patients one died shortly after the first course of chemotherapy. The others completed 3–9 courses after irradiation; their survival after reoperation reached 9–14–25 months, which proved to be longer than the time before the second surgical intervention. In the sub-group of malignant gliomas two patients died within 9 and 15 months of re-operation, but completed 3–5 courses of chemotherapy as well as irradiation. Four patients are alive now 15–33 months after reoperation (Fig. 1). The average survival time in reoperated cases was 16 and 24 months – depending on the primary histology.

Twenty patients were treated by chemotherapy only. With six patients we used a combination of CCNU and PCB therapy. Two of the three glioblastomas responded with clinical improvement and simultaneously, an objective regression of the tumour was demonstrated by radiological control. The disease remained stable in the third patient. Survival times from the beginning of treatment were 5–8–10 months. Three malignant gliomas treated by the same schedule showed a better response. Two of them are still alive after 26 and 29 months, and only one died with unchanged radiological findings five months after the start of treatment. The number of courses varied between two and ten (Fig. 2).

A combination of BCNU and DBD has been used in 14 patients. Seven died after the first course; they all had glioblastomas or high grade astrocytomas, either proven by hisology at the earlier operation or they had to be considered as such, according to radiological investigations at the time of recurrence. Out of the remaining cases we observed clinical improvement and objective regression in one glioblastoma and three malignant glioma patients. Three of them are at present alive after 5–16 months and one died after 21 months. Survival times of patients with stable disease were 5, 9 and 16 months, respectively.

Toxicity

No severe toxic side-effects have been observed during treatment with any kind of chemotherapy. None of the patients died because of drug toxicity and treatment had not be stopped in either case. The milder toxic complications were different in the two chemotherapeutic regimens. CCNU + PCB therapy caused only minor myelotoxicity which could be balanced by transitory drug reduction in some cases. On the other hand, nearly all patients complained of nausea and occasional vomiting, due mainly to PCB. In two cases PCB had to be stopped after 6–8 courses because of skin rashes. BCNU, given in intravenous infusion was followed in some cases by mild nausea. The orally administered DBD was always well tolerated. A transitory myelosuppression has been observed in all cases but WBC and platelet count became normal during the rest between courses. A dose reduction of 25% was necessary in one case after the third course.

Discussion

A comparison of the results of different treatment regimens is always difficult. This is usually due to the heterogenous histology of tumours treated and many individual factors such as the location and extension of tumours, the patients' condition at the beginning of treatment etc. Although, our thirty patients have been treated by different methods, they are perhaps more comparable, since all recurrences were with supratentorial gliomas with a proven histology.

In ten suitable cases of our present material we performed reoperation first, in order to remove as much tumour mass, as possible. After irradiation, treatment was continued with chemotherapy (CCNU + PCB). This combined treatment seemed to be more effective than our previous efforts. Regarding individual cases survival times were longer than before reoperation in all but two cases. On the other hand, survival times exceeded one year in 70%, and two years in 40% of cases. The small number of cases is not enough for statistical evaluation, but for the sake of comparison, we refer to our previous results with a larger number of reoperated low grade glioma recurrences where the corresponding percentages were 46% and 18.5% only (1). Taking into consideration that our present material consisted of primary glioblastomas as well, we have to consider this result as a promising possibility for treatment under similar conditions.

The majority of our cases was unsuitable for repeated operation, so that only chemotherapy has been used. Of the various chemotherapeutic combinations reported recently, the most frequently used drug had been PCB, beside nitroso-urea derivatives (8, 9, 11, 17). All these cytostatics are cyclus non-specific agents and proved to be effective in monotherapy as well (6, 7, 10, 18). Our fourth compound, DBD has been similarly regarded as an alkylating agent (4) and has had some effect against human gliomas in monotherapy (5).

Furthermore the combination of CCNU and PCB has been used for treatment of re-operated gliomas in six cases of inoperable recurrences. Recently, we changed to BCNU and DBD therapy in treating the same kind of regrowths, partly because of intolerance of some patients to PCB. The total response rate was 65%, with a mean survival time of 13 months, which is among the highest so far reported.

Our results are remarkable from several points of view. This supports the idea that a combination of cyclus non-specific agents, such as CCNU and PCB or BCNU and DBD could be more active against glioma recurrences, than the use of cyclus-specific drugs. Even using relatively strong myelotoxic drugs a careful selection of dosage and continuous monitoring of patients can prevent severe toxic side-effects.

In appropriate cases reoperation – through removal of a larger mass – can create a more favourable basis for further conservative treatment. With our material the longest survivals were achieved in the group of reoperated patients, particularly with originally low grade gliomas.

In both groups of cases – combined forms of treatment or chemotherapy only – we found a more favourable response with primary low grade gliomas. The poorest results was obtained with glioblastoma recurrences. This observation is consistent with other similar experiences (3), and therefore has to be taken into consideration in patients' selection as well as in the evaluation of the effects of drugs.

Conclusions

In appropriate cases of recurrent supratentorial gliomas reoperation should be performed first, in order to reduce the tumour mass. Reoperation followed by irradiation *and* chemotherapy resulted in longer survivals than reoperation alone or combined with irradiation. Combination of two cyclus non-specific agents seemed to be more effective against gliomas, than the use of cyclus-specific drugs.

Primary low grade gliomas responded better to either form of therapy, than high grade tumours. Each form of treatment might also be tried with glioblastomas, but a considerable lower response-rate could be generally expected.

References

1. Afra, D., Müller, W., Benoist, G., Schröder, R.: Supratentorial recurrences of gliomas. Results of reoperations on astrocytomas and oligodendrogliomas. Acta Neurochir. *43*, 217–227 (1978)
2. Afra, D., Norman, D., Levin, V.A.: Cyst in malignant gliomas. Identification by computerized tomography. J. Neurosurg. *53*, 821–825 (1980)
3. Bloom, H.J.G.: personal communication
4. Chiuten, D.F., Rozencweig, M., Von Hoff, D.D., Muggia, F.M.: Clinical trials with the hexitol derivatives in the U.S. Cancer *47*, 442–451 (1981)
5. Eckhardt, S. (ed.): Dibromducitol. Budapest: Medicina 1982
6. Fewer, D., Wilson, C.B., Boldrey, E.B., Enot, J.K.: Phase II study of 1-(2-chloroethyl)-3-cyclohexyl-1-nitrosourea (CCNU) NSC-79039 in the treatment of brain tumors. Cancer Chemother. Reports *56*, 421–427 (1972)

7. Fewer, D., Wilson, C.B., Levin, V.A.: Brain tumor chemotherapy. Springfield: Charles C. Thomas 1976
8. Gutin, Ph.H., Wilson, C.B., Kumar, A.R.V., Boldrey, E.B., Levin, V.A., Powell, M., Enot, K.J.: Phase II study of Procarbazine, CCNU and Vincristine combination chemotherapy in the treatment of malignant brain tumors Cancer 35, 1398–1404 (1975)
9. Jellinger, K., Kothbauer, P., Volc, D., Vollmer, R., Weiss, R.: Combination Chemotherapy (COMP Protocol) and radiotherapy of anaplastic supratentorial gliomas. Acta Neurochir. 51, 1–13 (1979)
10. Kumar, A.R.V., Renaudin, J., Wilson, C.B., Boldrey, E.B., Enot, K.J., Levin, V.A.: Procarbazine-hydrochloride in the treatment of brain tumors. Phase II study. J. Neurosurg. 40, 365–371 (1974)
11. Levin, V.A., Crafts, D.C., Wilson, C.B., Schultz, M.J., Boldrey, E.B., Enot, K.J., Pischer, T.L., Seager, M., Elashoff, R.M.: BCNU (NSC-409962) and Procarbazine (NSC-77213) treatment for malignant brain tumors. Cancer Treatm. Reports 60, 243–249 (1976)
12. Levin, V.A., Hoffman, W.F., Pischer, T.L., Seager, M.L., Boldrey, E.B., Wilson, C.B.: BCNU – 5-Fluorouracil combination therapy for recurrent malignant brain tumors. Cancer Treatment Reports 62, 2071–2076 (1978)
13. Levin, V.A., Wilson, C.B., Davis, R., Wara, W.M., Pischer, T.L., Irwin, L.: A Phase III comparison of BCNU, hydroxyurea, and radiation therapy to BCNU and radiation therapy for treatment of primary malignant gliomas. J. Neurosurg. 51, 526–532 (1979)
14. Poisson, M., Philippon, J., van Effentere, R.: Cerebral pseudocysts following chemotherapy of glioblastomas. Acta Neurochir. 39, 143–149 (1977)
15. Reagen, T.J., Bisel, H.F., Childs, D.S., Jr., Layton, D.D., Rhoton, A.L., Jr., Taylor, W.M.: Controlled study of CCNU and radiation therapy in malignant astrocytomas. J. Neurosurg. 44, 186–190 (1976)
16. Rosenblum, M.L., Reynolds, A.F., Smith, K.A., Rumack, B.H., Walker, M.D.: Chloroethyl-cyclo-hexyl-nitrosourea (CCNU) in the treatment of malignant brain tumors. J. Neurosurg. 39, 306–314 (1973)
17. Seiler, R.W., Greiner, R.H., Zimmermann, A., Markwalder, H.: Radiotherapy combined with Procarbazine, Bleomycin and CCNU in the treatment of high-grade supratentorial astrocytomas. J. Neurosurg. 48, 861–865 (1978)
18. Walker, M.D., Alexander, E., jr., Hunt, W.E., McCarthy, C.S., Mahaley, M.S., Jr., Mealey, J., Jr., Norrhell, H.A., Owens, G., Ransohoff, J., Wilson, C.B., Gehan, E.A., Strike, T.A.: Evaluation of BCNU and/or radiotherapy in the treatment of anaplastic gliomas. A cooperative trial. J. Neurosurg. 49, 333–343 (1978)

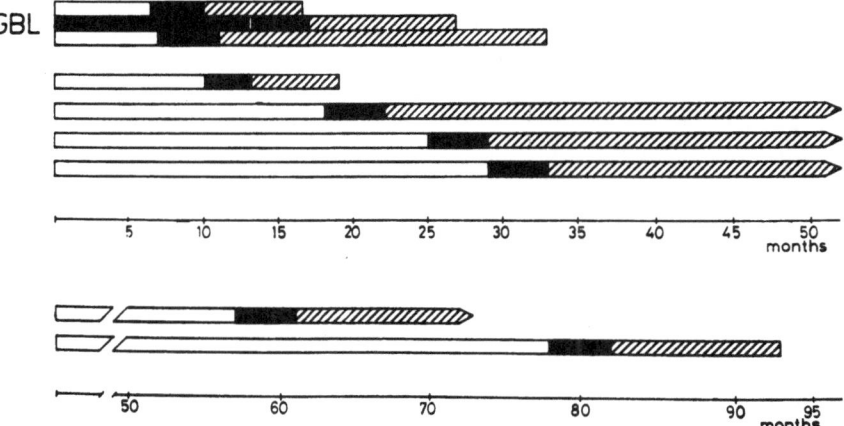

Fig. 1. Survivals of individual cases before and after reoperation and conservative treatment. *Open=* not irradiated; *black=* irradiated; *hatched=* chemotherapy; *arrow-shaped end of the file=* still alive; *GBL=* glioblastoma multiforme; *unmarked files=* lower grade gliomas

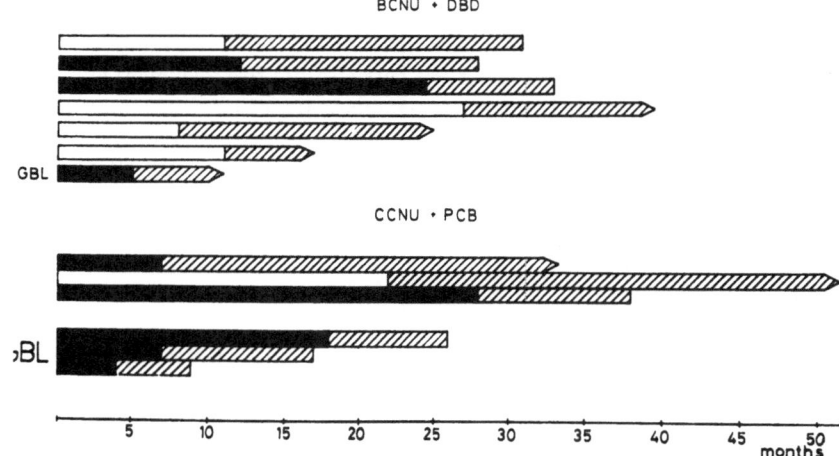

Fig. 2. Survivals of individual cases before and after chemotherapy. Abbreviations: see Fig. 1

Chemosensitivity Testing of Human Brain Tumours in Vitro *

M. Weizsäcker and M.L. Rosenblum

Introduction

A comparison of *in vitro* methods available to determine drug-induced cell lethality suggested that only clonogenic cell (colony formation) assays provide a reliable and dose-dependent index of cell kill (9). The development of monolayer and soft agar techniques for culturing human tumour cells has encouraged the use of this method (3, 7), but the small numbers of cells that can be obtained from a tumour biopsy and the intrinsic low colony forming efficiency (CFE) of these cells impart severe limitations on drug screening.

For an assay based on cells from biopsy specimens to be maximally useful, a large number of tumour cells that are representative of cells within the tumour must be available for chemosensitivity testing. Cells derived from five malignant glioma biopsy specimens were serially passed in culture to increase their CFE. We compared the response to BCNU of original and passaged cells. These results were compared to each patient's clinical response to 1,3-bis (2-chloroethyl)1-nitrosourea (BCNU) or 1-(2-chloroethyl)-3-cyclohexyl-1-nitrosourea (CCNU).

Materials and Methods

Tumour Cell Origin. Cells were dissociated from five tumour biopsy specimens (designated by numbers) histologically diagnosed as glioblastoma multiforme. However, tumour No. 160 demonstrated characteristics that suggest classification as an astroblastoma (L. Rubinstein, personal communication). All but one (biopsy No. 126) were taken from gliomas that had recurred after radiation therapy or chemotherapy.

Culture Procedures. The methods used to grow human brain tumor cells *in vitro* and to determine the CFE have been described (7). All CFE's were determined in Petri dishes to which 5×10^4 heavily x-irradiated (4000 rad) 9L rat brain tumour feeder cells were added.

* Supported by NCI Grant CA-13525, the Morris Stulsaft Foundation, and a grant from the Deutsche Forschungsgemeinschaft

Colonies grown from passaged cells of tumour No. 126 or 159 were picked from the bottom of Petri dishes with a sterile razor blade under an inverted microscope. Cells from these single colonies were grown on a 9L feeder cell layer.

Treatment with Chemotherapeutic Agents in Vitro. Single cell suspensions from tumour biopsy specimens were treated in spinner flasks at 37°C and pH 7.2–7.4 with graded concentrations of BCNU. After 2 hr of exposure, cells were washed with complete medium. Monolayer cultures derived from passaged cells of the tumour or from single colonies of these passaged cells were treated during the exponential phase of growth with similar doses of BCNU, after which cells were washed with medium and trypsinized. Passaged cells from tumour biopsy No. 126 were also treated with cis-platinum (Platinol, cis-platinum for injection, Bristol Laboratories, Syracuse, NY) for 1 hr and/or with dianhydrogalactitol (NSC No. 132313) for 2 hrs of exposure.

After treatment, cells were plated in Petri dishes, incubated at 37°C in a 5% CO_2 and 95% air atmosphere for 2–4 weeks, and stained with crystal violet. Twenty-five or more cells grouped together were counted as a colony. CFE's were determined for treated and untreated cells from 3–12 Petri dishes per test point. The surviving fraction (SF) of clonogenic tumour cells was defined as the ratio of the CFE of treated cells to the CFE of untreated cells. A response to BCNU *in vitro* was arbitrarily defined as SF ⟨ 0.5 (⟩ 50% cell kill) at the maximum clinically achievable tumour cell exposure dose of BCNU (2.5 μg/ml x 2 hrs or 8.5 μM; V.A. Levin, personal communication, 1980).

Clinical Data and Treatment of Tumours with Nitrosoureas. Age, sex, tumour location, and chemotherapy of given patients are summarized in Table 1. All patients were treated with a single iv dose of BCNU or a single oral dose of CCNU before evaluation. The *in situ* response of tumour therapy was assessed by UCSF criteria (5). *In situ* and *in vitro* tumour response were compared retrospectively.

Results

Effect of Culture Passage on the Colony Forming Efficiency. All CFE's of cells plated immediately after disaggregation from tumour biopsy specimens were smaller than 1% (Table 2). CFE's increased up to 1000-fold during the first five passages of all cell lines, reaching values over 10%.

Response to Chemotherapy in Vitro and Correlation to the in Situ Tumour Response. Tumour Biopsy No. 168. Survival curves for both original and cells passaged in culture demonstrated SF's of 1.21 and 0.85, respectively, at the maximum clinically achievable dose of BCNU; however, higher drug doses produced substantial cell kill (Fig. 1). The patient from whom the specimen was obtained had failed treatment with BCNU and CCNU before operation (Tables 1 and 3).

Tumour Biopsy No. 159. For both original and passed cells, cell kill at the maximum clinically achievable dose of BCNU was less than 50% (Fig. 2), but cell kill for both increased dramatically at higher drug doses.

Table 1. Clinical data for patients with glioblastoma multiforme from whom biopsy specimens were obtained for chemosensitivity studies

Tumour biopsy No.	Patient (years)	Tumour location	Nitrosourea therapy $(mg/m^2/dose)$
168	41 m	R parietal	BCNU (50); CCNU (100)
159	54 m	R parietal	BCNU (200); CCNU (100)
126	50 f	L frontal	BCNU (200)
167	50 f	L frontal	BCNU (200)
160	30 f	medulla	BCNU (180)

m= male; f= female

Table 2. *In vitro* plating efficiency (%) of original compared with passed human glioblastoma cells

Tumour biopsy No.	Original cells	Passage No. 1	2	3	4	5
168	0.163	–	–	13.97	–	–
159	0.101	2.08	–	–	2.70	–
126	0.149	–	1.67	16.23	–	17.02
167	0.009	–	–	–	–	7.66
160	0.008	–	–	14.20	–	–

Table 3. Correlation of the *in vitro* and *in situ* response to BCNU of human malignant gliomas

Tumour biopsy No.	*In vitro* response (SF at 2.5 $\mu g/ml$ x 2 h) Original cells	Passed cells	*In situ* response
168	1.21 (R)	0.85 (R)	R
159	0.54 (R)	1.07 (R)	R
126	0.03 [a] (S)	0.11 (S)	S
167	0.15 (S)	0.41 (S)	R
160	0.39 (S)	0.83 (R)	S

[a] BCNU dose: 4 *$\mu g/ml$ x 2 h*

Four "cloned" tumour lines could be derived from colonies of passaged cells from this tumour. All except clone 2 showed a similar pattern of sensitivity to BCNU when tested as exponentially growing monolayer cultures (Fig. 2). Cells of clone 2 were relatively resistant to BCNU at the high doses.

The tumour from which the biopsy was derived was "unchanged" after the first course of BCNU, but clearly failed with further therapy that included CCNU (Tables 1 and 3).

Tumour Biopsy No. 126: BCNU produced approximately 90% cell kill with both original and passaged cells; a further marked decrease in cell survival was noted with higher BCNU doses (Fig. 3). A clone derived from a colony of passage 3 of this tumour that was grown to monolayer culture showed almost the same pattern of response to BCNU (Fig. 3).

Passaged cells of this tumour were also treated with cis-platinum and dianhydrogalactitol. All drugs produced exponential-type survival curves. On a molar basis, dianhydrogalactitol was less cytotoxic than BCNU and cis-platinum, both of which were equally effective (Fig. 4).

In situ, the tumour responded to BCNU as predicted by the *in vitro* results (Tables 1 and 3). Chemotherapy and subsequently administered radiation therapy produced a 9-month progression-free interval after which the tumour recurred. Retreatment with BCNU could not halt tumour progression. At a second operation, a specimen was obtained from the recurrent tumour (designated No. 167). Surprisingly, original cells and cells passed in culture demonstrated more than 50% cell kill at the maximum clinically achievable dose of BCNU, despite the fact that the recurrent tumour was clinically resistant to BCNU (Table 3).

Tumour Biopsy No. 160: A difference between the sensitivity of original and passaged cells was found for this specimen. More than 50% cell kill could be achieved with the original cells, but less than 50% cell kill resulted from treatment of passaged cells at the maximum clinically achievable dose of BCNU (Table 3). However, the tumour from which the biopsy was derived responded to BCNU *in situ* (Tables 1 and 3).

Discussion

Only about half of patients harbouring recurrent gliomas respond to treatment with nitrosoureas (11). Nevertheless, drug toxicity to the bone marrow and the lungs may complicate alternative therapies. Therefore, preclinical tests of the chemosensitivity of human gliomas are urgently needed to predict response to chemotherapeutic agents *in situ.*

The chemosensitivity studies outlined have many potential problems; the assay employs enzymatic disaggregation, growth in medium supplemented with high concentrations of fetal bovine serum, and *in vitro* drug exposure. The monolayer cell cultures obtained may not be representative of the original tumour, and tumour cells may be contaminated by an overgrowth of non-tumour host cells.

The applicability of the colony formation assay is enhanced if the CFE of the tested cell population is relatively high: A variety of drugs can be tested, and the reproduceability of the results can be assessed. The CFE can be increased by using cells passaged in culture. However, it is important to show that the pattern of response to therapy is retained by tumour cells after a period of time in culture. The data presented here suggest that populations of malignant glioma cells are consistently responsive to BCNU, at least during early passages. Cells from other human tumours that were tested with different assays have shown similar results; the chemo- or radiosensitivities of a human melanoma or an ovarian carcinoma were the same when tested immediately after biopsy or after cryopreservation and several passages in agar diffusion chambers (10). Xenografted human tumours appear to retain the chemosensitivity of their original tumour type (6).

In these studies, *in situ* tumour response correlated with the *in vitro* response in four of five patients. These and previous studies (8) suggest that *in situ* tumour resistance can be predicted with more reliability than *in situ* tumour sensitivity. For instance, the tumour from which biopsy No. 167 was derived did not respond to BCNU *in situ,* but cells from the specimen responded to BCNU *in vitro.* Because at the time of recurrence this tumour showed large areas of low density on the CT scan, clinical failure may have been related to impaired drug delivery rather than to inherent cell resistance, which illustrates a major problem of predicting the *in situ* tumour response from *in vitro* data. The difference between the response of original and passaged cells of tumour biopsy No. 160 may have been caused by the overgrowth of a BCNU-resistant clone during passage.

Conclusion

Our criteria of *in vitro* tumour response (⟩ 50% cell kill) was chosen arbitrarily; the predictive value of this cell kill threshold must be substantiated by further clinical and experimental data. Because *in situ* tumour response is affected by changes in tumour size, assessed by radiographic and neurological examinations that have inherent errors (4), the correlation of *in vitro* and *in situ* results is even more difficult. Other systems to evaluate chemotherapeutic activity such as semi-solid agar techniques for studying stem cell survival (2) and *in vivo* methods to quantify changes in the size of human tumour implants placed under the renal capsule of rodents (1) should be developed to extend and validate our observations. However, the clinical usefulness of this stem cell assay for the individualization of patient treatment will depend on the development of more effective drugs for the treatment of malignant brain tumours.

References

1. Bogden, A., Kelton, D., Cobb, W., Esber, H.: A rapid screening method for testing chemotherapeutic agents against human tumor xenografts. In: Proceedings of the Symposium on the Use of Athymic (Nude) Mice in Cancer Research. Houchens, D.P., Ovejera, A.A. (eds), pp. 231–250. New York: Fischer 1978
2. Hamburger, A.W., Salmon, S.E.: Primary biopsy of human tumor stem cells. Science *197*, 461–463 (1977)
3. Hamburger, A.W., Salmon, S.E.: Primary bioassay of human myeloma stem cells. J. Clin. Invest. *60*, 846–854 (1977)

4. Hoffman, W.F., Levin, V.A., Wilson, C.B.: Evaluation of malignant glioma patients during the post-irradiation period. J. Neurosurg. *50*, 624–628 (1979)
5. Levin, V.A., Crafts, D.C., Norman, D.M., Hoffer, P.B., Spire, J.-P., Wilson, C.B.: Criteria for evaluating patients undergoing chemotherapy for malignant brain tumors. J. Neurosurg. *47*, 329–335 (1977)
6. Povlsen, C.E., Jacobsen, G.K.: Chemotherapy of a human malignant melanoma transplanted in the nude mouse. Cancer Res. *35*, 2790–2796, 1975
7. Rosenblum, M.L., Vasquez, D.A., Hoshino, T., Wilson, C.B.: Development of a clonogenic cell assay for human brain tumors. Cancer *41*, 2305–2314 (1978)
8. Rosenblum, M.L.: Chemosensitivity testing for human brain tumors. In: Cloning of human tumor stem cells. Salmon, S.E. (ed.), Alan Liss Co., New York, Chap. 20. Prog. Clin. Biol. Res. *48*, 259–276 (1980)
9. Roper, P.R., Drewinko, B.: Comparison of *in vitro* methods to determine drug induced cell lethality. Cancer Res. *36*, 2182–2188 (1976)
10. Selby, P.J., Steel, G.G.: Clonogenic cell survival in cryopreserved human tumor cells. Br. J. Cancer *43*, 143–148 (1981)
11. Wilson, C.B., Gutin, P.H., Boldrey, E.B., Crafts, D.C., Levin, V.A., Enot, K.J.: Single agent chemotherapy of brain tumors: A five-year review. Arch Neurol. *33*, 739–744 (1976)

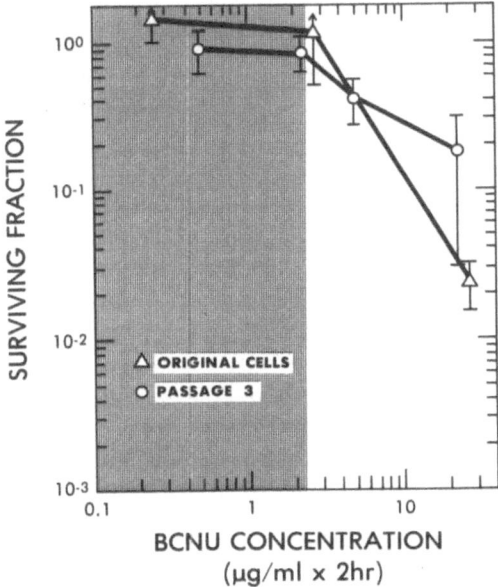

Fig. 1. Survival curves for original and passaged cells derived from tumour biopsy No. 168 after treatment with BCNU. The error bars represent standard deviations from the mean. The shaded area covers the clinically achievable dose range

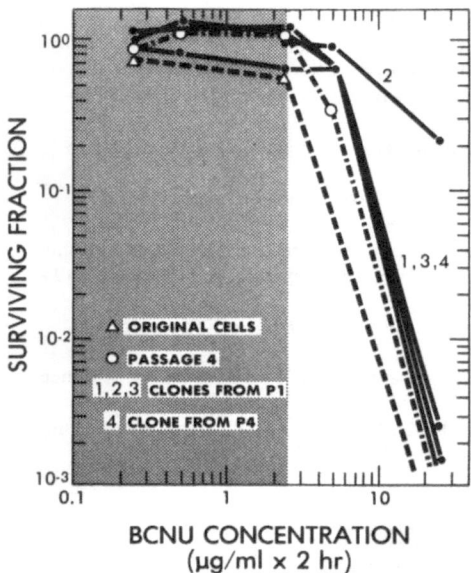

Fig. 2. Survival curves for original, passed, and cloned cells derived from tumour biopsy No. 159 after treatment with BCNU. The error bars represent standard deviations from the mean. The shaded area covers the clinically achievable dose range

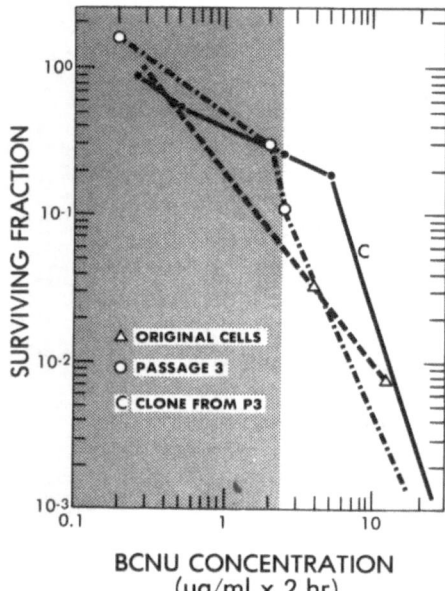

Fig. 3. Survival curves for original passaged, and cloned cells derived from tumour biopsy No. 126 after treatment with BCNU. The error bars represent standard deviations from the mean. The shaded area covers the clinically achievable dose range

150

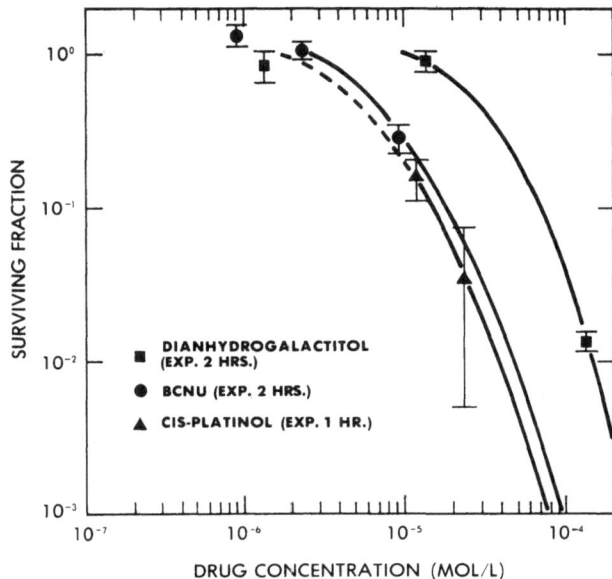

Fig. 4. Survival curves for passaged cells derived from tumour biopsy No. 126 after treatment with BCNU, cis-platinum, and dianhydrogalactitol. The error bars represent standard deviations from the mean

Hyperprolactinaemia: Results of Operation in Patients Selected on the Basis of Dynamic Endocrine Tests

G. Teasdale, J.A. Thomson, J.A. Ratcliffe, E.A. Cowden, D. McCruden, P. Macpherson, E. Teasdale, and D. Doyle

Introduction

In 1979 we suggested that dynamic endocrine tests would be useful in the detection of small prolactinomas, irrespective of radiological findings (1). Among our reasons for this approach were, first, the uncertainty about the significance of minor changes in the radiological appearances of the pituitary fossa, and second, the hope that optimum results would be obtained by an operation performed before a tumour had become large enough to produce a markedly abnormal fossa. Forty women thought to have an intrasellar prolactinoma, on the basis of abnormal prolactin dynamics, have now undergone trans-sphenoidal operation. We report the findings at operation and their relationship to the preoperative endocrine and radiological studies, and results of this method of management.

Patients Studied

The 40 patients underwent operation between July 1977 and December 1980. Thirty-seven patients had amenorrhoea and 22 had galactorrhoea; one patient had neither of these symptoms but was infertile. We have excluded from this review patients with evident extrasellar extensions who were treated in the same period. In this series, therefore, no patient had clinical or radiological signs of a suprasellar extension. After endocrinological studies had suggested a prolactinoma, each patient was given a detailed explanation of the advantages and disadvantages of the various methods of management. Each of these patients chose to undergo operation but, in the same period, several other patients opted for medical treatment.

Pre-Operative Endocrine Tests

After hyperprolactinaemia had been documented on several occasions, the effect of an intravenous injection of TRH (200 ug) and metoclopramide (10 mg) was determined (1). Anterior pituitary function was assessed by comined stimulation with insulin induced hypoglycaemia, TRH and GnRH.

Radiological Studies

The radiological techniques have been described by Teasdale et al. (7). All patients, in addition to plain skull films, had sagittal and coronal linear tomography (thickness of cut 0.27 cm). Twenty-five patients had unequivocally normal tomograms; two patients had borderline abnormalities, and only 13 patients had abnormal findings. In the latter group, the serum prolactin ranged between 620 and 7298 mU/L (mean 3,229 mU/L). Among patients with a normal pituitary fossa the serum prolactin ranged between 546 and 6204 mU/L (mean 1956 mU/L). Cavernous sinography was performed in each patient but abnormalities suggestive of pituitary expansion were seen in only seven patients, six of whom also had abnormal plain films or tomograms. Carotid angiography was performed in only one patient, in order to confirm the sinographic demonstration that one artery lay extremely close to the midline.

Operation

A unilateral, sub-labial, para-septal approach was used. The sella was inspected and its characteristics noted. The anterior wall of the fossa was removed, the dura diathermied and incised to display the gland as widely as possible. If the anterior surface of the pituitary was intact, the lateral surface of the gland was then mobilised, retracted medially and inspected or, if the exposure was limited by medially placed venous channels, the lateral surface was explored with a dissector and scoop. If this did not disclose a tumour, the gland was incised vertically in the midline and in the middle of each lateral lobe and horizontal extensions were made from each of these incisions. The size of any tumour cavity was estimated by comparison with 3mm or 5mm curettes. Unless there was only a small remnant of pituitary remaining, a 1mm layer of gland was removed from around the tumour cavity. Finally, the cavity was packed with patties soaked in absolute alcohol. If no tumour was discovered, biopsies were taken from the midline and from each lateral lobe.

Results

Operative Findings

In 35 patients there was a discrete tumour. Histological studies, including immunoperoxidase staining, confirmed in each case that the lesion was a prolactin producing adenoma, Per-operative smear biopsies were helpful in many cases in confirming the identification of tumour and normal tissue. In one of the remaining five patients there was a poorly demarcated region of softness and loss of the normal colour; the lesion was not identified as a tumour but histological studies showed intra-pituitary granulomata. In four patients there was no localised abnormality and histological studies of the pituitary biopsies showed only normal anterior pituitary features. In the other four patients we could not discover an abnormality, either at operation or on histological examination of the biopsies.

153

Relation of Operative Findings to Pre-Operative Endocrine and Radiological Studies

A tumour was found in each of the 13 patients whose tomograms had been clearly abnormal and in 22 of the patients with a normal fossa. The four patients with completely negative explorations, and the patient with a granulomata, each had a normal pituitary fossa. As a group the latter five patients had lower levels of prolactin than those with a tumour (Table 1). On the other hand, there was considerable overlap in the values of individual patients in all groups.

As previously reported (7), there was a close correlation between the radiologist's opinion of the pituitary fossa and the surgeon's findings. When the radiologist considered that the pituitary fossa was normal, the surgeon concurred in each case. Each of the 13 patients with a definitely abnormal tomogram had a tumour in an appropriate location. The average maximum diameter of the tumour in patients with an abnormal fossa (5.7 mm; range 3–10 mm) was slightly greater than in patients with normal tomograms (5.2 mm; range 2–10 mm) but the overlap was considerable.

Postoperative Endocrine Function

A week after operation the basal prolactin was measured and anterior pituitary reserve tested. Subsequent studies were performed three months later and at six month or yearly intervals, unless the patient was pregnant or declined for other reasons. Currently, the duration of follow-up varies between three months and four years (median 24 months).

Postoperative Basal Prolactin Levels in Patients with an Adenoma

When a tumour was found at operation, the basal serum prolactin concentration was normal (< 360mU/L) at three months or later follow-up, in 73% of patients. Surprisingly the presence or absence of tomographic abnormalities, did not influence the proportion of patients achieving normal values after operation (Table 2). Although the serum prolactin concentration and the estimated diameter of the tumour were, on average, greater in patients with post-operative hyperprolactinaemia, values in individual patients showed a wide range in the two groups (Table 3).

More important as a determinant of outcome of operation than its size, was the tumour's position in the gland. In 13 patients it was discovered when the gland was retracted medially, so that the tumour appeared to have eroded the surface of the lateral aspect of the gland. After operation only 46% of these patients had a normal basal serum prolactin concentration (Fig. 1). By contrast, normal prolactin concentrations were found in 91% of the remaining 22 patients, whose tumour was either on the anterior surface or enclosed within the gland (Fig. 1, Table 4). The poorer results with laterally placed tumours were not a reflection of tumour size. Sixty-one per cent of laterally eroding tumours were < 5mm in diameter, whereas 60% of tumours in other sites were between 5mm and 10mm in diameter.

154

Table 1. Relationship between tomographic and operative findings and pre-operative basal serum prolactin concentrations in 40 women with hyperprolactinaemia and impaired responses to TRH and metaclopramide

Tomograms	Operative findings	n	Basal prolactin mu/l	
			Mean	Range
Normal	No tumour	5	1639	706–3880
	Tumour	22	2027	540–6204
Abnormal	Tumour	13	3229	620–7298

Table 2. Relationship between tomographic and operative findings and post-operative serum prolactin (normal ⟨ 360mU/L)

Tomograms	Tumour at operation	Post-operative basal prolactin	
		Raised	Normal
Normal	No	3	2
Normal	Yes	6	16 (73%)
Abnormal	Yes	3	10 (77%)

Table 3. Pre-operative basal serum prolactin concentrations and tumour size in 35 patients found to have a tumour at operation; subdivided according to whether post-operative prolactin concentrations were normal (⟨ 360m U/L) or raised

	Post-operative prolactin	
	Normal (n= 26)	Raised (n= 9)
Basal PRL Pre-operation mean $\pm$ SE (range mU/L)	2176 $\pm$ 345 (546–6204)	3330 $\pm$ 637 (1581–7298)
Estimated maximum Diameter of tumour Mean (range mm)	5.2 (2–10)	6.1 (3–10)

Table 4. Relationship between position and size of tumour and outcome of operation in 35 patients with a microprolactinoma

Position of tumour	No. of patients	Tumour < 5 mm	Normal post-operative prolactin
Anterior or enclosed	22	9 (41%)	20 (91%)
Lateral surface	13	8 (62%)	6 (46%)

Patients Without a Tumour

The post-operative basal serum prolactin concentration was normal in the patient with a pituitary granuloma. In three of the four patients with negative explorations, the level did not change substantially, but in the remaining patient the serum prolactin concentration fell to normal immediately after operation, and it has remained normal over a follow-up of six months.

Anterior Pituitary Reserve

Clinically important changes in anterior pituitary function were rare. Two patients, both of whom had biochemical evidence of impaired growth hormone reserve before operation, now require cortisol replacement. Two other patients with a tumour, and two with negative explorations, have some biochemical evidence of reduced anterior pituitary reserve, but do not require replacement therapy. On the other hand, two patients who had biochemical evidence of reduced reserve (one growth hormone, one cortisol) before operation, have normal function post-operatively. No patient developed gonadotrophin deficiency as a consequence of the operation but several have impaired growth hormone reserve.

Fertility

Twenty-eight of 35 patients who were found to have a tumour have wished to become pregnant since the operation: 16 (64%) have conceived. These include three patients with post-operative levels that were still above the normal range, even though only one of these was taking bromocriptine at the time of conception. In addition, seven women who have not yet become pregnant, are ovulating, in each case without additional therapy. Thus, fertility was restored by the operation in 22 of the 28 women (75%). Seven of the women with a tumour have not yet attempted to become pregnant. The serum prolactin concentration is normal in all of these patients. Two of the women in whom no tumour was found, have also become pregnant. In one case this reflected the return of prolactin to normal after operation; in the other, bromocriptine treatment was used.

Complications

There were no persisting serious complications. One patient developed mild meningism one week after operation. Lumbar puncture showed an increased white cell count with a growth of penicillin resistant Staphylococcus aureus; treatment with cloxacillin resulted in rapid recovery. Pituitary function returned to normal and the patient became pregnant subsequently.

Discussion

The view that abnormal dynamic endocrine tests would be associated with high probability of finding a microprolactinoma, is supported by the present results. A tumour was found at trans-sphenoidal operation in 88% of 40 patients with an elevated prolactin level that showed little or no change in response to TRH or metaclopramide. By itself, the basal serum prolactin concentration was of limited value. The average level in the four patients whose pituitary appeared normal was lower than in those with a tumour but there was considerable overlap. Thus the lowest serum prolactin concentration (546 mU/L) was seen in a patient shown to have a tumour, and at the same time, 80% of patients with a tumour had basal serum prolactin concentrations below the value in one patient with a negative exploration (3880 mU/L).

The value of dynamic endocrine tests in the diagnosis of microprolactinomas has been questioned (5). It is important to scrutinise the criteria employed to assess responsiveness. In some patients with a tumour the serum prolactin concentration does increase in response to either TRH or metaclopramide. On the other hand, the magnitude of the increase, when expressed as a proportion of the basal serum prolactin concentration, is relatively small, and not the several fold rise that is seen in normal subjects or patients with functional hyperprolactinaemia (8). On the other hand, abnormal responses do not invariably predict the presence of an identifiable prolactinoma. The 10% of patients whose exploration was negative may in fact have harboured a minute microadenoma that we failed to recognise at operation. Without performing a total hypophysectomy, this possibility cannot be excluded and prolonged follow-up will be necessary to establish the truth.

Endocrinological tests were a more sensitive index of a prolactinoma than radiological investigations, but the latter were more specific. A tumour was found at operation in each patient in whom there was a distinct abnormality on either plain films or tomograms. It has been claimed, on the basis of autopsy material, that minor radiological abnormalities are not a reliable sign of the presence of a microadenoma (2). On the other hand, in the age range encountered in clinical practice, localised bulging with erosion, accurately predicted the presence of a tumour (7). Patients with abnormal tomograms tended to have a higher serum prolactin concentration and slightly larger tumours, but surprisingly, had no worse outcomes than patients with normal tomography and a tumour.

The major cause of persisting hyperprolactinaemia seemed to be local anatomical factors that precluded complete excision of the tumour. Infiltration into the dura is common in patients with pituitary adenomas (9). Only 37% of patients had a laterally placed tumour in contact with, and possibly infiltrating into, the dura of the cavernous sinus, but this group accounted for 78% of those whose prolactin remained high after operation.

The operation was followed by a high rate of restoration of fertility, judged by either the occurrence of pregnancy or the return of ovulatory menstrual cycles. This usually reflected return of prolactin to normal levels but two patients became pregnant without further therapy even though their prolactin levels remained slightly above the normal range.

Comparisons between the present results and those in other series can be made only with reservations about the consistency of criteria for diagnosis and for assessment of outcome. Schlechte et al. (6), in a recent review, found 'success' rates for surgical treatment of prolactin-secreting tumours ranging from 46% to 83%. They reported a return of menstruation in 66% of 30 patients with a microprolactinoma operated upon in their clinic. Fahlbusch (3) reviewed 111 patients with a microprolactinoma who underwent operation in either Milan, Munich or Paris and observed a normal serum prolactin concentration in 60% after operation. Hardy (4) found a microprolactinoma in 188 of 195 patients with a normal sized but usually asymmetrical fossa; and he reported that 77% of such patients had a normal prolactin concentration after operation, irrespective of the size of the tumour.

Exploration for a microprolactinoma, is technically demanding. Often the tumour is only 2–3 mm in its maximum diameter and difficult to expose because of overlapping intradural venous sinuses. It may lie in contact with, and infiltrate the walls of the cavernous sinus; injury to this tructure or its contents are a major hazard of trans-sphenoidal surgery. The long term results of the different methods of treatment have not yet been established. Until then, operative management may not be advisable as a routine particularly in patients with a normal fossa, but perhaps should be confined to centres in which special expertise in the endocrinology, radiology, pathology and surgery of hyperprolactinaemia, can be accumulated.

Summary

1. In 40 patients with amenorrhoea, galactorrhoea or infertility, and hyperprolactinaemia that was associated with little or no increase in response to TRH or metaclopramide, a microprolactinoma was found in 35 patients (88%) and in 81% of those whose tomograms were normal.
2. After operation, the basal serum prolactin concentration returned to normal in 75% of patients with a tumour, and in 70% of all patients. Although patients with a normal pituitary fossa had somewhat smaller tumours, this was not associated with an improvement in outcome.
3. Persisting hyperprolactinaemia was usually the consequence of surgically inaccessible infiltration of tumour into the dura of the medial wall of the cavernous sinus.

References

1. Cowden, E.A., Thomson, J.A., Doyle, D., Ratcliffe, J.G., Macpherson, P., Teasdale, G.: Tests of prolactin secretion in diagnosis of prolactinomas. Lancet I, 1155–1158 (1979)
2. Burrow, G.N., Wortzman, G., Rewcastle, N.B., Holgate, R., Kovacs, K.: Microadenoma of pituitary and abnormal sella tomograms in an unselected autopsy series. New Engl. J. Med (in press)
3. Fahlbusch, R.: Surgical failures in prolactinomas. In: Pituitary Adenomas, Biology, Physiopathology and Treatment. Derome, P.J., Jedynak, L.P., Peillon, F. (eds), pp. 273–284. Paris: Aesclepios
4. Hardy, J., Mohr, G.: Le prolactinome aspects chirurgicaux. Neurochirurgie 27, Suppl. 1, 41–60 (1981)
5. Lancet Editorial. Hyperprolactinaemia: pituitary tumour or not? Lancet I, 517–519 (1980)
6. Schlechte, J., Sherman, B., Halmi, N., Van Hilden, J., Chapler, F., Dolan, K., Granner, D., Duello, T., Harris, C.: Prolactin-secreting pituitary tumours in amenorrhoeic women: a comprehensive study. Endocrine Reviews 1, 295–308 (1981)
7. Teasdale, E., Macpherson, P., Teasdale, G.: The reliability of radiology in detecting prolactin-secreting pituitary microadenomas. Brit. J. Radiol. 54, 566–571 (1981)
8. Teasdale, G., Ratcliffe, J.G., Thomson, J.A., Cowden, E.A.: The prolactinoma problem. Lancet I, 925–926 (1980)
9. Wrightson, P.: Conservative removal of small pituitary tumours: is it justified by the pathological findings. J. Neurol. Neurosurg. Psychiat. 41, 283–289 (1978)

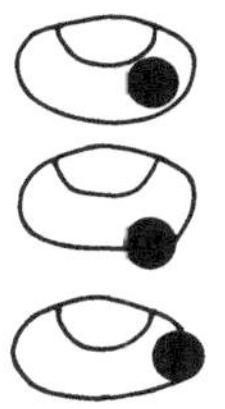

	Post-op. PRL	
	Normal	Raised
	16	2
	4	0
	6	7

Fig. 1. Position of tumour and result of operation

Immunohistochemical Classification of Pituitary Adenomas

A. Teramoto, T. Fukushima, K. Takakura, K. Sano, and R.Y. Osamura

Introduction

At the beginning of this century, Benda (1) and Erdheim (7) classified the anterior pituitary cells into eosinophilic, basophilic and chromophobic types according to the staining affinity of the cytoplasm. This classification was also applied to the pituitary adenomas, and for a long time it was considered to correlate with the endocrinological functions of adenomas. On the other hand, it was known that the classification could not always correspond to the hormonal functions; i.e., acromegaly or Cushing's disease were sometimes associated with chromophobe adenomas. Since the latter half of 1960, when the radioimmunoassay for anterior pituitary hormones was available, various kinds of functioning adenomas have been diagnosed endocrinologically. Moreover several cases of multihormonal adenomas were reported in the literature.

At present, pituitary adenomas are clinically classified by their functions, whereas pathologists still tend to separate them into classical entities. Thus, there exists a considerable gap between the clinical diagnosis and the pathological one. It is necessary to compose a new pathological classification of pituitary adenomas that reflects endocrinological features specifically. For this purpose the immunohistochemical techniques, such as immunoperoxidase method, are of great use.

We have studied the immunohistochemical characteristics of pituitary adenomas in 195 cases (22, 26–30). In order to establish the pathological classification of pituitary adenomas based on their functions, these cases were divided immunohistochemically into several groups.

Materials and Methods

The adenoma tissues were obtained by operation from a total of 195 cases, which were treated from 1976 to 1980. The tissue was fixed in 10% neutral formalin and embedded in paraffin. 4 μm sections were initially examined after haematoxylin and eosin (H–E) and PAS-orange G stainings for a general survey of the tissue.

Subsequently they were studied by Nakane's indirect peroxidase-labelled antibody method (18). The first step in the immunohistochemical staining was the incubation of the sections with rabbit antiserum to each of the human anterior pituitary hormones, such as anti-prolactin (1:500), anti-GH (1:1,000), anti ACTH (1:40) and anti-TSH (1: 500) (Ratio of dilution). All the antisera but anti-ACTH were supplied by NIAMDD.

 Modern Neurosurgery 1. Edited by M. Brock

The second step was the incubation with peroxidase-labelled goat anti-rabbit IgG (1: 40). After the immunologic incubation of each serum for 15 minutes and washing sections for 15 minutes in 0.01 M phosphate buffer, pH 7.6, the peroxidase reaction was done by 3,3'-diaminobenzidine 4 HCI (DAB) according to Graham and Karnovsky (8) for 4 minutes, the final concentration containing 20 mg DAB and 0.005% H_2O_2 in 100 ml Tris HCl buffer.

Double Staining Method (9). After the first immunostains, the tissue was incubated with 0.1 M glycine HCl, pH 2.2 for one hour. Then the antisera were removed from the section by elution, leaving the coloured reaction products. The second antigen was localized as stated above, using substrates that developed reaction products of different colours such as 4 Cl-1-Naphtol.

Mirror Section Technique. For the precise demonstration of the same cells in two consecutive paraffin sections, the method of mirror sections was used. The mirror sections were obtained by two consecutive sections mounted on the glass slides with the cut surfaces facing each other upward, so that the same surface of the sectioned cells could be stained by two different antibodies.

Results

The results of the observations on H-E and PAS-orange G stainings are summarized in Table 1. Prolactin (PRL) producing and non-functioning adenomas consisted of chromophobe ones for the most part. About three quarters of GH producing adenomas belonged to eosinophil or mixed eosinophil-chromophobe types. Basophil adenomas were found only in the cases of ACTH producing adenomas. On the other hand, both chromophobe and eosinophil adenomas were observed in all kinds of adenomas.

Immunohistochemically, 195 cases of pituitary adenoma were mainly classified into seven categories as shown in Table 2. Each of the PRL, GH and ACTH producing adenomas was subdivided into two types.

PRL Producing Adenomas (65 cases)
With immunostains, PRL producing adenomas could be separated into two types according to the proportions of PRL positive cells and the location of PRL in the cytoplasm.

a) Type I (55 cases) (Fig. 1 a,b). PRL was demonstrated in most tumour cells. Intracytoplasmic PRL was characteristically found as a small perinuclear mass. Clinically, the type I adenomas were found from microadenomas to large ones with suprasellar extensions. Serum PRL concentrations, ranged from 133 to 12,500 ng/ml, and increased significantly corresponding to the volume of the adenoma; i.e., mean serum PRL levels were 211 ng/ml in microadenomas, 1,509 ng/ml in small or intrasellar adenomas and 4,340 ng/ml in large adenomas. Statistical analysis revealed the significant correlation between serum PRL levels and the stages of tumour growth (R= 0.7979, P < 0.01).

b) Type II (10 cases) (Fig. 1 c,d). A few PRL positive cells were sparsely found in the type II adenomas. Intracytoplasmic PRL was demonstrated diffusely throughout the

161

Table 1. Conventional classification of 195 pituitary adenomas using haematoxylin and eosin and/or PAS orange G stainings

Function of adenoma \ Results of H-E stain	Chromophobe	Mixed	Eosinophilic	Basophilic	Total
PRL	58 (89)	2 (3)	5 (8)	0	65
G H + GH−PRL	18 (24)	30 (41)	26 (35)	0	74
ACTH + ACTH−PRL	11 (58)	0	2 (10)	6 (32)	19
TSH	2 (100)	0	0		2
Non-function	33 (94)	0	2 (6)	0	35
					195 cases
					(%)

Table 2. Immunohistochemical classification of 195 pituitary adenomas

Function of adenoma	Subdivisions in the immunohistochemical classification		No. of cases
PRL	Type I	55	
	Type II	10	65
G H	Diffuse type	26	
	Sporadic type	32	58
GH−PRL	−		16
ACTH	Diffuse type	7	
	Sporadic type	6	13
ACTH−PRL	−		6
TSH	−		2
Non-function	−		35
		Total	195

cytoplasm of each PRL positive cell, which resembled the non-tumourous PRL cells. Clinically, all of the type II adenomas showed moderate to large suprasellar extensions. Serum PRL levels were mildly elevated, ranging from 33 to 107 ng/ml (mean; 68.9 ng/ml).

GH Producing Adenomas (58 cases)
Immunohistochemically, GH producing adenomas were also divided into two groups according to the proportion of GH positive cells.

a) Diffuse Type (26 cases) (Fig. 2 a,b). GH cells, diffusely distributed, were the chief component of these adenomas, i.e., more than half of the adenoma cells were positive for GH.

b) Sporadic Type (32 cases) (Fig. 2 c,d). A few GH cells were found sporadically in this type of adenomas.

In either type of adenoma GH cells were round to polygonal in shape, with immuno-reactive GH throughout the cytoplasm. These findings were similar to those of GH cells in the anterior pituitary gland. Clinically, both types of adenoma were distributed from microadenomas to large tumours, although the former ones were associated with higher GH concentrations (mean; 164 ng/ml) than the latter (mean; 36 ng/ml). The difference of serum GH levels was statistically significant ($p < 0.01$); and was more prominent in the case of large adenomas.

GH-PRL Producing Adenomas (16 cases)

Sixteen cases among 74 GH producing adenomas (21.6%) were also positive for PRL. In an attempt to investigate the morphological relationship between GH and PRL cells, the double staining method was employed on the same section (Fig. 3a). Generally, each hormone was located in separate cells, while no definite rule existed as regards the number and location of the two kinds of cells.

In the next step, the mirror section technique was used for studying the possibility of dual hormone secretion by a single cell (Fig. 3b). In most instances the both hor-mones were demonstrated in separate cells as shown by the double stains, whereas a few cells were shown to contain both GH and PRL. In the double staining and mirror section methods, anti-GH and anti-PRL sera were absorbed with PRL and GH (5–10 μg/ml) respectively to avoid the effect of cross-reactivities.

Clinically, these adenomas were found from microadenomas to large ones. They were associated with acromegaly and occasionally with galactorrhoea.

ACTH Producing Adenomas (13 cases)

With immunostains, ACTH producing adenomas were subdivided into diffuse and spo-radic types.

a) Diffuse Type (7 cases) (Fig. 4a). Most adenoma cells showed the presence of ACTH. Usually, intracytoplasmic ACTH was demonstrated as granules throughout the cyto-plasm.

b) Sporadic Type (6 cases) (Fig. 4c). ACTH cells were demonstrated sporadically. Intra-cytoplasmic ACTH was distributed diffusely in the cytoplasm, while in some adenoma cells it was situated along the cell membrane. These adenomas sometimes contained a few small foci of ACTH cells which resembled those of the diffuse type.

Clinically, most of the adenomas associated with Cushing's disease belonged to the former type, while those with Nelson's syndromewere apt to be of the latter type.

ACTH-PRL Producing Adenomas (6 cases)

Six cases out of 19 ACTH producing adenomas (31.5%) were also positive for PRL. In every case ACTH cells were far more frequent than PRL cells, while no specific re-lation between two cell types could be found. With double staining and mirror section techniques, both hormones were demonstrated in separate cells. Clinically, ACTH-PRL producing adenomas were associated with Cushing's disease or Nelson's syndrome, and sometimes with galactorrhoea.

TSH Producing Adenomas (2 cases) (Fig. 4d)
By conventional stainings, these adenomas were chromophobe ones. With immunostains, many adenoma cells were positive for TSHβ. Both patients showed clinical and biochemical evidences of hyperthyroidism associated with mild elevation of serum TSH levels.

Non-Functioning Adenomas (35 cases)
As a rule, tumour cells were negative for every anterior pituitary hormone. However, a very few cells were sometimes positive for PRL, ACTH, or LH. Their clinical significance has yet to be elucidated.

Discussion

Though the conventional classification of pituitary adenomas roughly correlates with the endocrinological functions, it fails to provide the specificity for each of the anterior pituitary hormones. Hence the core of morphological studies on pituitary adenomas has been based on electronmicroscopy or immunohistochemistry. Horvath and Kovacs (12, 14) classified a large series of adenomas mainly from the ultrastructural findings and referred to some immunohistochemical observations. However, ultrastructural identification of cell types on purely morphological ground is hazardous at best; and in the case of any given cell, may be impossible (6). On the other hand, the immunohistochemistry has been used merely as a method to demonstrate the presence of hormones. Thus this may be the first report on the immunohistochemical classification of pituitary adenomas in a large series.

PRL producing adenomas were divided immunohistochemically into two types. The type I adenomas are more common and account for 84.6% of PRL producing adenomas. Since these tumours consist entirely of PRL cells and are distributed in every stage of tumour growth, they are regarded as the primary PRL producing adenomas. With electronmicroscopy, they are categorized as sparsely granulated cell adenomas (12), which are characterized by a few secretory granules with misplaced exocytosis, prominent Golgi apparatus and well-developed rough endoplasmic reticulum (ER) (22). With the use of immunoelectronmicroscopy, the authors demonstrated the presence of PRL in the cistern of the Golgi apparatus and rough ER (28, 30), which corresponds to "the perinuclear mass" seen in light microscopy. In the type II adenomas, PRL cells, the lesser component of the adenoma, show a close resemblance to those of the anterior pituitary gland. The type II adenomas cannot always be grouped with the densely granulated cell adenomas described by Horvath and Kovacs (12), since densely granulated cells in our cases are very scarce. Clinically, all of the type II adenomas showed marked suprasellar extensions, while serum PRL levels were mildly elevated as compared with the tumour volume. Hence it is suggested that the interruption of PRL inhibizing factors, caused by the damage to the pituitary stalk and/or hypothalamus, might activate the PRL secretion in originally non-functioning adenomas. For the present the type II adenoma has not been found in the smaller tumours.

GH producing adenomas were also divided into two types. GH cells of both types showed similar findings to those of non-tumorous GH cells. Since immunoreactive GH has been demonstrated on the secretory granules (30), GH positive cells in the light microscopy correspond to the densely granulated cells. Consequently, each of the immunohsitochemical types can be consistent with densely and sparsely granulated cell adenomas respectively. Clinically, both types are distributed from microadenomas to large ones. Though adenomas of the diffuse type are usually associated with higher serum GH levels than those of the sporadic type, exceptional cases are not rare especially in the micro- or small adenomas. Thus, it is assumed that a transitional or mixed type may exist.

It is known that 20-30% of acromegalic patients are associated with mild hyperprolactinaemia. Since such cases are found even in the stages of microadenomas, the aetiology of hyperprolactinaemia can be attributed to the adenoma itself. It has long been discussed, whether these two hormones are derived from a single cell (16), or from separate cells (2, 9, 10, 14, 34). Against the classical one cell-one hormone theory some examples of multihormonal cells are known, such as FSH-LH cells in the human pituitary gland (20) and GH-PRL cells in the rat pituitary adenoma (23, 25, 32). Several investigators, using the doubel staining method, have reported the simultaneous presence of two hormones. However, the technique is not adequate for this purpose, for the multihormonal cell does not always show the neutral tint between the colours of the two substates (28—30). In this study the mirror section technique revealed that a few cells could secrete both GH and PRL, although the respective hormones were usually present in separate cells.

It has been reported that adenomas associated with Nelson's syndrome are aetiologically similar to those of Cushing's disease. Landolt (16) stated that there was no basic difference in the ultrastructure of adenomas of the two syndromes. Immunohistochemically, ACTH producing adenomas were divided into diffuse and sporadic types, which corresponded mostly to the adenomas of Cushing's disease and Nelson's syndrome, respectively. Some transitional types can be observed; small foci of ACTH cells like those of the diffuse type are scattered in the adenomas of the sporadic type. Adenomas with Cushing's disease are generally assocatiated with a mild elevation of serum ACTH levels in spite of a higher proportion of ACTH cells. It may result from the poor autonomy of these adenomas. For example, Crooke's degeneration is found not only in the non-tumorous pituitary gland, but even in the adenoma itself (28, 30). It suggests that these adenoma cells are subject to the influence of the negative feedback system.

Authors have reported the presence of ACTH-PRL producing adenomas similar to GH-PRL producing adenomas, in which the respective hormones were detected in the separate cells. A lot of combinations in multihormonal adenomas were described in the literature; i.e., PRL and gonadotropin (3), PRL and TSH (5, 11, 31), GH and TSH (13), et al. (17, 24). Further study is required to assess the genesis and the clinical features of these multihormone producing adenomas.

Recently several cases of TSH producing adenomas have been reported (21, 31), although they are still rare. These adenomas are classified into two categories; primary TSH producing adenomas and those associated with long-standing hypothyroidism. Both of our cases belong to the former type. They were chromophobe by conventional stainings, while numerous adenoma cells were positive for TSHβ with immunostains.

The latter adenomas are regarded as a kind of hyperplasia of TSH cells and even of PRL cells. Similar genesis of pituitary adenomas is known in the cases of long-standing hypogonadism (4, 15, 33).

As a rule, non-functioning adenomas were negative for all of the anterior pituitary hormones, while a very few cells, one or two cells in a low power field of light microscopy, sometimes showed positive stainings for PRL, ACTH or LH. Although they should have originated from the adenoma itself, their clinical or pathological significances are not known.

Conclusion

In order to establish the pathological classification of pituitary adenomas, based on their endocrinological functions, 195 cases were studied by peroxidase-labelled antibody method. These adenomas were classified into seven groups; namely:
1. PRL,
2. GH,
3. GH-PRL,
4. ACTH,
5. ACTH-PRL,
6. TSH producing adenomas,
7. non-functioning adenomas.

According to the immunohistochemical findings, PRL, GH and ACTH producing adenomas were further separated into the subdivisions. The immunohistochemical classification revealed the specific correlation with the endocrinological functions.

References

1. Benda, C.: Beiträge zur normalen und pathologischen Histologie der menschlichen Hypophysis cerebri. Berl. Klin. Wochenschr. 36, 1205–1210 (1900)
2. Corenblum, B., Sirek, A.M.T., Hovath, E. et al.: Human mixed somatotrophic and lactotrophic pituitary adenoma. J. Clin. Endocrinol. Metab. 42, 857–863 (1976)
3. Cunningham, G.R., Huckins, C.: An FSH and prolactin-secreting pituitary tumor; pituitary dynamics and testicular histology. J. Clin. Endocrinol. Metab. 44, 248–253 (1977)
4. Danziger, J., Wallance, S., Handel, S. et al.: The sella turcica in primary end organ failure. Neuroradiol. 131, 111–115 (1979)
5. Duello, T.M., Halmi, N.S.: Pituitary adenoma producing thyrotropin and prolaction. An immunocytochemical and electron microscopic study. Virchows Archiv. A Path. Anat. Histol. 376, 255–265 (1977)
6. Duello, T.M., Halmi, N.S.: Ultrastructural-immunocytochemical localization of growth hormone and prolactin in human pituitaries. J. Clin. Endocrinol. Metab. 49, 189–196 (1979)
7. Erdheim, J.: Zur normalen und pathologischen Histologie der Glandula thyreoidea, parathyroidea und Hypophysis. Beitr. Pathol. Anat. 33, 158–236 (1903)
8. Graham, R.C., Karnovsky, M.J.: The early stages of absorption of injected horseradish peroxidase in the proximal tubules of mouse kidney. Ultrastructural cytochemistry by a new technique. J. Histochem, Cytochem. 14, 291 (1966)
9. Guyda, H., Robert, F., Colle, E. et al.: Histologic, ultrastructural, and hormonal characterization of a pituitary tumor secreting both hGH and prolactin. J. Clin. Endocrinol. Metab. 36, 531–547 (1973)

10. Halmi, N.S., Duello, T.: "Acidophilic" pituitary tumors. A reappraisal with differential staining and immunocytochemical techniques. Arch. Pathol. Lab. Med. *100*, 346–351 (1976)
11. Horn, K., Erhardt, F., Fahlbusch, R. et al.: Recurrent goiter, hyperthyroidism, galactorrhea and amenorrhea due to a thyrotropin and prolactin-producing pituitary tumor. J. Clin. Endocrinol. Metab. *43*, 137–143 (1976)
12. Horvath, E., Kovacs, K.: Ultrastructural classification of pituitary adenomas. Can. J. Neurol. Sci. *3*, 9–21 (1976)
13. Kourides, I.A., Ridgway, E.C., Weintraub, B.D. et al.: Thyrotropin-induced hyperthyroidism: use of alpha and beta subunit levels to identify patients with pituitary tumors. J. Clin. Endocrinol. Metab. *45*, 534–543 (1977)
14. Kovacs, K., Horvath, E.: Pituitary adenomas. Pathologic aspect. In: Clinical Neuroendocrinology: A Pathophysiological Approach. Tolis, G. et al. (eds.), pp. 367–384. New York: Raven Press 1979
15. Kovacs, K., Horvath, E., Rewcastle, N.B. et al.: Gonadotroph cell adenoma of the pituitary in a woman with long-standing hypogonadism. Arch. Gynecol. *229*, 57–65 (1980)
16. Landolt, A.M.: Ultrastructure of human sella tumors: Correlations of clinical findings and morphology. Acta Neurochir. Wien (Suppl.) *22*, 1–167 (1975)
17. Müller, O.A., von Werder, K., Scriba, P.C.: Hypersecretion of ACTH, growth hormone and prolactin in a patient with pituitary adenoma. Acta Endocrinol. Kbh. (Suppl. 215) *87*, 4–5 (1978)
18. Nakane, P.K., Pierce, G.B.: Enzyme-labeled antibodies: Preparation and application for the localization of antigens. J. Histochem. Cytochem. *14*, 929–931 (1966)
19. Nakane, P.K.: Simultaneous localization of multiple tissue antigens using the peroxidase-labelled antibody method. A study on pituitary gland of the rat. J. Histochem. Cytochem. *16*, 557–560 (1968)
20. Nakane, P.K.: Classification of anterior pituitary cell types with immunoenzyme histochemistry. J. Histochem. Cytochem. *18*, 9–20 (1970)
21. Nesbakken, R., Aanderud, S.: TSH-secreting pituitary adenomas – more frequent than hitherto recognized ? Abstracts of 32nd Annual Meeting of the Scandinavian Neurological Society (Linköping) 20–21 (1980)
22. Osamura, R.Y., Watanabe, K., Teramoto, A. et al.: Male prolactin secreting pituitary adenomas in humans studied by peroxidase-labeled antibody method. Acta Endocrinol. *88*, 643–652 (1978)
23. Richardson, U.I.: Establishment in culture of a multihormone-secreting cell strain derived from the MtT/F4 rat pituitary tumor. J. Cell Physiol. *88*, 287–296 (1976)
24. Scanarini, M., Mingrino, S.: Pituitary adenomas secreting more than two hormones. Acta Neuropathol. Berl. *48*, 67–72 (1979)
25. Tashijian, A.H., Jr., Bancroft, F.C., Levine, L.: Production of both prolactin and growth hormone by clonal strains of rat pituitary tumor cells: differential effects of hydrocrotisone and tissue extracts. J. Cell. Biol. *47*, 61 (1970)
26. Teramoto, A., Matsutani, M., Hirakawa, K. et al.: Immunohistochemical observations of the pituitary adenomas with the use of enzyme-labelled antibody method. On the cases with hyperprolactinemia. Neurol. Med. Chir. Tokyo *18*, 207–214 (1978)
27. Teramoto, A., Sano, K., Osamura, R.Y. et al.: Immunohistochemical observations of the pituitary adenomas with the use of enzyme-labelled antibody method. On the residual pituitary gland and "capsule" of the adenoma. Neurol. Med. Chir. Tokyo *19*, 895–902 (1979)
28. Teramoto, A., Sano, K.: Immunohistochemical studies on functioning pituitary adenomas. Abstracts of 32nd Annual Meeting of the Scandinavian Neurosurgical Society (Linköping) 22–23 (1980)
29. Teramoto, A.: Immunohistochemical studies on the functioning pituitary adenomas. Brain Nerve *32*, 1163–1174 (1980)
30. Teramoto, A.: Pathology of functioning pituitary adenomas with emphasis on the immunohistochemical classification. Brain Nerve *33*, 479–488 (1981)
31. Tolis, G., Bird, C., Bertrand, G. et al.: Pituitary hyperthyroidism. Case report and review of the literature. Am. J. Med. *64*, 177–181 (1978)

32. Ueda, G., Moy, P., Furth, J.: Multihormonal activities of normal and neoplastic pituitary cells as indicated by immunohistochemical staining. Int. J. Cancer *12*, 100–114 (1973)
33. Woolf, P.D., Schenk, E.A.: An FSH-producing tumor in a patient with hypogonadism. J. Clin. Endocrinol. *38*, 561 (1974)
34. Zimmerman, E.A., Defendini, R., Franz, A.G.: Prolactin and growth hormone in patients with pituitary adenomas. A correlative study of hormone in tumor and plasma by immunoperoxidase technique and radioimmunoassay. J. Clin. Endocrinol. Metab. *38*, 577–584 (1974)

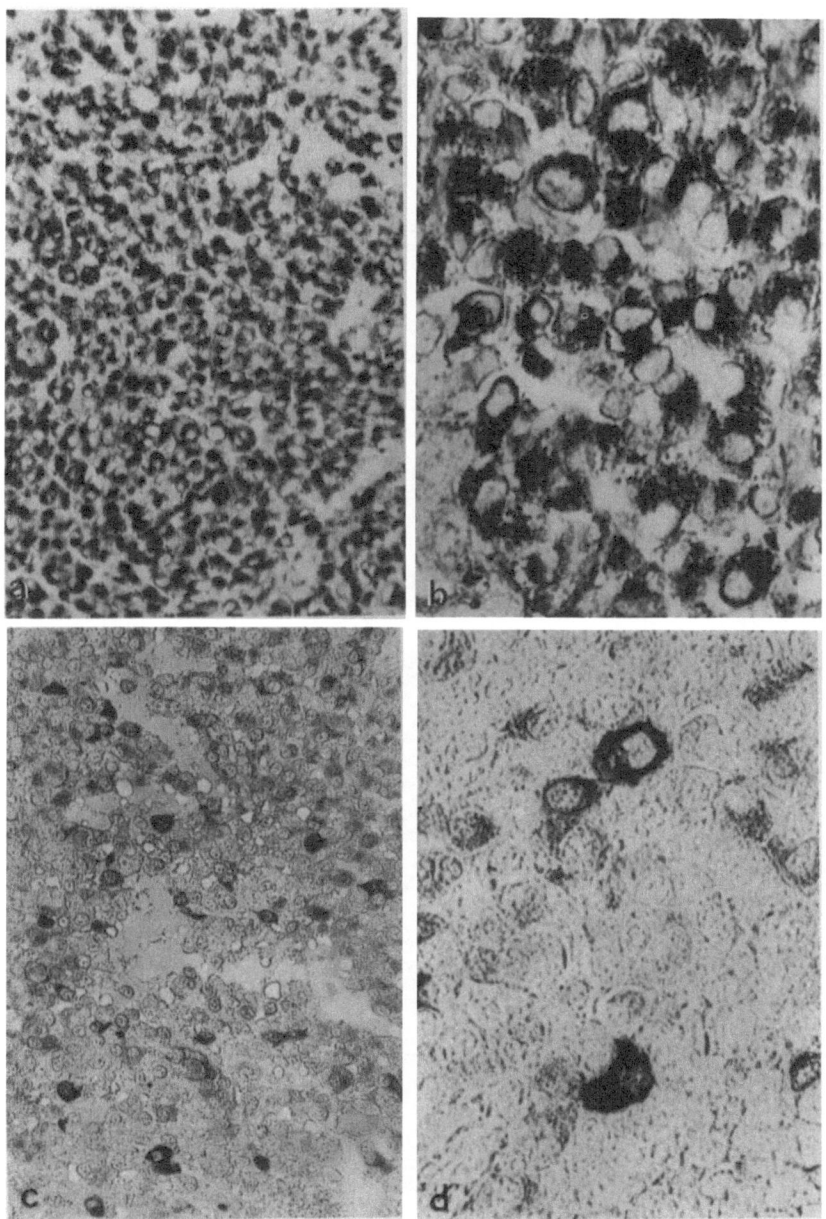

Fig. 1 a-d. PRL-producing adenoma. **a, b** Type I; **c, d** Type II.
a Most adenoma cells are positive for PRL. **b** Intracytoplasmic PRL is seen as a small perinuclear mass. **c** A few PRL cells are scattered in the adenoma. **d** Intracytoplamic PRL is distributed throughout the cytoplasm. Immunostains for PRL (**a, c** x100; **b, d** x 200)

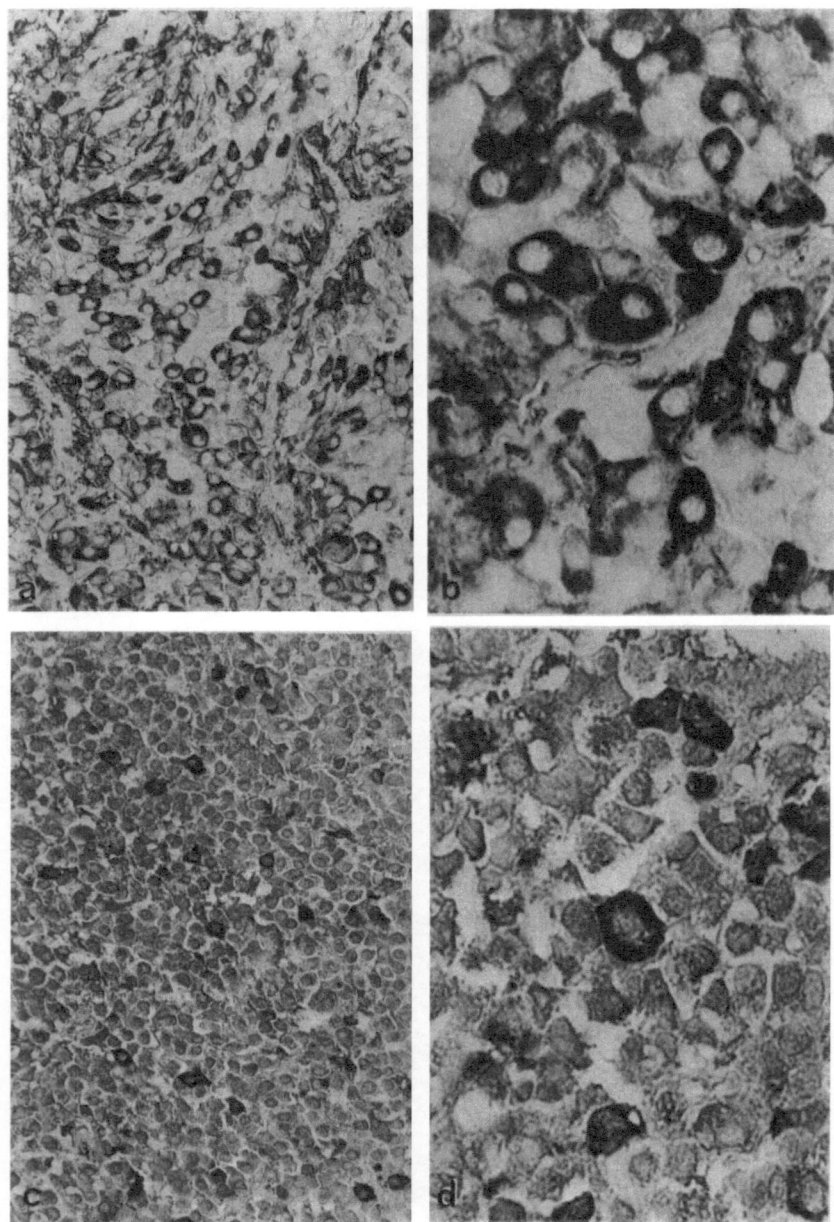

Fig. 2 a-d. GH producing adenoma. **a, b** diffuse type; **c, d** sporadic type. **a** GH cells, diffusely distributed, are the chief component of the adenoma. **b** Each adenoma cell contains GH throughout its cytoplasm. Reaction products are somewhat prominent at the periphery in some cells. **c** A few GH cells are found sporadically in the adenoma. **d** The distribution of intracytoplasmic GH is similar to that of the diffuse type. Immunostains for GH (a, c x100; b, d x200)

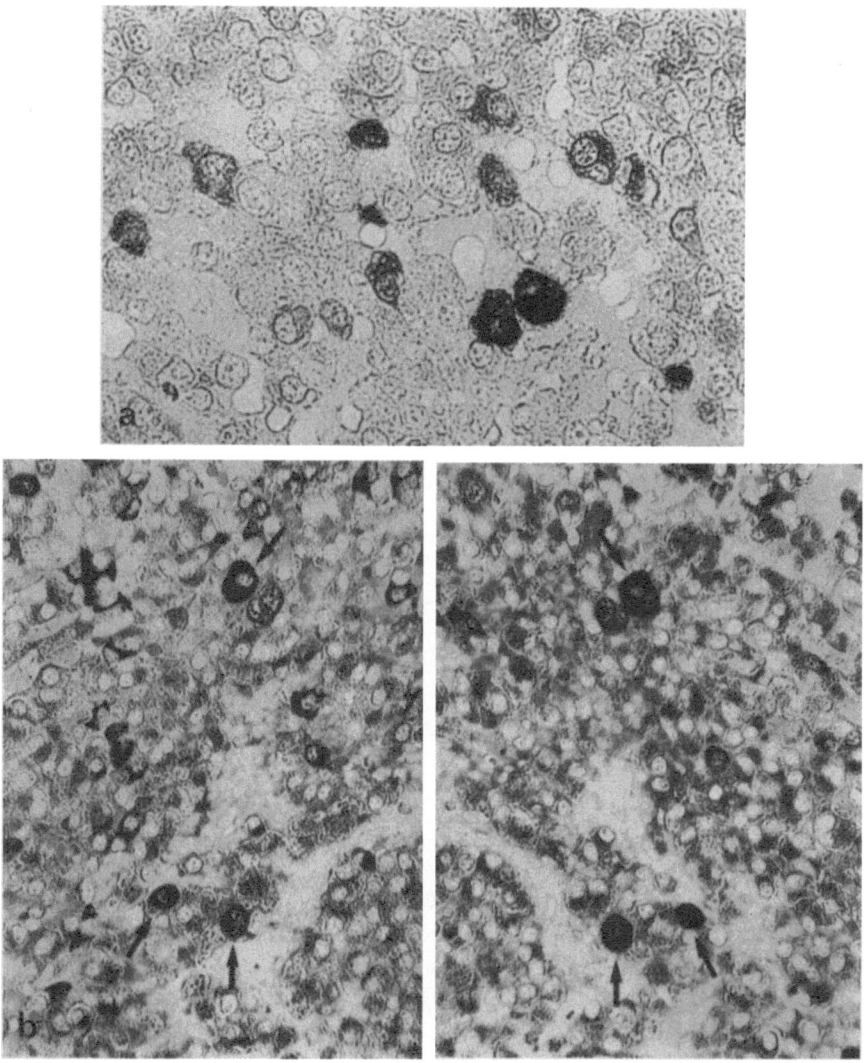

Fig. 3 a,b. GH-PRL producing adenoma. **a** Double staining for GH and PRL. Both hormones are usually demonstrated in separate cells. In this photograph, GH cells are dark ones, while PRL cells are light (x200). **b** Mirror section technique for GH (*right*) and PRL (*left*).Both hormones are found simultaneously in a few adenoma cells (*arrows*) (x200)

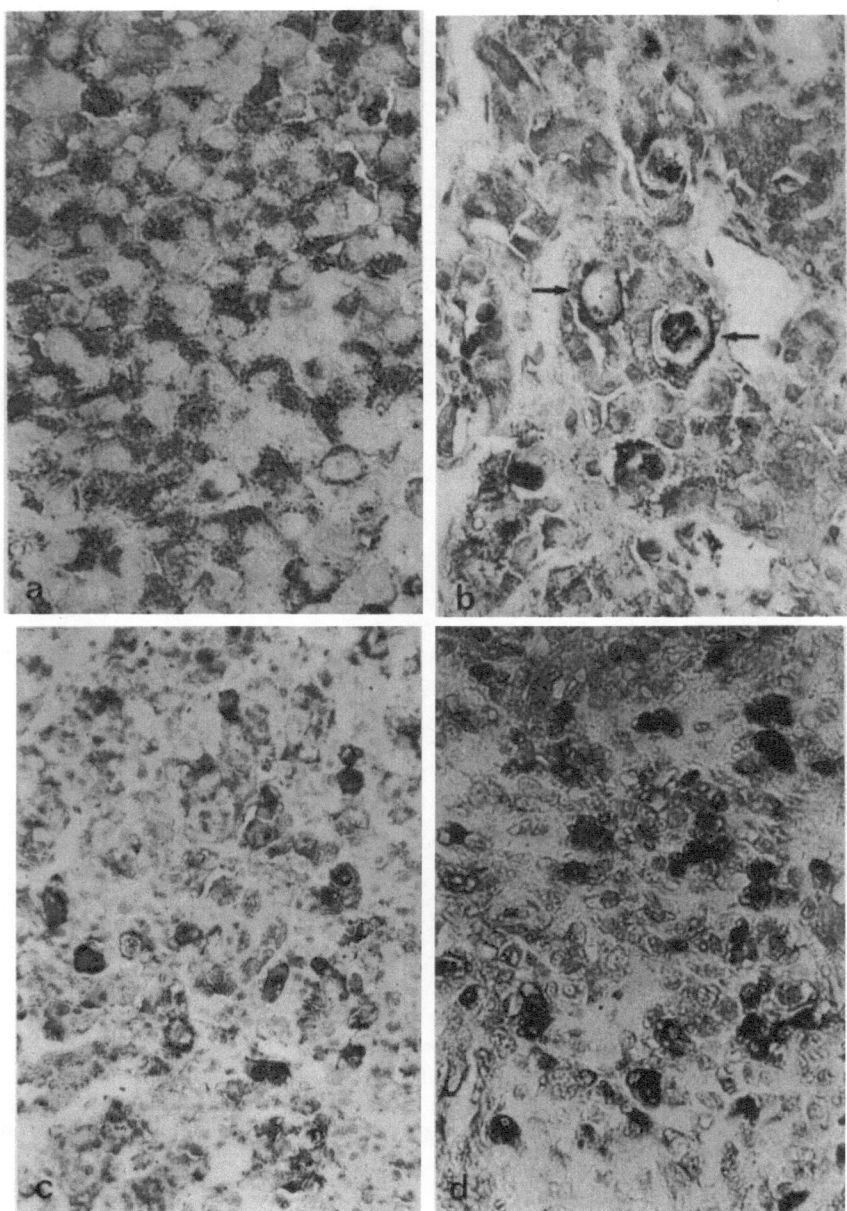

Fig. 4 a-c. ACTH producing adenoma. d TSH producing adenoma. a Diffuse type. ACTH is demonstrated as granules throughout the cytoplasm of most adenoma cells. b Crooke's cells in the non-tumourous pituitary gland of Cushing's disease. A small amount of ACTH is located near the nucleus or at the periphery in these cells (*arrows*). c Sporadic type. ACTH cells are scattered in the adenoma. Intracytoplasmic ACTH is distributed diffusely, whereas it is located at the periphery in some adenoma cells. d TSH producing adenomas. Many adenoma cells are positive for TSHβ. Immunostains for ACTH (a-c) and TSHβ (d) (x200)

Fifteen Years Experience with Transnasal Trans-Sphenoidal Operation for Pituitary Tumours

R.W. Rand

Introduction

Although Koenig in 1898 developed a bucco-nasal transnasal approach to the pituitary gland, operations using a superior nasal approach became more popular. For example, the Giordano superior nasal approach as modified by Schloffer in 1907 was used successfully in patients (10, 12). Moszkowicz (20) also modiefied Schloffer's operation by doing the procedure in two stages, trying to reduce the infection rate by making the entry into the sphenoid sinus at a second stage. A year later, Borchard used Schloffer's technique successfully in a patient. Hochenegg also described a superior nasal approach which Cushing used in three cases (9, 10). The operative mortality was reported to be 25–38% with these techniques due to uncontrolled infections.

Chiari (6) in 1912 proposed the transethmoidal approach to the sphenoid sinus in order to reach the floor of the sella turcica more directly. This was accomplished by a small incision about the inner border of the orbit and resection of the ethmoid sinuses. Kanavel in 1909 (17, 18) developed the inferior nasal approach to allow entry to the sphenoid sinus and the floor of the sella turcica. Success in patients followed. However, the mortality with this technique was 21%.

Hirsch (13) then introduced in the same year a two-stage operation utilizing a single nostril entrance and nasal septum resection under local anaesthesia and reported a successfully treated case. The procedure was modified so that it came more to the midline and an additional series of patients was operated upon (25). In 1926 100 cases were reported by this technique with the lower mortality of 12% (14). A sublabial approach was introduced by Halsted (10) in 1910 under the upper lip. The nasal septum was moved upward and laterally. The lower turbinates, vomer and perpendicular plates of the ethmoid were removed and the sphenoid sinus was entered successfully in two cases.

Cushing (9) combined this inferior nasal approach leaving the septum intact and removed the anterior wall of the sphenoid sinus in order to obtain entrance to the sella turcica. The high infection rate and the limited field of operative exposure as well as the substantial mortality led generally to the discontinuance of both the superior and inferior nasal approaches. Some surgeons including Cushing, however, did continue to use these procedures as an alternative to intracranial operations, if the chiasm was thought to be prefixed or if the patient was acromegalic.

Hirsch (15) remained the strongest advocate of the transnasal trans-sphenoidal operation and reported the results in 413 cases. Once antibiotic therapy had been developed the mortality in this series dropped to less than 2% using an endonasal approach to the sphenoid sinus between the septal membranes. The disadvantage of this operation was the narrow surgical exposure and other operations to the sphenoid sinus were described to improve visibility.

To improve the surgical exposure and manipulative ability of instruments, Bateman (4) developed a double approach to the sphenoid sinus which allowed him to view the area using the transethmoidal incision and sinus resection and manipulate the surgical instruments through the transnasal trans-sphenoidal approach. This operation, however, has never become popular (16).

Several European surgeons continued to use a transnasal trans-sphenoidal approach to the sella turcica for excision of pituitary tumours. This technique was improved by Hardy (11) using the sublabial transnasal trans-sphenoidal microsurgical operation employing the operative microscope to enhance the visual field by magnification and to improve the lighting (23). Furthermore, by performing a partial pneumoencephalogram during the operation, lateral fluoroscopy allowed the surgeon also to reach into the suprasellar recess safely to extract tumour tissue.

As a result of the efforts of Hardy and others the transnasal trans-sphenoidal operation, using the surgical microscope and closed television fluoroscopy has currently become more the standard operation, with antibiotic coverage to prevent infection, and special techniques to reduce the risk of cerebrospinal fluid rhinorrhea.

Certain aspects of the anatomy of the sphenoid sinus and sella turcica are worth consideration (1, 5). The sphenoid sinus varies significantly in length and height. The septum within the sinus may be thick or thin, in the midline or off to the side and can therefore mislead the surgeon (7). In the majority of situations the sphenoid sinus is pneumatized so that the floor of the sella turcica can be reached without drilling the sphenoid bone but in those instances where only slight aeration is present, drilling through the bone of the sella floor will be found to be necessary. In the lateral walls of the sphenoid sinus the carotid groove can be identified and it is important to recall that the medial wall of the optic canal is in the lateral portion of the upper part of the sphenoid sinus (8, 21).

Consequently, in the majority of patients done at UCLA Hospital, AP carotid angiograms are performed prior to operation to identify the position of the carotid arteries within the cavernous sinus and sphenoid sinus in order to be sure that arteriosclerosis or some other congenital changes have not caused the artery to lie close to the midline and also to rule out aneurysms simulating non-functional pituitary adenomas. In the future a direct carotid angiogram can be avoided by using intravenous digital computerized radiography which will show the carotid arteries quite well without doing an intra-arterial study. This technique will be used in the future at UCLA Hospital.

The sella turcica of course varies in size and shape normally and it changes especially with intrasellar tumours. If there is a microadenoma one may only see a thinning of the wall of the sella turcica usually in one side or the other with a small bulge. On the other hand the pituitary gland may harbour a microadenoma without any change in the size or shape, or calcification of the sella turcica, especially in Cushing's disease.

As CT brain and skull scanning has become more refined and sophisticated, such changes, including small micro-adenomas can be seen by using thin sections with high resolution and contrast.

From the point of view of the transnasal trans-sphenoidal operation the important vascular structures in the region are the carotid arteries laterally as well as the vessels in the surrounding dura mater and the cavernous sinuses. At times the pituitary tumour will actually invade the cavernous sinus and when it is removed there can be rather vigorous venous bleeding. This can be controlled by using such substances as Surgicel or muscle.

If the tumour is limited to the sella turcica this author tries to avoid producing a cerebrospinal fluid leak which entails repair of the floor of the sella turcica and therefore tends to prevent potential recurrent tumour growth coming inferiorly into the sphenoid sinus and it may go superiorly in the superchiasmatic area against the optic chiasm.

At UCLA Hospital prior to operation, the majority of patients harboring pituitary tumours receive a fairly extensive endocrine evaluation by members of the Department of Medicine, Division of Endocrinology. The routine endocrine evaluation includes FHS, LH, HGH, Cortisol, Prolactin, FT_4 Index, testosterone (male), oestrodiol (female) and glucose. Other special endocrine studies are ordered as seems indicated.

If the patient is showing any evidence of hypopituitarism either with a hypersecreting syndrome or in a non-functioning tumour, supplementary cortisone support is given prior to diagnostic radiographic studies such as carotid angiograms or pneumoencephalograms to overcome any excessive stress that may occur.

Operative Technique

Once the operation has been decided upon the patient is given the usual pre-operative medication for sedation and given a general anaesthetic with intubation while in a supine position on the operating room table. The oral cavity is packed to reduce the amount of blood going into the region of the superior portion of the larynx. The face and nasal cavities and oral cavities are prepared with antiseptic soap and the anterior portion of the right thigh or groin is prepared with an iodine solution in case a muscle and/or fat tissue is required to reconstruct the floor of the sella turcica to prevent a cerebrospinal fluid leak. If the patient has a suprasellar extension of the tumour then a small indwelling catheter is placed in the lumbar subarachnoid space in order to deliver increments of filtered oxygen to the supraoptic chiasm to outline where the microsurgical instruments may be passed safely into the suprasellar extension of the tumour.

We believe that preservation of the anterior portion of the septum is a critical part of the operation in order to preserve the appearance and function of the nose. Consequently, after appropriate draping, a 22 gauge needle is used to infiltrate the submucous superchondrial area with appropriate local anaesthetic solution with 100 to 200,000 epinephrine. This same solution is used to infiltrate the sublabial area.

The septum is approached through the right nares with a vertical incision made to the mucoperichondrium which is then elevated from the left side of the cartilaginous and bony septum preserving the right mucoperiosteum and blood supply to this area. The mucoperiosteum of the nasal fossae is elevated from both floors and the attachment of the septal membrane to the maxillary crest is sectioned. The cartilage is incised vertically at the junction of the bony nasal septum and then the mucoperiosteum is dissected bilaterally to the vomer of the sphenoid sinus.

A sublabial incision is made in a horizontal manner as has been described by others and subperiosteal dissection is performed to open into the septal spaces previously dissected. In this manner the serrated Hardy speculum which has been fashioned after Cushing and others is inserted through the sublabial opening between the septal membranes, pressing the preserved quadralateral cartilaginous plate to the right. The lower part of the middle turbinates may be outfractured in gaining adequate exposure but this has not caused any complication postoperatively in the patients.

A closed high resolution television fluoroscopy unit C-arm system is then activated in order to guide the speculum properly to the sphenoid sinus, which is then opened. Once this has been accomplished, the surgical microscope is introduced and further opening of the sphenoid sinus is carried out with resection of the septa of the sinus and the mucous membrane. As much of the mucous membrane as possible is preserved in case a small cerebrospinal fluid leak requires repair.

The speculum can be moved into the sphenoid sinus if the opening is wide enough, nicely exposing the floor of the sella turcica. Occasionally it may appear, especially in acromegalic patients, that there is an infection in the sphenoid sinus. Under these circumstances the operation should be discontinued at this time, cultures taken, appropriate antibiotics given and the patient treated conservatively until the infection is under control.

The surgical findings at the floor of the sella turcica depend on the size and shape of the intrasellar tumour and its influence on the surrounding structures. At times no remaining osseous floor remains, and at other times, if the tumour is very small in one area within the pituitary gland it may be quite normal. In those instances where the floor of the sella is paper-thin this bone is removed and aspiration is carried out using a disposable spinal needle. If dark fluid is obtained it indicates that there has been a previous hemorrhage in the tumour. If the posterior wall of the sphenoid sinus is particularly thick then high speed drilling is required. On the other hand, the usual floor of the sella can be opened with small chisels and then using an angled punch to enlarge it to its widest diameters.

Generally the dura is opened in a vertical and then horizontal manner and specimens of the tissue are obtained for frozen section, electronmicroscopy and permanent sections for special hormone staining. The dura can then be opened in a more circular manner and using intensified light the contents of the sella turcica can be quite readily viewed at higher magnification (19). Thus appropriate surgical resection of the tumour is carried out. If the tumour has basically occupied the entire sella causing it to be ballooned, one can expect that any residual normal pituitary tissue would be found posteriorly and superiorly in the region of the pituitary stalk. Naturally, every effort is made to preserve any residual normal pituitary tissue in this situation.

In those instances where one is looking for a microadenoma and there is no gross tumour detectable upon opening the dura, it would then be necessary to open the pituitary gland horizontally. Rather than open both sides of the dura of the sella this author limits the opening to the suspected side and removes the microadenoma using special microtechniques including the cryoprobe, which can destroy any residual cells in the bed of the pituitary gland.

One technique that has been quite useful when there is a suprasellar extension is to use a specially designed curved cryoprobe which employs compressed nitrogen as a coolant. This cryoprobe can be attached to the inferior surface of residual tumor in the suprasellar space and once an adherence is adequate the mass can be pulled down into the sella viewing the procedure on closed circuit television. This technique has been highly successful in bringing suprasellar tissue into the sella for subsequent resection.

In my opinion even with a radical excision of a pituitary tumour mass within the sella and this is especially true in a suprasellar position, total removal is not accomplished as small areas of pituitary adenoma will remain. In order to try and decrease the risk of recurrence of the tumour, another special cryoprobe is used to freeze the internal boundaries of the sella turcica with overlapping cryogenic lesions to $-90^{\circ}C$ or below.

Even then it may be necessary to give postoperative radiation to reduce the risk of recurrence of the tumour. It is well established in the literature that in tumours that occupy a large extent of the sella turcica, especially those with suprasellar extensions, a recurrence will generally occur unless some type of postoperative radiation is used.

In the future since we now have acquired the Leksell Stereotactic ^{60}Cobalt Gamma Radiation Unit we shall be giving certain selected pituitary tumours primary radiation without a transnasal operation (2, 3). In other situations this type of one-dose highly collimated gamma radiation will be used in patients postoperatively to take the place of the previous radiation techniques using other ^{60}Cobalt sources and linear accelerators (22, 24).

Discussion of Results

During the 15 years between 1966 and 1981, 203 transnasal trans-sphenoidal operations have been done for pituitary tumours. In this group of patients there were slightly more females than males due to the preponderance of prolactinomas which are more common in females than males. The ages varied from 16 to patients in their 70's with an average age around 40 years. Approximately 14% of these patients suffered from acromegaly due to increased growth hormones secreted by the adenoma. In the early years prior to the diagnostic techniques of detecting prolactin the majority of the patients were classified as non-secretory pituitary adenomas but with more sophisticated endocrine tests the classification of prolactinoma became more common. With the advent of Bromocriptine[R] there has been a decrease in the number of patients operated upon for prolactinomas because an arrest, if not a cure, of a number of these adenomas has been achieved by the use of various doses of Bromocriptine, even up to 25 grams per day. Although this drug may indeed not produce a cure there have been reliable reports in the literature of definite shrinkage of the tumour mass with improvement of the endocrinopathy syndrome and the neurological deficits such as bitemporal hemianopsia. We have seen dramatic improvement in some cases. A total of thirty additional patients underwent transnasal trans-sphenoidal operations for craniopharyngioma, hypophysectomy for metastatic breast cancer and some unusual conditions such as intrasellar angiofibroma and meningioma.

The postoperative course for pituitary tumour patients has been fairly benign in the majority of individuals although one patient did develop a persistent cerebrospinal fluid leak in spite of reconstruction of the sella floor. Meningitis developed and death subsequently occurred due to vascular cerebritis with rupture of vessels. Another patient who was shown preoperatively to have a small aneurysm on the anterior cerebral artery died in the recovery room from rupture of the aneurysm which was attached to the dome of the suprasellar mass of the pituitary adenoma. It would have been more prudent in retrospect to have done this case by craniotomy in order to treat the cerebral aneurysm first and then do a decompression of the pituitary tumour. In the majority of our patients AP angiograms have been performed to determine the position of the internal carotid artery and to rule out large aneurysms in the region of the sella which might be mimicking a pituitary tumour. In actual practice this has worked out well without complication. The newer techniques of digitalized computer angiography may replace standard angiography in this situation.

Every effort was made to avoid re-building the floor of the sella in patients with large pituitary tumours so that the suprasellar contents could prolapse into the sella and thus limit the field of postoperative radiation. Therefore, although radical resection of these tumours was performed a total resection was not attempted because of the inability to do such an operation with piecemeal removal of tumour tissue and the risk of producing a serious cerebrospinal fluid leak. This would necessitate rebuilding the floor of the sella with muscle and cartilage. Approximately one-third of the patients had to have some reconstruction of the floor of the sella because of the risk of cerebrospinal fluid leak. This was done by a technique similar to that described by Hardy.

Cerebrospinal fluid rhinorrhea is a complication in approximately 8% but is usually transient and controlled by the use of lumbar punctures postoperatively if the floor of the sella had been reconstructed. If not a subsequent operation was performed to rebuild the floor of the sella in a few patients.

In the early years prior to CT brain scanning, pneumoencephalograms were performed in the vast majority of patients using a partial technique often performed as an outpatient. With the advent of CT brain scanning and particularly with the newer techniques using colour coding and three dimensional reconstruction, there have been fewer cases in which a partial pneumoencephalogram has been needed.

The operative mortality has been less than 2%. In one patient there was a death due to myocardial infarction and in another patient an arrest occurred when the patient wished to have a general anaesthetic to remove the nasal packing. This was the patient's request. Ordinarily the packing is removed readily without any anaesthetic or even narcotic.

The transnasal trans-sphenoidal approach to pituitary tumours has replaced the transfrontal craniotomy in the majority of patients with pituitary tumours. This author believes that the transnasal trans-sphenoidal procedure should be considered and used in the majority of patients including those with suprasellar extensions. However, tumours which have been extremely long-standing with potential severe adherence to the hypothalamus and mesencephalon so that inversion of the diaphragm sella will not occur may be better served by a transfrontal trans-sphenoidal operation.

The majority of pituitary tumours are quite resectable using the trans-sphenoidal operation because of their soft consistency and especially with the advent of special probes to help displace the tumour tissue into the sella turcica from the suprasellar position. The cryosurgical probe can also destroy residual tumour tissue in the walls of the cavernous sinus.

In addition, midline small craniopharyngiomas and cystic pituitary lesions can be managed satisfactorily by the transnasal trans-sphenoidal approach. This has been accomplished in several of our patients.

There remain, however, some patients where a transfrontal operation is definitely indicated. This is particularly useful if it is combined with a transfrontal trans-sphenoidal operation pushing the mucous membrane of the sphenoid sinus away to allow a greater access to the sella turcica, in those cases where the optic chiasm is pre-fixed and danger to vision may be predicted if manoeuvres are made to the optic nerve or optic chiasm.

We have been pleased by the special surgical techniques in managing the nasal septum preserving the quadrilateral cartilaginous plate. With this technique we have neither observed nasal deformities such as "saddle nose" nor been troubled by septal defects causing discomforting nasal symptoms.

If residual tumour tissue cannot be managed by the use of a cryoprobe and thus avoid postoperative radiation, this author continues to recommend postoperative radiation in those situations where it is evident that tumour tissue was probably left behind. This dose should not exceed 180 rads tumor dose per day.

This programme of postoperative radiation is in contrast to the microadenoma where one can dissect out the neoplasm and then freeze the base of the tumour. In these situations postoperative radiation may indeed not be necessary because we have followed patients after stereotactic cryohypophysectomy for over 17 years without evidence of recurrence of their tumour after profound freezing of the tumour tissue.

With the arrival of the Leksell Stereotactic ^{60}Cobalt Gamma Unit to UCLA Hospital from Stockholm, Sweden, we shall be treating some microadenomas, particularly those causing acromegaly and Cushing's disease by this successful technique (22, 24). This treatment is unique in that the radiation can be delivered at one dose up to 7000 to 10,000 rads to the microadenoma via 179 needle sources thus reducing radiation to the entire brain as ordinarily is done with conventional radiation.

Conclusion

The transnasal trans-sphenoidal operation using microneurosurgical and closed television fluoroscopy is the preferred surgical technique for microadenomas and intrasellar tumours. Stereotactic cryosurgery is an excellent alternative in these situations. Stereotactic ^{60}Cobalt Gamma radiation is especially satisfactory in Cushing's disease with a normal sella turcica. For suprasellar extensions the transfrontal trans-sphenoidal approach is an alternate to the transnasal trans-sphenoidal approach in selected cases.

References

1. Alyea, O.E.V.: Sphenoid sinus — anatomic study with consideration of the structural characteristics of the sphenoid sinus. Arch. Otolaryngol. *34*, 225–253 (1941)
2. Backlund, E.O., Rähn, T., Sarby, B., de Schryver, A., Wennerstrand, J.: Closed Stereotaxic Hypophysectomy by means of ^{60}CO Gamma Radiation. Acta Radiologica Therapy Physics Biology *2*, 545–555 (1972)
3. Backlund, E.O., Rähn, T., Sarby, B., Wennerstrand, J.: Stereotaxic Gammahypophysectomy. Acta Neural Scand. *48*, 261–262 (1972)

4. Bateman, G.H.: Trans-sphenoidal hypophysectomy, a review of 70 cases treated in the past two years. Trans. Am. Acad. Ophthalmol. Otolaryngol. *66*, 103–110 (1962)
5. Bergland, R.M., Ray, B.S., Torack, R.M.: Anatomical variations in the pituitary gland and adjacent structures in 225 human autopsy cases. J. Neurosurg. *28*, 93–99 (1968)
6. Chiari, O.: Über eine Modifikation der Schlofferschen Operation von Tumoren der Hypophyse. Wien, Klin. Wochenschr. *25*, 5–6 (1912)
7. Congdon, E.D.: The distribution and mode of septa and walls of the sphenoid sinus. Anat. Rec. *18*, 97–116 (1920)
8. Cope, Z.V.: The internal structure of the sphenoidal sinus. J. Anat. Physiol. *51*, 127–136 (1917)
9. Cushing, H.: The pituitary body and its disorders, p. 298. Philadelphia: J.B. Lippincott Co. 1912
10. Halstead, A.E.: Remarks on the operative treatment of tumors of the hypophysis. Surg. Gynecol. Obstet. *10*, 494–502 (1910)
11. Hardy, J., Wigser, S.M.: Trans-sphenoidal surgery of pituitary fossa tumors with televised radio-fluoroscopic control. J. Neurosurg. *23*, 612–619 (1965)
12. Heuer, G.J.: The surgical apparoach and the treatment of tumors and other lesions about the optic chiasm. Surg. Gynecol. Obstet. *53*, 489–518 (1931)
13. Hirsch, O.: Diskussion in: Offizielles Protokoll der K.K. Gesellschaft der Ärzte. Wien Klin. Wochenschr. *22*, 473 (1909)
14. Hirsch, O.: Tumeurs hypophysairés basée sur 100 cas apérés par l'auteur d'apres sa propre méthode endonasale. La Presse Med. *1*, 578–580 (1926)
15. Hirsch, O.: Pituitary tumors, a borderland between cranial and trans-sphenoidal surgery. N. Engl. J. Med. *254*, 937–939 (1956)
16. James, J.A.: Transethmosphenoidal hypophysectomy. Arch. Otolaryngol. *86*, 256–264 (1967)
17. Kanavel, A.B.: The removal of tumors of the pituitary body by an infranasal route. J.A.M.A. *53*, 1704–1707 (1909)
18. Kanavel, A.B.: A consideration of final results in hypophyseal surgery. Surg. Gynecol. Obstet. *16*, 541–548 (1913)
19. Kaplan, H.A., Browder, J., Krieger, A.J.: Intercavernous connections of the cavernous sinus. J. Neurosurg. *45*, 166–168 (1976)
20. Moszkowicz, L.: Zur Technik der Operationen an der Hypophyse. Wien Klin. Wochenschr. *20*, 792–795 (1940)
21. Peele, J.C.: Unusual anatomical variations of the sphenoid sinus. Laryngoscope *67*, 208–237 (1957)
22. Rähn, T., Thorén, M., Hall, K., Backlund, E.O.: Stereotactic radiosurgery in Cushing's syndrome: Acute radiation effects. Surg. Neurol. *14*, 85–92 (1980)
23. Rand, R.W.: Microneurosurgery. 2nd ed. St. Louis: C.V. Mosby Co. 1978
24. Thorén, M., Rähn, T., Hall, K., Backlund, E.O.: Treatment of pituitary dependent Cushing's syndrome with closed stereotactic radiosurgery by means of [60]Co Gamma Radiation. Acta Endocrinologica *88*, 7–17 (1978)
25. West, J.M.: The surgery of the hypophysis from the standpoint of the rhinologist. J.A.M.A. *54*, 1132–1134 (1910)

Complications of Trans-Sphenoidal Microsurgery for Pituitary Adenoma

E.R. Laws, Jr.

During the past 15 years, radical changes have taken place in the diagnosis and management of pituitary adenomas (1). Pituitary tumours are being detected and treated much more frequently than in the past. Treatment, which once consisted of craniotomy or radiation therapy, is now primarily by trans-sphenoidal microsurgery or medical therapy. At present, approximately 96% of the pituitary tumours treated surgically at our institution are approached trans-sphenoidally rather than by craniotomy.

Although the mortality and complication rates for most large series of craniotomy for pituitary adenoma were quite acceptable (12), the prospect of such an operation for the patient and the referring physician is still terrifying. The trans-sphenoidal approach is more acceptable psychologically and has proved to be considerably safer for the patient. This is a review of the complications encountered during a nine year period in the management of nearly 800 patients with pituitary adenomas using trans-sphenoidal microsurgery.

In previous reports (9, 10), we have grouped the potential complications into various categories.

Intracranial complications consist of hypothalamic injury (6), intracranial vasospasm, injury to intracranial branches of the circle of Willis, ischaemic or haemorrhagic stroke, meningitis, and complications related to extension of a large tumour into the anterior or middle fossa (5). These complications are the most common cause of operative mortality (2, 4).

Carotid artery complications may also be fatal or lead to serious disability. They include laceration, perforation, avulsion and occlusion of the cavernous carotid artery, rupture of an unrecognized carotid aneurysm (8, 11, 12), and spasm provoked by manipulation or damage to the vessel.

Complications involving the *visual system* may occur in a variety of ways. The optic nverves and chiasm may be traumatized directly or may be injured by interference with their blood supply. They may be compressed by muscle or other agents used to pack the sella and obtain haemostasis, and they may be damaged by prolapse into the secondary empty sella. The instruments used for surgery may produce fractures of the orbit or optic foramen which can result in visual loss.

The *cavernous sinus* is a potential source of several complications, with haemorrhage being the most common. The cranial nerves running within the cavernous sinus may be traumatized or avulsed. Air emboli through this venous channel have been reported (13).

Complications involving the *sella turcica* itself may occur, and are usually related to its anatomy (1). Variations in structure can lead to difficulties in approach to a conchal sella or shallow sella, and a very large sella may be a factor in haemorrhagic complications (5). CSF rhinorrhoea usually occurs through the sella, and can lead to meningitis it not promptly repaired.

Sphenoid sinus and nasofacial complications are usually less serious. Postoperative mucocele (19) or pyocele can occur, as can severe sinusitis. The retractor can fracture the hard palate and distort the teeth. Postoperative nasal septal perforations and nasal deformities can be uncomfortable and disfiguring. Epistaxis and wound haematomas are also unpleasant complications.

Endocrinologic complications include failure to cure a hypersecreting pituitary endocrinopathy, damage to preoperative normal endocrine function, and electrolyte disturbances related to diabetes insipidus or inappropriate ADH secretion.

Material and Approach

The records of all patients who have been treated by trans-sphenoidal microsurgery from November 1972 to June 1982 were reviewed, and current follow-up data were collected. There were 785 patients with pituitary adenomas treated, and the various types of pituitary adenoma are presented in Table 1. Approximately 30% of the cases had large tumours with suprasellar extension and visual loss. Nearly 50% had microadenomas (tumours $\leq$ 10 mm in diameter). Of the larger tumours, approximately 10% were partially cystic and about 6% were firm "fibrous" tumours.

Results

There were four fatalities in this series, a case mortality rate of 0.5%. Three of the fatalities occurred in patients with non-functioning adenomas, two of whom had undergone prior craniotomy. One of these deaths was attributed to hypothalamic injury, one to haemorrhage in an extensive tumour involving the parasellar region and middle fossa, and a third fatality occurred as a result of injury to the cavernous carotid artery. The last patient who died had a prolactin adenoma previously treated by craniotomy and radiation therapy. He too developed haemorrhage into the intracranial portion of the tumour.

Non-fatal complications encountered are described in Tables 2 and 3.

Among the non-functioning adenomas, there were two cases with vascular occlusion resulting in strokes, one of which was transient. There were three cases of subarachnoid haemorrhage, one resulting in a stroke, one in decreased visual acuity, and the third associated with meningitis, obstructive hydrocephalus and eventually a CSF shunt procedure. There were six cases of postoperative CSF rhinorrhoea, all of which were successfully treated. Visual loss occurred in five of these patients, in one case associated with an optic nerve infarct and in another with a third nerve palsy. Four of these patients regained their vision. One patient had an early postoperative haemorrhage requiring reoperation. Less serious complications in the group consisted of one patient with

Table 1. Trans-sphenoidal operations for pituitary adenoma (Mayo Clinic 1972–1981)

Type of adenoma	No. of patients	No. of operations
"Non-functioning"	209	218
Prolactin	311	319
Acromegaly	149	155
Cushing's	84	85
Nelson-Salassa	29	30
Other	3	3
Total	785	810
Operative mortality	4/810	0.5%
Case mortality	4/785	0.51%

Table 2. Trans-sphenoidal operations for pituitary adenoma; serious complications (non-fatal)

Stroke	4	
CSF rhinorrhoea	12	(1.5%)
Meningitis	2	
Loss of vision (4 transient)	6	
Third nerve paralysis	1	
Sixth nerve paralysis	1	
Vascular injury (2 carotid, one anterior cerebral)	3	
Total serious complications	29	(3.6%)

Table 3. Trans-sphenoidal operations for pituitary adenoma; less serious complications

Transient third nerve palsy	2	
Transient sixth nerve palsy	1	
Excessive bleeding	6	
Permanent diabetes insipidus	10	(1.2%)
Symptomatic electrolyte disturbance	3	
Severe sinusitis	2	
Nasal septal perforation	3	
Total	27	(3.3%)

a transient third nerve palsy, three cases of permanent diabetes insipidus and one patient with a delayed electrolyte disturbance.

Among the prolactin adenomas, one patient suffered a subarachnoid haemorrhage associated with stroke and permanent diabetes insipidus. One carotid artery injury occurred in a patient with a microadenoma and was repaired intraoperatively. One case of CSF rhinorrhoea occurred in a patient with an invasive tumour treated by bromocriptine and was also associated with a sixth cranial nerve palsy. Cerebrospinal rhinorrhoea occurred in three other cases and was managed successfully by prompt reoperation. Less serious complications in this group included one patient with a transient third nerve palsy and two with permanent diabetes insipidus.

Among the acromegalics, there were two arterial injuries. In one, the carotid was lacerated and repaired intraoperatively, and in another, the anterior cerebral artery was lacerated and clipped trans-sphenoidally. The latter patient also developed permanent diabetes insipidus. There were three cases of CSF rhinorrhoea, two in patients with gigantism. Significant intraoperative bleeding was encountered in three patients, causing the procedure to be abandoned permanently in one and temporarily in another. Two other patients developed permanent diabetes insipidus, two had significant postoperative bleeding, one had severe sinusitis, one had a nasal septal perforation, and two developed late electrolyte imbalance.

There were no significant complications among the patients with Cushing's disease.

Among the patients with Nelson-Salassa syndrome, one patient had permanent diabetes insipidus, and one had a symptomatic nasal septal perforation.

One patient with an FSH adenoma developed a nasal septal perforation.

Discussion

It is evident from the results that the size of the tumour is a very important factor in the risk of complications. There were no fatal complications among the microadenomas treated, and the number of serious problems was very small (Table 4). The other factor clearly predisposing patients to complications was a previous operation for pituitary tumour. Three of the four operative deaths occurred in patients who had had previous craniotomies. Prior operation was a factor of 12 of the 28 serious complications and in 7 of the 12 patients who developed postoperative CSF rhinorrhoea.

Careful adherence to basic surgical principles will help in avoiding serious complications. Pre-operatively, the endocrine status of the patient should be carefully documented, hormonal deficiencies and electrolyte imbalances should be corrected, and the patient should be adequately prepared for operation. In addition, thorough assessment of the surgical anatomy should be performed with appropriate radiologic studies and physical examination. During the operation, the anatomy should be respected, and techniques should be used which carefully dismantle and reconstruct the nasal structures and the base of the skull. The midline approach should be maintained, as well as continual orientation of the instruments in relation to the sella. Postoperatively, careful attention to steroid replacement and fluid and electrolyte balance are essential.

The benign nature of the trans-sphenoidal approach to the sella was emphasized by Norman Dott and Gerard Guiot (3) when most pituitary tumours were still being trea-

Table 4. Pituitary microadenomas (380 patients)

Mortality	0
CSF rhinorrhoea	3
Carotid artery injury	1
Excessive bleeding	1
Permanent diabetes insipidus	4
Nasal septal perforation	1

ted by craniotomy. The low incidence of serious complications reported here and in other large series confirms this impression, and challenges us to do even better in the future.

Conclusions

Trans-sphenoidal microsurgery for pituitary adenomas can be accomplished with a mortality rate of approximately 0.5%.

No mortality has accompanied trans-sphenoidal removal of more than 300 pituitary microadenomas.

Serious complications are more likely to occur in patients with large tumours and in those who have had previous surgical treatment for their pituitary tumours.

References

1. Bergland, R.M., Ray, B.S., Torack, R.M.: Anatomical variations in the pituitary gland and adjacent structures in 225 human autopsy cases. J. Neurosurg. *28*, 93–99 (1968)
2. Deborsu, F.L.: Difficultés de la voie transphénoïdale de l'opération de l'adénome de l'hypophyse. Neurochirurgia (Stuttg). *1*, 209–215 (1959)
3. Guiot, G.: Trans-sphenoidal approach in surgical treatment of pituitary adenomas: General principles and indications in non-functioning adenomas. In: Excerpta Medica International Congress Series, No. 303, pp. 159–178. Amsterdam: Excerpta Medica 1973
4. Guiot, G., Cheibani, G.: Risques et problèmes de l'exérése trans-sphénoïdale des adénomes hypophysaires. Nouv. Presse Med. *1*, 2117–2119 (1972)
5. Guiot, G., Derome, P., Demailly, P., Hertzog, E.: Complications inattendue de l'exérése complète de volumineux adénomes hypophysaires. Rev. Neurol. (Paris) *118*, 164–167 (1968)
6. Halstead, A.E.: Remarks on the operative treatment of tumors of the hypophysis. Surg. Gynecol. Obstet. *10*, 494–502 (1910)
7. Hardy, J.: Trans-sphenoidal surgery of hypersecreting pituitary tumors. In: Excerpta Medica International Congress Series, No. 303, pp. 179–193, Amsterdam, Excerpta Medica 1973
8. Jordan, R.M., Kerber, C.W.: Rupture of a parasellar aneurysm with a coexisting pituitary tumor. South Med. J. *71*, 741–742 (1978)
9. Laws, E.R., Jr., Kern, E.B.: Complications of trans-sphenoidal surgery. Clin. Neurosurg. *23*, 401–416 (1976)
10. Laws, E.R., Jr., Kern, E.B.: Complications of trans-sphenoidal surgery. In: Clinical management of pituitary disorders. Tindall, G.T., Collins, W.F. (eds.), pp. 435–445. New York: Raven Press 1979

11. Lippmann, H.H., Onofrio, B.M., Baker, H.L. Jr.: Intrasellar aneurysm and pituitary adenoma: Report of a case. Mayo Clin. Proc. *46*, 532–535 (1971)
12. Maccarty, C.S., Hanson, E.J., Jr., Randall, R.V., Scanlon, P.W.: Indications for and results of surgical treatment of pituitary tumors by the transfrontal approach. In: Excerpta Medica International Congress Series, No. 303, pp. 139–145. Amsterdam, Excerpta Medica 1973
13. Newfield, P., Ablin, M.S., Chestnut, J.S., Maroon, J.C.: Air embolism during trans-sphenoidal pituitary operations. Neurosurgery, *2*, 39–42 (1978)
14. Schoen, D.: Mukozele des Keilbeines nach Hypophysektomie. Fortschr. Geb. Roentgenstr. Nuklearmed. *112*, 114–116 (1970)
15. Svien H.J., Kennedy W.C., Kearns, T.P.: Results of surgical treatment of pituitary adenoma: The factor of the excessively enlarged sella. J. Neurosurg. *20*, 669–674 (1963)
16. White, J.C., Ballantine, H.T., Jr.: Intrasellar aneurysms simulating hypophyseal tumors. J. Neurosurg. *18*, 34–50 (1961)

The Surgical Treatment of Craniopharyngioma

L. Symon, V. Logue, and J. Jakubowski

Series published over the past twenty years give ample evidence of the tendency of craniopharyngioma to recur and its generally poor prognosis (2, 3, 7, 14–16, 20). Kramer (11)
(11) has claimed that minimal surgical intervention to establish the diagnosis, followed by
by radical radiotherapy, is the treatment of choice (12, 19). This view has not gained uni-
universal acceptance, and notable surgeons, particularly Matson (14, 15), and Sweet (21),
have maintained a steadfastly aggressive attitude to excision, an attitude which the operating microscope has encouraged.

We have used a variety in the treatment of craniopharyngioma. Simple subfrontal exploration to establish the diagnosis and partially remove the tumour if it were accessible
beneath the optic nerves, or for tapping cysts, has sometimes been modified to allow an
interhemispheric approach with division of the lamina terminalis (6, 10), or an extended
approach with access into the temporal fossa behind the carotid artery. However the increased precision of information given by the CT scan makes exploratory operative in
the region of the chiasm less frequent than before, and accurate assessment of the probable nature of the lesion justifies a more extensive radical approach.

This review is based on the developing experience of two surgeons in one clinic between 1954 and 1979. One hundred cases have been operated upon. The age and sex incidence of this group of cases is shown in Table 1. In the early years a simple subfrontal
exploration was usual, and radical excision was only occasionally possible in those tumours which were particularly favourable with a very high placement of the chiasm. Increasingly effective removal of the postero-superior part of craniopharyngiomas was gradually achieved by a route which gained access behind the optic nerves, first by an extended fronto-temporal approach, but more recently by a radical temporal approach.

Pre-Operative Investigation

a) Endocrine/Metabolic. Pituitary hypothalamic function should be elucidated in a full
pre-operative work-up. The key to endocrine management however, is the use of large
doses of dexamethasone and control of the inevitable diabetes insipidus by judicious
doses of DDAVP. Under these circumstances, many clinics may prefer to place the patient on high steroid dosage pre-operatively, and to defer detailed endocrine investigation until the postoperative period when the degree of impairment of pituitary hypothalamic function may be assessed in detail.

Table 1. Age and sex distribution (100 craniopharyngiomas)

	0–10	10–20	20–30	30–40	40–50	50–60	60–70	70	
Male	3	4	12	12	15	11	4	2	63
Female	2	7	7	5	9	2	5	–	37
	5	11	19	17	24	13	9	2	100

b) Radiological. The plain x-ray in craniopharyngioma shows calcification in between 80 and 100% of craniopharyngiomas in children, with a large proportion of adults (between 25% and 50%) showing detectable calcium. The characteristic shortening of the dorsum sellae has also been well described. *Computerized tomography* (17) shows a characteristic picture of mixed attenuation lying predominantly in the suprasellar region, often with lacunae of lower density to suggest a cystic component, and usually irregularly enhancing on the injection of contrast medium. The extent and direction of spread of the tumour, its spread sub-frontally or through the tentorium into the posterior fossa is readily and conveniently determined by CT. Except in the relatively uncommon adult case with papilloedema (18) (less than 8% in the current series of 94 cases), the most specific information as to the extent of the tumour and its relation to the third ventricular structures and the brain stem is obtained by *air encephalography.* While the air encephalogram will outline the size, shape and situation of the mass, its relationship to major arteries can only be determined with confidence by careful *arteriography.* Bilateral carotid angiography with magnification studies, and vertebral angiography, is necessary to show the position of the terminal carotid branches and their relationship to the mass.

Surgical Approaches

Where the tumour mass is in the third ventricle, and the extent of the tumour through the foramen of Monro and into the lateral ventricle clearly precludes an attempt to remove it from below, a transventricular approach by a right post-frontal parasaggital craniotomy may be used to attack the craniopharyngioma through the foramen of Monro, a manoeuvre suggested first by Dott (13). Alternatively an approach may be made through the lamina terminalis, as advocated by Hoffman et al. (6) and more recently by King (10).

The Radical Temporal Approach to Craniopharyngioma

Most craniopharyngiomas in adults are found in the floor of the third ventricle, the postero-inferior portion of such tumours presenting in the interpeduncular cistern. A considerable quadrant of the mass is available for early excision, through limited access between the branches of the posterior communicating artery, or below the posterior communicating artery itself. Where the operation is performed for visual failure, and this type of craniopharyngioma appears likely, the radical temporal operation is appropriate and with the advent of the operating microscope, has become the approach of choice. An extended sphenoidal wing approach is used, with a small resection of the anterior two centimetres of the temporal lobe. The inner end of the Sylvian fissure is opened, and dissection pursued behind the carotid artery, along the tentorial edge. Removal of the uncus by secondary suction gives access to the interpeduncular fossa. The presenting lower pole of the craniopharyngioma with the posterior communicating artery, its thalamo-perforating branches and the third nerve lateral to it and in their own separate arachnoid, are then evident. It is at this stage usually possible to dissect the third nerve clear, and preserve it although some transient third nerve palsy is very frequent. The posterior cerebral artery and the top of the basilar artery and its branches are defined. If the tumour is of a lesser size, and visible only as a protrusion through the floor of the third ventricle, it may be necessary to develop the small triangular space between the internal carotid artery and its anterior choroidal branch anteriorly, and the posterior communicating artery and its anterior thalamo-perforating branches below and posteriorly. It is unwise to divide either the posterior communicating artery or its thalamo-perforating branches except in the clear knowledge that this may result in a small infarct in the basal ganglia or hypothalamus. The usual sequela is a fluctuating hemiparesis for some days which then improves. The posterior communicating artery being an early branch of the carotid artery, can usually be mobilised forward, leaving a portion of capsule available for access between it and the anterior thalamo-perforating artery. After interior decompression of the tumour, the third ventricle may be transgressed just in front of the mamillary bodies.

The optic tract is scarcely adherent to the edge of the mass, but if the mass is extremely large, a transient homonymous field defect may occur. The nuclear masses on the floor of the third ventricle appear to be substantially separated by the craniopharyngioma. Although the tumour itself is apparently invasive as has been pointed out by many authors (4, 5, 23, 22) careful histological examination reveals that there is a layer of condensed glial reaction to the mass in which dissection may be safely pursued without actual transgression of the nuclear masses in the walls of the third ventricle.

Adhesions to the vascular structures on the contralateral side, to the posterior communicating artery, internal carotid or thalamo-perforating arteries are visible as the tumour is folded forwards and downwards out of the third ventricle. The tumour may be adherent to the diaphragma sellae or the internal carotid artery on one or both sides, and is almost invariably densely adherent to the anterior third ventricle in the region of the posterior part of the optic chiasm. Here, the preservation of a line of the top of the capsule, and the excellent exposure of the ipsilateral optic nerve and optic tract, enables calculation of the line of the chiasm and under reasonable magnification, sharp dissection of the tumour from the posterior aspect of the chiasm. Adhesions to the carotid complex constitute the usual cause of the abandonment of the radical procedure and conversion to a subtotal excision.

A craniopharyngioma which is almost completely cystic is unsatisfactory for radical excision by any route, since every movement of dissection of the wall is accompanied by considerable disturbances of the third ventricular structures. Lesser operations for such craniopharyngiomatous cysts are probably advisable. Any solid portion of the tumour having been removed, we now insert a large gauge (5 mm internal diameter) rubber or silastic tube with several side holes, anchored to the dura along the sphenoidal wing, its free end lying within the cavity of the cyst, and the tube brought out along the sphenoidal wing to a Rickham reservoir in the temporal muscle. Aspiration of the cyst through the Rickham reservoir may be followed by connection to the pleural cavity through a wide bored tube. Adequate drainage of such cases for periods of up to five years without further trouble has been possible.

Results

More radical excision occasions fewer recurrences with a slightly higher initial mortality. Primary radical excision in this series has been performed in 19 cases with a mortality rate of 10.5%. Secondary radical excision, that is a radical excision after one or more previous interferences with the tumour, has been carried out in seven cases with a mortality rate of 28.5%. From this group of 26 cases, 20 patients are still alive without recurrence, the follow-up ranging from two years to over 20 years (76%). Cases operated on in the past two years have not been included in the present study. Four patients have survived more than 20 years without recurrence, two patients more than ten years, seven between four and eight years, and seven between two and four years. With a less radical operation, 34 cases were treated with an operative mortality of 3%. Recurrence, however has taken place in 15 of these cases (44%) and only 26 of these cases now survive. Therefore the percentage of survivors at this time is the same as for apparently more radical operation, although presumably further recurrence is to be expected in the less radical group.

Where a considerable portion of the tumour is known to have been left behind (22 cases in the current series), the operative mortality of 23% is somewhat higher, although this includes many cases early in the series. Only ten of these cases now survive, five having survived re-operation, and five requiring no further operation. This represents 22.7% of the original group. Exploration with biopsy and a shunt procedure was performed in 19 cases, but only nine patients now remain alive. Only three of the original 19 cases survived without further surgery, although the mortality of the original operation was only 12%.

Conclusion

Throughout this review, the use of the term complete excision has been avoided. It seems that the best that can be hoped for in any operation for a craniopharyngioma is maximal removal of accessible tumour at the time of the primary exposure. If, after 25 years the tumour has not recurred, then perhaps it has been completely removed. Assessment of the extent of radical excision may either be by CT scanning or by post-operative air encephalography, of which the latter is by far the most effective (Fig. 1).

Backlund (1) and his associates in Sweden have further given unequivocal CT scan evidence of reduction in size of craniopharyngiomas following stereotactically controlled radiotherapy but the complete eradication of such tumours by radiotherapeutic means has not been described. Only total removal of the tumour will prevent early or late recurrence, and to us it seems that a radical operation with the use of the microscope and appropriate hormonal replacement, represents the best and most hopeful means of cure at the present time.

References

1. Backlund, E.-O.: Stereotactic radiosurgery in intracranial tumours. In: Advances and technical standards in neurosurgery, Vol. 6. Krayenbühl, H. (ed.), pp. 3–37. Berlin, Heidelberg, New York: Springer 1979
2. Banna, M.: Review article. Craniopharyngioma: based on 160 cases. Brit. J. Radiol. 49, 206–223 (1976)
3. Bartlett, J.R.: Craniopharyngiomas – a summary of 85 cases. J. Neurol. Neurosurg. & Psychiat. 34, 37–41 (1971)
4. Ghatak, N.R., Hirano, A., Zimmerman, H.M.: Ultrastructure of craniopharyngioma. Cancer 27, 1465–1475 (1971)
5. Grcevic, N., Yates, P.O.: Rosenthal fibers in tumors of the central nervous system. J. Pathol. 73, 467–472 (1957)
6. Hoffman, H.J., Bendrick, E.B., Humphreys, R.P., Buncic, J.R., Armstrong, D.L., Jenkin, R.D.T.: Management of craniopharyngioma in children. J. Neurosurg. 47, 218–227 (1977)
7. Katz, E.L.: Late results of radical excision of craniopharyngiomas in children. J. Neurosurg. 42, 86–90 (1975)
8. Kahn, E.A., Gosch, H.H., Seeger, J.F., Hicks, S.P.: Forty-five years experience with craniopharyngiomas. Surg. Neurol. 1, 5–12 (1973)
9. Kerr, A.S.: Craniopharyngiomata – Proc. Soc. Brit. Neurol. Surgeons. J. Neurol. Neurosurg. Psychiat. 31, 646–650
10. King, T.T.: Removal of intraventricular craniopharyngiomas through the lamina terminalis. Acta Neurochir. 45, 277–286 (1979)
11. Kramer, S., McKissock, W., Concannon, J.P.: Craniopharyngiomas treated by combined surgery and radiation therapy. J. Neurosurg. 18, 217–226 (1960)
12. Kramer, S., Southard, M., Mansfield, C.M.: Radiotherapy in the management of craniopharyngiomas, further experiences and late results. Am. J. Roentgenol. 103, 44–52 (1968)
13. LeGros Clarke, W.E., Beattie, J., Riddoch, G., Dott, N.M.: "The Hypothalamus" Oliver and Boyd. 1938
14. Matson, D.D.: Craniopharyngioma. Clin. Neurosurg. 10, 116–129 (1962)
15. Matson, D.D., Crigler, J.F.: Management of craniopharyngioma in childhood. J. Neurosurg. 30, 377–390 (1969)
16. Michelson, W., Mount, L.A., Redadin, J.: Craniopharyngiomas: a 39 year study. Acta Neurologia Latino Americana 18, 100–106 (1972)
17. Naidich, T.P., Pinto, R.S., Kushner, B.A., Lin, J.P., Kricheff, I.I., Leeds, N.E., Chase, N.E.: Evaluation of sellar and parasellar masses by computed tomography. Radiology, 120, 19–99 (1976)
18. Ross Russell, R.W., Pennybacker, J.B.: Craniopharyngioma in the elderly. J. Neurol. Neurosurg. Psychiat. 24, 1–13 (1961)
19. Sharma, U., Tandon, P.N., Saxena, K.K., Shinghal, R.M., Barvah, J.D.: Craniopharyngiomas treated by a combination of surgery and radiotherapy. Clin. Radiol, 25, 13–17 (1974)

20. Svolos, D.G.: craniopharyngiomas: a study based on 108 verified cases. Acta Chir. Scand. (Suppl.) *404*, 8–44
21. Sweet, W.H.: Radical surgical treatment of craniopharyngioma. Clin. Neurol. *23*, 52–79 (1976)
22. van der Bergh, R., Brucher, J.K.: L'abord transventriculaire dans les craniopharyngiomes du troisième ventricule. Neurochirurgie *16*, 51–65 (1970)
23. Zülch, K.J.: Brain Tumors; their biology and pathology, 2nd ed, p. 228–233. New York: Springer 1965

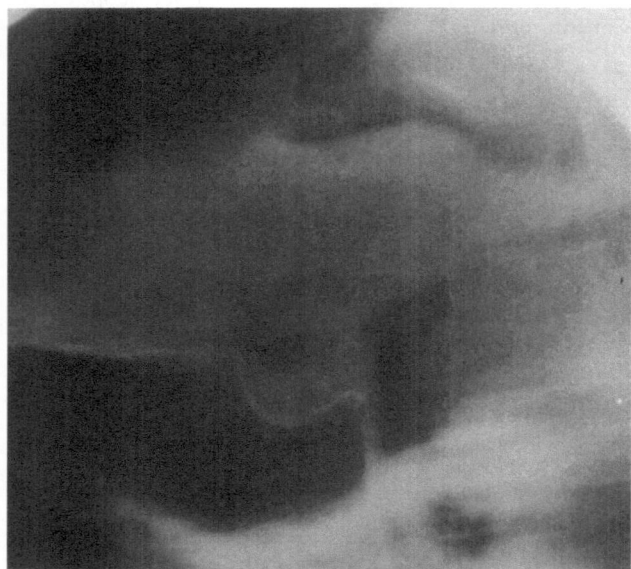

Fig. 1a

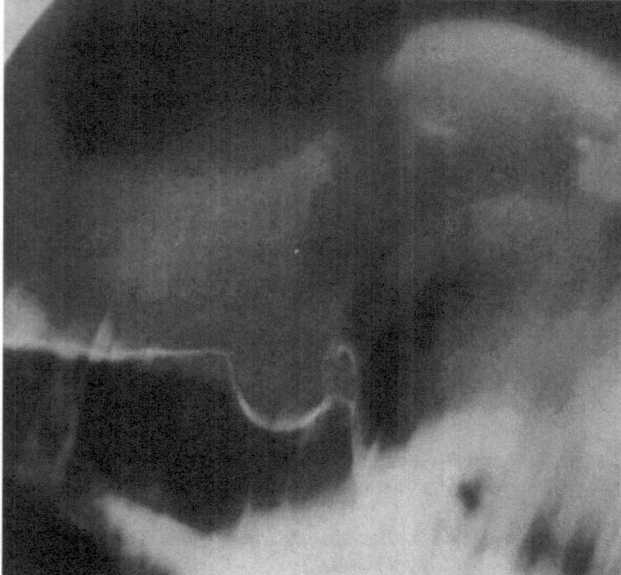

Fig. 1b

Trans-Sphenoidal Microsurgery in the Management of Non-Pituitary Tumours of the Sella Turcica

F. Grisoli, F. Vincentelli, P. Farnarier, J. Gondim-Oliveira, and
R.P. Vigouroux

The advantages of a rhinoseptal approach in the neurosurgical management of pituitary tumours are now well accepted. It was its harmlessness, rapidity and selectivity towards pituitary tissue which led us to choose it instead of any other one. This trans-sphenoidal approach can also be used for several non-pituitary tumours providing that they are also in relation to the sella. The origin of these tumours may thus be intrasellar, suprasellar, infrasellar or even lateral to the sella. Schoffer (1907) tapped a cystic craniopharyngioma by endonasal puncture and Halstead (6) (1909) performed the first trans-sphenoidal approach to a dysembryoplastic tumour. From 1975 to 1980 we operated on 279 pituitary adenomas by the trans-sphenoidal approach. During the same period, the same technique was used for 27 non-pituitary tumours of the sella turcica area (Table 1). Primary or secondary empty sella, benign purely intrasellar cysts and total hypophysectomy for metastatic breast carcinoma were excluded from this series. The 27 cases are divided into: 11 craniopharyngiomas, three chordomas, one chondroma, two dermoid cysts, seven sphenoidal tumours, two giant arachnoidal cysts and one glioma of the suprasellar area invading the skull base.

Craniopharyngiomas

First described in 1904 by Erdheim, this type of tumour has been studied in many papers which have not completely answered the problems of their surgery and evolution. We here present 11 patients (9 males, 2 females) with a sellar craniopharyngioma, who were operated on by the trans-sphenoidal approach. There are few children in this series since only six patients were under 20 years of age and only 2 were under 15 years. (The average age was 23.) Clinical features were, in all the cases, a tumour syndrome with a syndrome of endocrine deficiency. The 11 patients had severe hedaches, and three of them had intracranial hypertension with papilloedema. There was a decrease in visual acuity and field changes in seven of them. In three cases of large suprasellar extensions, an oculomotor palsy was noted (hemiplegia was also encountered in one case). Endocrine deficiency was noted in all patients, with panhypopituitarism in nine cases and an amenorrhoea-galactorrhoea syndrome in two cases. True diabetes insipidus was observed in five cases only (Table 2).

Neuroradiological examinations were carried out as follows: plain X-rays, hypocycloidal tomography, CT scan and, more rarely, pneumoencephalography. Various bone

Table 1. Breakdown of cases operated on using the trans-sphenoidal approach

---

Pituitary tumors (n = 279)

Non-secreting	36
Prolactinomas	160
Acromegalic	65
Cushing adenomas	18

Non-adenomatous sellar tumours (n = 27)

Dysembryoplastic tumours

Craniopharyngiomas	11
Dermoid cysts	2
Chordomas	3
Chondroma	1

Sphenoidal sinus tumours

Mucocele	1
Cylindromas	2
Adenocarcinomas	2
Metastases	2

Intra- and suprastellar arachnoidal cysts	2
Glioma invading the sellar region	1

Excluded from this study were cases of empty sella, intrasellar benign cyst and hypophysectomy

---

distortions of the sellar floor were observed: two normal sella turcica, six vezina grade I or II distortions, three grade III or IV distortions. Plain X-ray examination showed five cases of intra- or suprasellar calcification which helped in the diagnosis. CT scan was always positive and showed a variable suprasellar extension in nine cases (Fig. 1). Guiot encephalographical classification adapted to these suprasellar extensions allowed us to describe three type A cases, four type B and two type C. Among these 11 patients, two had already been operated on by a sub-frontal approach four and five years before, a third one with ventriculoperitoneal shunt, and a fourth one with a sub-frontal approach had also undergone a stereotaxic tapping of a cyst and interstial irradiation. These 11 patients thus had a trans-sphenoidal approach, with TV control and under the microscope according to the technique of Guiot and Hardy. In two cases calcifications were found which had not been seen on the X-rays or the tomograms. Twice a clear liquid cyst was emptied and three times a cyst with cholesterol crystals; in two cases clear and cholesterol cysts were encountered together. As far as completeness of removal is concerned, even if the tumours were easily excised we could never be sure of removal of the capsule.

Death unhappily occurred ten days postoperatively for the polyoperated case which was a pre-operative stage II coma with a right hemiplegia. The surgical indication was the presence of a very large suprasellar and intrasellar cyst. Concerning the other cases no postoperative rhinorrhoea, meningitis or increase of endocrine signs was noted. The tumour syndrome always improved rapidly; the seven patients with field changes recovered their vision. It must be noted, however, that these field changes recovered less rapidly and less completely than in pituitary adenomas. The present perspective is of 39 months in mean (extremes: 5 and 72). Two suprasellar recurrences of tumour were observed after three and five years.

Other Tumours

1. Chondroma (1 case). A 30-year-old man having undergone the removal of a suprasellar tumour (chondroma), was re-admitted to hospital because of recurrence of headaches and facial neuralgia (V2). Clinical features: panhypopituitarism, superior temporal quadranopsia, sella turcica type III with unhomogeneous calcifications on the X-ray (Fig. 2), type A suprasellar extension on CT scan. Operation showed a fleshy, calcified tumour, the posterior part of the sella turcica had completely disappeared, there was an aperture in the clivus dura and by the trans-sphenoidal route the basilar trunk and superior cerebellar arteries were visible. There were no immediate postoperative complications: improvement of visual signs, disappearance of facial neuralgia, no increase in the pituitary syndrome. Five years later visual field was still normal, and the patient was healthy under replacement treatment.

2. Chordomas (3 cases). These three patients (28, 48 and 63 years old) had the same clinical features, i.e. a long evolutionary period, several hospital admissions and, at the time of surgical treatment, headaches together with decrease of visual acuity and oculomotor palsies. One of the patients complained of facial neuralgia and another one had a cerebellar syndrome. Radiological features: in all three cases sellar distortions, in two cases clivus calcifications, in two cases the basilar trunk was shifted back markedly (Fig. 3). CT scan alone was unable to confirm the diagnosis. The trans-sphenoidal route certainly never resulted in a total removal of tumour but it always permitted a decompression sufficient for improvement and later for disappearance of the clinical syndrome. Postoperative radiotherapy was performed in all cases. The duration of follow-up was more than five years in the three cases. Little is known about the spontaneous evolution of chordomas, so that it is not possible for us to assert if the good result is due to the operation or due to a spontaneous remission. In view of these considerations the trans-sphenoidal approach must be choosen rather than the more damaging intracranial one.

3. Dermoid Cysts (2 cases). These two cases were completely different: one endocrine syndrome, one purely ophthalmological syndrome.

Case 1: A 38-year-old female had developed an amenorrhoea-galactorrhoea syndrome two years earlier and had recent diabetes insipidus. Plain radiological examination showed a type II sellar distortion. Endocrine results showed hyperprolactinemia reacting to TRH. Operation was easy; normal pituitary tissue was identified and preserved. Clinical signs rapidly disappeared; present follow-up: six years.

Table 2. Summary of cases of craniopharyngioma

Age at operation (years)	Sex	Symptoms	Tumour Vezina grade	Guiot class.	Calcif- ication	Prior treatment	Length of follow-up (months)	Remarks
22	M	Headache, PHP, VF	II	A			5	Vision improved, no DI GF
18	M	Headache, PHP, VF, oculomotor	III	C		Shunt (x2)	72	Vision improved, no DI GF
40	M	Headache, PHP, DI	II	O	Calc		48	GF
27	M	Headache, PHP, VF, somnolence, hemiplegia	0	B		Craniotomy Radiation		Death 10 days after
13	M	Headache, PHP, DI, growth reaction	0	B	Calc		48	GF
12	M	Headache, PHP, DI	II	B	Calc		30	GF
28	F	Headache, AG, VF	I	O			60	Vision improved, recurrence, craniotomy
17	M	Headache, PHP, DI, VF, growth retardation	II	A			36	Vision improved, GF
16	M	Headache, PHP, DI	II	B	Calc	Craniotomy	36	Recurrence, craniotomy

20	F	Headache, PHP, VF, diplopia	IV	C	Calc	Craniotomy	36	Vision improved, no DI,, GF
28	M	Headache, PHP, VF	III	A			12	Vision improved, no DI, GF

PHP= panhypopituitarism; AG= amenorrhoea-galactorrhoea syndrome; DI= diabetes insipidus; VF= visual failure; O= normal sella; I and II= enclosed tumours; III and IV= invading tumours; A= in the chiasmatic cistern; B= compressing the third ventricle; C= reaching the foramen of Monro; GF= good follow-up; M= male; F= female

197

Case 2: A 25-year-old male with a progressive decrease of visual acuity, without any headache and without any endocrine syndrome. On admission visual acuity was 3/10 in right and left eyes, and there was bitemporal hemianopsia. Plain X-ray examination showed a type II sellar distortion and a suprasellar calcified shell. On CT scan a low density round mass could be observed which displaced the third ventricle backwards and extended to the frontal horns (Fig. 4). The operation permitted emptying of the tumour but the calcified wall could not be removed. Nevertheless, visual acuity rapidly improved: vision in right and left eyes was 9/10 one month later. Present follow-up: 6 months.

4. Mucocele (1 case). This kind of tumour seldom concerns the neurosurgeon but they sometimes expand, mainly intracranially.

Our patient was a 51-year-old male with signs of intracranial hypertension (severe headaches and horizontal diplopia); no endocrine signs were noted. Plain X-rays showed total destruction of the sella turcica and opacity of the whole sphenoidal sinus. The pre-operative diagnosis was chordoma. Sphenoidal approach: total removal of mucocele was easily performed. Present follow-up: 6 years.

In the management of mucocele with suprasellar extension an intracranial subfrontal approach seems contra-indicated because of the high risk of postoperative meningitis.

5. Cylindromas (Adenoid Cystic Carcinoma) (2 cases). Cylindromas of the skull base are tumours with a potential for malignant evolution. They originate mostly from the lacrimal glands and ethmoidal area, and are seldom located in the sphenoid sinus. We had to operate on two patients, using the trans-sphenoidal approach (note that despite their malignancy these tumours often had a slow evolution varying from several years to some decades).

Case 1: a 40-year-old female admitted after headaches and amenorrhea-galactorrhea syndrome. X-ray examination showed a tumour of the sphenoid sinus with destruction of sellar floor. Endocrine tests: a rather high prolactin rate reacting under TRH. Pre-operative diagnosis was pituitary adenoma. During the operation a tough white well-encapsulated tumour filling the whole sphenoid sinus was discovered.

Case 2: a 57-year-old male complaining of supra-orbital headaches and of a typical V 1 facial neuralgia, without endocrine syndrome and visual signs. Tomographs and CT scan showed an intrasphenoidal neoplasm invading the cavernous sinus, which enhanced after contrast injection. Pre-operative diagnosis was primary or secondary malignant tumour. At operation the tumour presented the same macroscopic characteristics as in case 1.

From a surgical point of view these tumours are similar to meningiomas with a well visible and separable capsule. These two patients, despite postoperative radiotherapy, suffered a cavernous and subtemporal recurrence of tumour several years later and had to undergo craniectomy. Present follow-up for these two patients: six years without metastasis. These tumours have a high risk of local recurrence. This local malignancy must lead one to perform many surgical reoperations allowing sometimes a long survival.

6. Epidermoid Carcinoma of the Sphenoid (2 cases). This involved two male patients (58 and 61 years old) with the same clinical features: headaches, facial neuralgia and oculomotor palsy. Radiological findings: these tumours filled the sphenoid sinus with marked destruction of sellar floor. Operation consisted only of a large decompression with biopsy, in both cases. Despite radio- and chemotherapy the two patients died 6 and 8 months later.

7. Metastasis (2 cases). We excluded from this study metastases of breast carcinomas found during hypophysectomies and true metastases which had not been operated on.

Case 1: a 58-year-old female operated on two years earlier for a hypernephroma.

Case 2: a 74-year-old male with a prevalent metastasis and who was later shown to have a bronchial carcinoma.

In both cases clinical data evolved acutely: headaches, decrease of visual acuity, oculomotor palsy and diabetes insipidus. A complete destruction of the sellar region was observed with a high density sellar and bicavernous lesion visible on CT scan. Operation was undertaken in order to obtain decompression and to help diagnosis. As with the epidermoid carcinomas, the result was bad after a short time in spite of radiotherapy.

8. Intra- and Supra-sellar Arachnoid Cysts (2 cases). These observations concerned two male patients (60 and 62 years old) with severe headaches and a marked visual syndrome without endocrine signs. Radiologically it was noted that sellar volume was increased slightly and that a large intracranial extension displaced the third ventricle floor upwards. On the CT scan this suprasellar expansion had a low density. Cyst emptying by a transsphenoidal approach was very easy and very good results were obtained after 4 and 5 years, respectively.

9. Glioma of the Sellar Region (1 case). This observation involves a very rare invasion of the skull base by a glial tumour. A 19-year-old male with retardation of growth and delayed puberty took opthalmological advice because of a great decrease of visual acuity and for recent headaches, without diabetes insipidus. Ophtalmological data: vision 1/20, R.E., 1/40 L.E. and papillitis. X-rays showed enlargement of the sella turcica with localized invasion. CT scan showed a very large non-cystic, partly calcified suprasellar tumour which obstructed the foramina of Monro. Clinical and radiological conclusions suggested a craniopharyngioma. Operation gave histological data which corrected the diagnosis. The patient was then shunted and operated by craniectomy and submitted to radiotherapy. The tumour probably originated from the floor of the third ventricle. Present follow-up: 3 years and 6 months. Headaches recovered but visual acuity did not improve.

Discussion

From 1975 to 1980, 279 pituitary adenomas were operated on (F.G.). The relatively few postoperative complications (death: 1 case= 0.35%) led us to follow Rougerie, Hardy and Laws and to extend the use of the trans-sphenoidal approach. We operated on 27 patients without CSF fistula meningitis or increase in endocrine signs. One patient died but he had presented with a craniopharyngioma and in a bad state of health.

He had been submitted to previous operation and suffered from intracranial hypertension with alteration of consciousness and hemiplegia. It appears that craniopharyngiomas with sellar involvment can be operated on by the trans-sphenoidal approach. This operation helps the treatment of the clinical tumour syndrome (particularly visual signs). As far as the tumour capsule is concerned, we were never sure of the total removal of the tumour, as compared to Hardy. Considering unforeseeable spontaneous evolution and the possible radiosensitivity of these tumours (14), and the risks of "at all costs" tumour excision by craniectomy, the trans-sphenoidal approach should be chosen whenever possible. This opinion is strengthened by the fact that histological examination did not confirm total tumour removal.

For chondromas and chordomas the surgical approaches do not seem to be as much discussed as for craniopharyngiomas. We think, like Rougerie (17) and Hardy (10, 12), that tumour removal must be as complete as possible using the less damaging approach: the trans-sphenoidal one.

In benign or malignant tumours originating from the sphenoid sinus, whatever the degree of intracranial extension, the trans-sphenoidal approach allows total removal of mucoceles, a radical removal of cylindromas and a biopsy of primary or secondary carcinomas in the sellar region.

Using the trans-sphenoidal approach we were able to operate on tumours which were very different in nature, in extent or in evolution. These lesions could often have been dealt with by craniectomy according to data in the literature but the trans-sphenoidal approach could well be the first choice for a surgical intervention.

References

1. Alonso, W., Black, P.: Transoral trans-sphenoidal approach for resection of clival chordomas. Laryngoscope *81*, 1628–1691 (1971)
2. Bartlett, J.R.: Craniopharyngiomas. Summary of 85 cases. J. Neurol. Neurosurg. Psychiat. *34*, 37–41 (1971)
3. Calvet, J., Claux, J.: Les craniopharyngiomes – le traitement par voie basse. Rev. Otoneuroopht. *27*, 121–128 (1955)
4. Derome, P.: Les tumeurs sphéno-ethmoïdales. Possibilité d'exérèse et de réparation chirurgicale. Neuro-Chirurgie *18*, Suppl. 1, 4–164 (1972)
5. Falconer, M.A., Bailey, I.C., Duchen, L.W.: Surgical treatment of chordoma and chondroma of the skull base. J. Neurosurg. *29*, 261–275 (1968)
6. Halsteadt, A.E.: Remarks on the operative treatment of tumors of the hypophysis with report of two cases operated only an oronasal method. Trans. Amer. Soc. J. *28*, 73–93 (1910)
7. Hamberger, C.A., Hammer, G., Norlen, G., Sjogren, B.: Surgical treatment of craniopharyngioma. Radical removal by the trans-sphenoidal approach. Acta Otolaryngol (Stockh) *52*, 285–292 (1960)
8. Hamer, J.: Removal of craniopharyngiomas by sub-nasal trans-sphenoidal operation. Neuropediatric *9*, 312–319 (1978)
9. Hardy, J., Lalonde, J.L.: Exérèse par voie trans-sphenoidale d'un craniopharyngiome géant. L'Union Médicale du Canada *92*, 1124–1129 (1963)
10. Hardy, J., Bertrand, C., Maltais, R., Robert, F., Thierry, A.: Volumineux chondrosarcome calcifié de la région sellaire. Neurochirurgie *12*, 491–502 (1966)
11. Hardy, J., Vezina, J.L.: Trans-sphenoidal neurosurgery of intracranial neoplasm. In: Neoplasia in the central nervous system. Advances in neurology, vol. 15, Thompson, R.A., Green, J.R. (eds). pp. 261–274. New York: Raven Press 1976

12. Hardy, J., Grisoli, F., Leclerq, T.A., Marino, R.: L'abord trans-sphenoidal des tumeurs du clivus. Neurochirurgie *23*, 287–297 (1977)

13. Kerm, E.B.: The trans-septal approach to lesions of the pituitary and parasellar regions. Laryngoscope *89*, 1–34 (1979)

14. Kramer, S., Southard, M., Mansfield, C.M.: Radiotherapy in the management of craniopharyngiomas. Further experience and late results. Am. J. Roentgen *103*, 44–52 (1968)

15. Laws, E.R.: Trans-sphenoidal microsurgery in the management of craniopharyngioma. J. Neurosurg. *52*, 661–666 (1980)

16. Laws, E.R., Kern, E.B.: Complications of trans-sphenoidal surgery. Clin. Neurosurg. *23*, 401–416 (1976)

17. Rougerie, J., Guiot, G., Bouche, J., Trigo, J.C.: Les voies d'abord des chordomes du clivus. Neurochirurgie *13*, 5, 559–570 (1967)

18. Shapiro, K., Till, K., Grant, D.N.: Craniopharyngiomas in Childhood. J. Neurosurg. *50*, 617–623 (1979)

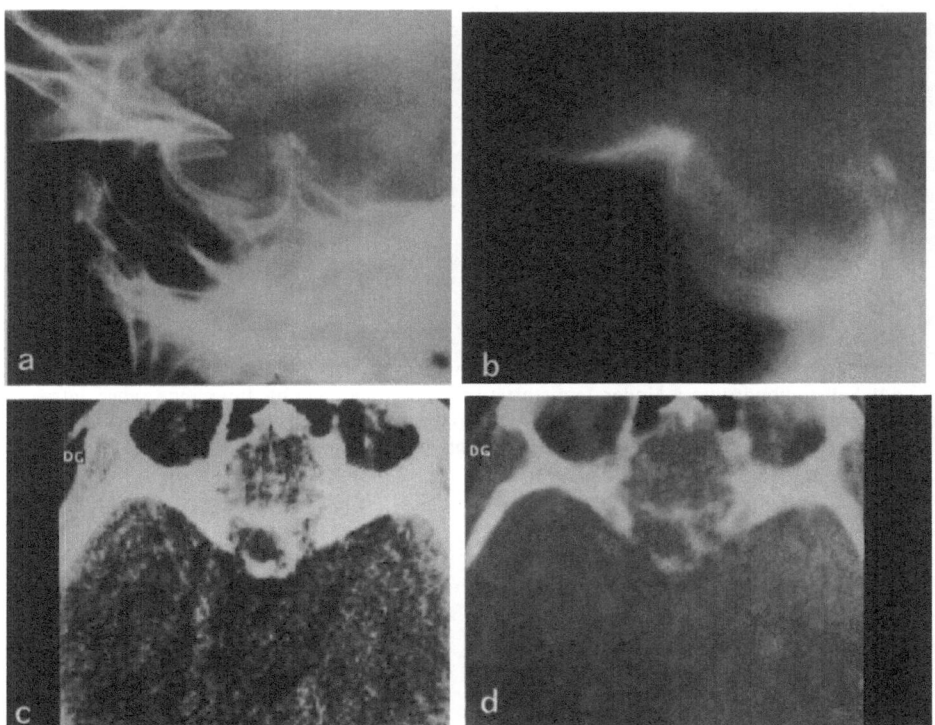

Fig. 1 a-d. Sellar and suprasellar craniopharyngioma. **a** Lateral view: distortion of sella turcica. **b** Lateral tomography: enlarged sella without changes in floor, intracellar calcification. **c, d** CT scan: suprasellar calcification with probable intratumoral cyst

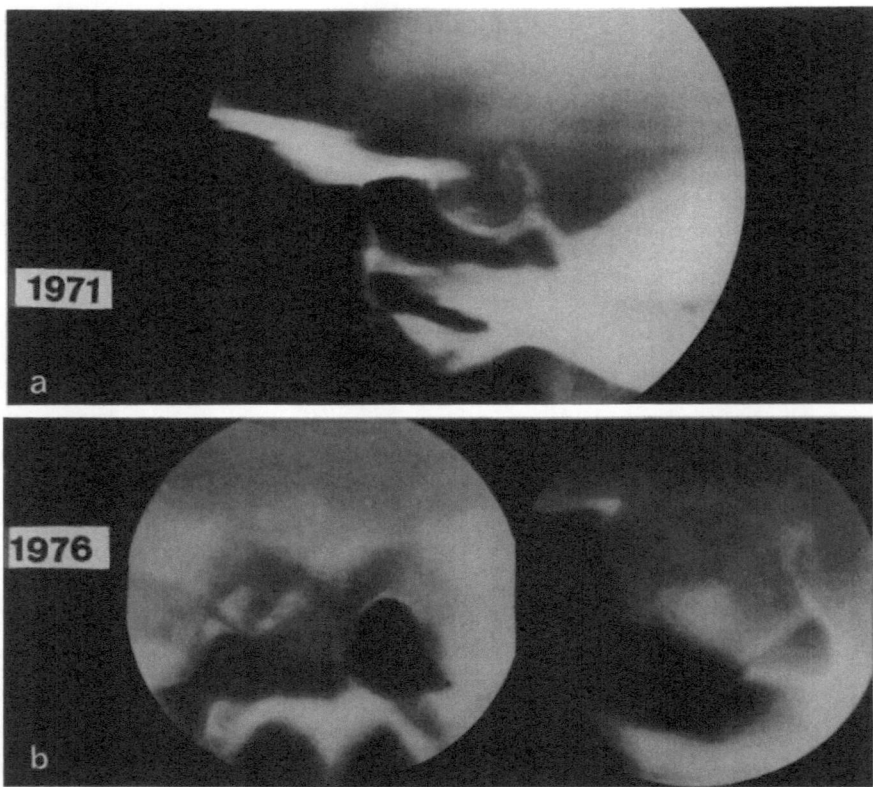

Fig. 2 a,b. Sellar chondroma. **a** Moderate distortion of sella turcica, double floor appearance, intrasellar calcifications. Patient operated on by a subfrontal approach at this time. **b** Five years later the sellar floor was broken down by the tumour with many non-homogeneous calcifications

202

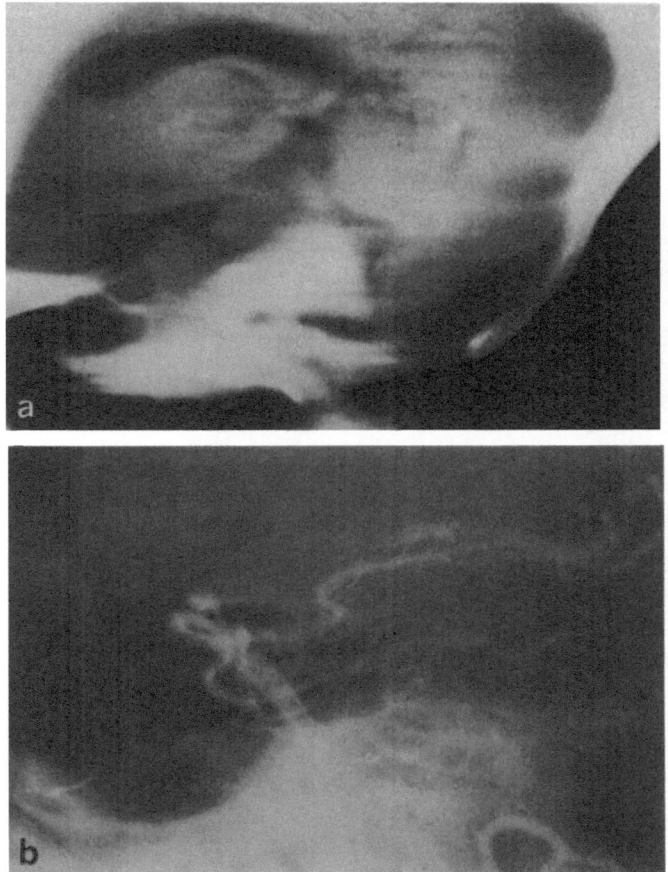

Fig. 3 a,b. Clivosellar chordoma. **a** Pneumo-encephalography: thickening of clivus, filling of the pre-pontine cistern and shift of brain stem. **b** Vertebral angiography: basilar trunk is shifted backwards by clivus tumour

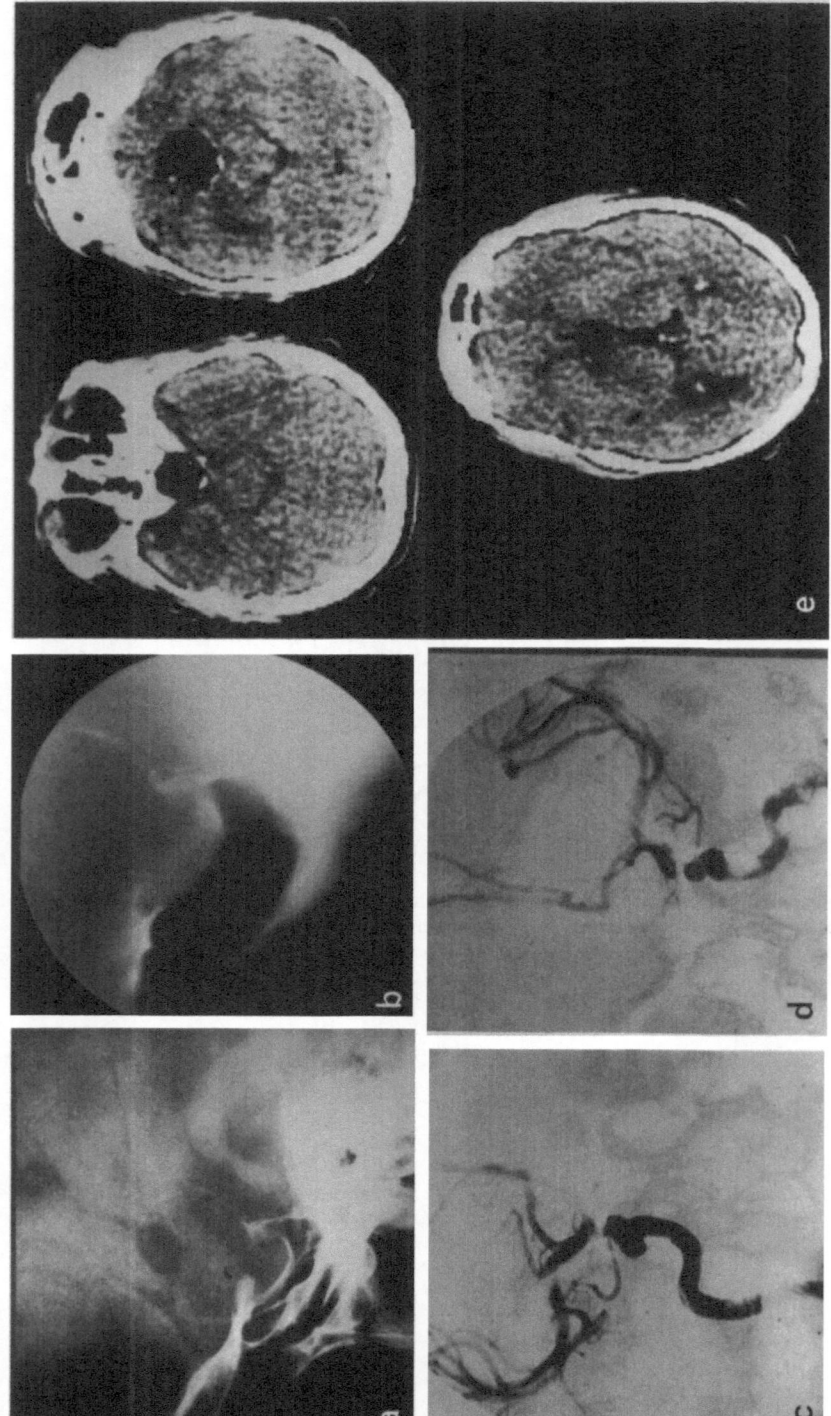

Fig. 4 a–e. Sellar and suprasellar dermoid cyst. **a,b** On lateral view and tomograms, floor of sella turcica was lower than normal but sella seemed enlarged upwards. Above the dorsum sellae the thin calcified shell of the cyst must be noted. **c,d** Bilateral carotid angiography on frontal seriographies confirms the existence of a suprasellar extension. **e** CT scan: low density (fat density) sellar and suprasellar tumour, covered behind by a round calcified shell

Microsurgical Anatomy of the Third Ventricle *

I. Yamamoto, A.L. Rhoton, Jr., and D.A. Peace

Introduction

The third ventricle is located in the centre of the head, below the corpus callosum and the body of the lateral ventricle, above the sella turcica, pituitary gland and midbrain and between the cerebral hemispheres, thalami and hypothalami. It is intimately related to the circle of Willis and its branches, and the great vein of Galen and its tributaries. Tumours in the region of the third ventricle are among the most difficult to expose and remove. Twenty-five cadaveric brains were examined in detail to evaluate the surgically important relationships of the walls of the third ventricle (1, 2).

Neural Relationships

The third ventricle has a roof, a floor and an anterior, posterior and two lateral walls (Fig. 1).

Roof. The roof of the third ventricle extends from the foramen of Monro to the suprapineal recess. The roof has four layers: one neural layer formed by the fornix, two thin membranous layers of tela choroidea and a layer of blood vessels between the sheets of tela choroidea. The upper layer of the anterior part of the roof of the third ventricle is formed by the body of the fornix and the posterior part of the roof is formed by the crura and the hippocampal commissures.

The tela choroidea forms two of the three layers in the roof below the layer formed by the fornix. The tela choroidea consists of two thin, semiopaque membranes derived from pia mater, which are interconnected by loosely organized trabeculae. The final layer is a vascular layer located between the two layers of tela choroidea. The vascular layer consists of the medial posterior choroidal arteries and their branches and the internal cerebral veins and their tributaries. Parallel strands of choroid plexus project downward on each side of the midline from the inferior layer of tela choroidea into the superior part of the third ventricle.

The lateral margin of the roof is formed by the cleft between the lateral edge of the fornix and the superomedial surface of the thalamus. This narrow cleft between the

* Supported in part by the National Institutes of Health, Grant No. NS 10978-03

fornix and the thalamus, which in its entirely is C-shaped, is called the choroidal fissure. The choroid plexus of the lateral ventricle is attached along this fissure. The fornix forms the outer margin of the C-shaped fissure and the thalamus forms the inner margin. In the body of the ventricle, the choroidal fissure is limited by the body of the fornix superiorly and by the thalamus inferiorly; in the atrium by the crus of the fornix posteriorly and the pulvinar anteriorly; and in the inferior horn by the fimbria of the fornix below and the striae terminalis and thalamus above. The tela choroidea forming the pedicle of the choroid plexus of the third ventricle is continuous through the choroidal fissure with the choroid plexus in the lateral ventricle.

Floor. The floor extends from the optic chiasm anteriorly to the orifice of the aqueduct of Sylvius posteriorly. The anterior half of the floor is formed by diencephalic structures and the posterior half is formed by mesencephalic structures. The structures forming the floor from anterior to posterior include the optic chiasm, the infundibulum of the hypothalamus, the tuber cinereum, the mamillary bodies, the posterior perforated substance and most posteriorly the part of the tegmentum of the midbrain located above the medial aspect of the cerebral peduncles. The optic chiasm is located at the junction of the floor and the anterior wall of the third ventricle.

Anterior Wall. The anterior margin of the third ventricle extends from the foramen of Monro above to the optic chiasm below. Only the lower two-thirds of the anterior surface is seen on the external surface of the brain; the upper one-third is hidden behind the rostrum of the corpus callosum. The part of the anterior wall visible on the surface is formed by the optic chiasm and the lamina terminalis. When viewed from within, the boundaries of the anterior wall from above downwards are formed by the columns of the fornix, foramen of Monro, anterior commissure, lamina terminalis, optic recess and the optic chiasm. The foramen of Monro is located at the junction of the roof and the anterior wall.

Posterior Wall. The posterior wall of the third ventricle extends from the suprapineal recess above to the aqueduct of Sylvius below. When viewed from anteriorly and within the third ventricle, it consists, from above to below, of the suprapineal recess, the habenular commissure, pineal body and its recess, the posterior commissure and the aqueduct of Sylvius.

When viewed from posteriorly, the only structure in the posterior wall is the pineal body. The pineal gland projects posteriorly into the quadrigeminal cisterns and is concealed by the splenium of the corpus callosum above, the thalami laterally and the lamina quadrigemina plate and the vermis of the cerebellum inferiorly.

Lateral Wall. The lateral walls are not visible on the external surface of the brain, but are hidden between the cerebral hemispheres. Each is formed by the hypothalamus inferiorly and the thalamus superiorly.

Arterial Relationships

Each wall of the third ventricle has surgically important arterial relationships (Fig. 2): The posterior part of the circle of Willis and the apex of the basilar artery are below the floor; the anterior part of the circle of Willis and the anterior cerebral and anterior communicating arteries are intimately related to the anterior wall; the posterior cerebral, pericallosal, superior cerebellar and choroidal arteries pass adjacent to the posterior wall; both the anterior and posterior cerebral arteries send branches into the roof; and the internal carotid, anterior choroidal, anterior and posterior cerebral and anterior and posterior communicating arteries give rise to perforating branches that reach the walls of the third ventricle.

Venous Relationships

The deep cerebral venous system is intimately related to the walls of the third ventricle (Fig. 3). It represents a formidable obstacle to the operative approaches to the third ventricle, especially in the region of the pineal gland where the internal cerebral vein and the basal vein of Rosenthal converge on the great vein of Galen. The internal cerebral vein originates from multiple tributaries at the foramen of Monro and courses posteriorly in the roof of the third ventricle, between the two layers of the tela choroidea. It unites with its fellow from the opposite side to form the great vein of Galen.

The great vein, after being formed by the union of the internal cerebral veins, passes posteriorly to join the straight sinus. The major tributaries of the great vein are the internal cerebral and basal veins, but it also receives blood from numerous other veins in the region. The basal vein originates on the surface of the anterior perforated substance by the union of multiple veins. It courses around the cerebral peduncle and the pulvinar to join the great vein of Galen or the internal cerebral vein in the quadrigeminal cistern. The internal cerebral, basal and great veins drain the walls of the lateral and third ventricles, the periventricular white and grey matter, the corpus callosum, thalamus, septum pellucidum, upper midbrain, choroid plexus of the lateral and third ventricles and the superior part of the cerebellum.

Discussion

The operative approaches to the third ventricle are divided on the basis of whether they are suitable for reaching the anterior or posterior part of the third ventricle (2). The approaches suitable for lesions within or compressing the anterior portion of the third ventricle are the trans-sphenoidal, subfrontal, frontotemporal, subtemporal, anterior transcallosal and the anterior transventricular. The approaches suitable for reaching the posterior portion of the third ventricle are the posterior transcallosal, posterior transventricular, occipital transtentorial and the infratentorial supracerebellar (Fig. 4). The selection of the best operative approach for a given tumour of the third ventricle depends on the site of origin, path of growth and location of the tumour, the site of compression of the third ventricle, and whether there is ventricular obstruction.

The most common third ventricular tumours begin in the pituitary gland and grow upward to compress the anterior inferior part of the third ventricle. The trans-sphenoidal approach is preferred for all those tumours involving the anterior inferior part of the third ventricle that are located above a pneumatized sphenoid sinus and extend upward out of an enlarged sella turcica. The subfrontal intracranial approach is used for those tumours involving the anterior inferior part of the third ventricle that are not accessible by the trans-sphenoidal route because they do not extend into the sella turcica, are separated from the sella by a layer of neural tissue, are located entirely within the third ventricle, extend upward out of a normal or small sella or are located above a non-pneumatized (conchal) type of sphenoid sinus. The subfrontal approach permits exposure of the tumour by four routes: subchiasmatic, opticocarotid, lamina terminalis and transfrontal trans-sphenoidal. The subchiasmatic approach is used most commonly because the subchiasmatic space is usually enlarged by the tumour. The opticocarotid route is selected if parasellar extension of the tumour widens the interval between the carotid artery and the optic nerve and the tumour cannot be reached by the subchiasmatic approach. The lamina terminalis approach is selected for tumours located above the sella turcica, below the foramen of Monro in the antero-inferior part of the third ventricle, if the tumour has pushed the chiasm into a prefixed position and has distended and stretched the lamina terminalis so that the tumour is visible through it. The transfrontal trans-sphenoidal approach is selected if the sphenoid sinus is pneumatized and the tumour does not stretch the lamina terminalis or widen the opticocarotid space and a prefixed chiasm blocks the subchiasmatic exposure.

The anterior transcallosal approach is suitable for lesions located in the anterosuperior part of the third ventricle or if the tumour extends out of the superior part of the third ventricle into one or both lateral ventricles near the foramen of Monro. The transcallosal approaches are easier than the transventricular approaches to perform if the ventricles are of a normal size or are minimally enlarged. The anterior transventricular approach is suitable for approaching tumours in the anterior superior part of the third ventricle, especially if the tumour has a major extension into the anterior part of the lateral ventricle on the side of the approach. It is more difficult to expose the anterior part of the lateral ventricle on the side opposite the craniotomy through the transventricular than through the transcallosal approach. The transventricular approach enters the lateral ventricle in a favourable location for exposing the superior half of the anterior part of the third ventricle by the subchoroidal approach or for biopsy or removal of the tumour through an enlarged foramen of Monro. The subchoroidal approach is suitable for exposing tumours in the anterior two-thirds of the superior half of the third ventricle in the area below the roof and posterior to the foramen of Monro.

The frontotemporal and subtemporal approaches are similar except that the subtemporal approach may be used to expose the parasellar region as far posteriorly as the interpeduncular region and basilar bifurcation. These approaches are used if the tumour is centred lateral to the sella, extends into the middle cranial fossa or appears to be approachable through the space between the optic nerve and carotid artery anteriorly and the oculomotor nerve posteriorly.

Tumour in the posterior part of the third ventricle may be approached from above the tentorium, through the posterior part of the lateral ventricle, through the corpus callosum, or along the medial surface of the occipital region or from below the tentorium through the supracerebellar space. The infratentorial supracerebellar approach is preferred for most tumours in the pineal region because the deep venous system which caps the dorsal and lateral aspects of pineal tumours does not obstruct access to the tumour. The approach is best suited to those tumours which are in the midline and which grow into both the posterior part of the third ventricle and into the posterior fossa, displacing the lamina quadrigemina plate and the anterior lobe of the cerebellum. The infratentorial supracerebellar approach is not well suited to the tumour which has a significant extension above the tentorium or grows from the thalamus or corpus callosum into the third ventricle. The occiptial transtentorial approach is preferred for tumours centred at or above the tentorial edge if there is not a major extension of tumour to the opposite side or into the posterior fossa and for those located above the great vein of Galen. The posterior transcallosal approaches would be used only for tumours that have a major upward extension into the posterior part of the corpus callosum or if the tumour appears to arise in the corpus callosum above the great vein of Galen and extends into the posterior part of the third ventricle. The posterior transventricular approach provides adequate exposure of the atrium and posterior portion of the body of the lateral ventricle and would be the preferred approach to a tumour involving the posterior part of the third ventricle if it extends into the posterior part of the thalamus or involves the atrium of the lateral ventricle or the glomus of the choroid plexus.

General Operative Principles

These principles apply to all of the operative approaches discussed above.

1. Incisions in neural tissue and sacrifice of neural structures should be minimized. It is impossible to reach the cavity of the third ventricle without incising some neural structures. The brain may be retracted to expose an external wall of the third ventricle but then the wall must be incised to reach its cavity. The fornix and lamina terminalis are common sites of incision in the wall of the third ventricle. In other cases, the cerebral cortex or corpus callosum is incised to reach the lateral ventricle and then another neural incision is frequently needed to expose the third ventricle adequately from the lateral ventricle. The consequences of injury to the neural structures incised in reaching the third ventricle are reviewed elsewhere (1, 2).

2. The arteries that pass over the tumour capsule to neural tissues should be preserved. Any vessel that stands above the surface of the capsule should be dealt with initially as if it were a vessel supplying the brain. An attempt should be made to displace the vessel off the tumour capsule using a small dissector after the tumour has been removed from within the capsule. Numerous arteries are exposed in removing tumours of the third ventricle: the posterior part of the circle of Willis and the apex of the basilar artery are below the floor; the anterior part of the circle of Willis and the anterior cerebral and anterior communicating arteries are intimately related to the anterior wall; the posterior cerebral, pericallosal, superior cerebellar and choroidal arteries pass adjacent to the posterior wall; both the anterior and posterior cerebral arteries send branches into the roof; and the internal carotid, anterior choroidal, anterior and posterior cerebral

and anterior and posterior communicating arteries give rise to perforating branches that reach the walls of the third ventricle. Only infrequently should any of these be sacrified in removing a tumour. Occlusion of these major trunks or their perforating branches at the anterior part of the circle of Willis is likely to result in disturbances in memory and personality, and occlusion of those at the posterior part of the circle of Willis is more likely to result in disorders of the level of consciousness and of extraocular movement.

3. The number of veins sacrificed should be kept to a minimum because of the undesirable consequences of their loss. Obliteration of the deep veins, including the great, basal and internal cerebral veins and their tributaries and the bridging veins from the cerebrum and cerebellum to the dural sinuses is unavoidable in reaching and removing some tumours. Before sacrificing the bridging veins, one should try placing them under moderate or even severe stretch, accepting the fact that they may be torn, if it will allow satisfactory exposure and yield some possibility of the veins being saved. Before sacrificing the basal, internal cerebral and great veins, try working around them or displacing them out of the operative route or try dividing only a few of their small branches which may prevent displacing the main trunk out of the operative field.

References

1. Yamamoto, I., Rhoton, A.L., Jr., Peace, D.A.: Microsurgery of the third ventricle, Part I: Microsurgical anatomy. Neurosurgery 8, 334–356 (1981)
2. Rhoton, A.L., Jr., Yamamoto, I., Peace, D.A.: Microsurgery of the third ventricle, Part II: Operative approaches. Neurosurgery 8, 357–373 (1981)

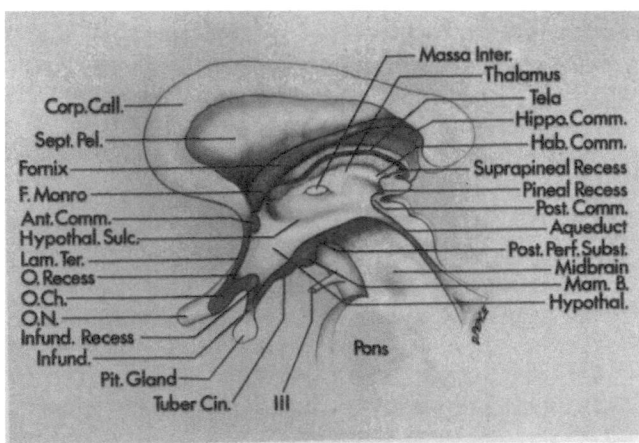

Fig. 1. Midsagittal section of the third ventricle. The floor extends from the optic chiasm *(O.Ch.)* to the aqueduct of Sylvius and includes the lower surface of the optic chiasm, the infundibulum *(Infund.)*, the infundibular recess *(Infund. Recess)*, the pituitary gland *(Pit. Gland)*, the tuber cinereum *(Tuber Cin.)*, the mamillary bodies *(Mam. B.)*, the posterior perforated substance *(Post. Perf. Subst.)*, and the part of the midbrain anterior to the aqueduct. The anterior wall extends from the optic chiasm to the foramen of Monro *(F. Monro)* and includes the upper surface of the optic chiasm, the optic recess *(O. Recess)*, the lamina terminalis *(Lam. Ter.)*, the anterior commissure *(Ant. Comm.)*, and the foramen of Monro. The roof extends from the foramen of Monro to the suprapineal recess and is formed by the fornix and the layers of tela choroidea *(Tela)*, between which course the internal cerebral vein and the medial posterior choroidal artery. The hippocampal commissure *(Hippo. Comm.)*, corpus callosum *(Corp. Call.)*, and septum pellucidum *(Sept. Pel.)* are above the roof. The posterior wall extends from the suprapineal recess to the aqueduct and includes the habenular commissure *(Hab. Comm.)*, pineal gland, pineal recess, and posterior commissure *(Post. Comm.)*. The oculomotor nerve *(III)* exits from the midbrain. The hypothalamic sulcus *(Hypothal. Sulc.)* forms a groove between the thalamic and hypothalamic *(Hypothal.)* surfaces of the third ventricle. [See Yamamoto, I. et al. (1)]

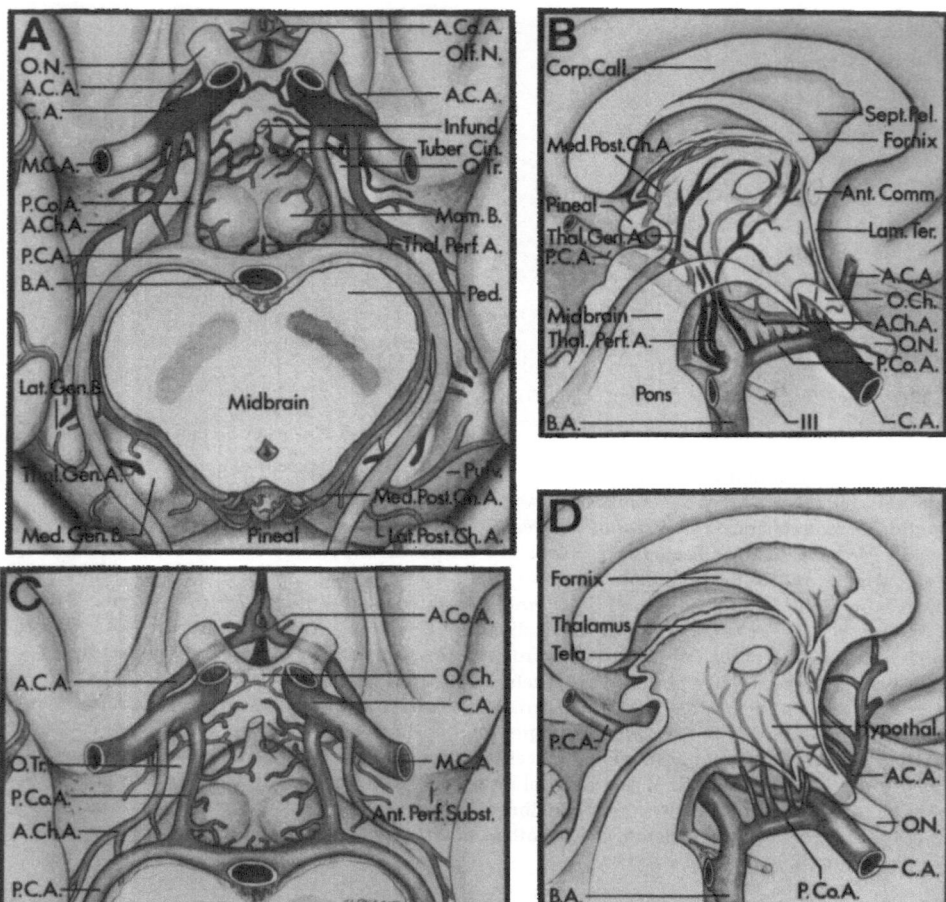

Fig. 2 A–D. Arterial relationships of the third ventricle. **A** and **C** are inferior views of the floor of the third ventricle, and **B** and **D** are midsagittal sections through the third ventricle. **A** and **B** show the relationship of the main trunks and perforating branches of the following arteries to the third ventricle: internal carotid *(C.A.)*, anterior choroidal *(A.Ch. A.)*, basilar apex *(B. A.)*, posterior cerebral *(P. C. A.)*, medial posterior choroidal *(Med. Post. Ch. A.)*, lateral posterior choroidal *(Lat. Post. Ch. A.)*, thalamoperforating *(Thal. Perf. A.)*, and thalamogeniculate *(Thal. Gen. A.)* arteries. **C** and **D** show the relationships of the main trunks and perforating branches of the following arteries to the third ventricle: anterior cerebral *(A. C. A.)*, anterior communicating *(A. Co. A.)*, and posterior communicating arteries. The olfactory *(Olf. N.)* and optic *(O. N.)* nerves are anterior to the floor of the third ventricle. The structures in the floor are the optic chiasm *(O. Ch.)*, optic tracts *(O. Tr.)*, infundibulum *(Infund.)* tuber cinereum *(Tuber Cin.)*, and mamillary bodies *(Mam. B.)*. The midbrain and cerebral peduncles *(Ped.)* are inferior to the posterior half of the floor. The anterior perforated substance *(Ant. Perf. Subst.)* is lateral to the optic tracts. The lateral geniculate *(Lat. Gen. B.)* and medial geniculate *(Med. Gen. B.)* bodies are attached to the lower margin of the thalamus near the pulvinar *(Pulv.)*, lateral to the midbrain. The structures in the anterior wall of the third ventricle are the anterior commissure *(Ant. Comm.)*, lamina terminalis *(Lam. Ter.)*, and optic chiasm. The corpus callosum *(Corp. Call.)* and septum pellucidum *(Sept. Pel.)* are above the roof of the third ventricle. The roof is formed of the two layers of tela choroidea *(Tela)*, the fornix, and a vascular layer composed of the internal cerebral veins and the medial posterior choroidal arteries. The oculomotor nerve *(III)* comes out of the midbrain. [See Yamamoto, I. et al. (1)]

212

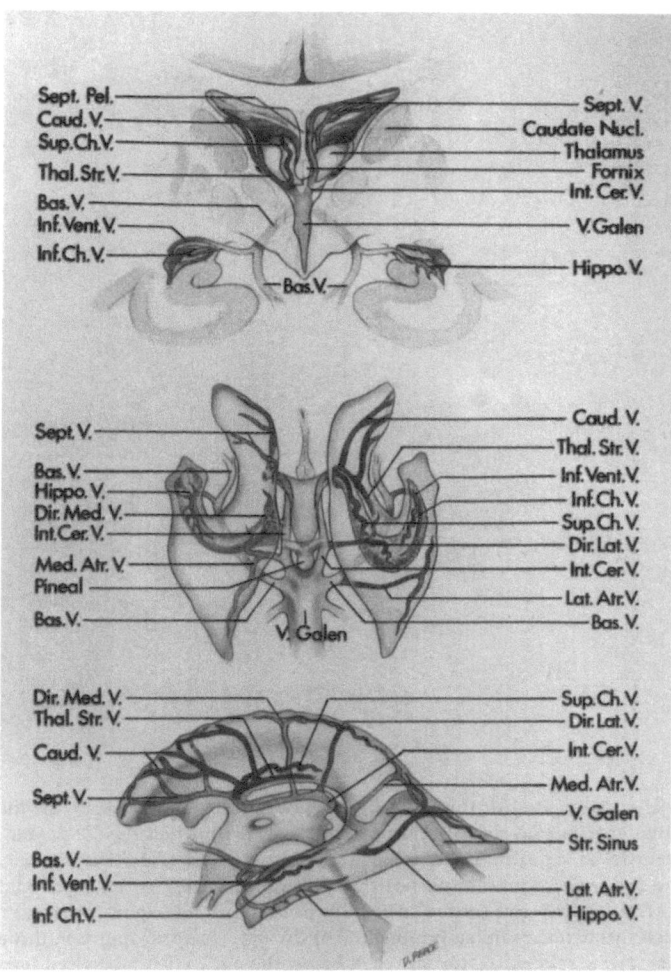

Fig. 3. Schematic drawing of the deep venous system of the cerebral hemispheres. *Top:* Anterior view of a cross section of the cerebrum through the third ventricle and the frontal and temporal horns of the lateral ventricles. *Middle:* Superior view of veins in the lateral and third ventricles. *Bottom:* Lateral view of veins draining the lateral and third ventricles. The drainage of the lateral ventricle is divided into a medial and a lateral group of veins that drain into the three major deep veins: internal cerebral *(Int. Cer. V.)*, basal *(Bas. V.)*, and great *(V. Galen)* vein of Galen. The lateral group in the frontal horn and body is composed of the caudate *(Caud. V.)*, thalamostriate *(Thal. Str. V.)*, and direct lateral *(Dir. Lat. V.)* veins; in the atrium it is the lateral atrial vein *(Lat. Atr. V.)*; and in the temporal horn it is the inferior ventricular vein *(Inf. Vent. V.)*. The medial group in the anterior horn and body is formed by the septal *(Sept. V.)* and direct medial *(Dir. Med. V.)* veins; in the atrium it is the medial atrial vein *(Med. Atr. V.)*; and in the temporal horn it is the hippocampal veins *(Hippo. V.)*. The superior choroidal veins *(Sup. Ch. V.)* drain into the thalamostriate and internal cerebral veins, and the inferior choroidal veins *(Inf. Ch. V.)* drain into the inferior ventricular vein, which in turn drains into the basal vein. The great vein of Galen drains into the straight sinus *(Str. Sinus)*. The thalamostriate vein runs in the groove between the thalamus and the caudate nucleus *(Caudate Nucl.)*. The septal veins cross the septum pellucidum *(Sept. Pel.)* and fornix. [See Yamamoto, I. et al. (1)]

213

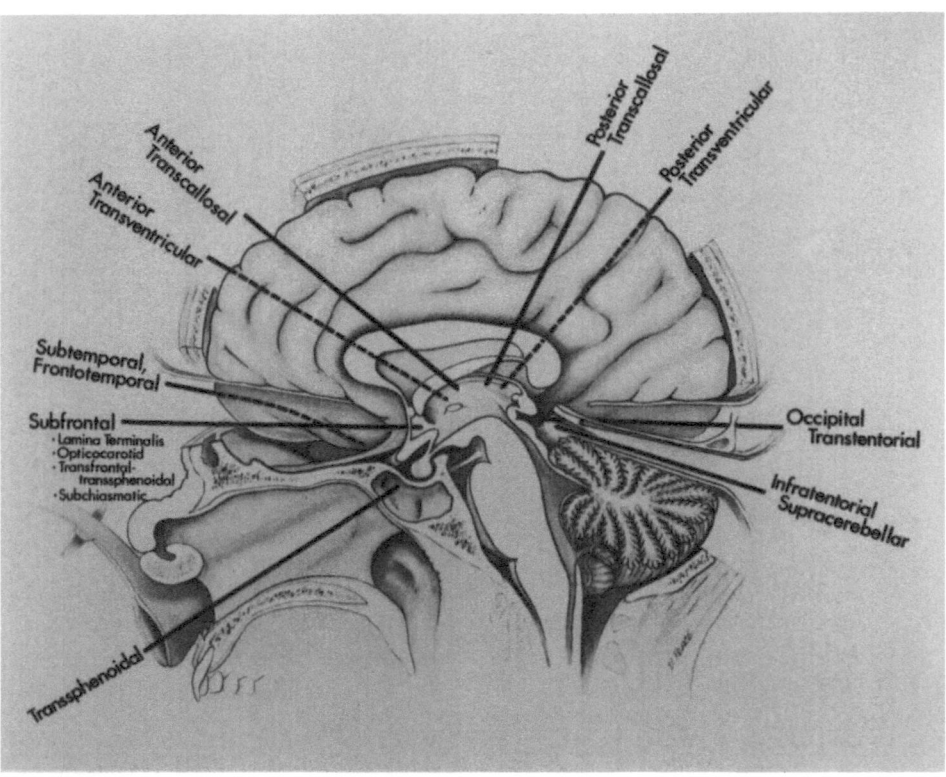

Fig. 4. Midsagittal view of the head shows the operative approaches to the third ventricle. The approaches that are directed along or near the midline are shown as *solid lines,* and those that approach the third ventricle away from the midline are shown as *dotted lines.* The midline or near-midline approaches to the anterior inferior part of the third ventricle are the trans-sphenoidal and the subfrontal. The subfrontal operative route is divided into four different approaches: (a) the lamina terminalis approach through the lamina terminalis; (b) the opticocarotid approach through the opticocarotid triangle; (c) the subchiasmatic approach below the optic chiasm between the optic nerves; and (d) the transfrontal trans-sphenoidal approach through the planum sphenoidale and sphenoid sinus. The approaches to the floor and anteroinferior part of the third ventricle that are directed off the midline are the subtemporal and the frontotemporal. The approaches to the anterosuperior part of the third ventricle in the region of the foramen of Monro are the anterior transcallosal and the anterior transventricular, and occipital transtentorial. The infratentorial supracerebellar approach is directed below the tentorium cerebelli to the posterior part of the third ventricle. [See Rhoton, A.L. et al. (2)]

214

Surgical Strategies in the Management of Tumours of the Anterior Third Ventricle

J.L. Antunes, K. Muraszko, D.O. Quest, and P.W. Carmel

No other area of the central nervous system harbours a wider variety of pathological entities than the sellar-suprasellar region. Lesions that develop in this area are intimately related to the anterior portion of the third ventricle and either originate from its walls or grow from adjacent structures (10).

Classification

Lesions of the anterior third ventricle can be divided into two main groups (Fig. 1).

1. *Primary intraventricular lesions* — These arise from structures that form the ventricular wall and are attached to it by a pedicle of variable width. They include *colloid cysts, choroid plexus, ependymomas, papillomas, congenital tumours (epidermoids, dermoids, teratomas), craniopharyngiomas, meningiomas,* and *gliomas.* Most of these tumours grow principally into the ventricular cavity and have a limited extension beyond their point of attachment. Non-neoplastic lesions include *ependymal cysts, mycotic granulomas* and *vascular malformations.*

2. *Secondary intraventricular lesions* — These are lesions which originate from structures adjacent to the ventricular wall. They include *craniopharyngiomas, pituitary adenomas* with suprasellar extension, *optic nerve-hypothalamic gliomas, epidermoid* and *dermoid tumours, meningiomas* and other rare neoplastic processes such as *lipomas* or *haemangiomas.* Secondary deposits from tumours such as *medulloblastomas, germinomas* and other primary neoplasms are also found in this area. Infrequently *sarcoidosis, histiocytosis-X, congenital arachnoidal cysts,* or large *intracranial aneurysms* can present as mass lesions in this situation.

Surgical Goals

The goals of surgery for lesions in this area are usually threefold:
1. to make a specific histological diagnosis;
2. to relieve pressure on local structures by removing the bulk of the lesion or if possible, by excising it totally;
3. to unblock the spinal fluid pathways.

In instances where a functioning pituitary adenoma is present, removal of the tumour may lead to the cure of the associated endocrinopathy. When a clinical syndrome consistent with hypothalamic dysfunction is present pre-operatively, surgical removal of the underlying lesion is less likely to resolve this dysfunction.

A number of surgical approaches to the anterior third ventricle have been devised. They are not mutually exclusive but rather complement each other, and although each surgeon may have his preferred route, he must be familiar with the various alternatives. For example, a surgeon who plans to approach a tumour beneath the optic chiasm may be forced, in the presence of a prefixed chiasm, to open the lamina terminalis or go through the planum sphenoidale or sphenoid sinus. Although there are a number of papers describing the different surgical techniques — which were recently summarized by Rhoton et al. (11) — little has been written on the morbidity of each approach, and how each succeeds in accomplishing the goals originally set forth.

Pre-Operative Evaluation

Before a surgical procedure for a third ventricular tumour is undertaken, careful evaluation of the possible nature of the lesion is essential. Although the clinical manifestations are of utmost importance, precise planning depends on a detailed radiographic evaluation. The relationship of the tumour to the optic apparatus, hypothalamic structures, and the vascular structures at the base are of particular interest. Changes in size and shape of the sella turcica and adjacent bony structures, patterns of growth within the basal cisterns, determination of the point of origin or attachment of the lesion and its blood supply, also have to be considered.

Computerized tomography with horizontal and coronal cuts is now an indispensable diagnostic tool and has largely replaced air contrast studies. However, air contrast is still useful, when one is trying to demonstrate a small lesion in the suprachiasmatic area, at the foramina of Monro, or when the cause of an obstructive hydrocephalus is not apparent. Computerized metrizamide cisternography may also add important information. Angiography is required in order to define the blood supply of the tumour, to exclude the presence of a vascular lesion, and to demonstrate the venous drainage system.

A full neuro-endocrine workup should be obtained. Pre-operative recognition and treatment of associated endocrine dysfunctions such as hypoadrenalism or hypothyroidism are crucial, as is the detection of a hypothalamic syndrome.

Management of associated hydrocephalus is a major pre-operative decision. If a transcortical or transcallosal route is planned, the dilated ventricles may facilitate the exposure. In contrast, a subfrontal approach will be made much more difficult. Pre-operative shunting has been advocated by some, particularly when it is expected that the operation will not unblock the spinal fluid pathways. Post-operative ventricular drainage is a useful adjuvant in the management of these lesions and may obviate the need for shunting in some cases.

Surgical Approaches

1. Trans-Sphenoidal Approach

This extra-axial route allows a simple and direct approach to intra-sellar tumour with dorsal extensions, but is of limited value if these are anteriorly, laterally, or posteriorly placed. It is useful for large pituitary adenomas and certain dumb-bell craniopharyngiomas. Intracapsular removal of the lesion is usually possible, allowing good decompression of the optic pathways. Approach to the suprasellar area is difficult in the presence of a normal sella. Possible complications of the trans-sphenoidal procedure include injruy to the neurovascular structures of the base, and cerebrospinal fluid leaks and infection. These are probably more common than when the operation is performed for pituitary microadenomas.

2. Dorsal Approaches

In these operations tumours of the anterior third ventricle are approached dorsally through the lateral ventricle or corpus callosum. They are indicated for lesions in the dorsal part of the third ventricle, particularly when they arise at the foramina of Monro, or for primarily intra-ventricular tumours. Lesions that extend beyond the walls of the ventricle may occasionally be followed through an opening into the lamina terminalis. Identification of precise landmarks, usually the venous drainage system and choroid plexus, are essential. The various routes include:

a) Transcallosal In this procedure a small (2–3 cm) opening is made into the corpus callosum exposing the lateral ventricle (Fig. 2). This approach has the advantage of not violating the cerebral cortex, thus reducing the incidence of post-operative seizures. Good visualization of both lateral ventricles and both walls of the third ventricle is obtained by opening the septum pellucidum. This manoeuvre exposes both foramina of Monro and establishes a communication between the lateral ventricles which is crucial. The transcallosal procedure can also be carried out in the presence of normal ventricles.

b) Transcortical In this operation the lateral ventricle is entered through an incision in the frontal lobe, usually in the mid-frontal gyrus. Although the anterior and contralateral walls of the third ventricle are well visualized, the exposure of the ipsilateral wall is limited. It is more difficult when the ventricles are small, and it carries a higher risk of seizures than the transcallosal operation.

Both the transcallosal and transcortical operations expose the foramina of Monro, but it is sometimes necessary to enlarge the foramen. Steps described to enlarge this foramen include excising one of the fornices (11), or removing the anterior tubercle of the thalamus (4). It can also be enlarged by coagulating the thalamo-striate vein and carrying the dissection posteriorly between the thalamus laterally and the choroid plexus and internal cerebral vein medially (6, 14). Although Hirsch (6) claims that interruption of the thalamo-striate vein is without danger, it may on occasion lead to a haemorrhagic infarction of the basal nuclei. Busch (2) and more recently Ciric (3) have advocated a midline approach by incising the septum pellucidum, finding a plane of cleavage between the two fornices and opening the tela choroidea in the midline between the two internal cerebral veins (Fig. 3). Another approach to the dorsal aspect of the third ventricle is a subchoroidal route (15) in which the roof of the ventricle is entered between the fornix and choroid plexus above and the thalamus below, until the internal cerebral vein is exposed. The right fornix and choroid plexus are then displaced medially and the remainder of the tela incised. Additional room may be created by dividing the thalamostriate vein and extending the opening to the foramen of Monro.

Among the possible complications of these procedures are cortical collapse with accumulation of subdural effusions, and injury to the fornices. Severe gastrointestinal haemorrhage following transcallosal procedures was originally described by Long et al. (8) but has not been mentioned in other series (1, 12, 13). The neuropsychological effects of the limited section of the anterior corpus callosum have been found to be minimal (5), but memory deficits when both fornices are damaged is reported.

3. Basal Approaches (Fig. 4)

In these operations the lesions are exposed from below, along the anterior base of the skull. They are ideally suited for lesions which grow from the sellar-suprasellar region and secondarily invade or displace the anterior third ventricle. They are essentially extra-axial approaches, through a subfrontal route or a fronto-temporal route; the optic nerve and carotid artery are the crucial landmarks in both instances. The subfrontal approach, usually through a frontal craniotomy (or more rarely through a bifrontal flap) allows a better exposure of both optic nerves, but does not give good access underneath the ipsilateral optic nerve and tract. The fronto-temporal route, opening the Sylvian fissure, is the most direct route to the parasellar region and also allows visualization of the retrosellar area. Once the supra-sellar area is exposed, dissection and excision of the lesion may take different paths:

a) Subchiasmatic. This is the more commonly used.

b) Opticocarotid. This is, in our experience, an excellent approach for tumours in this area, particularly craniopharyngiomas. The dissection proceeds between the optic nerve and tract medially, the carotid artery laterally, and the anterior cerebral artery as it runs horizontally from the carotid bifurcation, posteriorly. This is also an effective alternative when the chiasm is prefixed.

c) Lamina Terminalis. This approach is useful for dealing with tumours totally within the third ventricle, which distend the lamina terminalis. The landmarks for this exposure are not always well defined and possible complications of the operation include damage to hypothalamic structures and to the vascular supply to the optic chiasm and hypothalamus (7, 14).

d) Lateral to the carotid artery between the carotid and the third nerve.

e) Transfrontal trans-sphenoidal, described recently by Patterson et al. (9) useful for cases in which the optic chiasm is prefixed. It requires the removal of the tuberculum sellae and anterior wall of the sella turcica after opening the sphenoid sinus. Tumours within the third ventricle can be removed by exposing them above the optic apparatus through the lamina terminalis and beneath the chiasm.

4. Subtemporal Approach

This route offers a more limited exposure to the anterior third ventricle but it may be used for lesions centred lateral to the sella or extending into the middle cranial fossa, or for a tumour that extends from the floor of the third ventricle into the interpeduncular fossa.

5. Needle Biopsy

Needle biopsy of an anterior third ventricular tumour has been gaining support since the advent of computerized tomography. Although it may be helpful for diagnostic purposes, it will rarely constitute a definitive form of treatment.

Clinical Material

We have reviewed 100 cases of primary and secondary anterior third ventricle tumours operated on the Neurological Institute of New York in the past two decades (Table 1). We excluded from this analysis patients with pituitary adenomas and optic nerve gliomas, since these raise different surgical problems. We did not include patients who were operated through the trans-sphenoidal approach, since in our institutuion this operations has been of limited use for the lesions considered in this series, and we were primarily interested in evaluating the morbidity and mortality of the dorsal and basal approaches. One patient included in this series had a transcallosal and a subchiasmatic approach performed at the same procedure. The results of our analysis are summarized in Tables 2–4.

Conclusions

With good operative technique the mortality of operations on anterior third ventricular tumours is quite low. The four patients with colloid cysts that died were operated on early in this series; in two instances the tumour was not found at operation, and the two other cases died of uncontrollable increased intracranial pressure before adequate shunting devices were available.

Transcallosal and transcortical procedures are both safe and effective procedures, but the latter seems to deal more effectively with the associated hydrocephalus. When this is caused by an intraventricular glioma it is usually not relieved by a direct surgical approach. It is of interest to note that two of the cases, in which only *one* fornix was transected, had profound memory deficits postoperatively.

The subchiasmatic approach alone or combined with the opticocarotid route deals effectively with the great majority of craniopharyngiomas. In only four cases was the optic chiasm so prefixed that another route had to be taken. In two patients who had previous subchiasmatic approaches, and had radiographic evidence of recurrence, no tumour was exposed when the same approach was used again suggesting that in these situations opening the lamina terminalis is the effective alternative. Diabetes insipidus,

Table 1. Nature of lesion

	No.
Craniopharyngioma	38
Colloid cyst	37
Glioma	13
Ependymal cyst	4
Dysgerminoma	2
Granuloma	1
Ependymoma	1
Inflammatory adhesions	1
Venous angioma	1
Giant aneurysm	1
Tuberous sclerosis	1
Total	100

Table 2. Transcallosal approach

Cases		Complications	
Colloid cyst	9	Postoperative shunt	3
Glioma	5	Postoperative shunt	4
		Memory loss	1
		Hemiparesis	1
		SIADH	1
Craniopharyngioma	2	Postoperative shunt	1
		Meningitis	1
Ependymoma	1	SIADH	1
Other, tuberous Sclerosis, granuloma, Ependymal cyst, Venous angioma Adhesions	5		
Total	22		

frequently transient, is to be expected in the majority of the cases in whom an aggressive surgical policy is adopted.

Table 3. Transcortical approach

Cases		Complications	
Colloid cyst	28	Deaths	4
		Seizures	2
		Hemiparesis	1
		Memory deficit	1
		Postoperative shunt	1
Glioma	6	Postoperative shunt	3
		Hemiplegia	1
		Death	1
Ependymal cyst	2	Subdural hygroma	1
Craniopharyngioma	1	Postoperative shunt	1
Giant aneurysm	1	Postoperative shunt	1
Dysgerminoma	1	Meningitis	1
Total	39		

Table 4. Basal approaches

Cases			Complications	
Craniopharyngioma	Subchiasmatic	23	Diabetes insipidus	17
			Increased visual deficit	5
			Postoperative shunt	2
			Hemiparesis	1
			Meningitis	1
	Optico-carotid	5	Diabetes insipidus	4
			Increased visual deficit	1
	Subchiasm and Optico-carotid	3	Diabetes insipidus	1
	Lateral carotid	3	III nerve palsy	1
	Subtemporal	1	III nerve palsy	1
	Lamina Terminalis	1	Hemiparesis Hypernatraemia	1
Glioma	Subchiasmatic	2		
Dysgerminoma	Subchiasmatic	1	Hypernatraemia – Shunt	1
Ependymal cyst	Subchiasmatic and optico-carotid	1	Subdural hygroma	1

References

1. Antunes, J.L., Louis, K.M., Ganti, S.R.: Colloid cysts of the third ventricle. Neurosurgery *7*, 450–454 (1980)
2. Busch, E.: A new approach for the removal of tumors of the third ventricle. Acta Psych. Neurol. *19*, 57–60 (1944)
3. Ciric, I.: Comment on paper by Antunes et al. (Ref. 1). Neurosurgery *7*, 454–455 (1980)
4. Ehni, G.: Comment on paper by Shucart and Stein (Ref. 12). Neurosurgery *3*, 343 (1978)
5. Geffen, G., Walsh, A., Simpson, D., Jeeves, M.: Comparison of the effects of transcortical and transcallosal removal of intraventricular tumours. Brain *103*, 773–788 (1980)
6. Hirsch, J.F., Zouaoui, A., Renier, D., Pierre-Kahn, A.: A new surgical approach to the third ventricle with interruption of the striothalamic vein. Acta Neurochir. (Wien) *47*, 135–147 (1979)
7. King, T.T.: Removal of intraventricular craniopharyngiomas through the lamina terminalis. Acta Neurochir. (Wien) *45*, 277–286 (1979)
8. Long, D.M., Chou, S.N.: Transcallosal removal of craniopharyngiomas within the third ventricle. J. Neurosurg. *39*, 563–567 (1973)
9. Patterson, Jr., R.H., Danylevich, A.: Surgical removal of craniopharyngiomas by a transcranial approach through the lamina terminalis and sphenoid sinus. Neurosurgery *7*, 111–117 (1980)
10. Pecker, J., Ferrand, B., Javalet, A.: Tumeurs du troisieme ventricule. Neurochirurgie *12*, 7–136 (1966)
11. Rhoton, Jr., A.L., Yamamoto, I., Peace, D.A.: Microsurgery of the third ventricle, Part 2: Operative approaches. Neurosurgery *8*, 357–373 (1981)
12. Shucart, W.A., Stein, B.M.: Transcallosal approach to the anterior ventricular system. Neurosurgery *3*, 339–343 (1978)
13. Stein, B.M.: Transcallosal approach to third ventricle tumors. In: Current techniques in operative neurosurgery. Schmidek, H.H., Sweet, W.H. (eds.), pp. 247–255. New York: Grune & Stratton (1977)
14. Stein, B.M.: Comment on paper by Rhoton et al. (Ref. 11). Neurosurgery *8*, 372–373 (1981)
15. Viale, G.L., Turtas, S.: The subchoroid approach to the third ventricle. Surg. Neurol. *14*, 71–76 (1980)

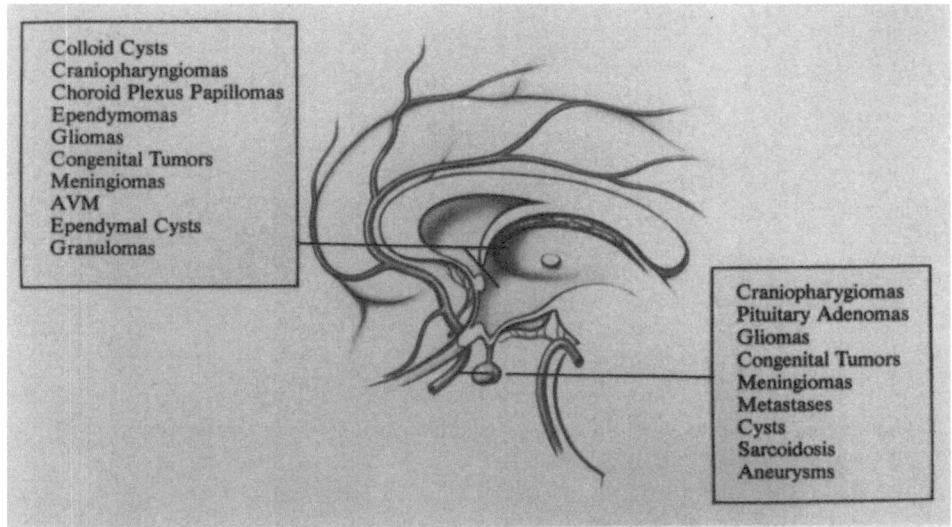

Fig. 1. Lesions of the anterior third ventricle

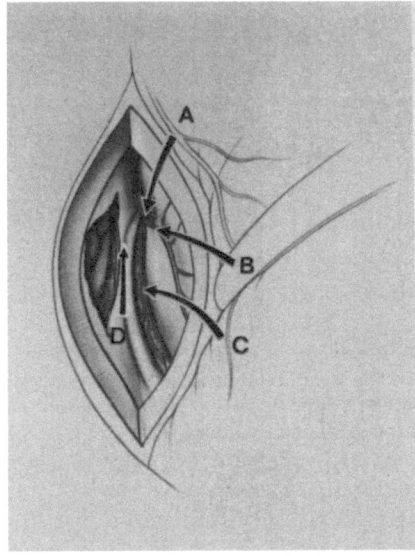

Fig. 2. Transcallosal approach to right lateral ventricle showing perforated septum pellucidum and retractor or mesial surface of the right hemisphere. Four approaches for enlarging the foramen of Monro and obtaining better access to the third ventricle are shown. *A* = sectioning ipsilateral column of the fornix; *B* = coagulation of thalamo-striate vein with dissection medial to the thalamus; *C* = subchoroidal route with retraction of fornix and choroid plexus medially; *D* = midline approach between the two fornices and internal cerebral veins

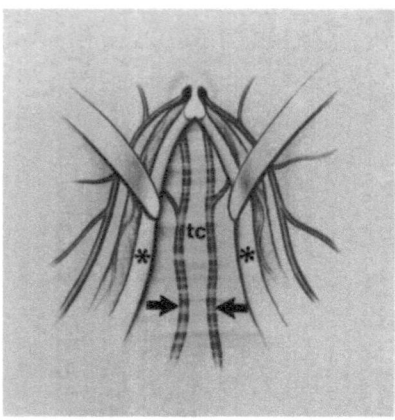

Fig. 3. Midline approach to the third ventricle. *tc*= tela choroidea; * *(asterisks)*= fornices; *arrowheads*= internal cerebral veins

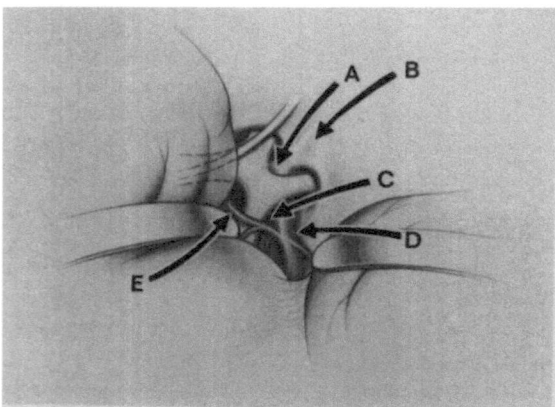

Fig. 4. Basal approaches showing optic chiasm, right internal carotid artery and retractors on right frontal and temporal lobes. *A*= Subchiasmatic; *B*= through tuberculum sellae − sphenoid sinus; *C*= between optic nerve and chiasm and internal carotid artery; *D*= lateral to internal carotid artery; *E*= through lamina terminalis

Posterior Third Ventricular Tumours

M. Sambasivan

Introduction

Variegated and interesting clinical features which occur as a result of a lesion in the posterior third Ventricle (Pineal region) make them neurological curiosities. But their location makes them accessible only with difficulty and thus they pose a challenge to the surgeon. Controversy exists regarding shunt and operation on the tumour versus shunt and radiotherapy without any operation on the tumour. On the basis of experiences in a personal series, approach to pineal region, removal or intraneoplastic decompression followed by radiotherapy — seems justifiable as well as beneficial.

Materials and Approach

At this centre we have seen 35 cases of posterior third ventricular tumour, who were subjected to operation, and tissue biopsy could be obtained. Eight cases were treated by modified Torkildsen's ventriculo-cisternal shunt/followed by radiotherapy. These have been excluded from this study, and were reported earlier (8).

Table 1 shows the age and sex incidence among the 35 cases. It is obvious that two-thirds of these cases were in the 11–20 age group. No case was encountered beyond the 40th year.

It can be seen from Table 2 that in all the cases the presenting symptom was headache. In 50% of them the headache was relieved by assuming certain postures, which the patient learned to adopt to get relief. Lying prone or in a knee forehead position gave relief from headache. In 37% of cases the headache came episodically and the relief was spontaneous. Headache described was of a 'bursting expansile' type.

More than the headache the visual difficulties made the patients seek medical attention. In 74% there was reduction in vision and 17% came to hospital after they had become blind.

Table 3 summarizes the signs noticed in these cases on admission in a decreasing order of frequency. It is obvious that many of the cases came for treatment at a late stage.

In all cases the diagnosis was made by positive contrast ventriculography, when filling defects could be demonstrated in the posterier third ventricle (see Fig. 1 for examples).

Table 4 represents the histopathological nature of the lesions as obtained from the biopsy material.

Table 1. Posterior third ventricular tumours; age and sex incidence (35 cases)

Age (years)	Male	Female	Total
0–10	1	1	2
11–20	12	8	20
21–30	5	3	8
31–40	4	1	5
Total	22	13	35

Table 2. Posterior third ventricular tumours; symptoms (35 cases)

	No. of cases	%
Headache	35	100
Postural relief	17	50
Intermittent attacks with relief	13	37
Morning headache	23	66
Diminution of vision	26	74
Double vision	18	57
Blind	6	17
Hearing Deficit	4	14
Unsteadiness	13	37
Precocious puberty	3	9
Diabetes insipidus	3	9
Other endocrine disturbances	3	9

Nineteen pinealomas were seen and this constitutes an incidence of 1.6% among the space-occupying lesions. The incidence of pinealomas appears to be highest in Japan, Araki (1) — reporting 4.5%.

Interesting Problems

One boy aged 11 years presented with papilloedema, unsteadiness and loss of upward gaze, precocious puberty and rapid deterioration in general health due to incessant vomiting. Conray ventriculogram, atrial shunt was performed as a first stage. Next day the patient became unconcious and became decerebrate. An upward coning was suspected and emergency approach to the tumour was done by Poppen's (13) technique. A teratoma impacted at the tentorial hiatus was excised. The patient made a satisfactory recovery and at seven year follow-up is well and doing college education.

Table 3. Posterior third ventricular tumours; signs on admission (35 cases)

	No. of cases	%
Papilloedema	23	66
Loss of upward gaze	21	60
Bilateral abducens lesion	12	34
Hippus	12	34
Convergent nystagmus	9	25
Bilateral pyramidal	9	25
Secondary optic atrophy	8	23
Gait ataxia	8	23
Unilateral sixth	7	20
Bilateral proptosis	6	17
Loss of convergence	6	17
Hearing deficit	5	14
Bilateral cerebellar	5	14
Unilateral pyramidal	5	14
Metabolic problems	5	14
Endocrine problems	5	14
Primary optic atrophy	4	11
Extensor rigidity	2	5

Table 4. Posterior third ventricular tumours; histology (35 cases)

	No. of cases	Pinealoma atypical teratoma	Teratoma	Epidermoid	Glioblastoma	Ependymoma	Meningioma	Others
Sano, K.	80	47	12	3	11	7	–	–
Yonemasu et al.	44	26	12	2	2	2	–	–
Obrador, S.	164	89	16	6	28	–	21	4
Bookallil, A.J.	21	11	2	–	1	3	–	4
Sambasivan, M. (Present series)	35	19	5	1	4	3	1	2 (Medullo-Blastoma)

A patient with an epidermoid in the pineal region manifesting with renal glycosuria was reported by the author earlier (9). Another similar example of renal glycosuria was noted in a patient harbouring a teratoma in the pineal region, but this patient died in the postoperative period due to a bleeding diathesis and hence could not be studied in

227

detail. Two cases of pinealoma presented with diabetes insipidus and in both of them this subsided completely after operation on the pinealoma.

Results

Eleven cases were subjected to surgery by Poppen's technique. After the tumour operation ventriculo-cisternal shunt was performed. Two patients died postoperatively.

In 24 instances a preliminary ventriculo-atrial shunt was done. In this group three patients died in the postoperative period.

There has been a mortality of 14% (5 out of 35 cases).

Five teratomas (Fig. 2), a miningioma and a cholesteatoma could be excised. This constituted 20% of the lesions. The others were subjected to radiotherapy by Cobalt 60 — Teletherapy unit receiving a dose of 5000 to 6000 r.

Tumours excised

1. Teratoma	− 5	Operative Mortality − 1
		4 Surviving well
2. Meningioma	1	
		Both alive and well
3. Cholesteatoma	1	

Tumours decompressed + radiotherapy

4. Pinealoma	19	Operative Mortality 2
	17 alive and well	
5. Glioblastoma	4	Operative Mortality 1
		2 Died in 12 months
		1 Well at 6 months
6. Ependymomas	3	Operative Mortality 1
		2 Died − 12−18 months
7. Medulloblastomas	2 Died at 3−6 months	

Discussion

As early as 1948 Torkildsen (15), was advocating a palliative operation in the management of posterior third ventricular tumours, by ventriculo-cisternal shunt.

Cummin et al. (3), Taveras (14), Martin, B., Camins et al. (6), Carteri and Salar (4), and many others advocated CSF diversion shunts followed by radiotherapy to the

228

tumour without any histological verification. They maintain that direct operation produces severe morbidity and mortality and thus they prefer the former treatment.

Bookallil (2), reviewing a series of 49 cases prefers a shunt and radiotherapy for tumours and reserves direct a approach for younger and older patients, as well as for those who deteroirate after conservative management.

Hide (5), concludes that while CSF drainage and radiotherapy given good survival to patients with pineal region tumours, some excisable lesions are missed and they are subjected to unnecessary radiotherapy. Early direct attack is not preferred and he advocates stereotaxic biopsy.

Obrador (7), reviewing a series of 164 lesions suggest a preliminary shunt, a second stage direct approach using an — operating microscope and depending upon the nature of lesion radiotherapy on third stage. Stien B.M. (11), also advocates direct surgery, but preferred supracerebellar infratentorial approach.

Suzuki and Iwabuchi (12), and Sano (10), advocate a direct tumour approach after preliminary shunting. Reasonable diagnosis may be possible by CSF cytology, when a direct operation must be avoided.

The percent report emphasizes the need for a direct approach, so that excisable lesions can be removed and in others tumour bulk can be reduced thus allowing better tolerance of radiotherapy.

Conclusion

Direct operation on tumours of the posterior third ventricular region is the procedure of choice, so that the excisable tumours could be removed with success.

Direct operation allows a biopsy and a definitive tumour diagnosis is possible.

Direct operation helps in tumour reduction and if they are nonexcisable, subsequent radiotherapy is well tolerated giving better results.

References

1. Araki, C., Matsumoto, M.: Statistical reevaluation of Pinealoma and related tumours in Japan. J. Neurosurg. *30*, 146–149 (1969)
2. Bookallil, A.J.: Tumors of Pineal Region: a review of 49 cases. Fifth European Congress; Abstract 36, pp. 79–81 (1975)
3. Cummin et al.: Treatment of gliomas of third ventricle and pinealomas with special reference to radiotherapy. Neurology (Mineap) *10*, 1031–1036 (1960)
4. Carteri, A., Salar, G.: Neurosurgical treatment of pineal region tumors. Fifth European Congress; Abstract 30, p. 83 (1975)
5. Hide, T.A.H.: A rational approach to treatment of pineal tumours. Fifth European Congress; Abstract 42, pp. 90–92 (1975)
6. Martin, B., Camins et al.: Treatment of tumors of the posterior third ventricle and pineal region. Fifth European Congress; Abstract 37 (1975)
7. Obrador, S. et al.: Surgical management of tumours of pineal region. Fifth European Congress; Abstract 49 (1975)
8. Sambasivan, M.: Posterior third ventricular tumors. Present limits of neurosurgery. Avicenum 165–168 (1972)

9. Sambasivan, M., Nayar, A.: Epidermoid cyst of pineal region. J. Neurosurg. Psychiatry *37*, 1333—1335 (1974)
10. Sano, K.: Diagnosis and treatment of tumors of pineal region. Fifth European Congress; Abstract 55 (1975)
11. Stien, B.M.: Surgery of pineal tumors. Excerpta Medica *418*, 300, 120 (1977)
12. Suzuki, J., Iwabuchi, T.: Surgical removal of pineal tumors (Pinealomas and teratomas) Experience in a series of 19 cases. J. Neurosurg. *23*, 565—571 (1965)
13. Poppen, J.L.: The right occipital approach to a pinealomas — J. Neurosurg. *25*, 706—710 (1966)
14. Taveras, J.M.: Radiotherapy of brain tumors. Clin. Neurosurg. *7*, 200—213 (1961)
15. Torkildsen, A.: Should extirpation be attempted in cases of Neoplasm in or near the third ventricle of the brain? Experiences with a palliative method. J. Neurosurg. *5*, 249—275 (1948)

230

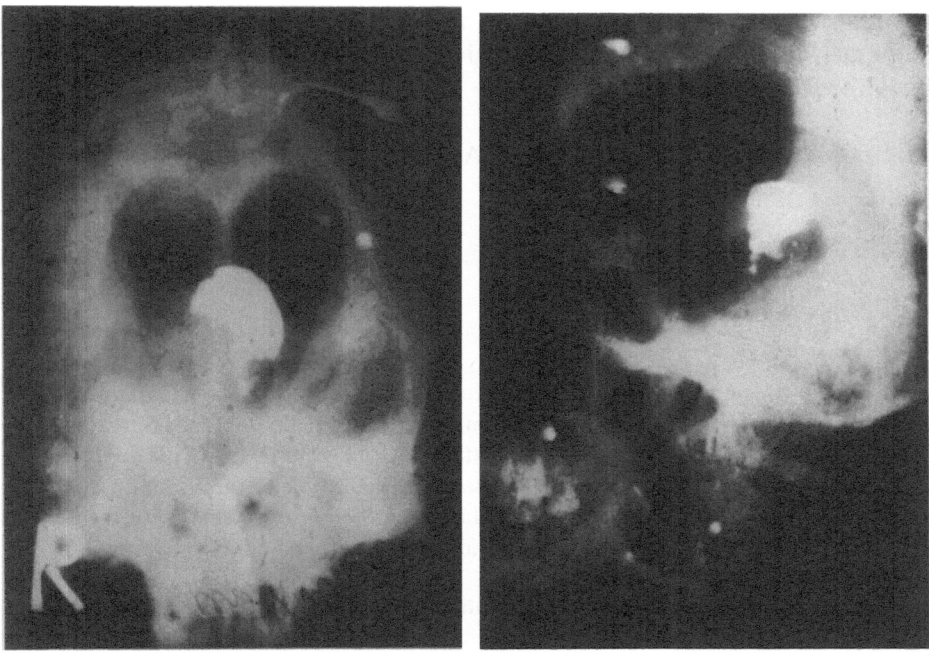

Fig. 1. Air and myodil ventriculograms showing filling defect in the posterior third ventricle

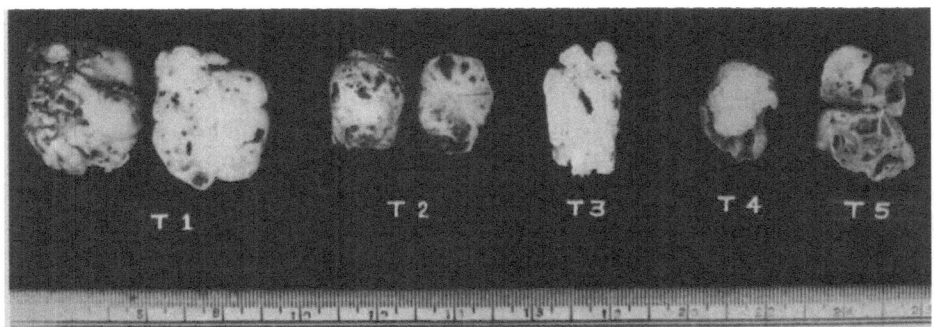

Fig. 2. Teratomas excised from the posterior third ventricle

231

Tumours of the Lateral Ventricles in Adults —
Pre-Operative Anatomical and Histological Diagnosis —
Surgical Implications

J. Philippon, M. Rivierez, D. Gardeur, A. Nachanakian, and B. Pertuiset

Tumours of the lateral ventricle, however different in their topography and histological nature, have certain characteristics in common the knowledge of which is of great importance to the neurosurgeon. Is removal partially or totally possible ? This depends first upon the type but also upon the exact location and especially the anatomical relation with the caudate nucleus, fornix and thalamus on their inferior side, with the corpus callosum on the superior. Is this relation simply a superficial adherence or a deep penetration ?

A second point concerns the effect of the tumour mass on the CSF flow from the lateral ventricles. Is there a unilateral or bilateral obstruction of the foramen of Monro? Is the obstruction due to a true tumoural invasion of the foramen or merely a displacement with distortion of the structure?

Material and Methods

Twenty-one tumours located in the lateral ventricles of the cerebral hemispheres were reviewed. The age at diagnosis varies from 21 to 63 years. It is not our purpose here to discuss the clinical signs but to try to define the main anatomical characteristics as shown by CT scan, and in some instances angiography, and to discuss the surgical considerations. From a topographical point of view, these lesions may be divided into those limited to the area of the interventricular foramina (seven cases), those of the body of the ventricle (11 cases), and tumours of the posterior part (three cases).

1. Tumours of the Intraventricular Foramina

Among the seven cases, there were two giant-cell astrocytomas, two astrocytomas, one neuroblastoma, one ependymoglioma, and one glioblastoma. Within this group, three typical cases are noteworthy.

Case 3. A 24-year-old male, with a clinical history of generalized seizures, complains of memory disturbances and intracranial hypertension. The CT scan revealed a lesion located mainly in the left frontal horn with posterior calcification, showing a massive homogeneous enhancement after contrast (Fig. 1A). The operation revealed a giant cell astrocytoma whose total removal was performed without problem.

Case 5. This 60-year-old woman had a three month history of frontal syndrome (trouble in walking, memory disturbances and incontinence). Neurological examination showed bilateral grasp reflexes. On CT scan, a hyperdensity was noted with slight enhancement after contrast, lateralized in the left ventricle; there was no widening of the septum pellucidum (Fig. 1B). On the lateral phlebogram there was an upward displacement of the septal vein and of the caudate vein (Fig. 1C). At operation, an astrocytoma arising from the head of the left caudate nucleus was found.

Septal tumours may have a similar clinical picture, as shown by our case 6.

Case 6. Clinical symptoms consisted mainly of memory disturbances, decreased attention capacity with loss of intellectual efficiency. This clinical picture was completed a few month later by temporo-spatial disorientation. The CT scan however was quite different (Fig. 2).

2. Tumours of the Ventricular Body

We have observed eleven cases of tumours developing predominantly in the ventricular body: eight were bilateral and quite symmetrical while only three were predominantly or strictly unilateral. An example of the first group is *case 14.*

This 29-year-old patient, was referred for an intracranial hypertension with pyramidal signs in the lower limb. CT scan showed a mass arising in both lateral ventricles, completely occupying the left frontal horn, spontaneously hyperdense with presence of calcification (Fig. 3). Angiography revealed that the main part of the mass was intraventricular.

Unilateral tumours are less frequent. Of our three cases only one, *case 17,* was strictly unilateral.

Two months before, this 27-year-old patient presented diplopia related to intracranial hypertension. The only focal sign at neurological examination was memory disturbances. The CT scan revealed a large, partially necrotic tumour on the left side. At angiography, the main features were the presence of arteriovenous shunts, and the fact that the tumour was completely situated above the plane of the internal cerebral vein.

3. Tumours of the Posterior Part (Ventricular Atrium)

Three cases were observed, two of which were meningioma.

Case 19. This 52-year-old woman had an abrupt onset of headache, with a syndrome of subarachnoid haemorrhage, followed a few days later by intracranial hypertension. The CT scan revealed the lesion located in the trigone of the ventricle (Fig. 4A). Angiography, showed vascular displacement and a large anterior choroidal artery, but otherwise no particular blush.

The last case was a choroid plexus carcinoma. Symptoms were marked by intracranial hypertension associated with moderate speech disturbances. Clinical signs consisted of a right hemianopia and aphasia. The possibility of a glioma was discussed after viewing the CT scan (Fig. 4B).

Discussion

Tumours of the lateral ventricles are relatively rare. They have in general been studied according to their anatomical pathology (1–3, 5) or more rarely in relation to their localisation (4, 7). The attempt to define their actual extent has been considerably facilitated by the use of the CT scanner.

1. Tumours in the Area of the Interventricular Foramen

Subependymal giant cell astrocytomas, typically associated with tuberous sclerosis, occur frequently in the region of the foramen of Monro. They are easy to recognize because of their characteristic appearance on CT scan: there is often subependymal calcification, the tumour itself has an antero-medial orientation; it may be bilateral and asymmetrical; with contrast there is massive enhancement. Surgical removal is usuallyally easy, as the tumour is pedunculated and the attachment to the caudate limited. The only difficulty may be due to a remote infiltration.

Not all tumours should be operated upon, however, as many of them are symptom-free: the only ones to be considered are those with intracranial hypertension.

Another group of tumours has some features similar to the giant cells astrocytomas: these are tumours originating from the head of the caudate nucleus which are also pedunculated and extend more or less in a upward direction. They generally develop asymmetrical, and the enlargement of the frontal horns is predominantly on the side of the tumour. This asymmetry associated with a septum of normal size eventually deviated as noted above is a strong indication of a strictly unilateral tumour.

Angiography may be helpful especially when considering the modifications of the deep veins in the lateral view; the septal vein is stretched and elevated in its first position which is unlikely to occur in septal tumours. On the antero-posterior view there is a displacement of the vein toward the contralateral side.

The diagnosis of the exact nature of these tumours, mainly astrocytomas and ependymogliomas, is based essentially on the CT scan.

Their surgical excision is usually easy through a unilateral transventricular approach. An infiltration of the head of the caudate nucleus may be removed without any problem (4).

Tumours of the septum and fornix area show a different radiological aspect: they are generally bilateral and more or less symmetrical. The septum is barely visible except at the extreme anterior part of posteriorly; the lateral part of the frontal horn may be free from the mass and completely laminated.

Likewise, in the tumours of the caudate area, the deep phlebogram may be helpful in showing a posterior and downward displacement of the deep venous angle, while septal veins are stretched downward or not visible.

The nature of the tumour varies widely; it is worth underlining the predominance of benign tumours. Laine and Blond (4) collected their own series using cases in the literature with a precise histological diagnosis. They observed 49 benign lesions, mainly astrocytomas and oligodendrogliomas, compared with 29 malignant tumours (ectopic pinealomas, glioblastomas, spongioblastomas, malignant ependymogliomas).

The main problem for the neurosurgeon concerns extension in a vertical direction, either upward to the corpus callosum or downward to the anterior commissure and anterior wall of the third ventricle, and laterally to the caudate. Coronal section on the CT scan may partially solve the problem.

Whatever the exact nature, a significant downward extension is an indication for incomplete removal. Metrizamide ventriculography may confirm the complete blockage of the interventricular foramina or the extension toward the anterior wall of third ventricle. It should be performed when this downward extension is not evident on the CT scan.

However, the exact anatomical extension can only be fully appreciated at operation; operation is always necessary except for the case with extensive invasion. Surgical exposure though a unilateral transfrontal approach is generally sufficient. After removal of the homolateral part of the mass — as complete as possible — (a superficial invasion of the caudate may be excised) the next step concerns the contralateral extension. This may be explored after division of the septum in a tumour-free zone if possible. Otherwise, with large tumours, the resection must start at the anterior crus of the fornix (4).

Another problem concerns the attitude toward ventricular dilatation; the persistance of non-functioning foramina should lead to CSF diversion, generally unilateral. When tumour removal has been very partial, a bilateral diversion may be necessary, particularly if the communication between the two frontal horns is uncertain.

2. Tumours of the Ventricular Body

Intraventricular ependymoglioma present a very constant picture on the CT scanner. The tumour is in general bilateral: their extent in our series, as often noted in literature, is considerable, occupying sometimes half or two-thirds of the ventricular cavities on both sides. Their aspects is almost always the same; they are microcystic, sometimes with calcification and with a marked enhancement after injection. There is no peritumoural oedema. Oligodendrogliomas have a similar appearance and are impossible to recognize before operation (6).

When performed, arteriography shows signs of ventricular dilatation with stretching of subependymal veins. The internal cerebral vein is displaced downward and the septal vein may also be displaced, depending upon the anterior extension (3).

Tumoural filling is often present and projects above the ventricular floor. It is present in about one third of the cases (3); the existence of an homogeneous tumour vascularization without any arteriovenous shunt suggests the presence of an ependymoma rather than of a glioblastoma. Another difference is related to the appearance on the CT scan; the mass is localized on one side of the ventricular system and is heterogeneous.

The inferior extension can be appreciated on the lateral phlebogram but is mainly seen on the coronal section of the CT scan. Visualization of the third ventricle, and more rarely of the inferior part of the lateral ventricle, are valuable elements from which one may assume a location remote from the basal nuclei (Fig. 5). This fact is usually impossible to affirm with large tumours filling the ventricular system completely. The upward extension toward the corpus callosum, however less dramatic, must be evaluated on the coronal section. It is not of such great importance for operation as thalamic invasion.

Surgical exploration seems to us always necessary, with the few exception of tumours extending mainly into the deep structures and secondarily into the ventricular lumen, explaining the importance of precise topographical diagnosis.

Pre-operative CSF shunting is unlikely; in bilateral tumours the ventricular cavity is very often divided into four different spaces, giving to the ventricle the appearance of a four-leaf clover. In the cases of tumours arising unilaterally with bilateral hydrocephalus, one has to think of the increasing risk of mass distorsion if the drainage is in the opposite free ventricle.

Operation has to be performed to remove the greatest part of the mass present in the cavity. It should be done bilaterally if necessary, usually through an unilateral transfrontal approach with division of the septum.

If the contralateral extension is large and there is an invasion of the foramen of Monro on the other side, removal will always be incomplete (4). The main problem after piecemal removal is to deal with the area of attachment more or less extensively. The microscope may be helpful.

3. Tumours of the Posterior Part

As reflected in this short series, meningiomas are predominant in this part of the ventricle: 72% in the series of 22 cases of Mani et al. (5). The CT scan normally shows a typical pattern: dilatation of the temporal and eventually of the occipital horns; the tumour is hyperdense and with marked enhancement after contrast injection. Zones of decreased density may coexist around the tumour and correspond to the peritumoural oedema. The presence of calcification is usual. Even if these indications are strongly in favour of meningioma, other tumours of the ventricle may have the same appearance, namely ependymogliomas. In our series, however, we have not observed such tumours in this location. Papillomas of the choroid plexus generally show a different picture; they are frequently associated with hydrocephalus. The ventricular dilatation involving all the ventricles (7) is due to the frequence of hydrocephalus from subarachnoid haemorrhage. Other rare tumours (vascular lesions) may be in relation with Sturge-Weber changes or are diagnosed at an older age. As regards the more malignant tumours (carcinomas) they often show transgression of the ventricular wall (7).

Angiography seems necessary; this may confirm suspicion of a meningioma with the classical changes in the choroidal arteries, mainly anterior choroidal but sometimes of the lateral posterior choroidal artery. A vascular tumour blush, if present, is another element, but not absolutely characteristic of meningioma. Other tumours may show the same apperance. Due to the fact that the posterior tumours are often operable, the main distinction concerns the tumour originating in the paraventricular area and seeming to extend into the lumen of the ventricle; these are mainly gliomas. On the CT scan, the existence of a heterogeneous appearance with zones of necrosis, and the limits of the mass evidently outside the ventricle is a fundamental point of distinction. As noted by Delandsheer (1) if the basilar vein of Rosenthal is always pushed downward in the lateral phlebogram by masses in this area, the changes in the internal cerebral and the vein of Galen are different. In the case of tumours originating from the pulvinar the structures are displaced upward with an increase in the curve of the vein of Galen. Another advantage of angiography is to show at times the characteristic injection of a glioblastoma: in our experience, such tumours should not be operated upon.

Conclusion

Intraventricular tumours are rare: but their occurence raises difficulties in their surgical treatment. CT scan has completely modified the appreciation of their anatomical extension.

It seems to us possible to distinguish three main categories in these lesions. Those located in the area of the interventricular foramina consist mainly of tumours originating from the caudate nucleus or the septum. Their removal is in general easier compared to the second group, tumours of the ventricular body, the size of which is much larger. They are mainly ependymogliomas and their growth, even if varying widely, is always particularly extensive toward the ventricular walls. Tumours of the trigone present fewer difficulties, as they are for the most part purely intraventricular, once the paraventricular gliomas have been recognized.

References

1. Delandsheer, J.M.: Les méningiomes du ventricule latéral. Neurochirurgie *11*, 32–46 (1965)
2. Fornari, M., Savoiardo, M., Morello, G., Solero, C.: Meningiomas of the lateral ventricles. Neuroradiological and surgical considerations in 18 cases. J. Neurosurg. *54*, 64–74 (1981)
3. Goutelle, A., Fischer, G.: Les épendymomes intra-crâniens. Neurochirurgie (Suppl. 1) *23*, 67–75 (1977)
4. Laine, E., Blond, S.: Les tumeurs trigono-septales. Neurochirurgie *26*, 247–278 (1980)
5. Mani, R.L., Hedgcock, M.W., Mass, S.I., Gilmor, R.L., Enzmann, D.R., Eisenberg, R.L.: Radiographic diagnosis of meningioma of the lateral ventricle. J. Neurosurg. *49*, 249–255 (1978)
6. Osborn, A.G., Daines, J.H., Wing, S.D.: The evaluation of ependymal and subependymal lesions by cranial computed tomography. Radiology *127*, 397–402 (1978)
7. Zimmerman, R.A., Bilanivk, L.T.: Computed tomography of choroid plexus lesions. J. Computed Tomography *3*, 93–108 (1981)

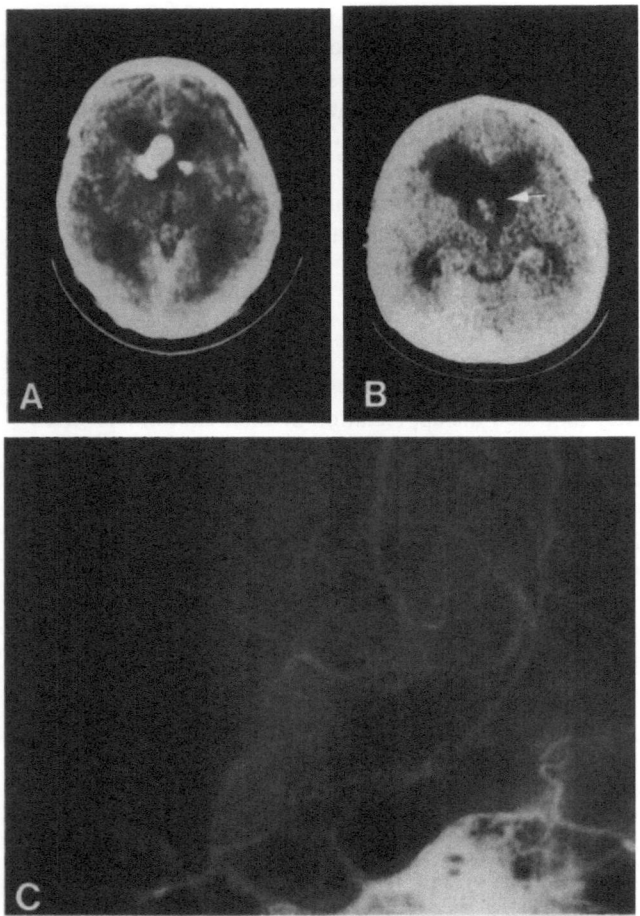

Fig. 1 A—C. Tumour of the interventricular foramina. A Case 3: giant cell astrocytoma of the left caudate nucleus in a case of tuberous sclerosis. Two calcifications are visible in front of the foramen of Monro: the tumour itself shows marked enhancement after IV contrast injection. As usual the mass has an anteromedial direction. In this case the ventricular dilatation is symmetrical. B Case 5: astrocytoma of the left caudate nucleus (CT after enhancement). Note the asymmetrical enlargement of the frontal horn with displacement of the septum (➡) and a transependymal resorption on the same side. C Case 5: lateral phlebogram in the same case as in B

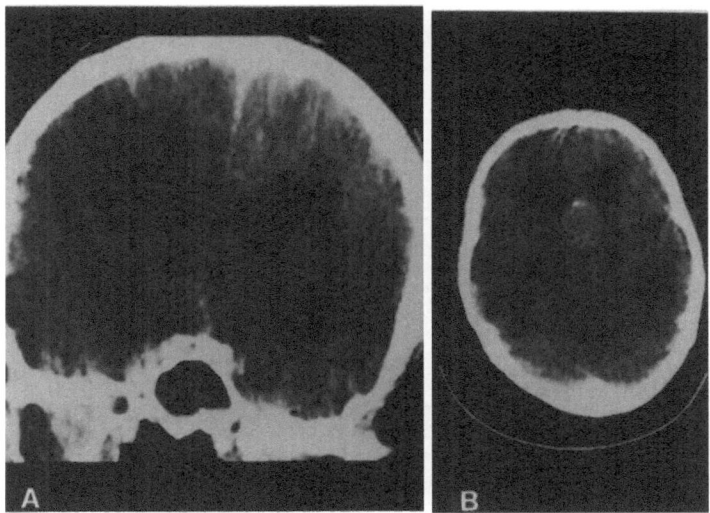

Fig. 2 A, B. Case 6: Septum pellucidum astrocytoma. On the coronal section (**A**) the septum is in the midline. Midline mass with microcalcification visible on the axial section (**B**). Note that the lateral walls of both frontal horns are visible, forming acute angles with the mass

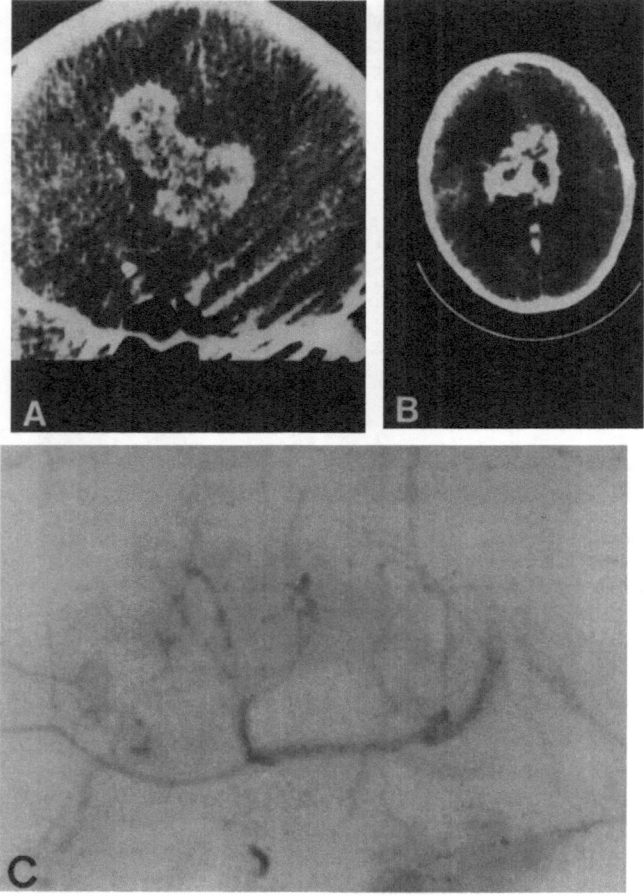

Fig. 3 A–C. Ependymoglioma of the lateral ventricle (case 14). A, B CT scan after injection. On the coronal section (A) one is able to note asymmetrical extension but the main part is in the midline. On the axial section (B) note the non-homogenous appearance with several hyperdense microcysts. Ventricular dilatation is asymmetrical. C Phlebogram in the same case. Tumour blush with a downward displacement of the septal and internal cerebral veins

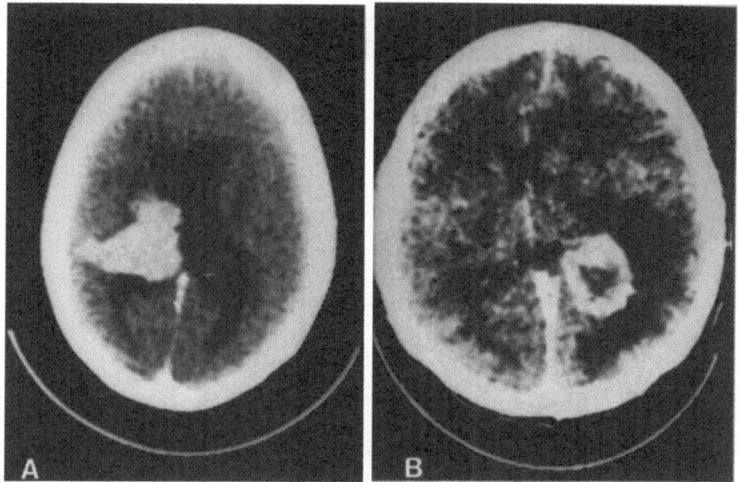

Fig. 4. A Case 19: meningioma of the ventricular trigone (CT after enhancement). There is large hyperdense and homogenous mass in the posterior part of the ventricle. **B** Case 21: choroid plexus carcinoma: ring-like enhanced mass of the left trigone. Note the entrapment of the temporal horn

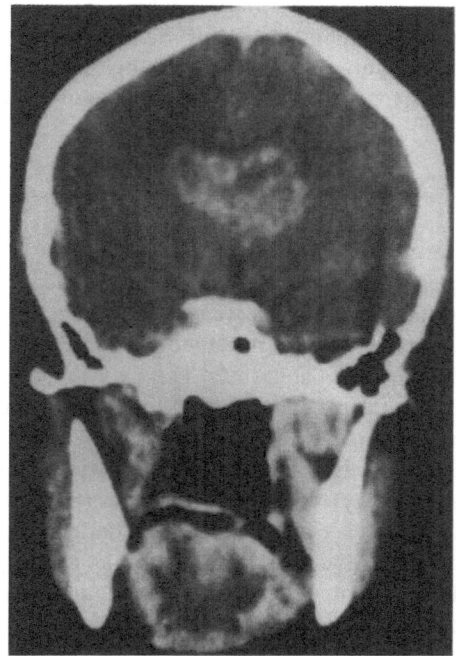

Fig. 5. Ependymoglioma (coronal section of CT scan after enhancement). The mass is well delineated from the corpus callosum *above* and the third ventricle *below*

Benign Tumours of the Lateral Ventricles —
Radiological and Surgical Considerations

M. Fornari, M. Savoiardo, G. Luccarelli, S. Giombini, C.L. Solero,
and F. Pluchino

Introduction

In spite of differences in their histological appearance tumours in the lateral ventricles
may be considered as a single group on account of the similar clinical picture and the
similarity of radiological and surgical approach (1, 5, 8).

Different problems arise in the case of anaplastic tumours and in the case of astrocytic
and oligodendroglial tumours which therefore have not been included in this series.
Eighty consecutive Malignancy Grade I intraventricular tumours (16) operated during
the last 20 years (1960–1980) have been considered in this study. Fifteen cases were
later on excluded because of the presence of some malignant dedifferentiation that was
recognized at retrospective histological review. Clinical features and neuroradiological
findings are presented. The surgical approaches and operative results are discussed.

Clinical Features

Out of the 65 cases finally considered 32 (49%) were ependymoma, 19 (29%) were meningioma, 8 (12%) were papilloma and 6 (10%) were epidermoid tumour. No clear pre-
dilection for either sex was found in case of ependymoma and epidermoid tumour; on
the contrary females prevailed (74%) in the case of meningioma and males prevailed
(87%) with the papillomas. The data concerning the mean age and the distribution of
patients in decades, according to different tumour type, are summarized in Fig. 1. Symptoms (Table 1) were extremely vague and in most of the cases of ependymoma, meningioma and papilloma were consistent with increased intracranial pressure (headache, dizziness, vomiting). Most of the patients (83%) with epidermoid tumour complained of epileptic seizures. Focal neurological deficits (contralateral motor deficits, visual field defects, incoordination of limbs, ataxia, tremor, speech difficulty, contralateral sensory deficits) were poorly recognized by the patients and often were only found at neurological
examination (Table 1), because of their mild nature.

Papilloedema was most frequently found in case of ependymoma probably because of
the particular location of these tumours which frequently obstructed the foramina of
Monro. The mean duration of the clinical history was short (6–10 months) in case of
epidermoid tumour and ependymoma and was less than 12 months also in 11 cases of
meningioma.

Diagnostic Investigations

The neuroradiological investigations performed in our series obviously included different kinds of examinations; moreover the quality of the angiograms improved over the years and Computerized Tomography (CT) study was only available since 1976. However, we think that several conclusions can be drawn from the review of the neuroradiological investigations performed in this series. The results obtained in each group of tumour will be first described and a comparison will then be made of the different clues which can help in reaching a pre-operative specific diagnosis.

Meningiomas

They form the largest, most homogeneous group, which has been already reviewed (6). The limited value of skull X rays and the limited value of the now obsolescent examinations as pneumoencephalography and ventriculography has been already pointed out. The examinations that we consider necessary are CT and angiography.

CT has been performed in the last four cases of the present series. In all the cases the tumour was hyperdense, although in one case it contained small hypodense areas and in another a few calcifications. In all the cases the tumour enhanced and its intraventricular location in the trigone was easily recognized either because of the dilatation of the entrapped occipital or temporal horn or because of the adherence of the tumour to the choroid plexus displaced anteriorly and medially (Fig. 2a). Hypodensity in the white matter surrounding the trigone, consistent with oedema, was a prominent feature in two cases. Angiography was remarkable in the fact that on carotid studies performed in 18 cases, tortuosity and displacement of the anterior choroidal artery were observed in 17, and in all of them this artery supplied a pathological circulation of variable extent and intensity. No participation in the pathological circulation was ever seen from the anterior or middle cerebral arteries. The great importance of stereoscopic views for recognizing the entire course of the anterior choroidal artery and its supply to the tumour vascularity has been stressed (Fig. 2b) (6). Unfortunately the atrial veins are not often demonstrated in meningiomas of the trigone, therefore the unquestionable demonstration of a complete intraventricular location, i.e. tumour blush surrounded by the atrial veins, was observed in only four cases. Vertebral angiography was performed in eight cases, but visualization of the posterior choroidal arteries was obtained in 12 instances: in four, the posterior cerebral artery filled at carotid angiography. The most common finding was reversal of the curvature of the lateral posterior choroidal artery, displaced forward with anterior convexity on lateral view (10 out of 12 cases). The lateral posterior choroidal arteries always contributed to the pathological circulation of the tumour, but in only one case (Fig. 2) was the tumour blush demonstrated at vertebral angiography more extensive than that seen on carotid angiograms.

Table 1. Symptoms (*above*) and neurological signs (*below*) at time of admission (65 cases)

	32 Ependymoma (%)	19 Meningioma (%)	8 Papilloma (%)	6 Epidermoid (%)
Epileptic seizures	22	11	25	83
Focal neurological deficits	25	42	25	16
Headache and/or vomiting	ʼ71	63	75	–
Mean duration of clinical history (months)	6	36	10	6
Mental deterioration	40	57	87	33
Focal deficits	78	90	100	100
Papilloedema	86	36	62	16

Ependymomas

They form the largest group of this series, but they have a more widespread distribution within the lateral ventricles. In our series of 32 cases, two were located in the frontal horn, five in the cella media, 11 developed in both these compartments but were particularly centred on the foramen of Monro, 12 were in the trigone and two in the temporal horn. Pneumoencephalography and ventriculography were performed in 19 cases and in 16 they demonstrated the intraventricular location of the tumour, and outlined the entire contour of the tumour in 13 cases.

In most of the cases skull X-rays demonstrated signs of increased intracranial pressure and tumour calcifications in six cases.

CT was performed in only three cases, and in two showed an isodense lesion and in one a hyperdense lesion; in all cases the tumour enhanced after contrast medium injection (Fig. 3a).

Carotid angiography was performed in 26 cases. In 18 it showed definite signs of an enlarged ventricle, but in only 13 cases did it show a pathological circulation within the ventricle; therefore, all the other five cases lacked a clear demonstration of the tumour. It is important to recognize the arteries which supply the pathological circulation: tumour vascularity originated from the choroidal arteries in only four cases: in two of them solely from the lateral posterior choroidal or from the posterior and anterior choroidal arteries, while in the other two cases there was a contribution to the pathological circulation from branches of the anterior and of the middle cerebral arteries. The most common origin of the pathological circulation in ependymoma of our series was from the perforating lenticulo-striate arteries of the middle cerebral artery and from the medial striate arteries of the horizontal segment of the anterior cerebral artery (seven cases) (Fig. 3 b,c). In the other instances the origin of the pathological circulation was either not well defined or was from branches of the middle cerebral artery along the insula or from the pericallosal or posterior cerebral arteries, indicating some infiltration of the parenchyma surrounding the ventricle. The posterior cerebral artery was shown eight times by carotid angiography. In another two cases vertebral angiography was performed: in one of these a significant contribution to the pathologic circulation was demonstrated.

Papillomas

Skull X-rays demonstrated signs of increased intracranial pressure in six out of eight cases (widening of sutures in five and sellar changes in a 16–year–old boy). Calcifications were seen in one case, in which they outlined the whole tumour which was located in the temporal horn. Pneumoencephalography and ventriculography were performed each in one patient, and showed the intraventricular location of the tumour.

No CT studies were available. Carotid angiography was available in six patients and in five showed tumour vascularity originating from the anterior and/or posterior choroidal arteries. In one of these, in whom the tumour was very large, the anterior cerebral and the posterior cerebral arteries contributed to the tumour circulation. No tumour circulation was seen in the heavily calcified tumour located in the temporal horn. In six cases the papilloma was in the trigone, while in the last one, not studied with angiography, it was located in the cella media. As with meningiomas, the tumour circulation was usually better evident and more uniform in the venous phase (Fig. 4).

Epidermoids

In only two of six cases the skull X-rays showed sellar changes consistent with increased intracranial pressure; in one of these, calcifications were also demonstrated. In five cases pneumoencephalography was performed and in four it showed the intraventricular mass lesion with the typical polylobulated contour of a cauliflower-like mass, indicative of the nature of the lesion.

CT was performed only in the last case: the low density of the lesion with negative attenuation values was the most diagnostic point (Fig. 5). Carotid angiography was performed in four cases and always showed an avascular mass lesion, undistinguishable from unilateral ventricular dilatation of whatsoever origin.

Surgical Treatment and Results

The location of the 65 intraventricular tumours according to the different tumour type is schematically represented in Fig. 6.

Total removal of the tumour was achieved in all the cases. Regarding the surgical approach no particular difficulty arose in removing the tumours located in the frontal horn and in the cella media of the lateral ventricle (20 cases: 18 ependymoma, two epidermoid) by the most direct route, that is through a transverse or longitudinal cortical

incision of the frontal lobe. In 11 cases of ependymoma the tumour was closely involved
with the foramen of Monro having sometimes expanded through it into the third ventricle. The five tumours located in the temporal horn (two ependymoma, one meningioma,
one papilloma and one epidermoid tumour) were reached by a straight incision along
the posterior portion of the middle temporal gyrus. In 40 cases (12 ependimoma, 18 meningioma, seven papilloma, three epidermoid tumour) the tumour was situated in the
trigone.

These tumours were mainly removed by a sagittal paramedian incision in the parietal
cortex, at a distance of 3 to 4 cm from the interhemispheric fissure and extending for
4 to 5 cm from 1 cm behind the postcentral fissure as far as the parieto-occipital fissure.

The operative mortality was 12.5% (four cases) in the group of ependymoma, 21%
(four cases) in the group of meningioma, 25% (two cases) in the group of papilloma and
16% (one case) in the group of epidermoid tumour. The total mortality was 16.9% (11
cases).

The mean duration of clinical follow-up study was about seven years. Five recurrences
were seen in the group of ependymomas (16%).

Discussion and Conclusions

In the evaluation of tumours of the lateral ventricles, CT has taken the place of pneumoencephalography and ventriculography. Pneumoencephalography or ventriculography
often demonstrated the intraventricular location of the tumour and, in some epidermoid
tumour, even predicted the nature of the lesion. However, there is no need to stress the
superiority of CT in demonstrating the full extent of the intraventricular tumours, with
their possible infiltration of the ventricular walls and extension into the surrounding
parenchyma.

Angiography retains its value for two reasons: because it shows the vascularity of the
tumour itself, which is often an important diagnostic feature, and also because it demonstrates to the neurosurgeon the surrounding vascular anatomy.

Different intraventricular tumours may present with similar CT and angiographic findings (1, 6). However, the comparison of the results of our observations offers a few
diagnostic clues. First of all, epidermoid tumours can be eliminated from further consideration because, apart from the extremely rare cases of hyperdense epidermoid tumours (2), they typically present as hypodense lesions with often negative attenuation
values. The other three types of tumour considered in this series, i.e. ependymoma,
meningioma, papilloma, may have very similar attenuation values and very similar enhancement on post-contrast CT. However, site, angiographic findings and age are important diagnostic features.

Eighteen out of 19 meningioma of our series were located in the trigone, even if they
presented sometimes some extension into the cella media or into the temporal horn.

A similar location was predominant for papilloma because both of these tumours
develop from the choroid plexus, even if from different components of it (15). Therefore, the origin of the tumour circulation is the same and angiography does not offer
specific elements for the differential diagnosis. However, the mean age of the menin-

gioma patients was 44 years, with no case in the first decade of life, while the mean age of the patients with choroid plexus papilloma was five years with only two cases above the age of ten.

The ependymomas develop mainly in the frontal horn or in the cella media with a high concentration in the region of the foramen of Monro, therefore causing a striking ventricular dilatation also of the frontal horn, which is uncommon in meningiomas (6). In addition, the choroidal arteries rarely contributed to the tumour vascularity, which most often originated from perforating lenticulo-striate arteries because of the most frequent anterior location of the ependymoma and their origin from the ependymal layer of the floor of the ventricle. Finally, even if we included in our series only malignancy grade I ependymoma which apparently had a completely intraventricular location, some contribution to the tumour vascularity from the cortical branches of the anterior and middle cerebral arteries, indicating some extent of infiltration of the periventricular brain parenchyma, was sometimes observed. In conclusion, the combination of various CT elements and of angiographic findings together with the location of the tumour, the age of the patient and other clinical features, and mainly the length of the clinical history, can offer determinant or at least highly indicative elements for a specific pre-operative diagnosis.

In this series the tumours were mostly found (40 cases, 62%) in the trigonal region. Many different surgical approaches to this ventricular region have been used in the past by different authors, including a resection of the occipital lobe (12), a straight or curved incision in the lower posterior portion of the parietal lobe (11, 14), a straight incision along the posterior portion of the second temporal gyrus (4), a linear parieto-occipital paramedian incision (3), an interhemispheric approach by incision of the splenium and posterior portion of the corpus callosum and removal of the tumour through the choroid fissure (7) (Fig. 7).

In our experience the parieto-occipital paramedian route appears the safest surgical approach as it allows the sparing of the optic radiations, which lie inferolaterally to the ventricle, and it never causes severe speech or motor deficits (6). In spite of the reported risk of post-operative disconnection syndrome (10), the removal of the tumour by an approach through the corpus callosum appears extremely promising, especially if performed with the aid of the ultrasonic suction device, but we have not yet had any personal experience of this route (6, 8).

The temporal route and the approach through the corpus callosum may allow a prior access to the supplying vessels (to the anterior choroidal and to the postero-lateral choroidal arteries respectively) provided that these arteries are not displaced and hidden behind the tumour (6).

The occlusion of the choroidal arteries becomes possible even with the parieto-occipital paramedian approach as soon as the tumour is reduced in size and mobilized to expose its supplying vessels. However, microneurosurgical technique allows a piecemeal removal of the tumour with minimal bleeding in most of the cases. Only in the case of an extremely hemorrhagic papilloma could "en bloc" removal of the tumour, after occlusion of the vascular pedicles, be preferred (13): nevertheless, in our series the surgical mortality was mainly due to post-operative intraventricular haematomas which occurred mostly in cases operated in the earlier years by tumour removal "en bloc". The dissection of the tumour from the ventricular walls must always be performed very carefully by microsurgical technique in order to recognize and coagulate the draining veins entering the subependymal venous system and to prevent damage to the surrounding tissues. In fact in case of large tumours the normal ependymal layer of the ventricle disappears and the tumour is closely adherent to a gliotic surface layer (14) of the periventricular white matter. This lack of a clearly defined plane between tumour, ependymal layer and surrounding tissue is quite often found in case of ependymoma, and gives additional difficulties in the removal of this type of tumour.

References

1. Bernasconi, V., Cabrini, G.P.: Radiological features of tumors of the lateral ventricles. Acta Neurochir. *17*, 290–310 (1967)
2. Braun, I.F., Naidich, T.P., Leeds, N.E., Koslow, M., Zimmermann, H.M. Chase, N.E.: Dense intracranial epidermoid tumors. Computed tomographic observations. Radiology *122*, 717–719 (1977)
3. Cramer, F.: The intraventricular meningiomas: a note on the neurologic determinants governing the surgical approach. Arch. Neurol. *98* (1960) (Abstract)
4. Delandsheer, J.M.: Les méningiomes du ventricule latéral. Neurochirurgie *11*, 3–57 (1965)
5. De la Torre, E., Alexander, E., Jr., Davis, C.H., Jr., Crandell, L.: Tumors of the lateral ventricles of the brain: report of eight cases, with suggestions for clinical management. J. Neurosurg. *20*, 461–470 (1963)
6. Fornari, M., Savoiardo, M., Morello, G., Solero, C.L.: Meningiomas of the lateral ventricles. Neuroradiological and surgical considerations in 18 cases. J. Neurosurg. *54*, 64–74 (1981)
7. Kempe, L.G., Blaylock, R.: Lateral trigonal intraventricular tumors. A new operative approach. Acta Neurochir. *35*, 233–242 (1976)
8. Kempe, L.G.: "Letter to the Editor". J. Neurosurg. *54*, 848–849 (1981)
9. Lakke, J.P.W.F.: Report on 16 intraventricular brain tumors: a clinical study. Europ. Neurol. *2*, 158–174 (1969)
10. Levin, H.S., Rose, J.E.: Alexia without agraphia in a musician after transcallosal removal of a left intraventricular meningioma. Neurosurgery *4*, 168–174 (1979)
11. Migliavacca, F.: Meningiomi dei ventricoli laterali. Chirurgia *10*, 249– 268 (1955)
12. Olivecrona, H., Tönnis, W.: Handbuch der Neurochirurgie, Vol. 4. S. 175–177. Berlin, Heidelberg, New York: Springer 1967
13. Raimondi, A.J., Gutierrez, F.A.: Diagnosis and surgical treatment of choroid plexus papillomas. Child's Brain *1*, 81–115 (1975)
14. Wall, A.E.: Meningiomas within the lateral ventricles of the brain. J. Neuropathol. *17*, 367–381 (1958)
15. Zimmerman, R.A., Bilaniuk, L.T.: Computed Tomography of choroid plexus lesions. CT: The Journal of Computed Tomography *3*, 93–103 (1979)
16. Zülch, K.J.: Historical development of the classification of brain tumors and the new proposal of the World Health Organization (WHO). Neurosurgical Review *4*, 123–127 (1981)

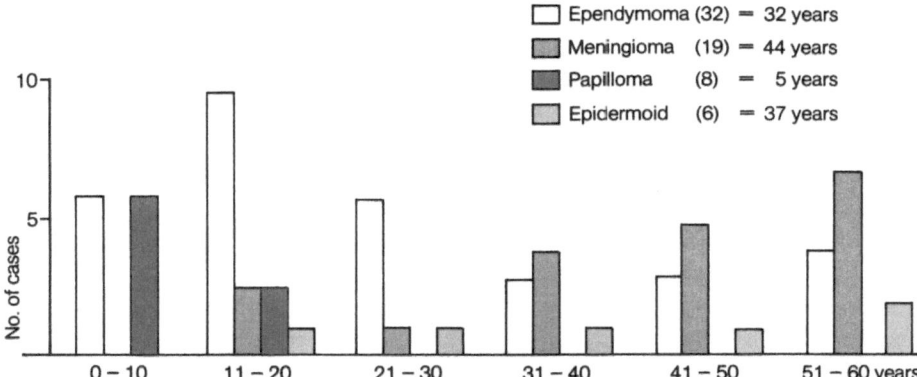

Fig. 1. Age at time of presentation of 65 patients with benign tumours of the lateral ventricles, according to different tumour types

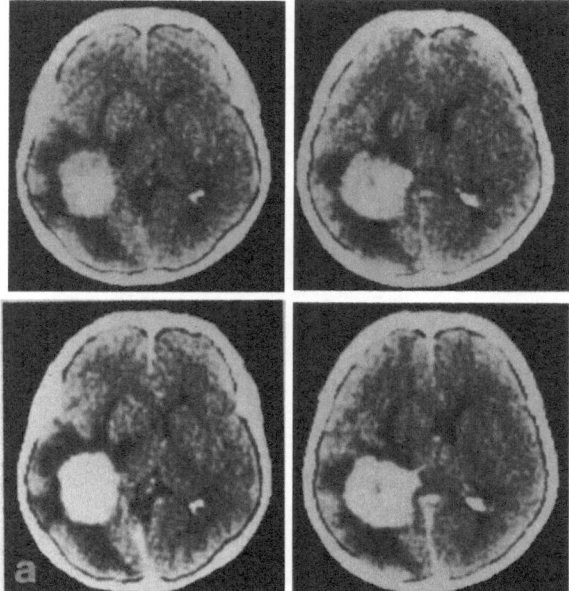

Fig. 2 a-e. Meningioma of the left ventricle. a Precontrast (*above*) and postcontrast (*below*) CT studies show a hyperdense, enhancing mass in the trigone, surrounded by oedema. On the lower right image, adherence of the meningioma to the choroid plexus is recognizable. The frontal horn and the cella media are not dilated

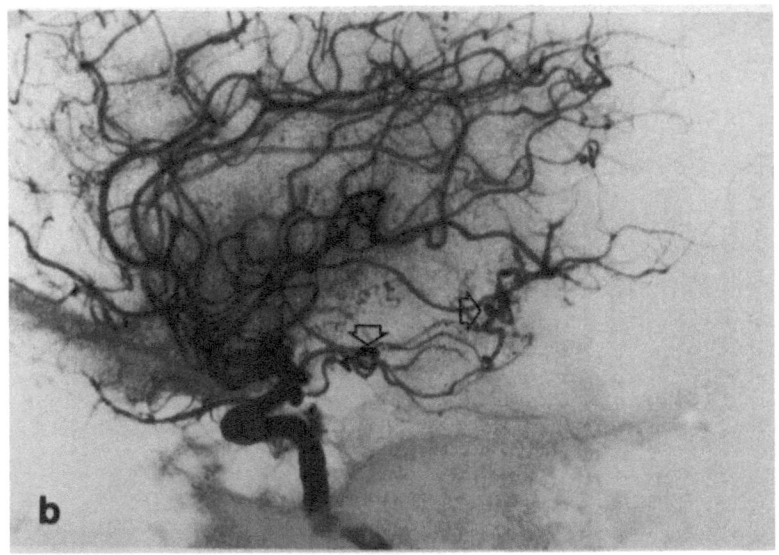

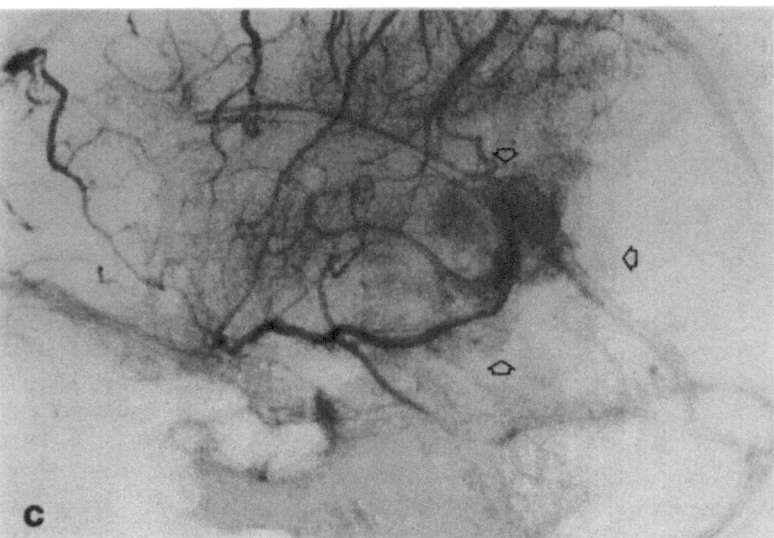

Fig. 2. b,c Carotid angiography, lateral view. The anterior choroidal artery (*arrows*), enlarged and tortuous (**b**) surrounds the anterior aspect of the tumour and supplies pathological circulation persisting in the venous phase (*arrows*) (**c**). **d,e** Vertebral angiography, lateral view. An irregularly dilated lateral posterior choroidal artery (**d**) supplies a uniform tumour blush more evident in the venous phase (*arrows*) (**e**), of larger extension than that seen on carotid angiography. In this case only, a possible contribution to the tumour vascularity from branches other than the choroidal arteries was seen, namely from tiny vessels of the distal segment of the posterior cerebral artery

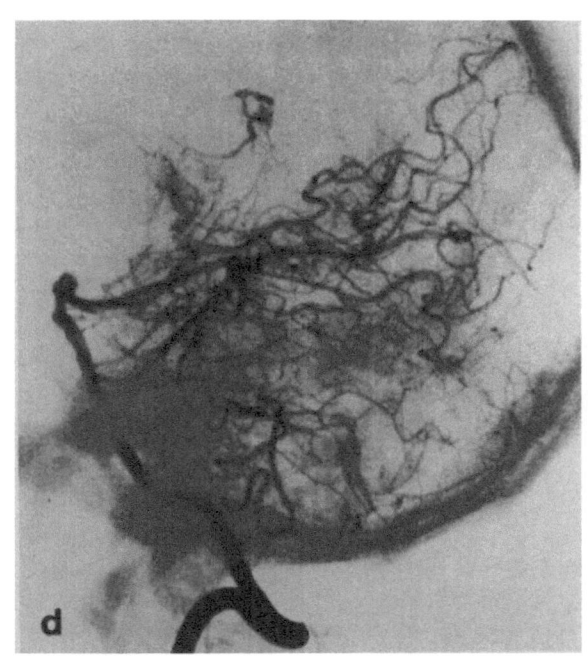

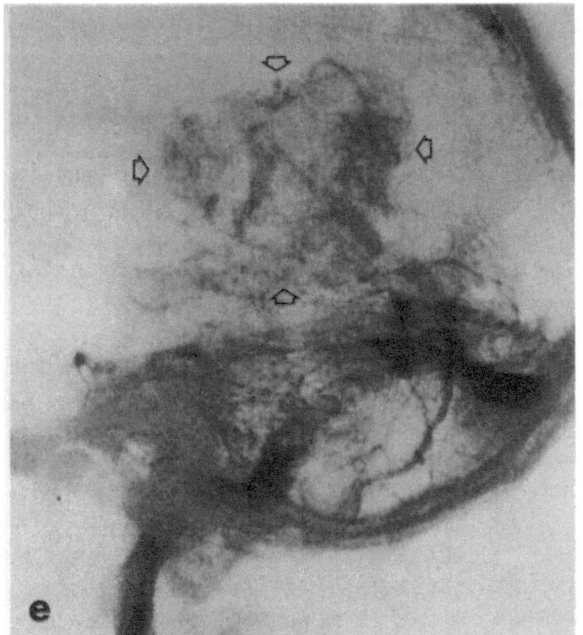

Fig. 2 d, e

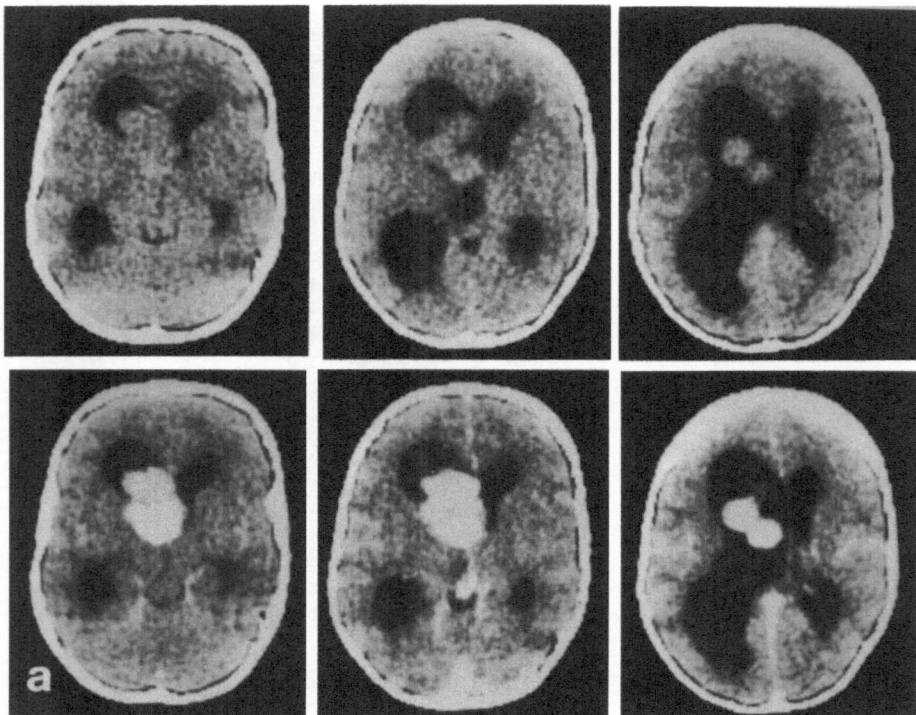

Fig. 3 a-c. Ependymoma of the left frontal horn and cella media. **a** Precontrast (*above*) and post-contrast (*below*) CT studies show a markedly enhancing, lobulated tumour, centred in the region of the foramen of Monro. **b, c** Carotid angiography, lateral view. The perforating lenticulo-striate arteries of the middle cerebral artery and the medial striate branches of the horizontal segment of the anterior cerebral artery (**b**) supply the tumour circulation, which, in the venous phase (**c**), appears surrounded by the subependymal veins, indicating the intraventricular location of the tumour

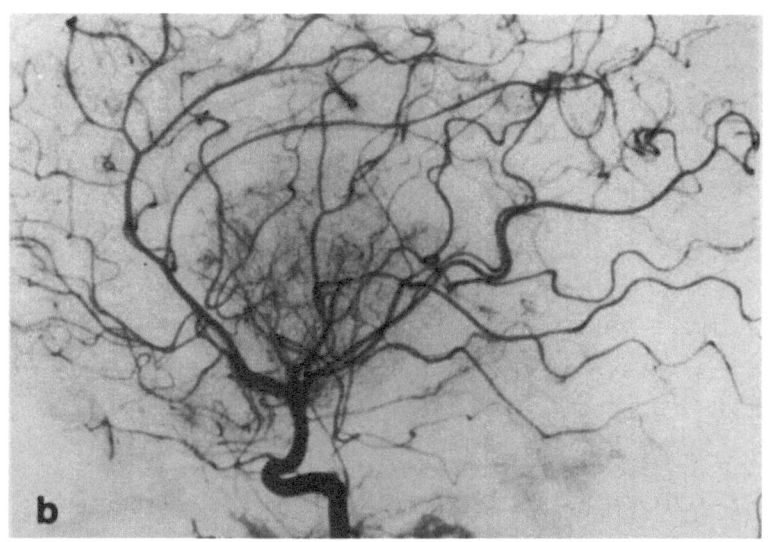

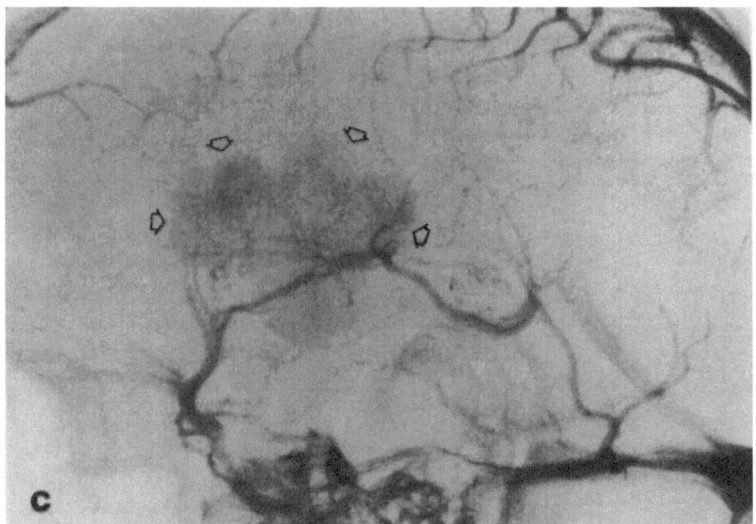

Fig. 3 b,c

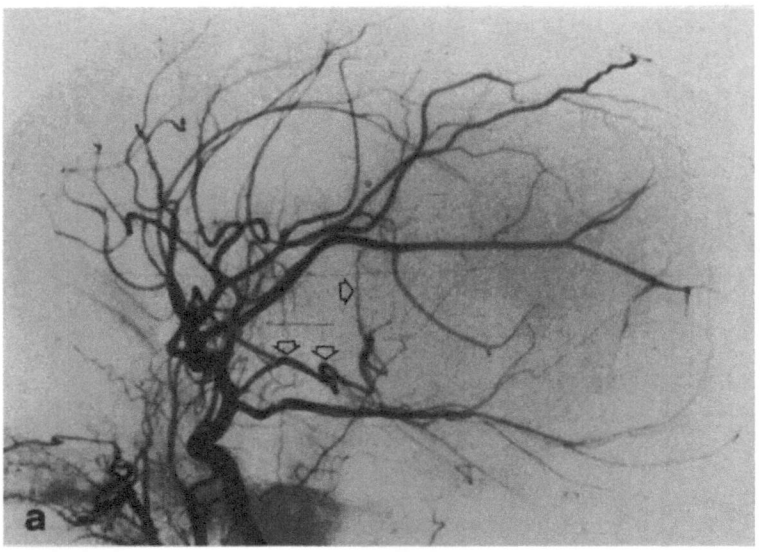

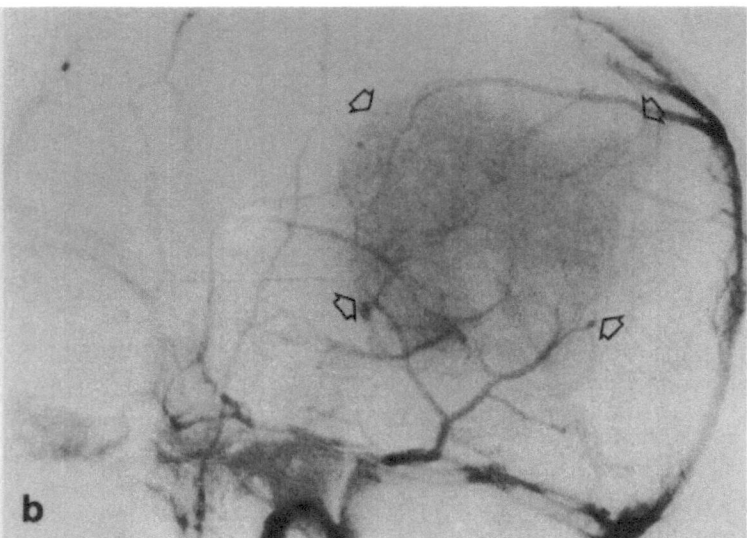

Fig. 4 a,b. Choroid plexus papilloma in an 11-month-old boy. Carotid angiography, lateral view.
The anterior choroidal artery (*arrows*) (**a**) is enlarged, accordeonated and displaced forward and upward in its plexual segment. The lateral posterior choroidal artery, faintly visualized, is displaced
forward and downward. Only these arteries contribute to the tumour circulation, well evident in
the venous phase (**b**). Differential diagnosis from a meningioma is made by the age of the patient

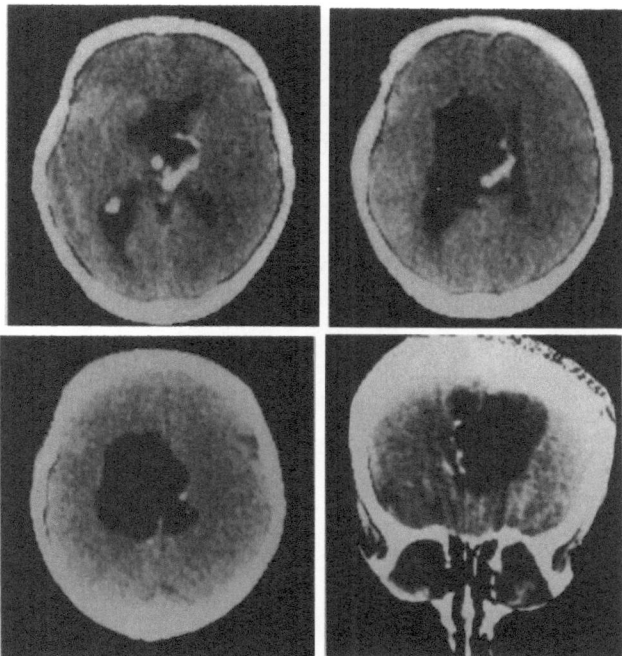

Fig. 5. Intraventricular epidermoid tumor. CT scan with the adjacent axial cuts and the coronal section (*lower right*) demonstrate a hypodense lesion with negative attenuation values, surrounded by a few calcifications. The epidermoid extends over the midline and involves the corpus callosum, with aspects very similar to those of a lipoma of the corpus callosum

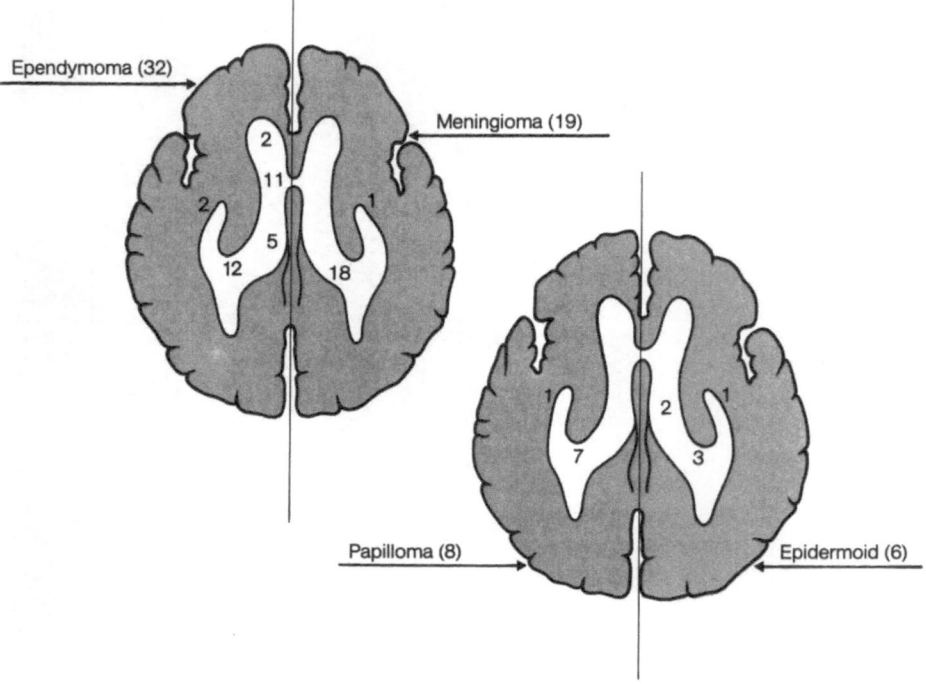

Fig. 6. Benign intraventricular tumours (65 cases) intraventricular location according to tumour type

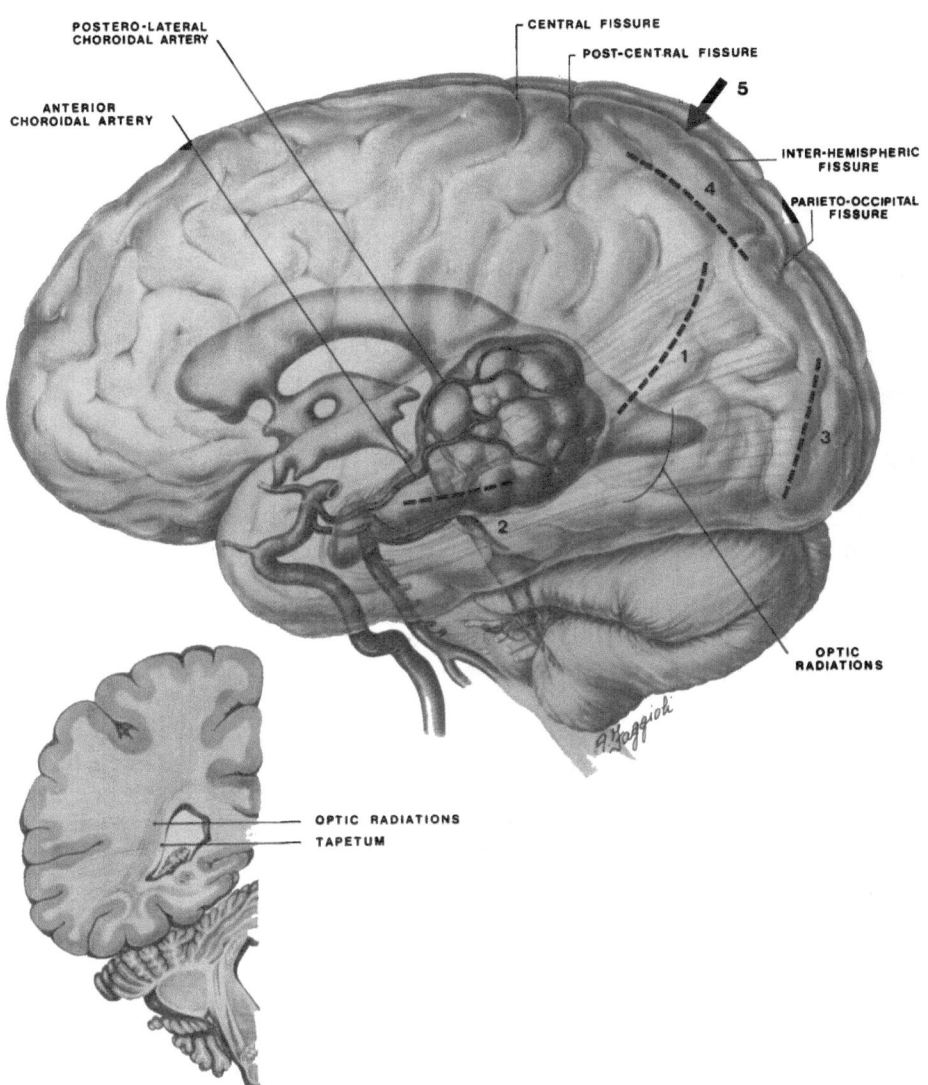

Fig. 7. Different surgical approaches to tumours located in the trigone of the lateral ventricle

257

Clinical Observations on 40 Cases of Tumours of the Fourth Ventricle in Adults

D.-K. Lin

Abstract

Forty cases of tumour of the fourth ventricle in adult were admitted to our hospital in a six year period. All of these patients were operated upon, with the tumour totally resected in 29 cases and subtotally resected in 11 cases. Three patients died in the early postoperative period from acute brain stem oedema (an operative mortality of 7.5%).

The other 37 cases were followed up for two to eight years. Up to now, 27 cases are still surviving; 15 of them have resumed their work; eight are living more or less normally and four must be taken care of by others. The essential points in diagnosis and treatment and the methods for improving the effectiveness of surgical excision are discussed.

Tumours of the fourth ventricle are not rare in adults over 16 years. Forty cases were admitted to our hospital from January 1972 to January 1978. Of these 37 were followed up for a period varying from two to eight years. Three died in the early postoperative period. Here is the analysis and discussion of the results of our treatment and follow-up.

Clinical Material

There were 17 male and 23 female patients. The age ranged from 16 to 52 years old with a mean age of 30 years old. The clinical course varied from 3 months to 5 years, i.e., from the onset of first symptom to the time of admission. All but three cases had symptoms and signs of intracranial hypertension at the onset. These three cases had dizziness and staggering of gait as the initial symptoms. Besides, there were 37 with headache, in 30 of whom they were frontal-occipital in nature, 21 had dizziness and vomiting, 8 had Bruns syndrome, 12 visual impairment and 17 staggering gait, 14 forced head posture and 4 had attacks of cerebellar fits. Neurological examination showed that there were 36 with papilloedema with retinal hoemorrhages in 8 of them, 4 secondary optic atrophy, 9 abducens nerve paralysis, 18 lateral nystagmus, 7 hypotonia, 10 ataxia, 12 positive Romberg sign, 17 neck rigidity and 2 positive Kernig sign. Skull X-ray showed that there were signs of intracranial hypertension in 21 cases. The diagnosis in all the 40 cases was confirmed by conray ventriculography.

Results of treatment and follow-up: All the 40 patients were operated upon with the tumour totally resected in 29 cases and subtotally resected in 11 cases. After operation deep X-ray therapy was given to 16 cases. Three patients died in the immediate post-operative period of acute brain stem oedema (giving an operative mortality of 7.5%). The histopthological types of tumour were: Ependymoma 19 cases, astrocytoma 9, plexus papilloma 5, simple cyst 4, haemangioblastoma 2 and medulloblastoma 1. The survived 37 cases were followed up for two to eight years. Among them ten died of tumour recurrence; the survival periods varied from 8 months to 4 years and 7 months. Up to now, 27 cases are still alive. Among them, nine have been followed up for five to eight years. Among these 27, there are 9 ependymomas, 7 astrocytomas, 5 plexus papillomas, 4 cysts, and 2 haemangioblastomas. Fifteen patients have resumed their work, 8 are living more or less normally and 4 must be taken care of by others.

Discussion

1. Diagnosis of Tumour of the Fourth Ventricle in Adults

This is made mainly on clinical grounds, but confirmatory neuroradiological examinations are considered to be indispensable before operation. As the tumour will obstruct the CSF circulation, hydrocephalus and intracranial hypertension is likely to be the first symptom. Since 37 cases had headache at an early stage and in most of them it was confined to the frontal-occipital region without specific localization, they were often erroneously diagnosed at the very beginning. Thus there were five cases diagnosed as hemicrania, three cases as occipital neuralgia. When the tumour had enlarged to a certain extent, cerebellar symptoms occurred or as a result of intracranial hypertension. Forced head posture and stiffness of neck generally occurred and these signs suggested the site of the lesion to be in the fourth ventricle. Tonsillar herniation was found in 16 cases during operation and in four of them the tumour had extended as low as the cisterna magna and in one even to the lower part of the second cervical vertebra. The findings in all these cases agree well with their clinical symptoms. There were eight cases had intermittent spells of severe headache, dizziness, vomiting and unconsciousness at an early period. Three of them were erroneously diagnosed in the other hospital as hysteria. This may be due to incomplete obstruction of the fourth ventricle in the early period, so that the tumour acts as a ball valve in the fourth ventricle. Whenever there is accumulation of CSF in the ventricle or when the position of patient's head is changed, typical attacks of Bruns syndrome occurred. We consider this sign to be a reliable feature for suspecting the diagnosis.

It is not difficult to suspect a typical case of tumour of fourth ventricle, but to judge the exact nature of the tumour merely on the basis of the clinical symptoms will be difficult. CT may help to locate a tumour in this situation but for determining its nature, vertebral angiography is of the utmost value. In case there is no such facility, positive contrast ventriculography is still considered to be a necessary diagnostic method. To sum up, the patterns of ventriculography in the 40 cases can be classified into the following three types:

1. Symmetrical enlargment of the part above the third ventricle, distension and shortening of aqueduct with upward shift accompanied with filling defect in the fourth ventricle (Fig. 1).

2. Compression and elevation of the fourth ventricle accompanied with filling defect (Fig. 2).
3. Partial or complete obstruction of the exit of the aqueduct with distension and angulation of its lower part. In some cases, there is a curved pressure mark on the aqueduct as well as on the posterior aspect of the fourth ventricle. In the A–P view, the fourth ventricle usually shows no lateral shift (Fig. 3).

The first two types described above suggest that the tumour lies within the fourth ventricle. This happened in 26 cases of the group. The histopathologic types of tumour were: ependymomas 14, plexus papillomas 5, cysts 4, haemangioblastoma 1, and astrocytomas 2. The third pattern suggests that the tumours lies at the top of the fourth ventricle. There are 14 cases among this group and the histopathologic types of tumour were: astrocytomas 7, ependymomas 5, haemangioblastoma 1, medulloblastoma 1. The last mentioned tumour is easily confused with a tumour of the vermis of the cerebellum and should be differentiated clinically.

2. Prognosis in Relation with Operation

Up to now, surgical excision of the tumour is still the only reliable treatment. The aims of excision are:
1. to relieve the brain stem and the cerebellum of the compression by the tumour;
2. to reduce the danger of chronic tonsillar herniation;
3. to restore the circulation of cerebrospinal fluid. Among the 27 survivor, there were 21 cases in which excision of the tumour was complete. This fact suggests that total excision of the tumour may play a role in the better prognosis. However, in its turn the total excision of the tumour depends upon several facts, as follows:

a) Special regard should be paid to the pre-operative preparation of the patients, since patients of this kind have usually failed to take food for quite a long time, and there may also be frequent vomiting. Therefore they are invariably suffering from varying degrees of dehydration and electrolyte disturbances, sometimes even undernutrition. This had a bad effect on the operative results. It is equally of importance before operation to take vigourous measures to release obstructive hydrocephalus or chronic tonsillar herniation if there is any. We advocate short term ventricular drainage, followed soon afterward by measures to correct water and electrolyte imbalance.

b) The prerequisite for the complete excision of a tumour is its good exposure during the operation, but the operative field is often rather narrow. The tumour is deeply seated and there are vital structures around the tumour. Should there be haemorrhage or inadvertent injury, the outcome is more serious. Thus the position of the patient is of prime importance to ensure a good operative exposure and successful excision. Before 1972, we operated on patients in the prone or lateral position. Because of the poor exposure, difficulties were frequently experienced. Since 1972, we have designed an operation chair, which allows a variable angle adjustment, and we are able to operate on a patient with his head in a hyperflexed position. This provides a favourable exposure, lessens the amount of bleeding and favours the complete excision of the tumour.

c) In the majority of the tumours of the fourth ventricle there are planes of cleavage between the tumour and the surrounding brain tissue, except for those tumours which are fixed to the floor of the ventricle. The dissection of the tumour is generally not difficult. It is customary for me to separated the tumour from its surrounding tissues from above downward and from left to right. By means of a small piece of cotton, it is easy to separate the tumour from its bed. It is also important to protect the normal neighbouring tissues from injuries, which may be caused by the instruments used during the operation. Except when the tumour is pedunculated and easily movable, it is generally wise to excise the tumour piecemeal. For those with broad bases, fixed to the floor of the fourth ventricle, the author rather prefers to leave a part of the tumour tissue behind than to remove it by force. Any inadvertent stimulus or injury to the floor of the fourth ventricle either from the instruments or by electrical coagulation will give rise to serious harmful effects. The author has experienced the failure of the operation in three cases, who died of acute brain stem oedema within 36–48 hours of the operation. If oozing occurs at the bottom of the tumour bed, it can usually be stopped by a hot compress with pieces of cotton pledget. Most patients have fever of above 39°C of unknown origin in the four nights period postoperatively. This is probably due to the stimulus of the vital centres in the floor of the fourth ventricle during the operation. In recent years the author has adopted the routine of postoperative ventricular drainage for three days to reduce the fever and to quiet down the alarming symptoms in the postoperative period. In the first or second postoperative day, there will usually be about 200 ml bloody CSF draining daily. The convalescence of the patient is thus enhanced. With the exception of benign tumour, all the patients should be given an intensive coures of radiation therapy no matter whether the tumour has been totally removed or not.

Summary

This article presents 40 cases of tumour of the fourth ventricle in adults admitted to our hospital in the period between Jan. 1972 and Jan. 1978. Among them there were 29 totally resected and 11 subtotally resected; 16 cases received postoperative irradiation in addition to excision. Three totally resected cases died of acute brain stem oedema shortly after operation giving an operative mortality of 7.5%. The remaining 37 cases all survived and were followed up for periods varying from 2 to 8 years.

There were ten cases died of tumour recurrence. Among the totally resected cases, 21 are still alive. The author analyses and discusses the factors of prognostic importance and clinical experiences in treating these tumour of the fourth ventricle. Characteristics of ventriculograms in such cases are presented.

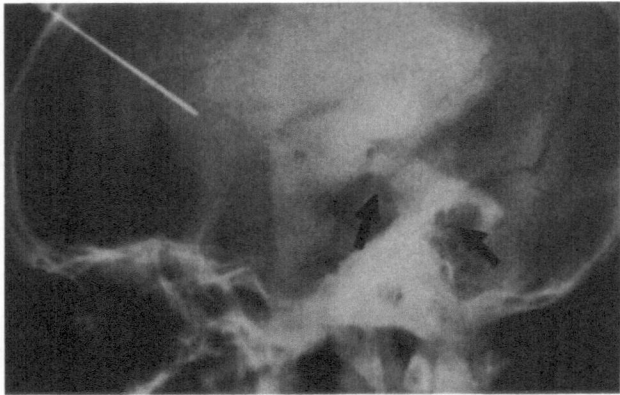

Fig. 1. Symmetrical enlargment of the part above the third ventricle, distension and shortening of aqueduct with upward shift accompanied by a filling defect in the fourth ventricle

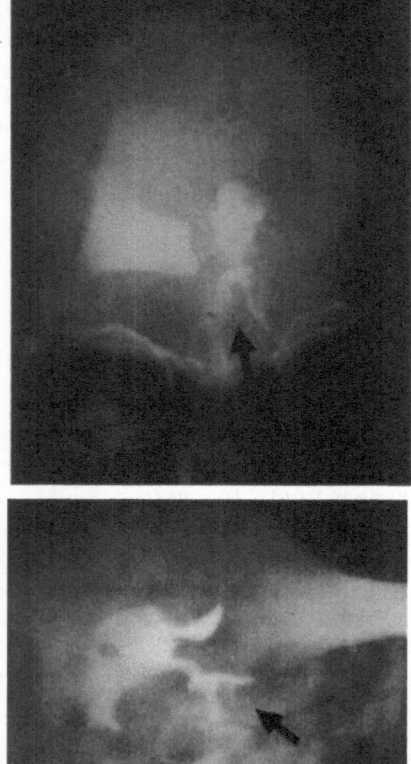

Fig. 2. Compression and elevation of the fourth ventricle accompanied by a filling defect

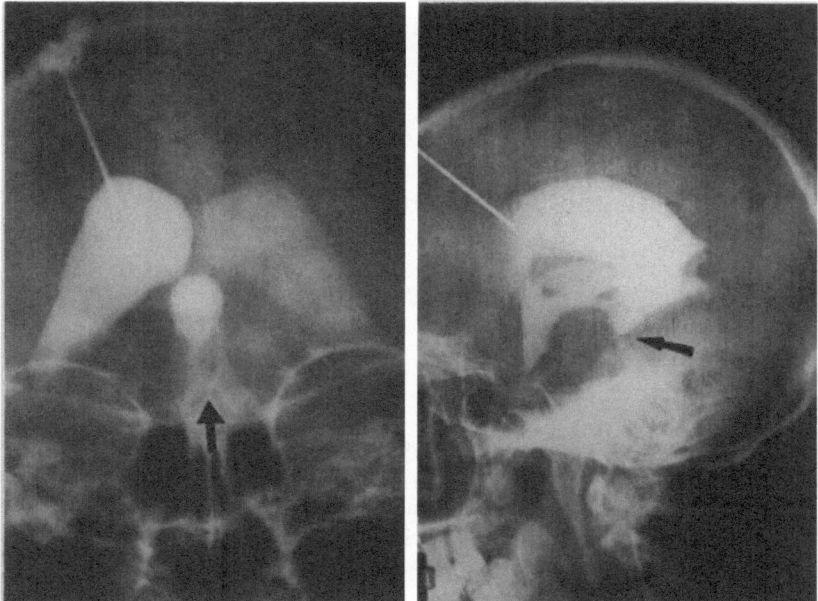

Fig. 3. Obstruction of the exit of the aqueduct with distension and angulation of its lower part, and a curved pressure mark on the aqueduct as well as on the posterior aspect of the fourth ventricle. In the A—P view, the fonrth ventricle shows no lateral shift

High Resolution CT Scan in Diagnosis of Lumbar Spine Lesions

A. Lifson, K.B. Heithoff, C.V. Burton, and Ch.D. Ray

Introduction

An epidemic of low back disability in the modern Western world is a widely recognized reality. While the majority of cases of low back pain can be successfully managed by preventive and conservative measures, by an improvement of the physical condition, education in proper body mechanics and dynamics, there is still a very significant number of patients for whom the solution of the question "to be or not to be" treated surgically is crucial, and whose clinical picture requires detailed morphological diagnosis. A complete understanding of lumbosacral anatomy is absolutely necessary in planning the surgical procedure which will give the best postoperative results and avoid the failed low back surgery syndrome.

The study of spinal anatomy in vivo first became possible after the introduction of X-rays by W. Konrad Roentgen in 1896 (18). Since that time a tremendous amount of knowledge has been accumulated about the radiographic anatomy of the spine, in normal and various pathological conditions. A number of contrast diagnostic methods, such as air and positive myelography, discography, venospondylography, and spinal angiography allowed visualization of spinal bony structures as well as the intraspinal subarachnoidal space, intravertebral discs, arterial and venous systems of the spine, and the spinal cord. The clinical importance of these studies for the diagnosis and delineation of a variety of pathological entities is well known.

Despite the sophistication of the above diagnostic methods, each of them has considerable limitations and negative features. Their complications, although extremely rare, can be very serious and even fatal. The above mentioned mehtods, as well as conventional radiography of the spine, can provide only antero-posterior, lateral, and oblique projections, being unable to display an axial view. The Toshiba unit which enabled one to perform axial tomography of the spine made a very significant contribution to the study of normal (8) and pathological (9, 17) bony anatomy of the spine. However, the relatively low resolution of this unit does not allow visualization of soft tissues, such as discs, nerve roots, epidural fat, etc.

Computerized tomography (CT) combines the safety of conventional radiography and the advantages of axial tomography. The high resolution of modern CT scanners makes the diagnostic accuracy of CT equal or even superior to the contrast studies. This method is now well recognized and is becoming more and more popular among medical groups specializing in lumbosacral spine pathology. Glenn (6) reported that the largest application of body CT in their practice, was in the lumbar spine. CT scanning is the leading diagnostic tool for lumbar spine pathology because it can identify and distinguish between the wide variety of lesions of the lumbosacral spine. There is an extremely high incidence of degenerative disc disease, facet joints disease, congenital and acquired stenotic conditions. At the same time, there is a relatively low incidence of intradural lesions which pose the greatest difficulties for CT diagnosis (7).

Material and Methods

The following conclusions are drawn from more than 4,000 cases examined by us and treated conservatively, and from 420 various surgical procedures performed on the lumbosacral spine, and about 7,000 CT lumbar scans.

Since 1978, the GE 8800 high resolution CT scanner was used in all cases. Filming techniques include magnification x2, and window settings (1000 and 300) which were used for the visualization of the bony structures and soft tissues, respectively. Non-tilted 5 mm thick contiguous scans with a scanning speed of 9.6 sec./slide were used. A lateral "Scout view", a computed radiograph, was employed in all cases for localization. Coronal, lateral, and oblique reconstructions were used in selected cases which required the solution of specific diagnostic problems.

During the initial nine months of experience, all lumbar CT scans were performed 3 to 4 hours after standard metrizamide myelography. The opacification of the cerebrospinal fluid (CSF) within the subarachnoidal space provided an excellent demonstration of the nerve roots and the dural sac on post-enhancement scans. It seemed that, when enhanced by intrathecal injections of metrizamide, CT scanning was the method of choice for the study of a variety of conditions involving the lumbosacral spine. However, the rapidly growing demand for CT scanning of the lumbar spine in many outpatients led to CT scanning of the lumbar spine without preliminary intrathecal injections of contrast medium. The non-enhanced CT scans proved to be diagnostically accurate and sensitive in a three month prospective study of 277 patients, providing the correct diagnosis in 40 of 44 patients operated on for herniated discs (91% accuracy). There was one false negative, and three false positives. All three false positives were in previously operated patients, there being no false positives in unoperated patients. Since May 1980, the majority of lumbar CT scans are being performed without enhancement. Our policy on very selective indications for enhancement has been outlined elsewhere (13).

Discussion

The greatest advantage of the third generation of CT scanners is their high resolution and their ability to show soft tissues. Our experience shows that the extradural portion of lumbosacral nerve roots, as well as ganglia, epidural veins, epidural fat, and protruding or freely extruded disc fragments can be easily shown by modern CT scanning technology. The presence of oily and dense, unabsorbed metrizamide or other contrast media within the spinal canal can make it much more difficult and in some cases even impossible to measure the attenuation values of various soft tissue structures which is crucial for the differentiation between nerve roots, discs, and fibrous tissue.

265

The normal anatomy of the lumbar spine in a CT image is well known (8). In the analysis of consecutive slices, special attention is paid to the configuration of the vertebral bodies, and intervertebral discs to evaluate for herniation of the disc nucleus. The anatomy of the posterior elements and the zygo-apophyseal joints in particular, is of paramount importance, since hypertrophy of the superior articular facets is the most frequent single cause or a contributing factor in the development of lateral spinal stenosis (11).

The capability of CT scanning to diagnose congenital and degenerative stenotic conditions of the lumbar spine is well recognized (3, 5, 11). High resolution CT scan provides direct visualization of nerve roots and ganglia and epidural perineural fat. This allows one to diagnose narrowings of the neural canal by direct measurements, and to visualize compressions and displacements of nerve roots or ganglia. A substantial decrease in the amount of epidural fat in non-operated patients without fibrosis is a very reliable sign of compression of the extradural portion of the nerve roots.

Despite the temptation to discuss separately disc herniations, zygo-apophyseal joint disease, and other conditions, it is worth-while mentioning that in the majority of cases we encountered a combination of the above findings, illustrating that lumbar degenerative disc disease is a complex entity involving all structures of the spine (Fig. 1). In many cases of congenital or degenerative narrowing of the lateral recesses, disc protrusions contributed to the compression of the nerve roots. Of special interest is the far lateral herniation of the disc into the lateral nerve root canal — a form of disc protrusion escaping myelographic diagnosis in many cases because there is compression of the nerve root beyond the ganglia, and no indentation of the dural sac (Fig. 2).

The importance and reliability of CT scan in the diagnosis of bony abnormalities of the lumbar spine has been well documented (3, 5, 9, 13). Our experience also showed the superiority of CT scanning over other diagnostic methods in demonstrating a variety of congenital and acquired (traumatic, degenerative, and iatrogenic) lesions of the lumbar spine. CT scan allows not only measurement of the various dimensions of the spinal and neurocanals, but, even more importantly, clarification of the interrelationships between the neural structures and normal and pathological bony structures. Clinical experience and operative findings showed that direct CT scan findings, such as a lack of epidural fat, visually documented compression of nerve roots in the subarticular space (subarticular stenosis) (3), enlargement of the nerve roots or ganglion due to post- or pre-stenotic oedema are diagnostically much more significant than a mere decrease in the width of neural foramina.

Congenital and acquired anomalies of the lumbar spine can provide an extremely challenging situation. Among them spondylolysis and resulting spondylolysthesis often require special coronal and lateral reconstruction techniques for a better understanding of the pathological anatomy and determination of the clinical significance of the pathology in terms of nerve root entrapment. Dynamic CT scanning with the spine in flexion and extension although technically quite cumbersome, can prove very useful in the diagnosis of dynamic stenosis and other position-related conditions.

CT scan is particularly valuable in the investigation of elderly patients with symptoms of chronic sciatic radiculitis, lumbar claudication, and other syndromes suggesting chronic lumbosacral spine disease. Only CT scanning allowed the demonstration of the entire gamut of pathological findings quite typical in this group of patients. Usually one sees multi-level involvement of the lumbosacral spine with marked degenerative and hypertrophic changes of zygo-apophyseal joints, a severe degree of degenerative disc disease with disc protrusion and even free extrusion. The combination may result in severe central and lateral spinal stenosis. Interest in the precise diagnosis of these conditions in old patients is anything but purely academic. As Wiltse et al. (19), who believe that age in not a contraindication for surgery, we found that elderly patients respond very favourably to extensive lumbar decompression with complete or nearly complete recovery from sciatic pain. We have performed two- and three-level total laminofacetectomy in a number of patients in their seventies and even eighties with excellent results. The routine use of the Tarlov position which dramatically reduces blood loss, microsurgical techniques, and early ambulation avoided postoperative mortality or morbidity in all cases.

High resolution CT scanning has become an absolutely necessary method in our practice in the evaluation of the so-called "failed low back surgery syndrome" (3), as well as in the previously discussed "virgin" backs. Burton et al. indicated that in cases of failed low back surgery one usually finds a variety of psychological, pathophysiological, and socioeconomic problems. However, in a very significant number of patients a well defined organic pathology can be found which, at least partially, can be corrected surgically. This improves a very pessimistic outlook for rehabilitation of such patients. The principal reason for failure of lumbar spine surgery is a wrong preoperative diagnosis and a lack of consideration of the fact that disc herniation is not the only cause of low back pain, and/or sciatic radiculitis. Kirkaldy-Willis and Yong-Hing found that among 225 patients operated on for herniated disc, 56% had lateral spinal stenosis. Burton et al. demonstrated that 53% of 500 evaluated patients with low back pain had lateral spinal stenosis. It is clear that any operation performed without CT scanning would have inevitably led to a failure in such cases (3).

In another group of patients with recurrence of pain, the postoperative problems were due to a variety of pathological events that occurred after the operative procedure. Among them are various pathomorphological changes which are either results of the progression of the lumbar degenerative disc disease (recurrence of disc herniation at operated levels, or new herniations at other levels, development of central or lateral spinal stenosis, progression of facet joint disease), or postoperative iatrogenic lesions such as: epidural fibrosis, stenosis due to overgrowth of fusion, instability of the spine, etc.

Reliable differentiation of the above-mentioned pathological conditions became possible only with the introduction of high resolution CT scanning. The diagnostic capabilities of myelography in previously operated patients are actually limited to visualization of a large disc protrusion or extrusion. Such myelographic symptoms as poor filling or amputation of the nerve root sheath do not have any significant diagnostic value since they may result from adhesive arachnoiditis or epidural fibrosis. In contrast to the views of some authors (11) that CT scan has only a limited value in postoperative cases because of difficulties in differentiation between fibrous tissue and disc density, our experience showed that such differentiation is possible on the basis of high resolution CT scanning with measurements of the attenuation values. In the majority of cases, soft tissue density of 90 to 120 Hounsfield units (HU) is compatible with herniated disc tissue. Lower density usually represents scar tissue (50–70 HU). In selected cases, a definitive diagnosis can be made only with re-scanning of the level of interest shortly after an intrathecal injection of 3 ml of metrizamide with a concentration of iodine about 190–210 mg/ml. This technique permits clear delineation of the nerve root sheath even if it is located within a mass of fibrous tissue (Fig. 3).

Repeat CT scans proved to be of very great value in following the development of post-operative fibrosis. It can also demonstrate unequivocally the potential of a free autogenous fat graft (10, 14) to protect the dural sac and nerve roots from epidural scarring (Fig. 4).

The capabilities of CT scanning in showing the problems resulting from spinal fusion were demonstrated by Burton et al. (3). We performed 78 reoperations for the failed low back surgery syndrome totally or partially related to previous fusions. The most frequent cause of recurrences of low back pain and sciatic radiculitis was an overgrowth of fusion, with entrapment of nerve roots or ganglia due to lateral spinal stenosis. This may be severe, is frequently multi-level and bilateral. A not infrequent combination of lateral stenosis with central stenosis and recurrent disc herniation, as well as frequent severe epidural fibrosis poses an extremely challenging surgical problem. Successful pre-operative separation and delineation of these entities is not possible without the comprehensive pre-operative information provided by high resolution CT scanning.

Conclusion

1. High resolution CT scan is an extremely valuable diagnostic tool for a variety of congenital and acquired pathological conditions of the lumbosacral spine.
2. The latest advances in CT technology allow visualization and differentiation of various bony and soft tissue structures within the spinal and neural canals.
3. The determination of attenuation values is frequently necessary in differentiating between the density of disc, fibrous tissue and nerve roots.
4. Enhancement with small amounts of metrizamide injected intrathecally is only indicated in very selected cases.
5. CT scan should be the first study in the diagnosis of the majority of pathological conditions of the lumbosacral spine.

References

1. Burton, C.V.: Computed tomographic scanning and the lumbar spine. Part I: Economic and historic review. Spine 4, 4, 353–355 (1979)
2. Burton, C.V., Heithoff, K.B., Kirkaldy-Willis, W., Ray, C.D.: Computed tomographic scanning and the lumbar spine. Part II: Clinical considerations. Spine 4, 4, 356–368 (1979)
3. Burton, C.V., Kirkaldy-Willis, W.H., Yong-Hing, K., Heithoff, K.B.: Causes of failure of surgery on the lumbar spine. Clin. Orthoped. & Related Res. 157, 185–193 (1981)
4. Carrera, G.F., Haughton, V.M., Syvertsen, A., Williams, A.L.: Computed tomography of the lumbar facet joints. Radiology 134 (1), 145–148 (1980)
5. Ciric, I., Mikhael, M.A., Tarkington, J.A., Vick, N.A.: The lateral recess syndrome. A variant of spinal stenosis. J. Neurosurg. 53, 433–445 (1980)
6. Glenn, W.V., Rhodes, M.L., Altschuler, E.M., Wiltse, L.L., Kostanek, C., Yu Ming Kuo: Multiplanar display computerized body tomography applications in the lumbar spine. Spine 4, 4, 282–352 (1979)
7. Hammerschlag, S.B., Wolpert, S.M., Carter, B.L.: Computed tomography of the spinal canal. Radiology 121, 361–367 (1976)

8. Jacobson, R.E., Gargano, F.P., Rosomoff, H.L.: Transverse axial tomography of the spine. Part I: Axial tomography of the normal lumbar spine. J. Neurosurg. *42*, 406–411 (1975)
9. Jacobson, R.E., Gargano, F.P., Rosomoff, H.L.: Transverse axial tomography of the spine. Part II: The stenotic spinal canal. J. Neurosurg. *42*, 412–419 (1975)
10. Keller, J.T., Dunsker, S.B., McWhorter, J.M., Ougkiko, C.M., Jr., Sounders, M.C., Mayfield, F.H.: The fate of autogenous fat grafts to the spinal dura; an experimental study. J. Neurosurg. *49*, 412–418 (1978)
11. Kirkaldy-Willis, W.H., Wedge, J.H., Yong-Hing, K., Reilly, J.: Pathology and pathogenesis of lumbar spondylosis and stenosis. Spine 3, *4*, 319–328 (1978)
12. Langenskjöld, A., Kiviluoto, O.: Prevention of epidural scar formation after operations on the lumbar spine by means of free fat transplants. Clin. Orthoped. & Related Res. *115*, 92–95 (1976)
13. Lifson, A., Heithoff, K.B., Burton, C.V., Ray, C.D.: High resolution CT scan of lumbosacral spine. International Workshop on contrast media in computed tomography. Berlin: Excerpta Medica (in print) 1980
14. Mayfield, F.H.: Autologous fat transplants for the protection and repair of the spinal dura. Clin. Neurosurg. 000, 349–361 (1980)
15. Meyer, G.A., Haughton, V.M., Williams, A.L.: Diagnosis of herniated lumbar disc with computed tomography. New Engl. J. Med. 21, *22*, 301 (1979)
16. Naidich, T.P., King, D.G., Moran, C.J., Sagel, S.S.: Computed tomography of the lumbar thecal sac. J. Comput. Assist. Tomogr. *4* (1), 37–41 (1980)
17. Post, M.J.D., Gargano, F.P., Vining, D.Q., Rosomoff, H.L.: A comparison of radiographic methods of diagnosing constrictive lesions of the spinal canal. J. Neurosurg. *48*, 360–368 (1978)
18. Roentgen, W.K.: On a new kind of ray. Sciences. *3*, 227–231 (1896)
19. Wiltse, L.L., Kirkaldy-Willis, W.H., McIvor, G.W.D.: The treatment of spinal stenosis. Clin. Orthoped. & Related Res. *115*, 83–91 (1976)

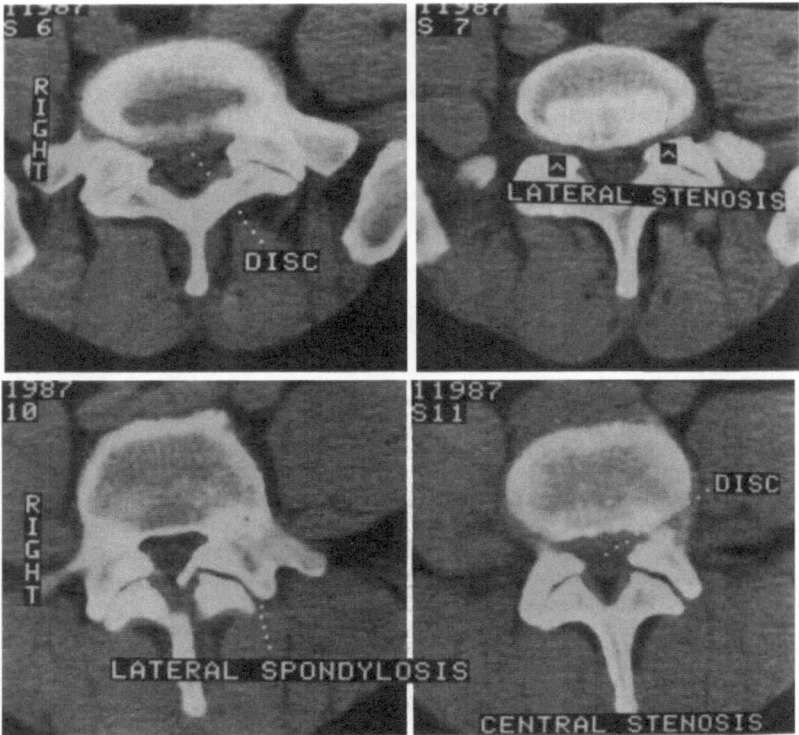

Fig. 1. CT scans of L5–S1 (*above*) and L4–L5 (*below*) levels. Bulging of L5–S1 disc with posterior displacement of S1 nerve roots, lateral spinal stenosis due to hypertrophy of superior articular facets with compression of L5 nerve roots at L5–S1 level. Lateral spondylosis, disc protrusion and central spinal stenosis at L4–L5 levels

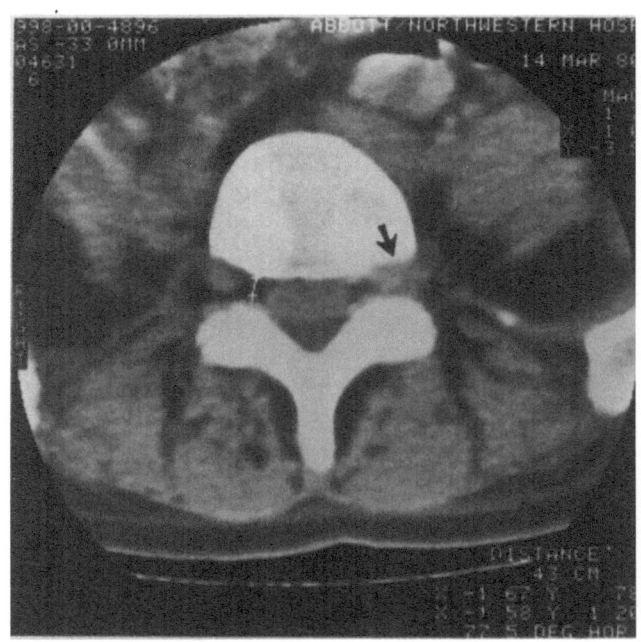

Fig. 2. CT scan of L4–L5 level. Lateral disc protrusion on the left. Compare with L4 nerve root on the right which is free of compression

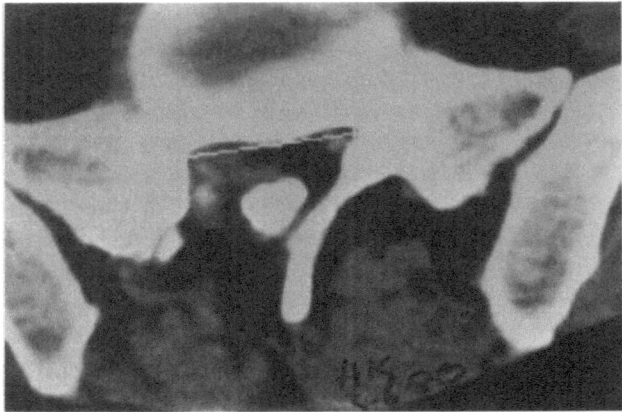

Fig. 3. CT scan of L5–S1 level of patient with failed low back surgery syndrome. Enhancement with intrathecal metrizamide. Posterior displacement of opacified S1 nerve root sleeve by herniated disc on the right

271

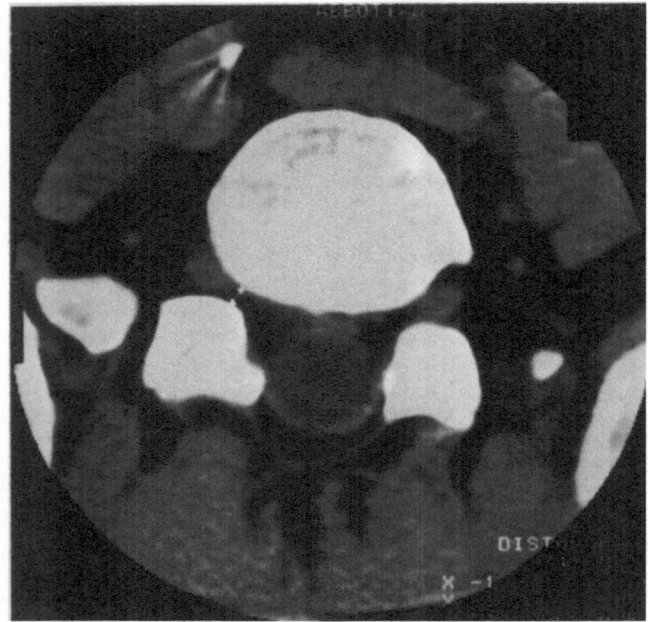

Fig. 4. CT scan one year after wide posterior decompression at L5–S1 level. Generous fat graft with newly formed pseudomembrane. No epidural fibrosis

Use of Hyperbaric Oxygenation for Spinal Cord Injury

M.H. Sukoff

In the United States alone, spinal cord trauma results in over 7,000 myelopathies yearly (21,44). The single most determining factor in the cord-injured patient is the initial severity of the injury. The grim prognosis of serious injuries may be improved inasmuch as there is probably a critical time period during which the progressive pathophysiological sequelae of the initial trauma can be modified (7, 8, 15, 70).

The natural variability in the severity of spinal cord trauma contributes to the complexity of understanding its pathogenesis. The problem is compounded by controversy regarding blood flow to the white matter after experimental injury (65). There is considerable evidence supporting the constancy of grey matter ischaemia subsequent to trauma (1, 3, 5, 6, 18, 20, 40, 49, 63). However, experimental evidence for both increased and decreased white matter spinal cord blood flow (SCBF) is available (3, 15, 19, 35, 36, 41, 53). The metabolic derangements attendant on traumatic myelopathies have been established (10, 32). The complexities of this pathogenesis notwithstanding, treatment concepts must take note of ischaemia, hyperaemia and the altered metabolism following spinal cord trauma. Accepted forms of treatment directed toward preserving or improving spinal cord function after trauma include skeletal realignment, blood pressure maintenance, Mannitol, Dexamethasone, and perhaps hypothermia (8, 16, 60, 65). These, and other less popular methods have generally been more successful in experimental trauma than when tried clinically (6, 13, 61).

The use of high pressure oxygen in a hyperbaric chamber (HBO) has received increasing attention for over a decade. Maeda in 1965, demonstrated that it increases the partial pressure of oxygen in the spinal cord (42). A rise in cerebrospinal fluid (CSF) PO_2 in patients was demonstrated in 1968 (18). Experimental evidence of the therapeutic potential of HBO was discussed by Hartzog (24). This was also suggested in 1972 by Kelly et al. (33). Subsequently, additional experimental and clinical evidence to support the use of HBO for spinal cord injury has been published (12, 13, 26, 27, 28, 29, 31, 39, 46, 67, 68, 69).

Our work includes both experimental and clinical studies suggesting that HBO should be considered as an ancillary form of treatment in traumatic myelopathy.

Materials and Methods

Experimental. Laminectomies were performed at the T−10 level in 20 anaesthetized, intubated, adult cats using the surgical microscope. It was determined that an 11.7 gm.

weight dropped through a 15 cm. tube on the intact dura produced a severe and reproducible neurological deficit. Seven animals were treated immediately after trauma by intermittent exposure to 100 % oxygen at 2 atmospheres for 30 minutes. Thirteen controls were untreated after their traumas. Neurological examinations were graded on the following scale: + 4:— plegic, no voluntary movement; + 3:— severely paretic, minimal movement, no weight-bearing or walking; + 2:— paretic, able to bear weight, occasionally walking possible; + 1:— nearly normal, weak walking possible (unsteady gait); 0:— normal.

All animals were killed on the third postoperative day.

The results indicate a beneficial result in the HBO group. No treated cat was plegic, whereas six of the 13 controls were. Five treated animals were "normal" and all but one could either walk or bear their own weight. Only two of the non-treated cats could do this and only one was considered "normal". The average neurological grade of the treated animals was 1.4. In the controls, it was 2.7.

Clinical. A series of 12 patients with traumatic myelopathies was subjected to the following protocol: initial evaluation in the shock-trauma unit (STU) including complete systemic and neurological examination. Respiratory function was assisted as necessary to maintain arterial PO_2 above 90 mm Hg. Problems outside the central nervous system were treated and blood pressure maintained between 100 and 130 mm Hg. systolic. X-ray films of the cervical spine were obtained in the lateral position and skeletal traction promptly utilized to maintain correct alignment in cases with fracture dislocation. Dexamethasone was given as was intravenous Mannitol as long as the blood pressure was in the ranges above 110 mm Hg systolic. Cisternal myelography or metrizamide-assisted computerized tomography (CT) was promptly obtained.

HBO treatments were performed in the Sechrist monoplace chamber (#2500B). The patients were nursed on the hyperbaric gurney. Skeletal traction, up to 35 pounds, can be constantly applied using the device (Fig. 1, 2) constructed for this purpose. The entire gurney maintaining the patient in constant skeletal traction with the weight device is simply slid into the hyperbaric chamber for treatment. No discontinuity of traction or untoward movements occur. Treatments consisted of 100 % oxygen at 2 atmospheres absolute (ATA) for 45 minutes every 4 to 6 hours for 4 days. If no response occurred by the tenth treatment, they were discontinued.

Case Reports

Case 1 (J.H., 20 years). This patient was taken to the hospital 10 hours after an altercation while drunk. Neurological examination revealed a flaccid tetraplegia with a C 7 sensory level. X-ray films of the cervical spine demonstrated a fracture of C 7. At myelography, a partial block at C 6—7 was present. HBO therapy was instituted 12 hours after trauma. The patient had been maintained in essentially the same position from the last myelography X-ray film through the initial HBO treatment. Repeat X-ray films at that time showed improvement with significant resolution of the partial block. Clinically, he showed no improvement until after anterior decompression and fusion which increased the functional strength of his hands.

Case 2 (M.H., 22 years). This patient sustained a T 12 fracture and an immediate flaccid paraplegia, as a result of a motorcycle accident. Metrizamide-assisted CT demonstrated a complete block at T 12. HBO was instituted 14 hours after injury. A modified costotransversectomy and Harrington rod fixation was also accomplished. There was no improvement in his paraplegia.

Case 3 (T.L., 25 years). An automobile accident resulted in a C 5—6 fracture with an immediate flaccid tetraplegia and a C 6 sensory level. Metrizamide-assisted CT showed cord swelling with no evidence of obstruction. Hyperbaric therapy was started four hours after trauma. She developed toe and foot movement during the first treatment and subsequently showed progressive improvement. The patient was neurologically intact one year later.

Case 4 (J.P., 25 years). Patient sustained multiple injuries including a flail chest as a result of an automobile accident. Neurological examination revealed a flaccid tetraparesis with a C 4 motor sensory level in a stuporous patient. There was minimal movement of both legs. Plane films of the cervical spine demonstrated a C 3—4 fracture and metrizamide-assisted CT showed no intraspinal obstruction. HBO was started six hours after the accident with marked improvement in his tetraparesis noted initially during the first treatment. It was discontinued after two days at which time the patient had functional movement of all extremities. Because of progressive pulmonary and systemic complications unrelated to HBO, sudden death occurred two days later.

Case 5 (J.R., 27 years). This patient sustained a gunshot wound of the chest and abdomen with an immediate flaccid paraplegia. CT demonstrated an intact spinous process with blood and metallic fragments at T 10 with no intraspinal haematoma or foreign body. He underwent abdominal and intrathoracic surgery. HBO therapy was started 11 hours after trauma with no improvement in his neurological status. The patient was transferred to a rehabilitation hospital in that condition one month later. Follow-up examination in six months revealed him to be fully ambulant with a mild paraparesis and a bladder that emptied satisfactorily to Crede.

Case 6 (H.M., 62 years). A patient with chronic rheumatoid spondylitis accidentally fell from a chair with immediate numbness and weakness of his extremities. Neurological examination revealed a severe, flaccid tetraparesis with a C 4 sensory level. Cisternal myelography demonstrated a high degree block at C 3—4. HBO was instituted three hours after admission with immediate improvement in his neurological status. He was discharged two weeks later, having attained his pre-injury motor capabilities.

Case 7 (D.E., 50 years). The patient fell while drunk, striking his forehead. Initial neurological examination revealed a flaccid tetraplegia with a C 6 level. X-ray film of the cervical spine showed severe spondylosis and no fracture. Cisternal myelography showed a high degree block at C 4—5. The patient's initial HBO treatment was instituted 12 hours after the trauma. He was discharged from the hospital two weeks later with no neurological improvement.

Case 8 (W.R., 71 years). The patient fell from a roof and developed immediate severe weakness of his arms and hands and mild weakness of the legs. Neurological examination revealed a moderately severe, flaccid tetraplegia, more marked in the upper extremities and particularly distally. X-ray films of the cervical spine revealed severe spondylosis and status post-operative decompressive laminectomy from C 5 to T 1. HBO treatments were started 22 hours after the trauma. The patient was discharged from the hospital within one month with a recovery of strength of approximately 50% in his upper extremities and somewhat greater in his legs.

Case 9 (C.G., 69 years). This patient was involved in an automobile accident with no loss of consciousness. Initial neurological examination revealed a flaccid tetraplegia with a C 6 motor and T 2 sensory level. X-ray films of the cervical spine revealed degenerative spondylosis. Cisternal myelography showed a high degree block at C 5—6. HBO was initiated nine hours after trauma. X-ray films immediately after HBO, with the patient in an unchanged position, demonstrated partial resolution of the high degree block. He remained neurologically stable and was transferred to a rehabilitation institute after two weeks.

Case 10 (G.W., 57 years). This patient accidentally fell while drunk, sustaining a frontal injury. Initial examination revealed a stuporous and apnoeic patient with grossly normal motor power of the lower extremities. He was unable to move his arms at the shoulders or distally, including the hands. Plane films of the cervical spine revealed a severe spondylosis, most marked at C 3—4 with subluxation. Cisternal myelography showed a high degree block at C 3—4 with cord oedema. HBO was instituted within 15 hours of the trauma. Improvement was noted during treatment sessions. He was discharged three weeks later with approximately 90% normal function of the upper extremities.

Case 11 (R.D., 66 years). This woman underwent decompressive laminectomy for a severe paraparesis secondary to metastatic breast cancer. Postoperatively, she was noted to have a flaccid monoplegia with some improvement of the other leg. HBO was initiated two hours postoperatively, with no improvement apparent during treatment. She was discharged from the hospital one month later improved, but not having achieved the preoperative status of the monoplegic leg.

Case 12 (M.A., 44 years). This patient was on anticoagulant treatment for chronic thrombophlebitis and experienced the sudden onset of low dorsal pain and subsequently a flaccid paraplegia. Myelography showed a complete extradural block at T 10. Ten hours after the onset of her paraplegia, a decompressive laminectomy for epidural haematoma was performed. There were no changes postoperatively. She underwent HBO two hours after operation with no improvement during treatment. The patient was transferred to a rehabilitation unit neurologically stable, one month later. Follow-up neurological examination in one year revealed no motor or reflex abnormalities. The patient was able to void normally.

Discussion

Theoretically, HBO possesses the capabilities of therapeutic assistance in the treatment of traumatic myelopathy. HBO has been shown to increase tissue PO_2 in normal and injured spinal cord (33, 42, 47, 48) and elevate CSF PO_2 (30). It can, therefore, be expected to mitigate any grey matter ischaemia. The degree of central cord cystic necrosis in experimental animals has been lessened by HBO (13, 68,69). Whereas, grey matter ischaemia is an accepted sequela of spinal cord trauma, the pathophysiological blood response in the white matter has yet to be well defined. Oedema (15, 64, 66) and hyperaemia (19, 35, 36, 40, 40) have been demonstrated in the experimental animal. This controversy has been considered by other authors (52, 54, 65). There is an inherent variability in the severity of experimental spinal cord trauma produced by certain methods (14, 22, 37). It has been shown that haemorrhages are more numerous and of greater magnitude in permanent experimental paraplegia (17).

White matter ischaemia does not occur in spinal cord injuries that can be expected to produce only transient paraplegia (41). Perhaps, therefore, the differences in the experimental lesions explain this controversy in white matter SCBF. There have been studies suggesting that the severity of the injury determines the effect on white matter SCBF (9, 11, 51, 52, 56). Credence, therefore, must be paid to the theory that one explanation for the discrepancy in white matter SCBF relates to the severity of the trauma (62). The greater the injury, the more likely it is that white matter SCBF will decrease initially and vice versa.

Autoregulation of SCBF is similar to that in the brain (34, 35, 55). The effects of systemic arterial blood pressure on SCBF have been investigated. Within limits, autoregulation is preserved. When they are violated, there is a tendency for SCBF to vary passively with blood pressure changes (36, 50, 53). White matter oedema probably occurs subsequent to the ischaemia and haemorrhage within grey matter (66). It has been shown that immediately after trauma, there is an extravasation of contrast material from vessels within the central grey matter (5) and that oedema can be expected to follow the ischaemia (38). White matter hyperaemia subsequent to trauma, reported by many authors (2, 35, 52), may be a consequence of vasoparalysis produced by direct injury to the spinal cord and its vasculature with vasomotor control disruption secondary to the neuronal injury (56). Therefore, in an experimental model that fails to respond to variability in blood pressure, differences in white matter SCBF can be expected (11, 54, 56).

If the concept that there is an early hyperaemic phase in the white matter and ischaemia in grey is accurate, then the use of HBO for traumatic myelopathy is well supported. It is well known that HBO possesses antioedema properties by causing vasoconstriction and reduced blood flow while at the same time increasing oxygen (57, 59). Its applicability for modifying the secondary effects of trauma on grey and white matter is (66), therefore, apparent. The work of Smith et al. (56), and Sandler (52) underscores the potential effectiveness of HBO in spinal cord trauma by hyperbaric's ability to mitigate the oedema by combating both hyperaemia and ischaemia. In this regard, the similarity of the vascular responses in both brain and spinal cord to trauma (56), suggests that the known properties of HBO against cerebral oedema (58) can also be applied to spinal cord oedema.

277

It has been suggested that the expanding central grey matter lesion produces a centrifugal pressure on circumferential white matter within the limiting leptomeninges and damage to the long white tracts takes longer than that to the central grey matter (63). Thus, there may be a period of time during which portions of white matter can be salvaged and long tract function preserved by various forms of treatment (15). If one object of treatment is to stabilize the pathological changes by reducing ischaemia (grey matter), and subsequent oedema (white matter), then HBO must be considered as an appropriate form of treatment.

Other hypotheses concerning the pathophysiology of traumatic myelopathies, suggest that major neurological deficits are not related directly to blood flow changes (3, 53). It has been demonstrated that damage to grey matter is greater than to white matter in irreversible injuries and that relative local tissue oxygen consumption is altered more than blood flow as evidenced by tissue hyperoxygenation and tissue acidosis (25).

These authors speculate that the reversibility of the lesion may be determined more by altering the metabolic disturbances than the blood flow. They conclude that the capacity of nervous tissue to maintain oxygen metabolism may hold the key to functional recovery. As has been suggested by others, HBO can restore viable tissue oxygen in damaged segments of the spinal cord. "It provides a substrate for aerobic metabolism and may be necessary for energy-dependent reparative processes. It appears to preserve and promote recovery of marginally injured neuronal structures. It is safe and can be considered as an adjunct in multimodality therapy of traumatic myelopathy" (26, 27).

The increased levels of PO_2 in injured spinal cords, may prevent neuropial dissolution in the damaged area (13). Gelderd et al. (13) demonstrated that HBO resulted in significant reduction of cavitations within the experimental spinal cord.transection as well as an increase in the number of regenerating nerve fibres. Severe tissue necrosis and reduced cavitation was also prevented in other experimental work (28, 69). This suggests the theory that HBO can retard neural tissue destruction until revascularization occurs (13).

The highly toxic hydroxyl-free radicals that may cause spinal cord cavitation in trauma, may be decreased by additional oxygen to the ischaemic spinal cord. Increased tissue oxygen can enable the available mechanisms to function by preventing a shift to metabolic pathways resulting in large quantities of the free radicals (13).

The safety of hyperbaric oxygenation has been discussed elsewhere and is considered to be satisfactory (4, 59). There were no complications from HBO in our series of patients. The dramatic improvement in three is impressive but only anecdotal. The myelographic findings of resolution of high degree intraspinal blocks immediately after treatment is of questionable significance and may be but a temporal phenomenon. It may, however, reflect anti-oedema properties of HBO. To this date, no clinical studies have proved the potential effectiveness of HBO for the traumatized cord. Previous encouraging reports have at best also been anecdotal (31). However, there are no studies of patients treated consistently within four hours of their injuries. Subsequent clinical trials utilizing double blind technique in patients whose treatments can be initiated within four hours are necessary before HBO can be considered a valid ancillary treatment for traumatic myelopathy. Our early treated patients did do well.

Summary and Conclusions

Theoretically, HBO is an excellent form of therapy for the acute spinal cord injury. It possesses three properties of potential application for reversing the pathological sequelae following trauma to the cord. HBO mitigates against the ischaemia found in grey matter by its known properties of increasing oxygenation. Oedema and hyperaemia of the white matter are, similarly, responsive to HBO's ability to reduce blood flow while increasing oxygenation. Furthermore, the damage resulting from breakdown of deprived oxygen-dependent enzyme systems may be modified by HBO. The metabolic dysfunctions that accompany spinal cord trauma may be of greatest significance in its pathogenesis.

Experimental evidence supports these concepts (24, 33, 68, 69). Clinical trials (28, 29, 31, 67), including the present one, have not been adequate to demonstrate the effectiveness of HBO for traumatic myelopathy. They have been primarily anecdotal. Additional clinical efforts are needed in this regard and are forthcoming (45).

References

1. Backe, L., Lee, J.C.: The effect of acute hypoxia in hypercapnia on the ultrastructure of the central nervous system. Brain *91*, 697 (1968)
2. Bingham, W.G., Goldman, H., Friedman, S.J., Murphy, S., Yashon, D., Hunt, W.E.: Blood flow in normal and injured monkey spinal cord. J. Neurosurg. *43*, 162–171 (1975)
3. Cawthon, D.F., Senter, H.J., Stewart, W.B.: Comparison of hydrogen clearance and ^{14}C-antipyrine autoradiography in the measurement of spinal cord blood flow after severe impact injury. J. Neurosurg. *52*, 801–807 (1980)
4. Clark, M.M., Fisher, A.B.: Oxygen toxicity and extension of tolerance. In: Hyperbaric Oxygen Therapy. Davis, J.C., Hunt, T.K. (eds.), pp. 61–77, Bethesda, MD: Undersea Medical Society, Inc. 1977
5. Dohrmann, G.J., Wick, K.M., Bucy, P.C.: Spinal cord blood flow patterns in experimental traumatic paraplegia. J. Neurosurg. *38*, 52–58 (1973)
6. Ducker, T.B., Hamit, H.F.: Experimental treatments of acute spinal cord injury. J. Neurosurg. *30*, 693–697 (1969)
7. Ducker, T.B., Perot, P.L., Jr.: Spinal cord oxygen and blood flow in trauma. Surg. Forum *22*, 413–415 (1971)
8. Ducker, T.B., Saloman, M., Danielle, H.B.: Experimental spinal cord trauma, III: therapeutic effect of immobilization and pharmacological agents. Surg. Neurol. *10*, 71–76 (1978)
9. Ducker, T.B., Saloman, M., Lucas, J.T., Garrison, W.B., Perot, P.L., Jr.: Experimental spinal cord trauma, II: Blood flow, tissue oxygen, evoked potentials in both paretic and paraplegic monkeys. Surg. Neurol. *10*, 64–70 (1978)
10. Enevoldsen, E.M., Jensen, F.T.: Autoregulation and CO_2 responses of cerebral blood flow in patients with acute severe head injury. J. Neurosurg. *48*, 689–703 (1978)
11. Fried, L.C., Goodkin, R.: Microangiographic observations of the experimentally traumatized spinal cord. J. Neurosurg. *35*, 709–714 (1971)
12. Gamache, F.W., Jr., Myers, R.A.M., Ducker, T.B., Cowley, R.A.: The clinical application of hyperbaric oxygen therapy in spinal cord injury: preliminary report. Surg. Neurol. *15*, 85–87 (1981)
13. Gelderd, J.B., Welch, D.W., Fief, W.P., Bowers, D.E.: Therapeutic effects of hyperbaric oxygen and dimethysulfoxide following spinal cord transections in rats. Undersea Biomedical Research *7*, 305–320 (1980)

14. Gerber, A.M., Corie, W.S.: Effect of impound or contact area on experimental spinal cord injury. J. Neurosurg. *51*, 539–542 (1979)
15. Goodkin, R., Campbell, J.B.: Sequential pathologic changes in spinal cord injury: a preliminary report. Surg. Forum *20*, 430–432 (1969)
16. Green, B.A., Kahn, T., Close, K.J.: Comparative study of steroid therapy in acute experimental spinal cord injury. Surg. Neurol. *13*, 91–96 (1980)
17. Green, B.A., Wagner, F.C., Bucy, P.C.: Edema formation within the spinal cord. Trans. Am. Neurol. Assoc. *96*, 244–254 (1972)
18. Griffiths, I.R.: Spinal cord blood flow in dogs. I. "Normal" flow. J. Neurol. Neurosurg. Psychiat. *36*, 34–41 (1973)
19. Griffiths, I.R.: Spinal cord blood flow after acute experimental cord injury in dogs. J. Neurol. Sci. *27*, 247–259 (1976)
20. Griffiths, IR.R., Trench, J.G., Crawford, R.A.: Spinal cord blood flow in conduction during experimental cord compression in normotensive and hypertensive dogs. J. Neurosurg. *50*, 353–360, (1979)
21. Haines, A.: Sexual function in spinal cord injuries. Urs. For. *4*, 9–10 (1976)
22. Hales, J.R.S., Yeo, J.D., Stabback, S., Fawcell, A., Kearns, R.: Effects of anesthesia and laminectomy on regional spinal cord blood low in conscious sheep. J. Neurosrug. *56*, 620–626 (1981)
23. Hart, B.G., Lee, W.S., Rasmussen, B.D., O'Reilly, R.R.: Complications of repetitive hyperbaric therapy. Proceed. Fifth Internatl. Hyperbaric Congress 1973, Vol. II. Trapp, W.G., Banister, E.W., Davison, A.J., Trapp, P.A. (eds.), pp. 867–873. Burnaby 2, B.C., Canada, Simon Fraser University 1974
24. Hartzog, J.T., Fisher, R.G., Snow, C.: Spinal cord trauma; effect of hyperbaric oxygen therapy. Proceed. of the Annual Cl. of Spinal Cord Injury Conf. *17*, 70–71 (1969)
25. Hayashi, N., Green, B.A., De la Torre, J.C., MOra, J., Kogurek: Alterations in local spine cord blood flow in tissue oxygen metabolism following experimental spinal cord injury in rats. Presented at the AANS meeting, Boston, April, 1980
26. Higgins, A.C., Nashold, B.S., Jr.: Effects of hyperbaric oxygen therapy on long tract neuronal conduction in the acute phase of spinal cord injury. Presented at the Undersea Medical Society Annual Scientific Meeting, Pacific Grove, California, May, 1981
27. Higgins, A.C., Nashold, B.S., Jr., Mullin, J.B.: The acute effects of hyperbaric oxygen therapy on long tract conduction in spinal cord injury. Presented at the AANS meeting, Boston, April, 1980
28. Holbach, K.H., Wassmann, H., Hoheluchter, K.L., Linked, D., Ziemann, B.: Clinical course of spinal lesions treated with hyperbaric oxygenation. Acta Neurochir. *31*, 297–298 (1975)
29. Holbach, K.H., Wassmann, H., Linked, D.: The use of hyperbaric oxygenation in the treatment of spinal cord lesions. Ur. Neurol. *16*, 213–221 (1977)
30. Hollin, S.A., Espinosa, O.E., Sukoff, M.H., Jacobson, J.H. III: The effect of hyperbaric oxygenation on cerebrospinal fluid oxygen. J. Neurosurg. *29*, 229–235 (1968)
31. Jones, R.F., Unsworth, I.P.: Hyperbaric oxygen in acute spinal cord injury in humans. Med. J. Aust. *2*, 573–575 (1978)
32. Kakari, S., Diaz, A., Decresciot, V., Tomasula, J., Flamme, E., Campbell, J.B., Ransohoff, J.: The role of lysozymes in the pathogenesis of traumatic paraplegia. Am. Soc. Neurochem. *139* (1974)
33. Kelly, D.L., Jr., Lassiter, K.R.L., Vongsvivut, A., Smith, J.M.: Effects of hyperbaric oxygenation in tissue oxygen studies in experimental paraplegia. J. Neurosurg. *36*, 425–429 (1972)
34. Kindt. G.W.: Autoregulation of spinal cord blood flow. Eur. Neurol. *6*, 19–23 (1971/1972)
35. Kobrine, A.I., Doyle, T.F., Martins, A.N.: Local spinal cord blood flow in experimental traumatic myelopathy. J. Neurosurg. *42*, 144–149 (1975)
36. Kobrine, A.I., Doyle, T.F., Rizzoli, H.V.: Further studies on histamine in spinal cord injury and post-traumatic hyperemia. Surg. Neurol. *5*, 101–103 (1976)
37. Koozekanani, S.H., Vice, W.M., Hashemi, R.M., McGhee, R.B.: Possible mechanisms for observed pathophysiological variability in experimental spinal cord injury by the method of Allen. J. Neurosurg. *44*, 429–434 (1976)

38. Lewin, M.G., Pappius, H.M., Hansebout, R.R.: Effects of steroids on edema associated with injury of the spinal cord. In: Steroids and Brain Edema. Reulen, H.J., Schurmann, K. (eds.), pp. 101. Berlin: Springer 1972
39. Linked, D., Holbach, K.H., Wassmann, H., Hoheluchter, K.L.: Electromyographic findings in spinal cord lesions treated with hyperbaric oxygenation. Proceed. of 1974 Annual Meet. Acta Neurochir. *31*, 298–299 (1975)
40. Locke, G.E., Yashon, D., Feldman, R.A., Hunt, W.E.: Ischemia in primate spinal cord injury. J. Neurosurg. *34*, 614–617 (1971)
41. Lohse, D.C., Senter, H.J., Kauer, J.S., Wohns, R.: Spinal cord blood flow in experimental transient traumatic paraplegia. J. Neurosurg. *52*, 335–345 (1980)
42. Maeda, N.: Experimental studies on the effect of decompression procedures and hyperbaric oxygenation for the treatment of spinal cord injury. J. Nara Med. Assoc. *16*, 429–447 (1965)
43. Martinez, L.J., Alderman, J.L., Kagan, R.S., Osterholm, J.L.: Spatial distribution of edema in the cat spinal cord after impact injury. Neurosurg. *8*, 450–453 (1981)
44. Miller, D.K.: Sexual counselling with spinal cord injured clients. J. Sex Marital Fair *1*, 312–318 (1975)
45. Myers, R.A.: Discussion: Use of HBO for acute spinal trauma. Sukoff, M.H. Presented at the Sixth Annual Conference of the Clinical Application of Hyperbaric Oxygenation, Long Beach, California, 1981
46. Nix, W., Capra, N.F., Erdmann, W., Halsey, J.H., Jr.: Comparison of vascular reactivity in spinal cord and brain. Stroke *7*, 560–563
47. Ogilvie, R.W., Ballentine, J.D.: Oxygen tensions in the deep gray matter of rats exposed to hyperbaric oxygen. Adv. Exp. Med. Biol. *37*, 299–304 (1973)
48. Ogilvie, R.W., Ballentine, J.D.: Oxygen tension in spinal cord gray matter during exposure to hyperbaric oxygen. J. Neurosurg. *43*, 156–161 (1975)
49. Osterholm, J.L.: The pathophysiological response to spinal cord injury. J. Neurosurg. *40*, 5–33 (1974)
50. Rawe, S.E., Perot, P.L., Jr.: Pressure response resulting from experimental contusion injury to the spinal cord. J. Neurosurg. *50*, 58–63 (1979)
51. Sandler, A.N., Tator, C.H.: The effect of spinal cord trauma on spinal cord blood flow in primates. In: Blood Flow and Metabolism in the Brain. Harper, A.M., Jennett, W.B., Miller, J.D. (eds.), pp. 22–26. Edinburgh: Churchill Livingstone 1975
52. Sandler, A.N., Tator, C.H.: Review of the effect of spinal cord trauma on the vessels and blood flow in the spinal cord. J. Neurosurg. *45*, 638–646 (1976)
53. Senter, H.J., Vaness, J.L.: Altered blood flow in secondary injury in experimental spinal cord trauma. J. Neurosurg. *49*, 569–578 (1978)
54. Senter, H.J., Vaness, J.L.: Loss of autoregulation in post-traumatic ischemia following experimental spinal cord trauma. J. Neurosurg. *50*, 198–206 (1979)
55. Smith, A.L., Pender, J.W., Alexander, S.C.: Effects of PCO_2 on spinal cord blood flow. Am. J. Physiol. *216*, 1158–1163 (1969)
56. Smith, A.J.K., McCreery, D.B., Bloedel, J.R., Chou, S.N.: Hyperemia, CO_2 responsiveness, and autoregulation in the white matter following experimental spinal cord injury. J. Neurosurg. *48*, 239–251 (1978)
57. Sukoff, M.H.: Central nervous system: review and update cerebral edema and spinal cord injuries. HBO Review *1*, 189–195 (1980)
58. Sukoff, M.H., Hollin, S.A., Espinosa, O.E., Jacobson, J.H. III: The protective effect of hyperbaric oxygenation in experimental cerebral edema. J. Neurosurg. *29*, 236–239 (1968)
59. Sukoff, M.H., Ragatz, R.E.: Use of hyperbaric oxygen for acute cerebral edema. Submitted to Neurosurgery
60. Wagner, F.C., Jr.: Management of acute spinal cord injury. Surg. Neurol. *7*, 346–350 (1977)
61. Wagner, F.C., Rawe, S.E.: Microsurgical anterior cervical myelotomy. Surg. Neurol. *5*, 229–231 (1976)
62. Wagner, F.C., Stewart, W.B.: Effect of trauma dose on spinal cord edema. J. Neurosurg. *54*, 802–806 (1981)
63. White, R.J., Albin, M.S., Harris, L.S., Yashon, D.: Spinal cord injury: sequential morphology and hypothermia stabilization. Surg. Forum *20*, 432–433 (1969)

64. Wolman, L.: The disturbance of circulation in traumatic paraplegia in acute and late stages; a pathological study. Paraplegia *2*, 213–226 (1965)
65. Yashon, D.: Pathogenesis of spinal cord injury. Orthop. Clin. North Am. *9*, 247–261 (1978)
66. Yashon, D., Bingham, W.G., Faddoul, E.M., Hunt, W.E.: Edema of the spinal cord following experimental impact trauma. J. Neurosurg. *38*, 693–697 (1973)
67. Yeo, J.D., Lawry, C.: Preliminary report on ten patients with spinal cord injury treated with hyperbaric oxygenation. Med. J. Aust. *2*, 572–573 (1978)
68. Yeo, J.D., McKinsey, B., Hindwood, B., Kindman, A.: Treatment of paraplegic sheep with hyperbaric oxygen. Med. J. Aust. *1*, 538–540 (1976)
69. Yeo, J.D., Stabback, S., McKinsey, B.: Study of the effects of hyperbaric oxygenation on experimental spinal cord injury. Med. J. Aust. *2*, 145–147 (1977)
70. Young, W., Tomasula, J., Decrescito, V., Flamme, E., Ransohof, J.: Vestibulospinal monitoring in experimental spinal trauma. J. Neurosurg. *53*, 64–72 (1980)

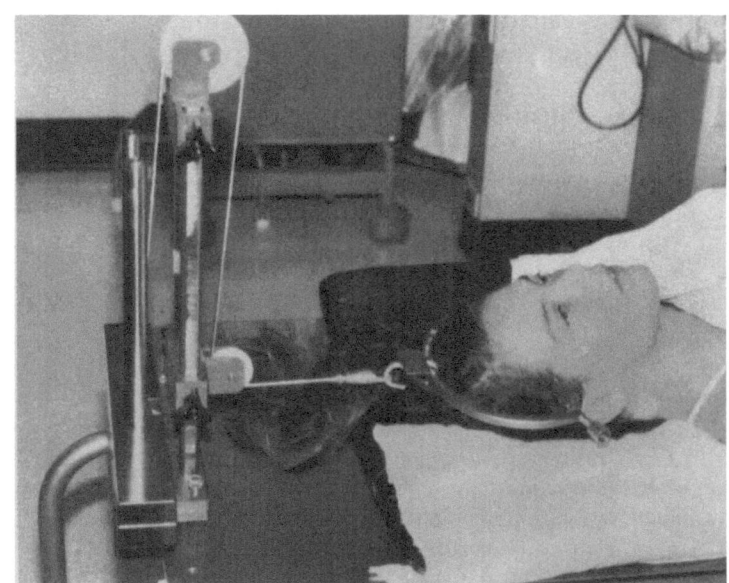

Fig. 1. HBO traction apparatus

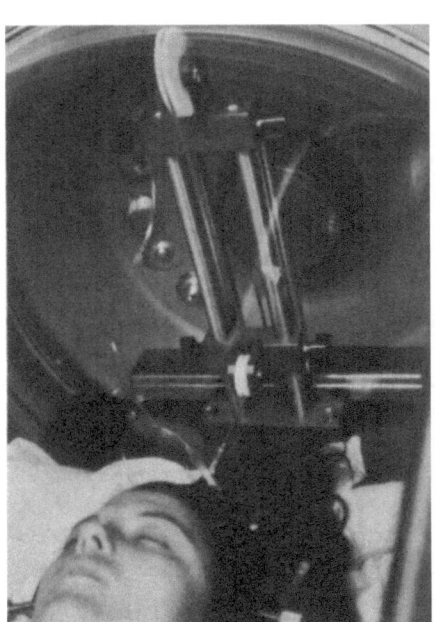

Fig. 2. Patient in HBO chamber with skeletal
traction

Anterior Cervical Discectomy Without Fusion: Comparison Study and Follow-Up

J.J. Guarnaschelli and A.J. Dzenitis

Surgical indications for cervical disc disease are well recognized, especially when limited to patients with nerve root compression involving a single level (mono-radiculopathy) (4, 16, 17, 19). The most frequent pathological finding is a 'soft' lateral disc extrusion, either alone or in combination with a lateral or midline spur. Patients with myelopathy, when associated with multiple level spondylotic changes, present a difficult challenge, and surgical results are usually less gratifying (14, 22).

Since the mid 1950's, the anterior surgical approach has rivaled the posterior approach with excellent results in most large series (2, 11, 15). Various anterior procedures have been used with a wide bony exposure, requiring an interbody fusion by bone graft. Although Hirsch, in 1960, was the first advocate of the anterior cervical discectomy without fusion, there has been a renewal of interest in this approach in recent years, especially with increasing use of microsurgical techniques (1, 3, 6–8, 10, 13, 20, 23). Controversy exists as to the best surgical procedure for patients with cervical radiculopathy and/or myelopathy, and their long-term results in clinical and radiographic follow-up (5, 9, 18, 21).

This paper deals with a retrospective study of 326 patients who underwent operation for cervical disc disease in the period from January 1974 to January 1981.

Case Material and Methods

Three hundred and twenty-six patients who had an operation for cervical disc disease from 1974 to 1981 were studied. Anterior cervical discectomy without fusion (ACD) was done in 175 patients; anterior cervical discectomy and fusion (ACD+F) in 76, and posterior cervical discectomy (PCD) in 75. Of the 326 patients, 297 (91%) had a radiculopathy alone, whereas 29 (9%) had a superimposed myelopathy.

The ratio of patients undergoing a cervical disc operation compared to a lumbar disc operation during this period was 326:1650 (16%) (Table 1). Sex distribution favored males 199:127 (61%), and the age incidence peaked between 40 and 60 years (65%). Most patients presented with clear cut nerve root compression involving a single nerve root (most commonly C7 – 49%). Excluded from this series were patients who were treated for traumatic fracture/dislocation, neoplasia, infection or severe rheumatoid disease.

 Modern Neurosurgery 1. Edited by M. Brock
© Springer-Verlag Berlin · Heidelberg 1982

Table 1. Clinical data of patient population

Ratio		
Cervical/lumbar disc operations	326:1650	(16%)
Sex		
Male	199	(61%)
Female	127	(39%)
Age		
Less than 40 years	86	(26%)
40–60 years	212	(65%)
More than 60 years	28	(9%)

Root

C4 –	1	C7 –	161
C5 –	14	C8 –	16
C6 –	107	Multiple–	27

Duration of presenting symptoms –	–	'Soft'	–	'Hard'
Less than 6 weeks		182		1
6 weeks – 6 months		100		3
More than 6 months		1		39

In all patients symptoms occurred spontaneously. There were no patients where disc rupture followed motor vehicular accidents, specific work related injuries, or was associated with mood disorders.

All patients had arm pain, signs of nerve root entrapment, and/or myelopathic findings that were refractory to a prolonged trial of bedrest, traction-immobilization, and analgesics. All patients had clinically correlated positive myelography, as the definitive diagnostic test, although recently high-resolution CT scans have been used as a confirmatory test with myelography (Fig. 1, 2). Discography or disc space injection to reproduce subjective complaints were not used in the investigation of any of our patients.

The majority of patients in our series presented with spontaneous onset of neck, shoulder and arm pain of less than six weeks duration. The most common cause of symptoms requiring surgical relief was a lateral, single level, 'soft' disc extrusion.

Results

Our surgical results are based on the criteria of Odom and others (12):

Excellent/Good: refers to relief of symptoms with return to full activity. *Fair:* refers to improvement with persistent limitation of activity. *Poor:* refers to no improvement or further deterioration. The follow-up period ranged from six months to a maximum of seven years. The median follow-up was three years.

Of the 297 patients with radiculopathy alone, excellent/good results occurred in 96% with ACD, 92% with ACD+F, and 83% with PCD, as shown in Table 2. In addition,

Table 2. Results (radiculopathy)

	Excellent/ Good	Fair	Poor	Total
ACD				
Single	145	3	2	
				167
Multiple	15	1	1	
ACD+F				
Single	46	4	0	
				61
Multiple	10	1	0	
PCD				
Single	55	7	1	
				69
Multiple	2	3	1	
Total				297

Table 3. Results (myelopathy)

	Excellent/ Good	Fair	Poor	Total
ACD				
Single	2	4	1	
				8
Multiple	0	0	1	
ACD+F				
Single	3	7	0	
				15
Multiple	4	1	0	
PCD				
Single	0	0	0	
				6
Multiple	1	3	2	
Total				29

two ACD patients with early 'poor' results were raised to an excellent/good category with an early surgical revision after identification and removal of residual lateral disc fragments.

Of the 29 patients with myelopathy, 2/8 ACD (25%) had excellent/good results, although 6/8 ACD (75%) were in the fair or above category (Table 3). Seven out of fifteen

ACD+F (47%) patients had excellent/good results although 15/15 (100%) were in the fair or above category. Procedures ranged from one to three levels. Of the group of patients who underwent an extensive posterior laminectomy and bilateral facetectomy, only 1/6 PCD (17%) had excellent/good results although 4/6 (66%) were in the fair or higher category.

Thus, for the 297 (91%) patients with single or multiple level nerve root compression, excellent/good results are obtained in 83% or above in each of three surgical approaches used: ACD (96%), ACD+F (92%), PCD (83%).

On the contrary, the series of 29 (9%) patients with myelopathy, have far fewer excellent/good results: ACD (25%), ACD+F (47%), PCD (17%). Although the progressive neurological deficit was arrested in all patients in this last group, the servere chronic symptoms were seldom reversed regardless of the three surgical approaches used. The exceptions occurred in those patients with acute onset of symptoms who were operated 'early' in the course of their disease: ACD − 2; ACD+F − 7; PCD − 1.

The duration of post-operative hospital stay was significantly less with ACD patients as compared to patients with ACD+F or PCD (Table 4). Ninety-eight out of 175 (56%) of ACD patients were home in three days and 161/175 (92%) within seven days, in contrast to 8/76 (11%) and 58/76 (76%) of ACD+F patients, or 7/75 (9%) and 52/75 (69%) of PCD patients respectively.

There was no mortality or major neuro-vascular morbidity in this series of 326 patients. Transient hoarseness occurred in three ACD and three ACD+F patients. Intervertebral disc space infection developed in one ACD patient. Donor site pain was common and three ACD+F patients required drainage of a seroma/haematoma. Thirty-four out of 175 (19%) ACD, 16/76 (21%) ACD+F, and 5/75 (7%) PCD patients complained of interscapular or shoulder pain for several days to a week, and required analgesics. Progression of neurologic deficit did not occur in any patient undergoing operation for myelopathy in the follow-up period.

Eleven out of three hundred and twenty-six (3%) patients have had a 'late' recurrent disc requiring surgical intervention (3 ACD, 2 ACD+F and 6 PCD). There was no recurrence at the same site. The maximum follow-up is seven years, the median follow-up is three years for all three groups.

Radiographic follow-up has been completed with dynamic flexion and extension studies at 3−6−12 month intervals in 80% of our ACD patients and 50% of our ACD+F patients. For ACD patients, narrowing of the disc space with slight anterior tilt is the most common finding (Fig. 3). 'Late' angulation deformity has not occurred in any ACD patient despite an apparent 'fibrous' rather than 'bony' union. For 17/167 (10%) ACD patients who underwent two level exposure, identical radiographic findings of narrowed disc spaces and slight anterior tilt occurred.

Surgical Techniques

When the anterior approach is used, proper exposure is essential in order to identify and remove the laterally extruded disc fragments. Radical removal of the disc is implicit for adequate decompression, and usually includes adjacent cartilage plates, posterior longitudinal ligament, and spurs if present. Only when the spinal dura, both nerve roots, and their axillae are visible is the decompression considered complete.

Table 4. Postoperative hospital stay

	Less than 3 days	4–7 days	More than 7 days	Total
ACD	98	63	14	175
ACD+F	8	50	18	76
PCD	7	45	23	75
Total				326

Magnified vision, using the operating microscope, or loupe and head light, is beneficial. When exposing the spinal canal through the disc space, an intervertebral spreader, small disc forceps, 1–2 mm Kerrison punches, small sharp curettes, and angled nerve hooks are essential.

Inadequate exposure of both nerve roots is the probable cause for residual lateral 'free' disc fragments (2 ACD patients), and transient contralateral shoulder and arm pain (4 ACD patients). Thus, in patients in whom an anterior cervical discectomy through the disc space does not provide adequate exposure, a wider decompression is performed, followed by fusion.

Most ACD patients, after removal of the intervertebral disc space spreader, had a disc space width (gap) of 5 mm or less. Patients with a disc space (gap) greater than 5 mm were fused. For those ACD+F patients, a bone graft was performed with either a dowel or interbody fusion (2, 15).

Eight out of 29 (28%) of our myelopathic patients underwent ACD. One ACD patient with severe myelopathy from a central 'soft' disc extrusion, developed an 'early' recurrence of symptoms after a six week symptom-free period. These symptoms were relieved after a fusion. Thus, patients with myelopathy, when approached anteriorly, are now fused as additional protection against cervical cord compromise.

Sixty-nine out of seventy-five (92%) PCD patients with radiculopathy underwent a hemilaminectomy and foraminotomy with removal of 'soft' lateral disc fragments or decompression for 'hard' bony spur. Six out of seventy-five (8%) PCD patients with myelopathy had an extensive, multiple-level decompressive laminectomy and bilateral foraminotomies. This group included patients with both an acute (3) and chronic (3) myelopathy.

Summary

In summary, the immediate results of pain relief and return of nerve root function are excellent for the majority of patients with cervical radiculopathy, regardless of the three surgical approaches used. In contrast, most patients with chronic, progressive myelopathy secondary to multiple-level spondylosis and ridging, have uniformly fair to poor results regardless of which of the three surgical procedures was used.

Our preferred approach for patients with cervical disc disease with nerve root compression without myelopathy, is the anterior cervical discectomy without fusion (ACD). The technical ease of the operation, relatively short hospital stay, and excellent clinical and radiographic results, make this approach most gratifying.

Our relative indications for anterior cervical discectomy with fusion (ACD+F) are:
1. A planned anterior cervical discectomy (ACD) does not provide adequate exposure for identification and removal of 'soft' lateral disc fragments. A wider bony exposure is performed, followed by a dowel or interbody fusion.
2. Patients with myelopathy, especially when there is a single level 'soft' or 'hard' central disc protrusion. A two or three level anterior approach, however, may occasionally be required.

Our preferences for the posterior cervical approach (PCD) include:
1. Patients with chronic, progressive myelopathy requiring a multiple level decompressive laminectomy and bilateral foraminotomies.
2. Patients with a C 8 radiculopathy, especially obese individuals, when exposure might be difficult.
3. Patients with suspected intradural/intra-medullary cord lesion.

References

1. Boldrey, E.B.: Anterior cervical decompression (without fusion). 25th Annual Meeting of American Academy of Neurological Sug. Key Biscayne, FL, Nov. 12, 1964
2. Cloward, R.B.: The anterior approach for removal of ruptured cervical discs. J. Neurosurg. *15*, 602–604 (1958)
3. Dunsker, S.B.: Anterior cervical discectomy with and without fusion. Clin. Neurosurg. *24*, 516–521 (1977)
4. Fager, C.A.: Management of cervical disc lesions and spondylosis by posterior approaches. Clin. Neurosurg. *24*, 488–507 (1976)
5. Guarnaschelli, J.J., Dzenitis, A.J.: Anterior cervical discectomy: comparison study and follow-up. Presented at 50th meeting Amer. Assoc. of Neurological Surg. Boston, Mass. April 9, 1981
6. Hankinson, H.H., Wilson ,C.B.: Use of the operating microscope in anterior cervical discectomy without fusion. J. Neurosurg. *43*, 452–456 (1975)
7. Hirsch, C.: Cervical disc rupture; diagnosis and therapy. Acta Orthop. Scand. *30*, 172–186 (1960)
8. Hoff, J.T., Wilson, C.B.: Microsurgical approach to the anterior cervical spine and spinal cord. Clin. Neurosurg. *26*, 513–528 (1978)
9. Lunsford, L.O., Bissonette, D.J., Jannetta, P.J., et al.: Anterior surgery for cervical disc disease. J. Neurosurg. *53*, 1–19 (1980)
10. Martins, A.N.: Anterior cervical discectomy with and without interbody bone graft. J. Neurosurg. *44*, 290–295 (1976)
11. Murphy, R.W., Simmons, C.H.J., Brunson, B.: Ruptured cervical discs. Clin. Neurosurg. *29*, 9–17 (1973)
12. Odom, G.L., Finney, W., Woodhall, B.: Cervical disk lesions. JAMA *166*, 23–28 (1958)
13. Robertson, J.T.: Anterior operations for herniated cervical disc and for myelopathy. Clin. Neurosurg. *25*, 245–250 (1977)
14. Robertson, J.T., Johnson, S.D.: Anterior cervical discectomy without fusion: long term results. Clin. Neurosurg. *27*, 440–449 (1980)
15. Robinson, R.A., Smith, G.W.: Antero-lateral cervical disc removal and interbody fusion for cervical disc syndrome. Bull. Johns Hopkins Hosp. *96*, 223–224 (1955)

16. Saunders, R.L., Wilson, D.H.: The surgery of cervical disk disease. Clin. Orthop. & Related Research *146*, 119—127 (1980)
17. Simeone, F.A., Rothman, R.H.: Cervical disc disease. In: The Spine, Vol. 1. Rothman, R.H., Simeone, F.A. (eds.), pp. 387—433, Philadelphia: Saunders 1975
18. Simmons, E.H., Bhalla, S.K.: Anterior cervical discectomy and fusion: a clinical and bio-mechanical study with eight year follow-up. J. Bone-Joint Surg. *51-B*, 225—237 (1969)
19. Stookey, B.: Compression of spinal cord and nerve roots by herniation of nucleous pulposus in cervical region. Arch. Surg. *40*, 417—432 (1940)
20. Susen, A.F.: Simple anterior cervical disectomy without fusion. 27th Annual Meeting, Amer. Academy of Neurological Surg. San Francisco, Calif. Oct. 17, 1966
21. Tew, J.M., Mayfield, F.H.: Complications of surgery of the anterior cervical spine. Clin. Neurosurg. *23*, 424—434 (1976)
22. Verbiest, H.: The management of cervical spondylosis. Clin. Neurosurg. *20*, 262—294 (1973)
23. Wilson, D.H., Campbell, D.D.: Anterior cervical discectomy without bone graft. J. Neurosurg. *47*, 551 (1977)

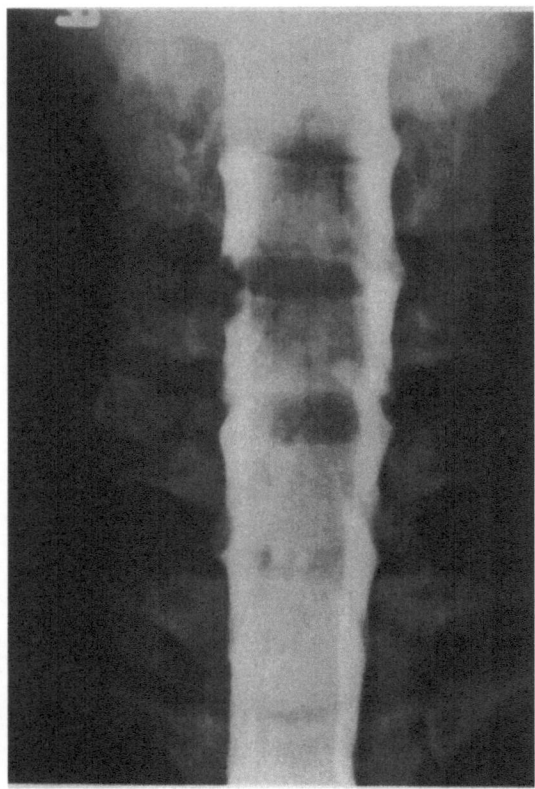

Fig. 1. Pantopaque myelogram showing right C 5—6 extra-dural defect

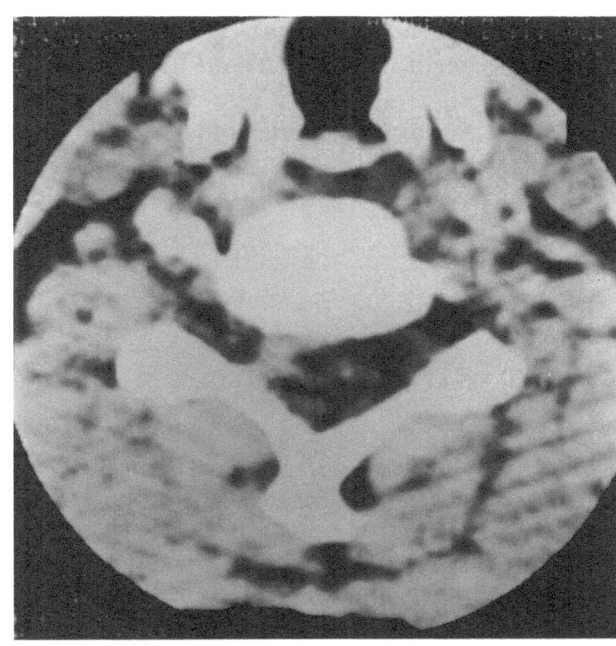

Fig. 2. CT scan showing right C 5—6 disc extrusion (same patient)

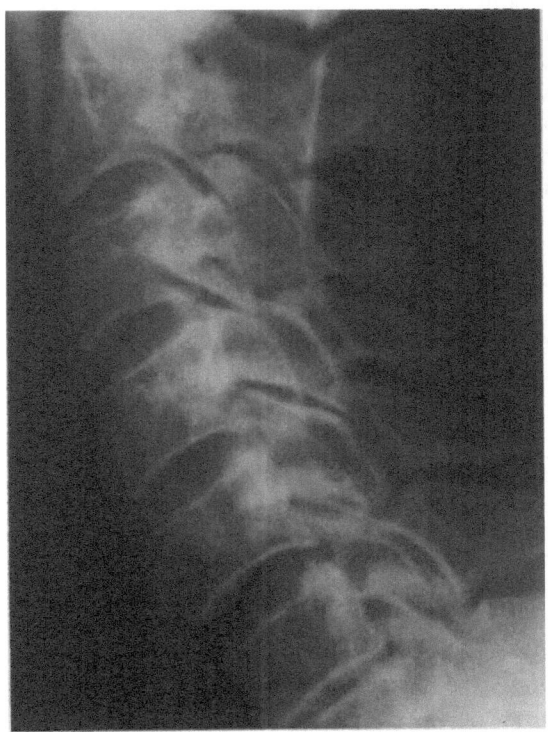

Fig. 3. Lateral X-ray of cervical spine (2 years postoperative) showing C 6—7 narrowing with slight anterior tilt

Cervical Spondylotic Myelopathy Treated by a Microsurgical Anterior Approach with or Without Interbody Fusion

S. Kadoya, R. Kwak, G. Hirose, and T. Yamamoto

Introduction

Surgical treatment of cervical spondylotic myelopathy has been less successful than operative treatment of cervical radiculopathy. These results of surgical treatment have led some authors recommended conservative treatment (5). Although it has been claimed that anterior disectomy with interbody fusion is a rational approach in terms of attacking directly the basic pathological process that causes the myelopathy and significant improvements have been reported after operative intervention (2, 6), it does potentially present the possibility of damaging the cervical cord, particularly when attempting to remove spondylotic osteophytes which frequently prove to be a main cause of the myelopathy (7). To help answer these conflicting questions we have performed a microsurgical anterior osteophytectomy with or without interbody fusion during the past six years and have carefully monitored the clinical status of these patients postoperatively. In this report, we briefly describe our operative procedures and present the neurological follow-up results which tend to emphasize the concept that an anterior osteophytectomy removing all those components compressing against the cervical cord and the roots is the treatment of choice for cervical spondylotic myelopathy.

Materials

Forty-three patients, 32 males and 11 females, with an average age of 55 years at the time of operation, were studied. Periodic neurological examinations were undertaken in the out-patient clinic and final follow-up periods for this study averaged 34 months (range 12 to 61 months). On the basis of the pre-operative neurological examination, 27 patients were suffering from radiculomyelopathy and 16 patients were diagnosed as having only myelopathy. Myelopathy was evaluated pre- and postoperatively according to the Nurick's grade (4), which is based on the degree of difficulty in walking. For examples, Grade 0: no myelopathy, Grade 1: signs of myelopathy but no difficulty in walking, Grade 2: slight difficulty in walking, Grade 3: difficulty in walking which prevented full-time employment or the ability to do all housework, Grade 4: able to walk only with some kinds of support, and Grade 5: chairbound or bedridden state. Either the Chi-square test or the Fisher exact probability test was used to evaluate the independence of the row and column scores.

Modern Neurosurgery 1. Edited by M. Brock

Operative Procedures

All 43 patients were operated by the senior author (S.K.). An anterior approach was undertaken using an operative microscope, and the degenerated disc was evacuated together with underlying hyaline cartilage plates. After this procedure all the compressing components, such as osteophytes, calcified ligament and herniated discs, were completely removed using fine curettes and the air drill. Extreme care was taken to minimize damage to the underlying nervous structures while both the cervical cord and the roots were freed of all compression (Fig. 1). When removing the osteophytic elements in the evacuated disc spaces the operating table was rotated to either side to get a clear view of the operation field. Autogenous iliac bone grafts were used for interbody fusion. Ten patients were not fused. The only reason for employing either fusion or non-fusion was the decision to perform these procedures consecutvely during 1978–1979. A single level was operated on in 23 patients (with fusion, WF. 17, without fusion, NF. 6); two levels were operated on in 17 (WF. 13, NF. 4) and three levels in three (WF. 3, NF. 0). A total of 70 discectomies was performed, in which the C5–6 interspace was operated on in 32 (WF. 28, NF. 4); C4–5 in 21 (WF. 16, NF. 5); C6–7 in 11 (WF. 10, NF. 1) and C3–4 in 6 (WF. 2, NF. 4).

Results

The follow-up grades for 43 patients are tabulated according to their initial grades in Table 1. At the time of thier initial pre-operative examination three (7%) were in Grade 1 category where the corticospinal tract involvement was minimal and their main neurological findings were those of radiculopathy. Eleven (26%) showed mild myelopathy (Grade 2). Twenty (46%) were in Grade 3, where their myelopathies were moderate in terms of moderately disturbed daily activities and not allowing full-time employment. Three (7%) required some kind of assistance for walking (Grade 4) and six (14%) were either either chairbound or bedridden (Grade 5). In the follow-up period all except four patients (9%) in Grade 3, showed improvement. Improvement in neurological scores by one grade was seen in 12 patients (28%), two grades in 24 (56%) and three grades in three (7%). As a result postoperatively, 34 patients (79%) were in Grades 0, 1, 2 and regained full daily activities and normal social living. It is most impressive to note that the severely affected patients (three in Grade 4 and six in Grade 5), whose outcome has been generally regarded as poor, recovered as well and four out of nine patients regained fulltime employment (Grade 2). No postoperative deterioration was encountered.

Four patients in Grade 3 remained unchanged. However, all these patients showed improvement by one grade post-operatively, but during a follow-up period of two to three years neurological deterioration appeared and consequently resulted in the initial neurological state (Grade 3). In three patients newly developed spondylotic changes in the adjacent interspaces and pseudoarthrosis were presumably responsible for the lack of improvement. One patient eventually suffered chronic renal failure.

Follow-up results were also evaluated in relation to fusion (WF. 33 patients) and non-fusion (NF. 10 patients) (Table 2). Postoperative improvement by one grade was experienced in eight WF and four NF patients. Improvement by two or three grades were documented in 23 WF and four NF. Between the WF and NF groups there was no significant

Table 1. Prognosis of cervical spondylotic myelopathy treated by microsurgical anterior osteophytectomy with or without interbody fusion. Myelopathy was evaluated by Nurick's grading (4). 39 out of 43 patients showed improvements of either 1, 2, or 3 grades

Follow-up grade	Initial grade 0	I	II	III	IV	V	Total
0		3	10	2			15
I			1	9			10
II				5	3	1	9
III				4		2	6
IV						3	3
V							0
Total	0	3	11	20	3	6	43

Table 2. Prognosis of cervical spondylotic myelopathy treated by microsurgical anterior osteophytectomy was evaluated separately between fusion and non-fusion groups. No significant differences in improvement rates were noted

Follow-up grade	With fusion 0	I	II	III	IV	V	Total		Follow-up grade	Without fusion 0	I	II	III	IV	V	Total
0		2	9	2	2		13		0		1	1				2
I			0	8			8		I			1	1			2
II				5	2	1	8		II					1		1
III				2		1	3		III				2		1	3
IV						1	1		IV						2	2
V							0		V							0
Total	0	2	9	17	2	3	33		Total	0	1	2	3	1	3	10

statistical difference in the improvement rates. The number of patients in Grade 0, 1, 2 at the initial and follow-up examinations was also tabulated between WF and NF groups, but again no statistical difference was found. It was concluded that improvement of cervical spondylotic myelopathy could result from anterior osteophytectomy irrespective of whether fusion was performed or not.

294

The cervical spinal canal was narrow in some of these cases. Actually six patients out of 43 showed a constitutionally narrow canal in which the anteroposterior diameters at C5 vertebra ranged from 11.5–12.0 mm (mean 11.7 ± 0.2). These measurements were made by the method of Burrow (1) in a cross table view of the cervical roentgenograms taken with a focus to film distance of 1.5 m (mean magnification factor: 1.17). We performed the same anterior osteophytectomy in these six patients who had a constitutionally narrow canal. Three patients were operated on at a single level and another three at two levels. All six patients showed improvement at the follow-up examinations. Improvement by three grades were recorded in two patients and two grades in four.

Table 3 summarizes postoperative complications. Partial graft extrusions were observed in two patients, and these were absorbed spontaneously. Pseudoarthrosis occurred in two patients, which contributed to neurological deterioration in one patient (Table 4). Cervical and upper arm pain was observed immediately after operation in six patients in whom no interbody fusion was performed. This was a relatively severe pain annoying the patients for a period of one to two months postoperatively, but had not been a part of the pre-operative symptomatology. In particular, one patient's pain continued for 23 months postoperatively, and finally we added an interbody fusion at the non-fusion site (C5–6). His pain was relieved to a modest degree. This kind of pain was not experienced in the fusion group. Postoperative cervical pain appeared in two patients of the fusion group, one and two years later respectively. It was mild and relieved by bed rest alone. Three patients complained of hoarseness, which was due to damage of the superior laryngeal nerve during the operative procedure.

Postoperative instability of the cervical spine was examined (Table 4). Pseudoarthrosis occurred in two patients and was assumed to be responsible for neurological deterioration in one patient. Spondylotic changes and retrolisthesis at adjacent levels of the operated disc spaces were observed in two and one patients respectively. These conditions significantly reduced neurological recovery. Accordingly, further operations on these disc spaces were scheduled, but refused by three patients. Only one patient, on whom C4–5 retrolisthesis had developped after C5–6 and C6–7 osteophytectomies with fusion, was operated 29 months after the first operation and again showed improvement.

Discussion

The surgical treatment for myelopathy has been less successful and as a consequence conservative approaches are still recommended (5). However, it is quite apparent that the main cause of cervical spondylotic myelopathy is spondylotic osteophytosis secondary to the disc degeneration, which affects the cervical cord, either by direct compression or vascular disturbance. This is the reason we adopted an anterior approach and performed a complete osteophytectomy. With meticulous care under an operating microscope and using fine instruments the risk of damaging the pathological cervical cord has been negligible. In our follow-up results based on 43 myelopathic patients, 39 showed improvement by either 1, 2, or 3 grades in the Nurick's system and 34 (79%) returned to their normal life activities. Even the most severely affected patients (Grade 4 and 5) recovered by 1, 2, or 3 grades. It was noteworthy that no patient was worsened postoperatively by the surgical procedures utilized for direct removing of osteophytes.

Table 3. Postoperative complications encountered in 43 cases

	No. of cases	%
1. Partial graft extrusion	2	3.6 (in 56 fusions)
2. Pseudo-arthrosis		
with fusion	2	6.1 (in 33 cases)
without fusion	0	0 (in 10 cases)
3. Cervical and upper arm pain		
with fusion	2	6.1 (in 33 cases)
without fusion	6	60.0 (in 10 cases)
4. Hoarseness	3	7.0 (in 43 cases)

Table 4. Postoperative instability of the cervical spine encountered during the follow-up period of an average of 34 months

	No. of cases	Neurological deterioration
1. Pseudo-arthrosis	2	1 [a]
2. Further spondylotic changes after anterior operation	2	2 [a]
3. Retrolisthesis at the adjecent level	1	1

[a] One patient showed two lesions

Anterior discectomy without interbody fusion has been regarded as an adequate treatment for radiculopathy due to a cervical disc hernia (3, 8), but this procedure without interbody fusion was not successful in our studies, simply because of newly developed postoperative cervical and neck pain. Myelopathy itself was relieved by anterior osteophytectomy without fusion. To eliminate the postoperative pain problem fusion was indicated. A patient with cervical spondylotic myelopathy combined with a constitutionally narrow spinal canal is generally regarded as a candidate for laminectomy. However, we prefer to perform a rather extensive anterior osteophytectomy removing a part of the posterior bony ridges of the vertebral body in patients with cervical spondylotic myelopathy and a narrow canal. The eventual neurological outcome was not much different from those cases not associated with a constitutionally narrow canal, and all ten patients showed apparent improvement. Further laminectomy may be expected in the future, but at present none of these cases exhibits signs and symptoms requiring such posterior decompression.

Conclusion

Anterior osteophytectomy employing the operating microscope was undertaken for cervical spondylotic myelopathy, regardless of the presence or absence of a constitutionally narrow spinal canal. In the follw-up evaluation 39 out of 43 patients showed improvement, and even nine severe myelopathic patients recovered as well. No postoperative deterioration was encountered as a result of the surgical procedures. The recovery rate of myelopathy was excellent both in the fusion and non-fusion groups, except for newly developed postoperative cervical and neck pain in the latter group. Now, we prefer doing interbody fusion.

References

1. Burrow, E.H.: The sagittal diameter of the spinal canal in cervical spondylosis. Clin. Radiol. *14*, 77–86 (1963)
2. Hakuba, A.: Trans-unco-discal approach. J. Neurosurg. *45*, 284–291 (1976)
3. Murphy, M., Gado, M.: Anterior cervical discectomy without interbody bone graft. J. Neurosurg. *37*, 71–74 (1972)
4. Nurick, S.: The pathogenesis of the spinal cord disorder associated with cervical spondylosis. Brain *95*, 87–100 (1972)
5. Lansford, L.D., Bissonette, D.J., Zorub, D.S.: Anterior surgery for cervical disc disease. Part 2: Treatment of cervical spondylotic myelopathy in 32 cases. J. Neurosurg. *53*, 12–19 (1980)
6. Phillips, D.: Surgical treatment of myelopathy with cervical spondylosis. J. Neurol. Neurosurg. Psychiat. *36*, 879–884 (1973)
7. Verbiest, H.: The management of cervical spondylosis. Clin. Neurosurg. *20*, 262–294 (1973)
8. Wilson, D.H., Campbell, P.D.: Anterior cervical discectomy without bone graft. Report of 71 cases. J. Neurosurg. *47*, 551–555 (1977)

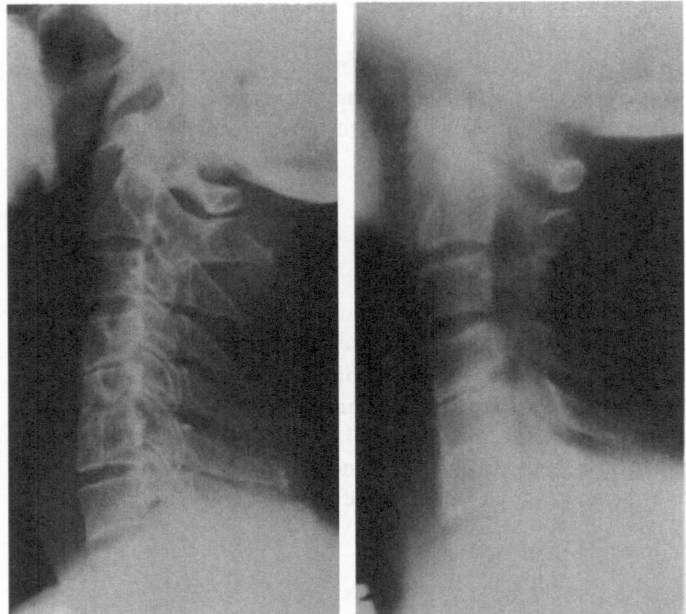

Fig. 1. Postoperative roentgenograms of anterior discectomy without interbody fusion (C4—5 and C5—6). *Left:* a cross table view; *right:* a laminagram. Note complete osteophytectomy including a part of bony ridges of vertebral bodies

Management of Paediatric Spinal Cord Injuries –
Analysis of Combined Survey

D.F. Dean, R.B. Morawetz, R.A. Sanford, R. Coulon, and J. Ransohoff

Abstract

One hundred-thirty-one cases of paediatric spinal cord injury, between the ages one and fifteen were analysed. Sixty-four had surgical procedures. Twelve of 24 tetraplegics subjected to operations improved. Seventeen of 27 paraplegics who were operated on remained the same. Of the 19 who improved with operations, six were normal, three had hand weakness, one became a Brown-Sequard, two were mild central cord injuries, two were walking paraplegics, two were improved tetraplegics and one tetraplegie became essentially a paraplegic.

Younger children, one to five, may present as a head injury, yet have a high cord innury. Delayed onset of deficit though rare is more common in the younger age group, less than five. There is a central cord injury of the lower thoracic area presenting initially as a complete lesion with bowel or bladder out, which will yet improve dramatically. Early computerized tomography of the spine and reduction is recommended after stabilization of airway, blood pressure and control of life threatening injuries.

Paediatric spinal cord injuries are uncommon (2, 4, 5, 10, 11). Review of hospital records for nine major medical centres in the United States and the Spinal Cord Injury Registry from the University of Maryland only identified 130 cases between birth and 15 years of age occurring between 1970 and 1979.[1] The study was undertaken to identify the results of treatment and discover any differences between conservatively and surgically managed cases.

Age and Sex

70% of the injuries occurred in males and 30% in females. 58% occurred in youths ages 13 to 15, 15% in children 9 to 12, 10% in the 5 to 8 year olds, and 18% in the 1 to 4 age group. This report does not cover birth trauma or the special problems of myelodysplasia or neoplasia.

---

[1] Departments of Neurological Surgery, University of South Alabama College of Medicine, Mobile, AL. University of Alabama, Birmingham, AL. University of Mississippi College of Medicine, Jackson, MS., Oschner Clinic, New Orleans, LA., New York University School of Medicine-Bellevue Hospital (NiNCDS Spinal Cord Center), New York, NY, Duke University, Durham, NC, Bowman Gray College of Medicine, Winston-Salem, NC, Grady Hospital-Emory University, Atlanta, GA

Cause of Injury

22% occurred in motor vehicle accidents in which the children were usually passengers, not drivers. 21% were caused by gunshot wounds reflecting the ready access of the American teenager to firearms. 13% resulted from diving accidents. 15% from sports or play and 8% from pedestrian accidents (Table 1).

Injury Site

In this series younger children tended to receive high cervical cord injuries, or an ill-defined cervical injury that usually presented as a central cord syndrome. Eight of 17 children five years and younger who received cervical injuries, had damage from C1—C3 whereas only two of 75 teenagers 13 to 15 had cord injuries here. In the children, the greatest number of injuries occurred between C3 and C5. 55% were located above C5—6. One pentaplegic girl was thrown into the windshield and suffered disruption of the cervical occipital ligaments. She ultimately required a diaphragmatic pacemaker. Of the 50 thoracolumbar injuries 25% occurred between T8 and L1. Most of the thoracic injuries were due to motor vehicle accidents, falls or gunshot. Moreover, several younger children suffered a thoracolumbar cord injury analagous to the cervical central cord injury. These children probably suffered a hyperflexion injury which usually presented with findings suggesting a complete cord injury with loss of sphincter control and a sensory level in the lower thoracic dermatomes. However, they improved dramatically.

Delayed Onset of Neurological Deficit

Thirteen patients presented with delayed neurological deficits. One 12-year-old had initially a weak arm which became plegic in hours. A 5-year-old fell at play and some two hours later had a similar deficit. Five children ages five and younger also had initial weakness worsening into a delayed paraplegia. Two of these were injured in car collisions, one was hit by a car and two fell at play and then worsened. There were only 18 altogether children of ages one to five with cervical injuries. The unusually high number of delayed neurological deficits (11) suggests either difficulty with the initial examination or a vulnerability to later cord oedema or haematomyelia not identified in the older teenager. ·

Presenting Neurological Condition

Unfortunately, uniform diagnostic or examining criteria had not been established at the nine medical centres, nor was the time of the injury or examination identified with exactness. Sixteen diagnostic categories were established retrospectively and are summarized by age groups in Table 2.

Thus, it can be seen that ten children ages eight and less presented as complete tetraplegics. Nineteen youngsters ages nine and older presented with complete tetraplegia usually from diving, sports or gunshot wound injuries. The former ten amounts to 28%

Table 1. Cause of pediatric cord injuries

	Unknown	0–4		5–8		9–12		13 –	15	Total	
		M	F	M	F	M	F	M	F	M	F
Collision MVA		2	7	2	2	3	3	6	4	13	16
Gunshot wounds		2		2		3		14	6	21	6
Diving						2		12	3	14	3
Fall, home or play		3		3		2	1	4	1	12	2
Other sports	1	1						10	1	11	2
Hit by motor vehicle		1	4	2		2		1	1	6	4
Motorcycle						2		3		2	3
Football								5		5	
Unknown	1	1						1	1	2	1
Fall, moving vehicle		1		1						2	
Play, school, etc.						1		1		1	1
Assault, knife									1		1
Fall, industrial	1									1	
Other injuries		1				1				1	1
Totals	2	12	11	10	3	12	8	57	18	91	39

M= male, F= female

of those from birth to eight years old whereas the latter is 20% of the 9 to 15 year olds. Ten children ages 11 to 15 experienced cervical central cord injury. On the other hand almost all those with incomplete tetraplegia were aged 14 or 15 (ten children).

The high preponderance of complete paraplegias in the 13 to 15 age groups reflects the popularity in the Southern states of hunting and fighting.

Diagnostic Studies

Normal plain radiographs were found in 21% of the cervical injuries, 33% of the thoracic injuries and 8% of the lumbar injuries. Dislocations and subluxations without fractures were seen in 20% of the cervical injuries. 5% of the thoracic and 8% of the lumbar injuries sustained fracture dislocations. Multiple compression fractures were seen in 4% of the cervical injuries, 7% of the thoracic injuries and 8% of the lumbar cases.

Table 2. Admitting neurological condition correlated by age of patient to cause of injury

Neurological condition	Collision MVA	Hit by car	Fall car	Motor-cycle	Foot-ball	GSW	Diving	Other sports	Assault	Fall play	Other
Anterior cord							13				
Improving arm plegia								15			
Brown Séquard	15	11			15	21/2		?	13		
Central cord	14, 15	11		15	14, 15	15	15(3)	14			
Mild paraparesis						6					15
Complete paraplegia	1,2,4,6 12(2) 15(2)	2,4,7 9	11/2 5	15(4)		9,11,13 14(2),13(6) 15(2)		14		7,11 15	15
Incomplete paraplegia		2				2,10,14 15(2)				12	
Transient paraplegia											14
Transient incomplete Quad delayed central Cord	2										
Complete quad	2,4(2) 5(3),61/2 15	5,7		15		6,14 15(2)	9,11,13 14(4),15(4)	14(2) 15(2)			
Incomplete quad	3,14(3), 15	11/2			14	14	14,15	15(2)			
Transient hemiparesis										2	
Initially weak, delayed Arm plegia	12									5	
Initially weak, delayed Paraplegia	2,5	3,7,13								3,5	11
Initially weak Delayed quad	11										10

Bullet fragments in or about the spinal canal were noted in 19% of the thoracic injuries, 5% of the cervical cases and 38% of the lumbar injuries. Ketamine anaesthesia in association with linear or polytomography was especially helpful in several centres. Only two cases benefited from the use of the fourth generation computed tomography of the vertebral canal, as it was not available for general use at the time of this study.

Myelograms on the other hand were definitely performed in 66 cases (51%). In those children who had the study, 26% were definitely normal. 6% demonstrated cord widening, 20% showed complete blocks, 11% incomplete blockage. Metrizimide was only used in a few cases, but no complications were observed from its use even in those under the age of two.

Outcome and Age

Outcome was assayed both in Frankel scoring and in the 16 clinical diagnoses (9). The results from the 13 children in the first two years showed three children remained sen- o-sori-motor useless paraplegics, one child stayed a sensori-motor useless tetraplegic, but six children improved from either a tetraparesis or incomplete paraplegia to a motor useful paraparetic or became normal.

At the other end of the age group, teenagers, 14 and 15, 23 remained unchanged paraplegics or tetraplegics (36%). However, 13 of this group had suffered gunshot wounds. If one excludes the gunshot wounds, then 20% of the older age group remained unchanged as against 31% of the youngest. In the group ages three to five (17 children) eight children ended complete motor-sensory, useless tetraplegics or paraplegics i.e. 47%. In the 25% in the age group 11 to 13, eleven or 44% remained paraplegic or tetraplegic. However, nine of these 11 children had received gunshot wounds. If the gunshots are excluded, then two of 14 or 14% in this age group remained motor-sensory useless.

Outcome and Operation

Sixty-four children had surgical procedures. Thirteen had anterior cervical fusions (predominantly in older teenagers and predominantly from New York University-Bellevue Hospital). Twenty-seven children underwent decompressive laminectomies, 16 had posterior fusions and six had laminectomy and fusion. One child had both an anterior and posterior fusion while another had an open reduction. Twelve children remained unchanged tetraplegics, 17 were unchanged paraplegics, six were normal and two died (3%). Three were left with hand weakness, two with mild central cord syndromes, one with a mild Brown-Séquard, two were mildly paraparetic and walking, three had moderate paraparesis but were walking with the aid of braces. Unfortunately, 12 of this series had inadequate follow-ups.

However, when improvement after operation was compared with results of no operation, in terms of Frankel scoring, the following was apparent (P = Para):

Frankel score No. of patients	PA-PD No.	PA-PC No.	PB-PD No.	PC-PD No.	PC-E No.	PD-E No.
Operation	3	2	–	2	1	1
No operation	4	1	1	1	1	2

Thus nine patients with injuries causing paraparesis had varying amounts of improvement after operation. Ten patients also improved without operation.

Cervical injuries fared somewhat differently (T= tetra):

Frankel score No. of patients	TA-PA	TA-TC No.	TA-TD No.	TB-PD No.	TB-PD No.	TB-E No.
Operation	1	1	–	–	–	–
No operation	1	2	1	1	3	1

Frankel score No.of patients	TC-TD	TC-PC No.	TC-PA No.	TC-E No.	TD-E No.	TD-PA No.
Operation	2	1	–	–	2	1
No operation	4	–	1	1	9	1

Site of Injury and Final Outcome

Cervical Region

Three children died from cord injuries at C1–2, one became normal, two were unchanged complete tetraplegics and complete paraplegics. Three became normal with injuries suffered at C2–3 and C3–4. On the other hand, 27 children suffered injuries at C4–5, four became normal, eight were unchanged tetraplegics, three were tetraplegics who improved to having functional hands and were essentially paraplegics, while three others were left with hand weakness. Two died. Twelve children sustained cervical cord injuries that were not localized. Four became normal, two were unchanged tetraplegics, one was left with a mild spasticity, one with a weak hand and arm and one died. Twenty-two children sustained injuries at C5–6. Two became normal, eight remained unchanged tetraplegics, three improved to mild spasticity. Only 11 children sustained injuries at C6–7, eight of these remained unchanged tetraplegics.

Thoracolumbar Injuries

Twenty-seven children sustained injuries from C7 to L3–4 and remained unchanged motor useless paraplegics (21% of the entire series.) Six children had moderate paraparesis but were walking with the aid of braces. Five became normal. One in this group died. Five had ill defined thoracic injuries and all did well, three becoming normal, one walking with mild paraparesis and one walking with braces with a moderate paraparesis.

Cause of Injury and Final Outcome

Thirty-one children were involved as passengers in motor vehicle accidents and four died. Only one became normal, six were left unchanged tetraplegics and six unchanged paraplegics. Three had hand weakness, one a severe central cord injury, and two with tetraplegia improved to motor useful paraplegics. Twenty-seven children sustained gunshot wounds of which only two became normal, 13 were unchanged paraplegics, one an unchanged tetraplegia, and two were mild paraparetics walking without aid of braces. While diving, 16 children sustained injuries resulting in six unchanged tetraplegics. Three became normal, two were left with hand weakness, one a mild central cord, another a Brown-Sequard, syndrome. Football and other sports accounted for 18 injuries of whom six were left as unchanged tetraplegics, seven became ultimately normal. Eleven children were struck by vehicles which resulted in one death, two normals and two unchanged paraplegics.

Comparison of Adults and Children with Frankel Scores

Cervical spinal cord injuries				Thoracic lumbar cord injuries			
Initial scores		Final scores		Initial scores		Final Scores	
Adults	Child	Adults	Child	Adults	Child	Adults	Child
A 54% (56%)	47%	44% (39)	42% [a]	A 70%	79%	59%	51%
B 16 (15)	10	6 (14)	1	B 11	4	9	None
C 20 (10)	15	6 (7)	7	C 8	10	4	6
D 10 (19)	28	33 (30)	25	D 11	12	20	26
E		10 (10)	17	E 1	None	8	8
				Unknown			8

[a] 10% children died

For the prior comparison the Frankel Scores for the adult series was reported by Maynard et al. (13). This series had also been correlated with Frankel's series, the percentages of which are in the parenthesis (9). Fewer children were admitted directly motor and sensory useless (A) 47% against 54% for the adults. But the final scores are amazingly similar for complete injuries, 44% for adults against 42% for children. The final scores for thoracolumbar injuries is also very similar.

Discussion

In most of the centres after immediate stabilization of airway, and blood pressure, immobilization was carried out. Most of the cervical injuries had tongs placed as soon as the diagnosis was assured and spine x-rays were taken. Myelograms were performed when no fractures were seen or in many complete injuries, but this varied. Treatment of central cord injuries seemed equally divided between early ambulation with cervical collar and three to six weeks in traction followed by ambulation in a brace. No difference in outcome could be detected.

The decision about whether an operation was indicated or not revolved around relieving complete blocks on myelogram, elevating indriven bone fragments and stabilization to allow for early ambulation and rehabilitation. As other authors have indicated, children as a group suffer higher cord injuries than adults. This is thought to be due to the more horizontal nature of the facets. However, the possibility of delayed deficit in the younger patients is alarming (1, 6). The lesson seems obvious. Judicious rest and observation after trauma is mandatory.

Twenty-seven children were admitted paraplegic and stayed paraplegic, but 13 of these were due to gunshot wounds. Decompressive laminectomy and wound debridement while perhaps limiting the likelihood of sepsis was not accompanied by any discernible neurological improvement. Twenty children (15%) were admitted tetraplegic and remained so. Only one of these was due to a gunshot. Twelve of the 20 had had operation.

While steroids may be of value, the study did not demonstrate this.

The deaths occurred in patients with multiple trauma, severe head injury, laceration of the jugular veins and carotid artery as well as penetrating gunshot wounds. Spinal cord infarction may play a part in the complete injury (1), but no autopsy analysis was available. Indeed spinal necropsy findings in children has been rarely reported (3). Previous detailed analyses of cervical and lumbothoracic paediatric spinal cord injuries have been made (5, 7, 8). Shock when it occurred was commonly accompanied by blood loss (12), but stress ulcers were uncommon. Initial nonrecognition of the spinal cord injury by emergency personnel or examining physicians happened in at least 8% of the children. Decubiti occurred in 19 patients, reflecting the vulnerability of the young person's skin.

Finally, the disheartening conclusion is that paediatric spinal cord injuries do not differ significantly from adult ones in their outcome. They experience both cervical and thoracic central cord injuries but are still left'with the same residua as adults. Indications for operation still remain 1. worsening neurological deficit, 2. stabilization, 3. debridement, and 4. correction of CSF fistulae.

Summary

1. Younger children, one to five, may present as a head injury yet have a high cord injury.
2. Delayed onset of deficit though rare is more common in the younger age group, under five.
3. One may see a central cord injury of the lower thoracic area presenting initially as a complete lesion with impaired bowel or bladder function, yet this will improve dramatically.
4. Evoked spinal cord potentials appeared to be diagnostic in the few done. When there is no conduction, there is no improvement.
5. Early computerized tomography of the spine and reduction of dislocation is recommended after stabilization of airway, blood pressure, and control of life threatening injuries.

6. Grading systems need to be standardized and nomenclature agreed upon. The time of examination after injury needs to be carefully documented.

References

1. Ahmann, P.A., Smith, S.A., Schwartz, J.F., Clark, D.B.: Spinal cord infarction due to minor trauma in children. Neurology *25*, 301–307 (1975)
2. Anderson, J.M., Schutt, A.H.: Spinal injury in children. A review of 156 cases seen from 1950 through 1978. Mayo Clinic Proc. *55*, 499–504 (1980)
3. Aufdemaur, M.: Spinal injuries in juveniles; necropsy findings in twelve cases. J. Bone Joint Surg. *56B*, 513–519 (1974)
4. Burke, D.C.: Spinal cord trauma in children. Paraplegia *9*, 1–14 (1971)
5. Burke, D.C.: Traumatic spinal paralyses in children. Paraplegia *11*, 268–276 (1973–1974)
6. Cheshire, D.J.E.: The paediatric syndrome of traumatic myelopathy without demonstrable vertebral injury. Paraplegia *15*, 74–85 (1977)
7. Dean, D.F., Morawetz, R.B., Sanford, R.A., Coulon, R., Ransohoff, J.: Management of Pediatric Spinal Cord Injury. Part I: Cervical injuries (in press)
8. Dean, D.F., Morawetz, R.B., Sanford, R.A., Coulon, R., Ransohoff, J.: Management of pediatric spinal cord injury. Part II: Thoracolumbar injuries (in press)
9. Frankel, H., Michaelis, L., Paeslack, V., Ungar, G., Walsh, J.J.: Closed injuries of the cervical spine and spinal cord: results of conservative treatment of vertical compression injuries to the cervical spine. Proceedings of 19th V.A. Spinal Cord Injury Conference. *10–73*, 28–32 (1977)
10. Hachen, H.J.: Spinal cord injury in children and adolescents: diagnostic pitfalls and therapeutic considerations in the acute state. Paraplegia *15*, 55–64 (1977–78)
11. Kewalramani, L.S., Tori, J.A.: Spinal cord trauma in children. Neurologic patterns, radiologic features and pathomechanics of injury. Spine *5*, 11–18 (1980)
12. LeBlanc, H.J., Nadell, J.: Spinal cord injuries in children. Surg. Neurol. *2*, 411–414 (1974)
13. Maynard, F.M., Reynolds, G.G., Fountain, S., Wilmot, C., Hamilton, R.: Neurological prognosis after traumatic quadriplegia. J. Neurosurg. *50*, 611–616 (1979)

A Scale for Evaluation of Acute Spinal Cord Injury

B. Chehrazi, F.C. Wagner, Jr., W.F. Collins, and D.H. Freeman, Jr.

Abstract

A sensitive and reproducible scale is presented for assessment of the severity of injury
and prognosis for recovery in patients with spinal cord injury. This scale provides for
numerical grading of selected functions below the level of spinal cord injury. The scale
is based on neurological examination and is easily adaptable to prospective as well as
retrospective studies. It provides for a reliable estimation of prognosis as well as comparison between effectiveness of different forms of treatment.

Application to a group of 37 patients with cervical spinal cord injury treated under
one protocol and assessed within twenty-four hours and again at one year from injury
provided a very clear objective idea of the patterns of recovery. Relative recovery from
the initial deficit measured as a "per cent recovery ratio" is presented as a sensitive analytical tool for comparison of effectiveness of different methods of treatment.

Spinal cord trauma continues to be a major cause of severe and persistent neurological
disability. Faced with the severe mortality following such injuries, the ancient Egyptians
instructed that the spinal cord injury "is an ailment not to be treated" (9). Early mortality remained close to 100% well into the nineteenth century (5). In the past forty years,
however, as the ability to prevent and treat the common complications of this injury has
improved, the mortality of such patients has decreased to less than 20% (24, 27). A large
number of the victims are young and continue to suffer from severe disability and require expensive medical and paramedical care throughout their lives (35). In search of more
effective treatment, the medical literature abounds with reports of various investigation-
al and clinical treatment protocols, the diversity of which has produced as much confu-
sion and controversy, as clarification and agreement in treatment of this injury (7, 16,
28, 29). This may be due to lack of any particularly effective therapy or at least in part
due to lack of a readily adaptable, sensitive and specific system of assessment of the
neurological injury and recovery. Interest in treatment of the critically injured patients
has increased over the past decade and so has the need for accurate measurement of
the severity of trauma and extent of recovery (17, 18). The time honoured descriptions
of complete or partial, sensory or motor paralysis are no longer adequate for evaluation
of the effectiveness of different methods of treatment (15).

An abundance of alternative methods for recording of the level of injury and the degree of improvement have been presented (3, 8, 11, 22, 23, 31). These systems are not

 Modern Neurosurgery 1. Edited by M. Brock

compatible (14, 32), and there is no agreement about what terms to use, and the ones in common use are not interpreted similarly by different workers (30). In practice, ambiguities and misunderstandings occur when the extent of recovery of patients treated by alternative methods is reported from different centres (36). Indeed, many clinicians retreat from any formal classification in favour of a general description of the patient's neurological state without clear guidelines as to what to record and how to describe it (1, 33). Partial sensory and motor paralysis covers a wide spectrum of neurological function and attempts to fit this spectrum into arbitrary and discrete categories to fit the data available in retrospective studies has resulted in artificial categories with indistinct boundaries which do not allow for any clear conclusions (2, 12, 13, 19, 23). Traumatic syndromes (4, 14, 31, 32) such as central cervical cord syndrome do not take into account the severity of damage and are complicated by the fact that often the individual patients may demonstrate fragments of more than one such syndrome. Classifications based on functional capabilities (1, 11, 23, 36) tend to place patients with similar abilities but differing neurological injuries in the same group. The emphasis of grading on ambulation results in decreased sensitivity to the deficit of patients with "central cord" injuries, and tends to confuse the outcome with the effects of rehabilitation and physical therapy. Classifications that measure only one aspect of the neurological function, such as the motor strength, although they tend to simplify the neurological assessment are insensitive to patients with a primary sensory deficit. Furthermore, the sensory function may have a more significant correlation with outcome (3).

There is a need for a clearly defined and readily applicable system that can adequately reflect the severity of the various types and levels of spinal cord injury. Based on our experience with assessment of patients in a prospective study at the Yale Spinal Cord Injury Study Centre and review of the literature, such a clinical scale has been evolved for assessing of the severity of impaired function after closed traumatic spinal cord injury.

Methods

The aspects of function which have been selected for examination are voluntary motor strength and response to pin prick, position and deep pain sensations, each being evaluated independently of the others. This scale facilitates grading of severity of the injury in a numerical fashion that yields to statistical analysis and prognostic evaluation.

In this scale, the segmental level of spinal cord injury is identified and clearly defined responses are measured distal to this level of injury and are graded according to a numerical scale which reflects the degree of retained function.

Level of Injury. The segmental level of injury is defined as the lowest spinal cord segment with intact sensory and motor functions (19, 26).

Motor Score. It has long been customary to use a gradation from 0 to 5 for recording of muscular strength in the following manner (4, 25, 26):
0 No contraction
1 Flicker or trace of contraction
2 Active movement with gravity eliminated

3 Active movement against gravity

4 Active movement against resistance

5 Normal power

The ten muscles shown in Table 1 were selected for examination based on the ease with which their contractions are identified, the range of spinal cord segments they collectively cover and their functional significance. The strength is measured in response to command as the response to a stimulus is not always easy to interpret, as a spinal reflex may cause extremities to move even in a recent spinal cord injury. The motor score is obtained by calculating the mean of the strength of all the muscles located below the level of injury. This mean is then rounded off to the first decimal point with the range of 0 to 5.0.

Sensory Score. Three modalities of sensory function, pin prick, position sense, and deep pain below the level of injury, comprise the sensory testing. For pin prick sensation, the response is graded between 0 to 2 with 0 indicating no sensation, 1 decreased or abnormal, and 2 intact sensation. The mean is obtained by dividing the sum of the responses from all dermatomes below the level of injury to the total number of such dermatomes tested (7, 20). The mean is then rounded off to the first decimal point and varies from 0 to 2.0. Position sense is tested in the little fingers and the big toes, using a 0 to 2 grading system as in the pin prick sensation. For injuries involving the cervical spine, the mean of the four measurements is then obtained and rounded off. With the level of injury at T 1 or below, only the two measurements from the toes are used for obtaining this mean. Deep pain sensation is graded either as 0 or 1 and is tested by compression of the big toe or the Achilles tendon. Patients who report any sensation and lateralize it correctly and reproducibly to either side are given a score of 1. If there is no evidence of retained function on either side, a score of 0 is given. The sum of the patients pin prick, position and deep pain scores forms that patients sensory score which ranges from 0 to 5.0.

Each patient's score on the Yale Scale for spinal cord trauma is then obtained by adding the motor and sensory scores. This scale is therefore a continuum with a range of 0 to 10.0. The follow-up examination is performed at a fixed interval, i.e., one year from the time of injury for all patients. The data from the initial and follow-up administration of this scale to a group of patients can then be presented descriptively as a curve, in which the initial Yale Scale Score (YSSo) is along the X axis and the score at follow-up after a fixed period of time (YSSi) is charted along the Y axis. Each point will then represent performance of an individual patient during the period of follow-up. The line of best fit through the points will contruct a performance curve for that group of patients.

In order to relate the amount of recovery to the initial functional loss due to injury, a per cent recovery ratio can be constructed for each patient by dividing the amount of actual change in the score (YSSi − YSSo) by the maximum possible improvement (10−YSSo) and multiplying by 100). This ratio represents an index of recovery of deficit for an individual patient or a norm for a group of patients under the same treatment.

Table 1. Muscles tested for evaluation of motor strength. Actions to be tested, peripheral innervation and representative spinal segment are included

Action to be tested	Muscles	Nerves	Cord segment
Abduction of arm	Deltoid	Axillary	C5
Flexion of forearm	Biceps	Musculocutaneous	C6
Extension of forearm	Triceps	Radial	C7
Flexion of first 4 fingers	Flexor digitorum superficialis profundus	Median Ulnar	C8
Opposition of metacarpal of thumb	Opponens pollicis	Median	T1
Hip flexion	Iliopsoas	Femoral	L1, L2
Knee Extension	Quadriceps femoris	Femoral	L3
Dorsiflexion of foot	Tibialis anterior	Deep peroneal	L4
Dorsiflexion of big toes	Extensor hallucis longus	Deep peroneal	L5
Plantar flexion of foot and big toes	Gastrocnemius flexor hallucis longus	Tibial	S1, S2

Application

Different observers were able to apply this scale with a high degree of consistency. When doctors and physician associates graded the same group of patients variations in scoring were limited to less than one point on the scale. This was in contrast to what happened when the observers were asked to judge the degree of usefulness of motor function for the same patients. Table 2 demonstrates the data acquisition and compilation form. A part of this scale may be untestable as limbs may be immobilized by splints or traction. In these instances, the mean is based on the muscles and dermatomes that can be tested. Patients who demonstrate rapid progressive improvement of neurological status within an hour of their hospital admission are tested repeatedly and the latest results obtained within the first eight hours of their admission are used for their initial score on the Yale Scale.

The application of this scale to an individual patient may be most easily demonstrated by the following case. A 17-year-old male was seen in the emergency room within one hour of an auto accident which left him with a fracture dislocation of C5 and C6. At the initial examination he had full strength in his deltoids and was intact to pin prick down to the shoulders and over the biceps. His level of injury was determined as C5.

311

Table 2. Data aquisition form for Yale Scale for spinal cord injury

Number _____   Date of injury _____

Name _____   Date of examination _____

Motor examination			Sensory examination					
Muscles tested	Strength [a] 0–5		Level of injury	Pin prick [b] 0–2		Position [b] 0–2		
	Right	Left		Right	Left	Extremity	Right	Left
Upper extremity						Upper		
Deltoid C5			C2					
Biceps C6			3			Lower		
Triceps C7			4					
Flexor digitorum			5					
superficialis & profundus C8			6			Total below the level		
Opponens pollicis T1			7			of injury		
			8					
			T1			Number of tests below		
Lower extremity			2			level of injury		
			3					
			4			Position sense		
Iliopsoas L1,2			5					
Quadriceps femoris L3			6			Deep pain [c]		
Tibialis anterior L4			7			0–1		
Extensor hallucis longus L5			8					
Gastrochemius			9			Lower extremities		
flexor hallucis longus S1,2			10			response to deep		
			11			pain		
			12					
			L1					
Total below the level of injury			2			Sensory score		
			3					
			4					
Number of muscles tested			5					
below the level of injury			S1					
			2					
			3					
			4					
			5					
Motor score								
			Total below the level of injury					
			Number of derma- tomes tested			Yale scale score		
			Pin prick					

[a] 0 No contraction
  1 Flicker or trace of contraction
  2 Active movement with gravity eliminated
  3 Active movement against gravity
  4 Acitve movement against resistance
  5 Normal power

[b] 0 Absent sensation
  1 Decreased or abnormal
  2 Intact sensation

[c] 0 Absent sensation or pain reportet only inconsistently
  1 Sensation reported correctly better than half the times

On motor testing, he had weakness of the biceps and brachioradialis against resistance on the right and was only antigravity on the left. He had no other motor function in the upper extremities. He could weakly adduct the lower extremities and could weakly wiggle his right toes and foot on the right, while the only movement on the left was a barely perceptible toe wiggle. Pin prick was intact over the right thumb and decreased on the index and middle fingers. Dull sensation was reported bilaterally in the perianal area and over the penis in response to pin prick. No other response was noted to pin prick testing. Position sense was absent in the small fingers and the left big toe. A diminished position sense was present in the right big toe. He correctly lateralized left toe compression while response to right toe compression was equivocal. He responded to cervical traction of up to 30 lbs. with good skeletal alignment. A myelogram demonstrated no soft tissue compression and he had no significant change in his neurological status during the first 3 hours after injury. The patient's performance is depicted in Table 3.

Based on 150 examinations performed on 42 patients, a comparison was made between the Yale Scale and two systems previously reported by Frankle (11) and Maynard (23). The result is presented in Table 4. It appears that a wide range of Yale Scale scores correspond with individual categories in these other classifications.

This scale was next applied to 37 patients with cervical spinal cord injury treated under the same protocol (6, 34). No correlation was present between the level of injury and score on the Yale Scale. No patient deteriorated. The performance curve was constructed for YSS on admission and at one year (Fig. 1). Patients with YSS_o of less than two on admission had very little improvement. These patients all had a "complete" injury on admission. The per cent recovery ratio for patients with initial scores of less than 2 had a mean of 6% while in patients with admission scores of greater than 2, this was 80% (6). The recovery ratio for patients with partial injury (YSS_o 2) was independent of their admission score.

Discussion

It is by no means our intention to deny the value of a detailed appraisal of the patients' spinal cord function in reaching a diagnosis and determining the proper form of treatment. However, repeated evaluations of function are usually made by relatively less experienced personnel. Therefore, there are good reasons for restricting the observations to those functions which can be reliably recorded and compared in a wide range of institutions in a fashion that comparison can be readily performed between different modes of treatment in the clinical setting. Apart from the practical use in the management of the recently injured patient, this scale allows the severity of injury to be defined precisely and reproducibly in a numerical fashion. In a comparison with the functional states reported from Stoke-Mandeville and San Jose, it appears that the Yale Scale provides for more precise assessment of the patients status and, therefore, may be used more accurately in follow-up of the neurological status, determination of prognosis and comparison of benefit of differing types of treatment. Patients treated in different ways may be compared by superimposing their curves of recovery. The finding of no statistically significant difference in the recovery ratio originally used by Lucas and Ducker (21) in

Table 3. Initial assessment of a patient with C5 level of severe spinal cord injury

Number _____   Date of injury _____

Name _____   Date of examination _____

Motor examination				Sensory examination					
Muscles tested		Strength [a] 0−5		Level of Injury	Pin prick [b] 0−2		Position [b] 0−2		
Upper extremity		Right	Left		Right	Left	Extremity	Right	Left
Deltoid	C5	5	5	C2	2	2	Upper	0	0
Biceps	C6	4	3	3	,,	,,			
Triceps	C7	0	0	4	,,	,,	Lower	1	0
Flexor digitorum				5	,,	,,			
superficialis & profundus	C8	0	0	6	2	0	Total below the level		
Opponens pollicis	T1	0	0	7	1	,,	of injury 1		
				8	0	,,			
				T1	,,	,,			
				2	,,	,,			
				3	,,	,, .	Number of tests below		
Lower extremity				4	,,	,,	level of injury 4		
				5	,,	,,			
Iliopsoas	L1,2	0	0	6	,,	,,	Position sense 0,3		
Quadriceps femoris	L3	0	0	7	,,	,,			
Tibialis anterior	L4	0	0	8	,,	,,	Deep pain [c]		
Extensor hallucis longus	L5	2	1	9	,,	,,	0−1		
Gastrocnemius				10	,,	,,			
flexor hallucis longus	S1,2	2	0	11	,,	,,	Lower extremities		
				12	,,	,,	response to deep		
				L1	,,	,,	pain 1		
				2	,,	,,			
				3	,,	,,			
Total below the level of injury 12				4	,,	,,	Sensory score 1,5		
				5	,,	,,			
				S1	,,	,,			
Number of muscles tested				2	,,	,,			
below the level of injury 18				3	1	1			
				4	1	1			
				5	1	1			
Motor score 0.7									

Total below the level of injury
9

[a] 0 No contraction
  1 Flicker or trace of contraction
  2 Active movement with gravity eliminated
  3 Active movement against gravity
  4 Active movement against resistance
  5 Normal power

[b] 0 Absent sensation
  1 Decreased or abnormal
  2 Intact sensation

[c] 0 Absent sensation or pain reported only inconsistently
  1 Sensation reported correctly better than half the times

Number of dermatomes tested
50

Pin prick 0,2

Yale scale score

2,2

314

Table 4. Comparison of the Stoke-Mandeville (Frankel) and San Jose (Maynard) classifications of spinal cord injury with the Yale Scale

Stoke Mandeville	Comparable YSS Range	Mean
A-Complete	0−3	0.7
B-Sensory only	2−5	3.3
C-Motor useless	3−7	4.4
D-Motor useful	6−9	8.0
E-Recovery	10	10
San Jose		
M-Motor incomplete	2−9	6.1
W-Walking	8−10	8.6

this preliminary application between patients with initially high scores and those with intermediate scores suggest that these patients may have a similar potential for recovery. In this schema, potentially all spinal cord injuries may be presented together on the same scale regardless of their level or severity of injury. Furthermore, although the initial score is of significant value in predicting actual score at a one year follow-up, the relative recovery of neurological deficit, per cent recovery ratio, may be independent of this initial score for patients with incomplete injuries. Whether the recovery ratio is a more sensitive and accurate way of determining the effect of different methods of treatment will require further testing by other spinal cord injury centres employing alternative treatment protocols.

References

1. Berard, E., Minaire, P., Girard, R. et al.: Results of rehabilitation in central cord syndromes. Paraplegia *14*, 259−261 (1977)
2. Bosch, A., Stauffer, E.S., Nickle, V.L.: Incomplete traumatic quadriplegia. A ten-year review. JAMA *216*, 473−478 (1971)
3. Bracken, M. et al.: Classification of the severity of acute spinal cord injury. Implications for management. Paraplegia *15*, 319−316 (1977−78)
4. Burke, D.C.: The neurological examination (spinal) Aust. Fam. Physician *8*, 119−128 (1979)
5. Carrolle, D.G.: History of treatment of spinal cord injury. Maryland State Medical Journal, 109−112 (1970)
6. Chehrazi, B., Wagner, F.C., Jr., Collins, W.F. et al.: A scale for evaluation of spinal cord injury. J.Neurosurg. *54*, 310−315 (1981)
7. Collins, W.F., Chehrazi, B.: Concepts of the acute management of spinal cord injury. In: Recent advances in clinical neurology. Edinburgh: Churchill-Livingstone (in press)
8. Dall, M.: Injuries of the cervical spine. Does the type of bony injury affect spinal cord recovery. South African Medical Journal, 1048−56 (1972)
9. Elsberg, C.: The Edwin Smith surgical papyrus and diagnosis and treatment of injuries to the skull and spine 5000 years ago. Annals of Medical History *3*, 271, 275 (1931)

10. Foerster, O.: The dermatomes in man. Brain *56*, 1–39 (1933)
11. Frankel, H.L.: The value of postural reduction in the initial management of closed injuries of the spine with paraplegia and tetraplegia. Paraplegia 7 (2), 179, 192 (1969)
12. Geisler, W.O., Jousse, A.T., Wynne-Jones, M.: Survival in traumatic transverse myelitis. Paraplegia *14*, 262–275 (1977)
13. Gjone, R., Nordlie, L.: Incidence of traumatic paraplegia and tetraplegia in Norway: a statistical survey of the years 1974 and 1975. Paraplegia *16*, 88–93 (1978)
14. Hardy, A.G.: Cervical spine cord injury without bony injury. Paraplegia *14*, 296–305 (1977)
15. Heiden, J.S.: Management of cervical spinal cord trauma in southern California, J. Neurosurg. *43*, 732–736 (1975)
16. Heyl, H.L.: Federal programs for the care and study of spinal cord injuries: Special report and editorial. J. Neurosurg. *36 (4),* 379–385 (1972)
17. Hunt, W.E.: Spinal cord injury and outcome. Neural trauma. New York: Raven Press 1979
18. Jennett, W.B.: Predicting outcome in individual patients after severe head injury. Lancet 1031–1034 (1976)
19. Jockheim, K.A.: Problems of classification in traumatic paraplegia and tetraplegia. Paraplegia *8*, 80–82 (1970)
20. Keegan, J.J., Garrett, F.D.: The segmental distribution of the cutaneous nerves in the limbs of man. Anat. Rec. *102*, 409–437 (1948)
21. Lucas, J.T., Ducker, T.B.: Morbidity, mortality, and recovery rates of patients with spinal cord injuries undergoing anterior decompressive procedure or fusion, or both. Surg Forum. *28*, 451–453 (1977)
22. Marar, B.C.: The pattern of neurological damage as an aid to the diagnosis of the mechanism of cervical spine injuries. J. Bone joint Surg. (Am) *56*, 1648–1654 (1974)
23. Maynard, F.M., Reynolds, G.G., Fountain, S. et al.: Neurological prognosis after traumatic quadriplegia. Three year experience of California Regional Spinal Cord injury Care System. J. Neurosurg. *50*, 611–616 (1979)
24. Meacham, W.F., McPherson, W.F.: Local hypothermia in treatment of acute injuries of the spinal cord. Southern Medical Journal *66*(1), 95–97 (1973)
25. Medical Research Council of the United Kingdom: Aids to the examination of the peripheral nervous system. Memorandum No. 45. London: Her Majesty's Stationary Office. 1943. (Palo Alto, CA: Pendragon House. 1978)
26. Michaelis, L.S.: International inquiry on neurological terminology and prognosis in paraplegia and tetraplegia. Paraplegia 7, 1–5 (1969)
27. Price, M.: Causes of death in 11 of 227 patients with traumatic spinal cord injury over period of nine years. Paraplegia *11(3),* 217–220 (1973)
28. Proceedings of the Nineteenth Veterans Administration Spinal Cord Injury Conference. Scottsdale, AZ, Oct. 29–31, 1973
29. Ransohoff, J.R.: Spinal cord injury: Current status and recent advances. Surgical Annals *4,* 91–101 (1972)
30. Ransohoff, J.: Cervical spinal cord injury; medical and surgical therapy. In: Proceedings of the nineteenth veterans administration spinal cord injury conference. Oct. 1973, pp. 1–6. Washington, D.C.: U.S. Gov't Printing Office 1977
31. Schneider, R.C., Crosby, E.C., Russo, H.R., et al.: Traumatic spinal cord syndromes and their management. Clin. Neurosurg. *20*, 424–492 (1973)
32. Shrosbnee, R.D.: Acute central cervical spinal cord syndrome – etiology, age, incidence, and relationship to orthopaedic injury. Paraplegia *14*, 251–258 (1977)
33. Sussman, B.J.: Fracture dislocation of the cervical spine: a critique of current management in the United States. Paraplegia *16*, 15–38 (1978)
34. Wagner, F.C., Jr.: Management of acute spinal cord injury. Surg. Neurol. *7(6)* (1977)
35. Webb, B.J., Berzins, E., Wingarder, T.S., Lorenzi, E.: Spinal cord injury: Epidemiologic implications, costs and patterns of care in 85 patients. Archives of Physical Medicine and Rehabilitation *60*, 335–340 (1979)
36. Young, J.S., Dexter, W.R.: Neurological recovery distal to the zone of injury in 172 cases of closed, traumatic spinal cord injury. Paraplegia *16*, 39–49 (1978)

316

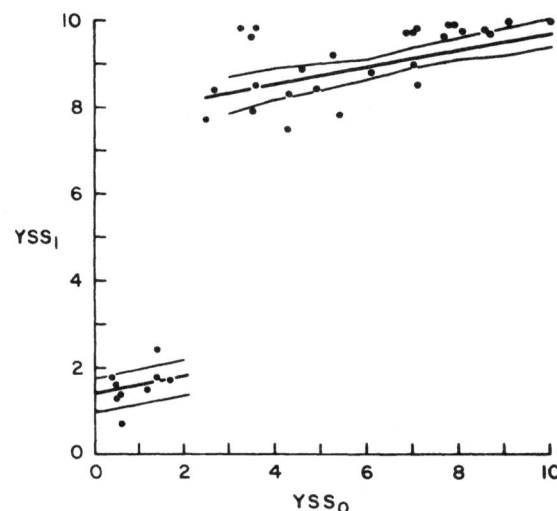

Fig. 1. Relationship between admission scores (YSSo) and follow-up scores at one year (YSS1) in patients with acute cervical spinal cord injury. Line of least squares and the 95% confidence limits are drawn

Patient Selection for an Extracranial–Intracranial Arterial Bypass

R. Deruty, J. Lecuire, Ph. Bret, and J. Capdeville

It has been fourteen years since the first extracranial intracranial bypass procedures (EIAB) were described (5). Such a procedure, consisting of an anastomosis between the superficial temporal artery and the middle cerebral artery, is now routinely performed (1, 2, 4). However, the indications for this operation are still controversial.

In order to select the patients for the EIAB procedure, three criteria are usually used: clinical history, angiographic lesions, or cerebral blood flow measurements. In our opinion, the clinical history comes first; the other two criteria are just accessory, as a means of confirming or refusing the indication, once the clinical history has suggested that the patient is a proper candidate.

Clinically two conditions are to be considered: the stroke and the relapsing ischaemic attack. As regards strokes, there has been no clear evidence so far the EIAB procedure is that of any value for the recovery of the patients: bypass operations in stroke patients only depend on personal opinion, and will not be discussed in this paper.

The relapsing ischaemic episodes are usually accepted as a better indication for the EIAB procedure; they will be the subject of this discussion.

Material and Approach

Basic Considerations

1. Two distinct clinical conditions are included inside the group of so-called "Relapsing Ischaemic Episodes", "The Transient Ischaemic Attacks" (TIA) in which recovery occurs within 24 hours, and "The Progressive Reversible Ischaemic Neurological Deficits" (PRIND) in which recovery occurs within a few days. We shall not separate these two conditions because, in both, the patient is asymptomatic at the time of operation.

2. The clinical history allows relapsing ischaemic episodes (both TIA and PRIND) to be classified in three categories:

The High Frequency Relapsing Ischaemic Episodes. In this category, a number of episodes occur, of the same clinical type, related to the same angiographic lesion, and separated by short intervals of time. These attacks may occur several times a day, a week, or a month.

The Low Frequency Relapsing Ischaemic Episodes. In this type, there are a few ischaemic episodes over a long period, usually several years; every episode has the same clinical features, and is related to the same angiographic lesion. For example, the patient may experience two to four or five similar episodes during ten or twelve years.

The Solitary Episode. The patient is usually admitted early after a fresh ischaemic episode, which is the first one of the type (should a similar episode be found to have occurred during the past, the clinical history would have to be classified into the "Low Frequency" category).

3. The outcome of the relapsing ischaemic episodes may be of three types:

Total disappearance of the attacks, either spontaneously or with medical treatment. Such a good outcome makes it particularly difficult to allocate to the "low frequency" group or to the "single episode" group; as we shall see later on, intervals up to twelve years were found in our series between two attacks.

Continuation of the ischaemic history, the attacks occuring at the same frequency without any improvement or deterioration.

Worsening of the clinical condition,with the onset of an acute stroke, or more rarely, of a progressive stroke.

4. Two kinds of vascular lesion related to the ischaemic accidents are to be described: the main lesion and the associated lesions.

The main lesion can be located at various sites: the cervical internal carotid artery, the carotid siphon, the intracranial carotid artery, the middle cerebral artery.
    In the cervical internal carotid artery, only a complete occlusion should be usually considered; a carotid stenosis in the neck should usually be treated directly, with an endarterectomy; in such a case, the bypass operation should be discussed only in those very infrequent cases, where direct operation is not feasible.
    The main lesion may either be single, or associated with other minor or major lesions.

The associated lesions are particularly frequent in the carotid artery:
They may be located on the same side as the main lesion, more distally: either siphon stenosis (tandem-lesions) or just recognizable atheromatous lesions.
They may be located contralaterally. Many combinations can be seen on the angiogram: bilateral carotid occlusion, occlusion plus stenosis, bilateral tandem lesions.
The carotid lesions may also be associated with vertebro-basilar atheromatous lesions.

5. Radioclinical Correlations. In most cases, the relapsing ischaemic episode is directly related to the territory of the artery with the main lesions (the affected side); for instance, a right carotid occlusion is responsible for a left hemiplegia. Such a condition may be called a *"direct" ischaemic episode.*
    Conversely, in some cases, the symptoms do not correspond to the affected artery; such a condition may be called a *"paradoxical ischaemic episode".* The mechanism responsible for such a paradoxical accident is usually an intracranial steal. The first type is a carotid steal; for instance a right carotid occlusion will be responsible for a right

hemiplegia; the second type is a carotid-vertebral (or carotid-basilar) steal, in which a carotid occlusion is responsible for vertebro-basilar symptoms.

Material

From 1972 to 1980, 70 patients have been operated upon with the EIAB procedure, of whom 24 had suffered from relapsing ischaemic accidents. Preoperatively, both carotid arteries were shown angiographically. Postoperatively an angiographic control was performed after two weeks. Amongst these 24 patients, nine had "high frequency" ischaemic attacks, six had "low frequency" attacks and nine had a "single ischaemic accident". Out of the "high frequency" group, only six patients were available for the follow-up study. We shall give some examples of the first two categories:

1. High Frequency Group

Case 1: Relapsing ischaemic history of the direct type. This 53-year-old right-handed man was admitted to hospital after a PRIND with aphasia and right hemiplegia. During the previous six months, he had suffered from about thirty TIA's of the same type.
   The angiograms showed:
— a left internal carotid occlusion in the neck;
— recognizable atheromatous lesions, in the right internal carotid artery, in the neck as well as in the siphon;
— good cross-filling through the anterior communicating artery from the right side to the left side.
   The patient was operated on in December 1978, on the left side. The bypass was demonstrated to be patent 15 days post-operatively. The ischaemic attacks completely disappeared, with a follow-up of two and a half years.

Case 2: Relapsing ischaemic history of the paradoxical type. This 58-year-old right-handed man was admitted after a two months history of TIA's in the vertebro-basilar circulation. About ten attacks had occured, with diplopia, loss of consciousness and drop-attacks.
   The angiograms showed:
— a right cervical internal carotid artery occlusion;
— recognizable atheromatous lesions in the left internal carotid artery;
— mild stenosis of both vertebral arteries at the ostium;
— filling of the right middle cerebral artery through the posterior communicating artery.
   The patient was operated upon in December 1979, on the right side. Patency of the bypass was demonstrated angiographically 15 days later. The ischaemic attacks completely disappeared, with an 18 months follow-up.

Case 3: Ischaemic episode of the direct type.

In 1966, this right-handed man had suffered with a PRIND, with aphasia and right hemiplegia. At this time, an angiogram had demonstrated a left internal carotid occlusion. Between 1966 and 1978 he remained free of symptoms. In 1978, when he was 50 years old he experienced two TIA's with right hemiplegia. A femoral catheterisation showed:
— a complete occlusion of the left internal carotid artery (already known since 1966)
— a normal right internal carotid artery;
— good cross-filling through the anterior communicating artery, from the right side to the left side.

Operation was performed in August 1978, on the left side, and patency of the bypass was demonstrated angiographically after 15 days. One year later, a second postoperative angiogram failed to show the bypass, which was probably occluded; despite this bypass occlusion, the patient remained asymptomatic.

Case 4: Relapsing ischaemic history of the direct type. In 1968, this right-handed man had suffered with one PRIND and three TIA's, consisting of aphasia and right upper-limb monoplegia. At the time, occlusion of the left middle cerebral artery was demonstrated. During the nine following years, he remained free of symptoms. In 1977, when he was 35 years old, he was admitted after a PRIND of the same type. A severe stenosis of the left middle cerebral artery was demonstrated on the angiograms. The patient was operated on in October 1977, on the left side, and the bypass was seen to be patent 15 days post-operatively.

Case 5: Relapsing ischaemic history of the paradoxical type. In 1975, this right-handed man experienced a TIA with a right hemiplegia, and a right internal carotid occlusion was found. The patient refused the bypass operation. In 1977, when he was 59 years old, he was admitted after a PRIND with aphasia and right hemiplegia. The angiographic lesions were the following ones:
— right internal carotid occlusion;
— recognizable atheromatous lesions on the left side;
— no right carotid filling through the posterior communicating artery.

The patient was operated on in January 1978, with postoperative patency of the bypass.

Case 6: Relapsing ischaemic history ending in a progressive stroke. In 1971, this right-handed man had an history of six TIA's with right hemiparesis. An occlusion of the left internal carotid artery was demonstrated on angiogram. The right carotid artery was normal. In 1974, he experience a PRIND with right hemiplegia. The same lesion was demonstrated on the left side; on the right side, there was evidence of atheromatous lesions. A bypass operation was discussed, but not carried out, because of refusal by the Neurologist.

In 1978, when he was 50 years old, he was readmitted with a progressive weakness of the right hand, and after a few weeks, complete palsy of the hand. The angiograms showed:

— occlusion of the left internal carotid artery;

— stenosis of the right carotid siphon;

— cross-filling from the right side to the left side through the anterior communicating artery.

The bypass was carried out in June 1978, on the left side. The recovery of the right hand occurred during the first few days postoperatively and the bypass was patent on the post-operative angiogram.

Discussion

1. High frequency relapsing ischaemic episodes are commonly accepted as the best indications for a bypass operation, because they are related to a low cerebral perfusion. In addition, in such a clinical condition, the surgical result can easily be assessed: either the attacks cease after operation or they still occur; the number of attacks and their frequency preoperatively offer a very good way of comparison for the post-operative period. Usually, the bypass operation is very effective in this group. Our experience correlates with this general idea: six out of nine of our patients were available for the follow-up. In the six of them, the attacks disappeared postoperatively.

2. Low frequency relapsing ischaemic episodes: Whether an extracranial/intracranial bypass should be performed for these is still controversial. We must consider separately the first three examples (cases 3—5) and the fourth one (case 6).

In the first three cases, the result of the bypass operation compared with the spontaneous evolution could not be assessed for a long time. The follow-up period should be at least as long as the pre-operative ischaemic history, that is up to twelve years for the first patient, and nine years for the second patient. Thus, we may find it difficult to support the surgical decision upon an asymptomatic follow-up period of just two or three years in such patients.

The ischaemic background of some of our stroke patients should be considered with the greatest attention. Besides the group of "reversible ischaemic episodes" we have operated on 45 patients who fit into a "stroke category". Amongst these 45 patients, nine, as far as we were able to record the ischaemic history, had previously suffered from such a low frequency relapsing ischaemic history. Thus, the risk of stroke in the group of "low frequency relapsing ischaemic episodes" appears to be real, and this is an argument for a by-pass to be carried out in these patients.

The fourth example (case 6) emphasizes another possibility of a poor outcome, in this category. This patient, after seven years, showed an impairment not only clinically as but also angiographically, as far as associated lesions were concerned. Such an outcome lends weight to our opinion for considering these patients as candidates for the EIAB operation.

Single Ischaemic Episode Category

In our opinion, in such patients, the clinical history by itself does not allow one to decide between surgical or medical treatment. In these patients the angiographic features and the cerebral blood flow (CBF) measurements should also be considered. Our experience in CBF measurement is too limited, and at the time the results appear rather difficult to be used. although some authors have found very a good correlation between the clinical history and the surgical results (3). Thus, we shall only discuss the angiographic features, in the internal carotid artery.

1. First Possibility. The main lesion, responsible for the symptom is unique. The contralateral carotid is normal; the cross-filling through the anterior communicating artery is good. Such a patient should not be operated on.

2. Second Possibility. Several lesions are shown: the main lesion (for instance occlusion of a carotid artery) is associated with obvious contralateral atheromatous lesions. Probably in such a pattern,the collateral blood supply, (which may be good at the time) may become more and more affected during the coming years. There is a risk of recurrence of ischaemic attacks, or of progress towards a stroke. In such a patient, a bypass operation should be considered.

In the cases with occlusion plus contralateral stenosis, it is a matter of personal opinion whether the contralateral carotid stenosis in the neck should be treated first, or whether a bypass on the affected side should be performed first.

Conclusion

In the patients presenting with a cerebral relapsing ischaemic history, due to non directly operable carotid lesions, we should consider an extracranial/intracranial arterial bypass as follows:
1. The patients with a high frequency relapsing ischaemic history should be operated on, whether the lesions be bilateral or not. The result of surgery is usually good.
2. The patients with a low frequency relapsing ischaemic history should probably be operated on. However the results cannot be clearly assessed due to the long interval between the pre-operative ischaemic attacks. A patient with a progressive mild stroke occurring after a long history of relapsing attacks should certainly be operated upon.
3. In our opinion, patients with a single relapsing ischaemic episode should probably be operated on if the angiograms demonstrate bilateral lesions namely, the main lesion, responsible for the symptoms, and the contralateral atheromatous lesions, affecting the collateral blood supply.

References

1. Austin, G.M.: Micro-neurosurgical anastomosis for cerebral ischemia. Springfield, Ill.: C.C. Thomas 1976
2. Peerless, S., McCormick, C.W.: Microsurgery for cerebral ischemia. Berlin, Heidelberg, New York: Springer 1981
3. Schmiedek, P., Gratzl, O., Spetzler, R., Steinhoff, H., Enzenbach, R., Brendel, W., Marguth, F.: Selection of patients for extra-intracranial arterial by-pass surgery based on rCBF measurements. J. Neurosurg. *44*, 303–312 (1976)
4. Schmiedek, P.: Microsurgery for stroke. Berlin, Heidelberg, New York: Springer 1977
5. Yasargil, M.G.: Microsurgery applied to neurosurgery. Stuttgart: Thieme 1969

Extracranial-Intracranial Bypass Operations in Patients with Stenotic Lesions of Major Cerebral Arteries

V. Olteanu-Nerbe, P. Schmiedek, and F. Marguth

According to reports by others (2, 3, 10, 11) as well as from our own experience (12) it is well known that stenotic lesions of major cerebral arteries may become occluded after a successful extracranial-intracranial arterial bypass (EIAB) operation. This has been explained on the basis of haemodynamic changes, particularly on changes of pressure gradients with decrease of the arterial pressure on both sides of the stenosis, resulting from the newly established blood supply to the brain.

The aim of this study was to find out whether successful bypass surgery can induce, by favouring occlusion of stenotic lesions localized in the area of the perforating arteries or of other main collaterals of the circle of Willis, a simultaneous decrease of blood flow through these vessels and thus possibly cause a new cerebral ischaemic episode.

Clinical Material

The study includes 31 patients, 19 men and 12 women. The ages ranged from 20 to 72 years. According to the site of the vascular lesion, cases were classified in the following three groups (Fig. 1a):

Group I comprised 12 patients with stenoses of the middle cerebral artery (MCA) before its major division (M1) or of its major primary branches (M2), in ten and two cases respectively.

Group II comprised nine patients with a stenosis of the internal carotid artery bifurcation (ICAB-S), three of them bilateraly.

Group III included ten cases with an internal carotid siphon stenosis (ICAS-S), in the area of the posterior communicating artery.

Because of bilateral cerebrovascular disease (CVD) in three cases a total of 34 EIAB operations were performed. All patients have been followed up postoperatively for a period of 5 to 50 months. With the exception of two cases one or several control angiograms were performed in all cases.

Pre-operative and postoperative regional cerebral blood flow measurements (rCBF) or perfusion scintigraphic studies were performed in 8 and 21 cases respectively.

Results

With one exception all anastomoses were patent at the time of the control angiographic study. A grading system from one to seven was used to evaluate the filling of the middle cerebral artery via the bypass. According to reports from the literature (1, 9) we have used Waddington's schema (14) regarding the MCA distribution areas.

Only ten patients of group I (Table 1) agreed to have postoperative angiographic evaluation, while two cases were examined by doppler sonography. With one exception all anastomoses were patent. In six cases, with a MCA filling score of three to six, the M1 or M2 stenotic lesions were found to be occluded on post-operative angiograms (Fig. 2a–d). In another three cases with filling scores of three, one and zero respectively, the degree of the MCA stenosis was increased as compared with preoperative findings. The clinical progress was good or excellent in nine patients, including all of those with secondary occlusions, whereas the results in the remaining three were fair. In one of these patients, with an excellent functioning bypass and a return to normal in his postoperative rCBF study, the increased M1 stenosis resulted in an infarct of the internal capsule with deterioration of his neurological deficit. The EIAB in the remaining two cases with new cerebral ischaemic episodes during the follow-up period was no patent or insufficient respectively.

All 12 microanastomoses performed in ten patients of group II (Table 2) were patent at the time of postoperative angiographic examination. In six cases, with a MCA filling score of one to three, the lesion was found to be unchanged as compared with the preoperative angiographic findings. In another four cases with filling scores of five and six, the ICAB was occluded, whereas in two cases, with scores of three and five respectively, the stenotic lesion was increased. In two cases who had bilateral bypass operations because of Moya Moya disease additional increase of the natural collateral blood supply could be seen. The clinical course was good to excellent in all but one case, who had a poor filling of the MCA through the bypass.

In six cases of group III (Table 3) the pre-operative vascular lesion remained unchanged. Of the remaining four lesions two reversed, one increased and one progressed to occlusion. The MCA filling score in this group varied from one to three.

Discussion

There are only a few comparable reports in the literature concerning the natural history of patients presenting with thrombotic lesions of the main trunk of the MCA (5, 7, 8, 13) or the ICA (4, 7) in the region of the circle of Willis.

Fischer (5) reported 40 cases of MCA trunk occlusion in which 87.5% presented with disabling deficits of moderate or severe degree. In the series of 59 patients analysed by Lascelles et al. (8) who had obstructive lesions at different levels of the MCA tree there were 75% who had a poor outcome.

Similarly the clinical course of obstructive lesions of the ICA within the circle of Willis seems to be more severe (4, 7) than those of ICA occlusion in its preophthalmic region (4). In our series there were 75% of cases with middle cerebral artery stenosis and 42% of patients with internal carotid artery bifurcation stenosis who presented

Table 1. Results in 12 cases with middle cerebral artery stenosis and EIAB

Case No.	Age (years) Sex	Preoperative vascular lesion	Clinical findings	Time after EIAB in months	Bypass patent (No. of areas filled)	Postoperative vascular lesion	Clinical result
1	39 M	L M1-S	smCS	50	Yes (5)	Occluded	Excellent
2	50 M	L M1-S	PRIND	36	Yes (5)	Occluded	Excellent
3	42 M	R M1-S	TIA	36	Yes (4)	Occluded	Excellent
4	46 F	L M1-S	smCS	23	Yes (6)	Occluded	Excellent
5	38 M	L M1-S	modCS	15	Yes (3)	Occluded	Excellent
6	54 M	R M1-S	smCS	10	Yes (6)	Occluded	Excellent
7	50 M	L M1-S	SIE	19	Yes (3)	Increased	Fair
8	65 F	R M1-S	smCS	8	Yes (1/0)	Increased	Fair
9	72 M	L M1-S	smCS	24	Yes (doppler)	N.D.	Excellent
10	55 F	L M1-S	TIA	16	Yes (doppler)	N.D.	Excellent
11	57 F	R M2-S R ICAS	modCS	32	No	Increased Increased	Fair
12	48 M	L M2-S	smCS	22	Yes (1)	Unchanged	Good

EIAB= extracranial-intracranial arterial bypass; M1-S= stenosis of the middle cerebral artery before major division; M2-S= stenosis of major primary branch of the middle cerebral artery; ICA-S= internal carotid artery stenosis; TIA= transient ischaemic attack; PRIND= prolonged reversible ischaemic neurologic deficit; SIE= stroke in evolution; smCS= small completed stroke; modCS= moderate completed stroke

Table 2. Results of 12 EIAB operations in nine cases with internal carotid artery bifurcation stenosis

Case No.	Age (years) Sex	Preoperative vascular lesion	Clinical findings	Time after EIAB in months	Bypass patent (No. of areas filled)	Postoperative vascular lesion	Clinical result
1	30 F	R ICAB-S	SIE	25	Yes (2)	Unchanged (increased nat. collat.)	Good
2	30 F	L ICAB-S	SIE	25	Yes (1)	Unchanged (increased nat. collat.)	Good
3	55 F	R ICAB-S	TIA	24	Yes (3)	Unchanged	Excellent
4	43 F	R ICAB-S	TIA	9	Yes (1)	Unchanged (increased nat. collat.)	Good
5	37 M	R ICAB-S	TIA	8	Yes (2)	Unchanged	Good
6	54 M	R ICAB-S	PRIND	5	Yes (1)	Unchanged	Fair
7	27 F	R ICAB-S	TIA	24	Yes (5)	Occluded	Excellent
8	55 F	R ICAB-S	smCS	24	Yes (6)	Occluded	Excellent
9	62 M	R ICAB-S	TIA	23	Yes (5)	Occluded	Excellent
10	34 M	L ICAB-S	SIE	18	Yes (6)	Occluded	Excellent
11	20 F	R ICAB-S	smCS	9	Yes (5)	Increased	Excellent
12	43 F	L ICAB-S	TIA	9	Yes (3)	Increased (increased nat. collat.)	Good

EIAB= extracranial-intracranial arterial bypass; ICAB-S= internal carotid artery bifurcation stenosis; TIA= transient ischaemic attack; PRIND= prolonged reversible ischaemic neurologic deficit; SIE= stroke inevolution; smCS= small completed stroke

Table 3. Results in ten cases with internal carotid artery siphon stenosis and EIAB

Case No.	Age (years) Sex	Preoperative vascular lesion	Clinical findings	Time after EIAB in months	Bypass patent (No. of areas filled)	Postoperative vascular lesion	Clinical result
1	24 M	R ICAS-S	smCS	42	Yes (3)	Unchanged	Excellent
2	53 M	R ICAS-S	TIA	37	Yes (1)	Unchanged	Excellent
3	66 F	R ICAS-S	TIA	14	Yes (2)	Unchanged	Excellent
4	65 F	L ICAS-S	TIA	8	Yes (3)	Unchanged	Good
5	58 M	R ICAS-S	smCS	8	Yes (1)	Unchanged	Good
6	63 F	L ICAS-S	TIA	6	Yes (3)	Unchanged	Excellent
7	44 M	R ICAS-S	TIA	36	Yes (1/2)	Reversed	Good
8	28 M	L ICAS-S	PRIND	34	Yes (2)	Reversed	Fair
9	66 M	L ICAS-S	smCS	48	Yes (1/2)	Increased	Good
10	52 M	L ICAS-S	TIA	8	Yes (3)	Occluded	Excellent

EIAB= extracranial-intracranial arterial bypass; ICAS-S= internal carotid artery siphon stenosis; TIA= transient ischaemic attack; PRIND= prolonged reversible ischaemic neurologic deficit; smCS= small completed stroke with a slight or moderate completed stroke (CS) at the time of admission to the hospital.

Our results also show that after an EIAB procedure in 11 cases (32%) a secondary occlusion of the pre-operative stenotic lesion occurred (Abb. 1b). This percentage rises to 75% in patients presenting with MCA stenoses. This finding seems to be in direct relation to the quality of the MCA filling through the bypass and to the time elapsed since operation. Changes in these angiographic findings however did not affect the clinical course in any of these eleven cases.

There was only one patient presenting with an M1 stenotic lesion in whom, during thte follow-up period, an increase of the stenosis occurred and who got worse neurologically after the bypass operation in spite of excellent function in the new anastomosis. A follow-up computer tomographic scan showed that he had an infarction in the strategic area supplied by his perforating arteries.

In contrast to our results Mizukami (11) reported that in three of nine patients of his series, presenting with similar vascular lesions as our groups, after MCA occlusion secondary to a bypass operation, a permanent deterioration of his neurological condition occurred. In all his cases however, filling of the middle cerebral artery via the Bypass was proved to be poor at the time of the postoperative examination.

In conclusion, in patients with stenotic lesions of major cerebral arteries the EIAB operation seems to be effective in the prevention of cerebral ischaemia even if angiographically demonstrated stenotic lesions progress to occlusion. In rare cases, as demonstrated by one of our patients, even a successful operation may result in worsening of the neurological symptoms because of impaired blood flow within the deep area of the middle cerebral artery territory.

References

1. Ausman, J.I., Latchaw, R.E., Lee, M.C., Ramirez-Lassepas, M.: Results of multiple angiographic studies on cerebral revascularization patients. In: Microsurgery for stroke. Schmiedek, P., Gratzl, O., Spetzler, R.F. (eds.), pp. 222–229. New York, Heidelberg, Berlin: Springer 1977
2. Chater, H.L., Weinstein, P.R.: Progression of middle cerebral artery stenosis to occlusion without symptoms following superficial temporary artery bypass: case report. In: Microvascular anastomosis for cerebral ischemia. Fein, J.M., Reichman, O.H. (eds.), pp. 268–271. New York, Heidelberg, Berlin: Springer 1974
3. Donaghy, P.: Evaluation of extracranial intracranial blood flow diversion. In: Microsurgical anastomosis for cerebral ischemia. Austin, G.M. (ed.), pp. 256–274. Springfield, Ill.: Thomas 1976
4. Fischer, M.C.: The natural history of carotid occlusion. In: Microsurgical anastomoses for cerebral ischemia. Austin, G.M. (ed.), pp. 194–201. Springfield, Ill.: Thomas 1976
5. Fischer, M.C.: The natural history of middle cerebral artery trunk occlusion. In: Microsurgical anastomosis for cerebral ischemia. Austin, G.M. (ed.), pp. 146–154. Springfield, Ill.: Thomas 1976
6. Grand, W.: Microsurgical anatomy of the proximal middle cerebral artery and the internal carotid artery bifurcation. Neurosurgery 7, 215–218 (1980)
7. Heilbrun, M.P., Anderson, R.E.: Preoperative evaluation of STA-MCA anastomosis candidates with rCBF studies. In: Microsurgery for stroke. Schmiedek, P., Gratzl, O., Spetzler, R.F. (eds.), pp. 202–213. New York, Heidelberg, Berlin: Springer 1977
8. Lascelles, R.G., Burrows, E.H.: Occlusion of middle cerebral artery. Brain 88, 85–96 (1965)

9. Lathchaw, R.E., Ausman, J.I., Lee, M.C.: Superficial temporal-middle cerebral artery bypass. A detailed analysis of multiple pre- and postoperative angiograms in 40 consecutive patients. J. Neurosurg. *51*, 455–465 (1979)
10. Merei, T.F., Bodosi, M.: Microsurgical anastomosis for cerebral ischemia in ninety patients. In: Microsurgery for stroke. Schmiedek, P., Gratzl, O., Spetzler, R.F. (eds.), pp. 264–270. New York, Heidelberg, Berlin: Springer 1977
11. Mizukami, M., Kawase, T., Nagata, K.: Pitfalls in extra and intracranial arterial anastomosis. Presented at: Fifth international symposium on microvascular anastomoses for cerebral ischemia: Vienna-Austria, September 14–17, 1980, in press
12. Olteanu-Nerbe, V., Schmiedek, P., Gratzl, O., Marguth, F.: Late follow-up studies in a selected group of patients with extra-intracranial bypass. In: Microsurgery for stroke. Schmiedek, P., Gratzl, O., Spetzler, R.F. (eds.), pp. 276–280. New York, Heidelberg, Berlin: Springer 1977
13. Waddington, M.M., Ring, B.A.: Syndromes of occlusions of middle cerebral artery branches. Angiographic and clinical correlations. Brain *91*, 685–696 (1968)
14. Waddington, M.M.: The normal anatomy of the middle cerebral artery. In: Microsurgical anastomosis for cerebral ischemia. Austin (ed.), pp. 133–145. Springfield, Ill.: C.C. Thomas 1976

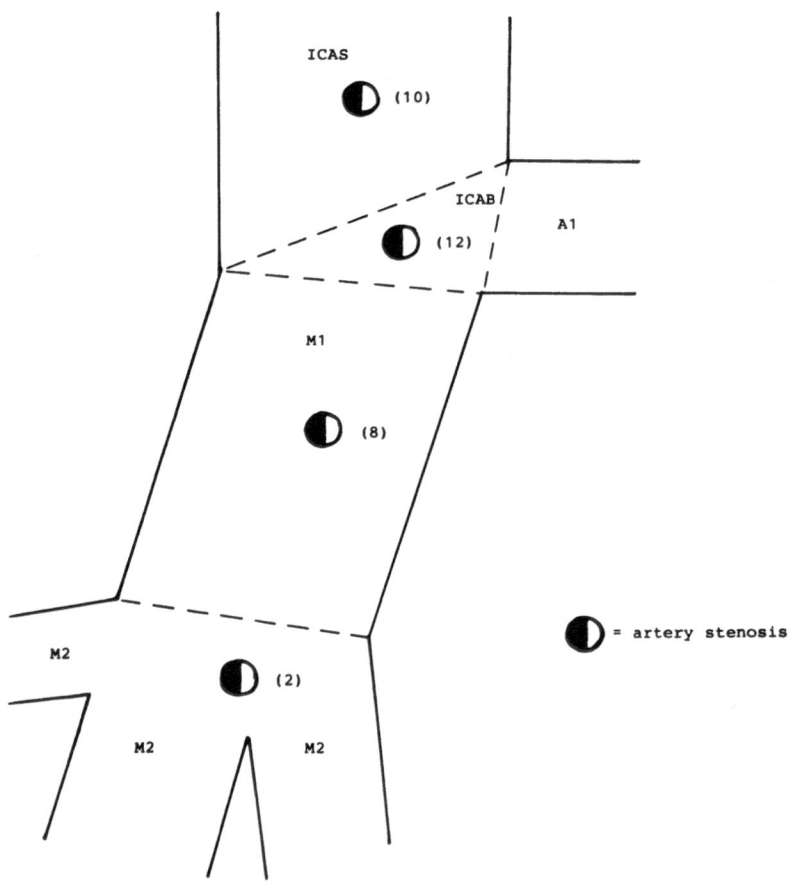

Fig. 1 a

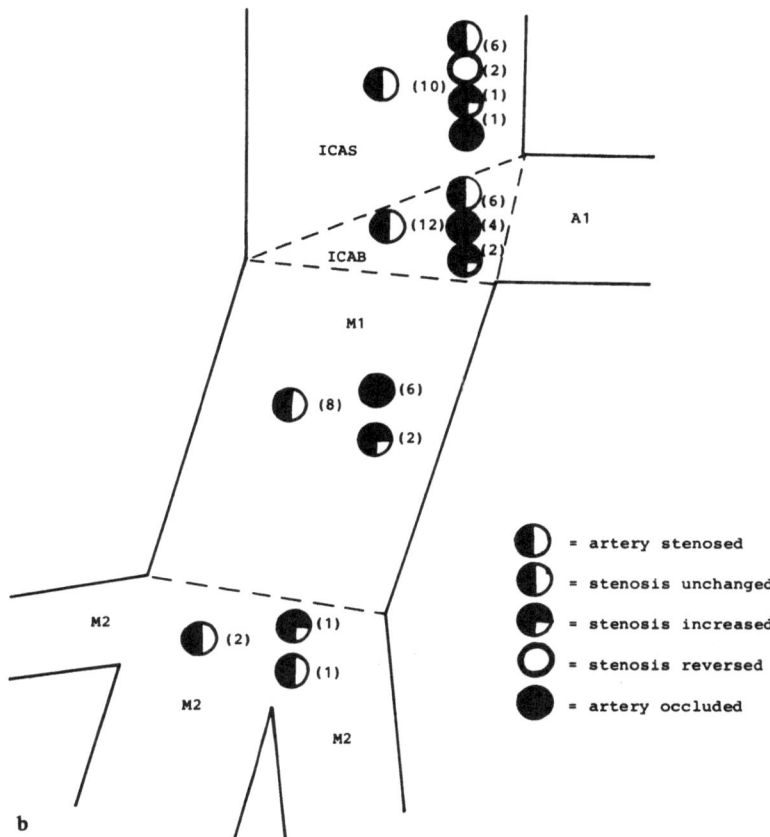

ICAS

ICAB

A1

M1

M2   M2   M2

(10)   (6)
        (2)
        (1)
        (1)

(12)   (6)
        (4)
        (2)

(8)   (6)
       (2)

(2)   (1)
       (1)

= artery stenosed

= stenosis unchanged

= stenosis increased

= stenosis reversed

= artery occluded

b

Fig. 1. a Pre-operative angiographic findings (adapted from Grand) (6). ICAS= internal carotid artery siphon; ICAB= internal carotid artery bifurcation; M1= middle cerebral artery before major division; M2= major primary branch; A1= part one of the anterior cerebral artery. **b** Postoperative angiographic findings

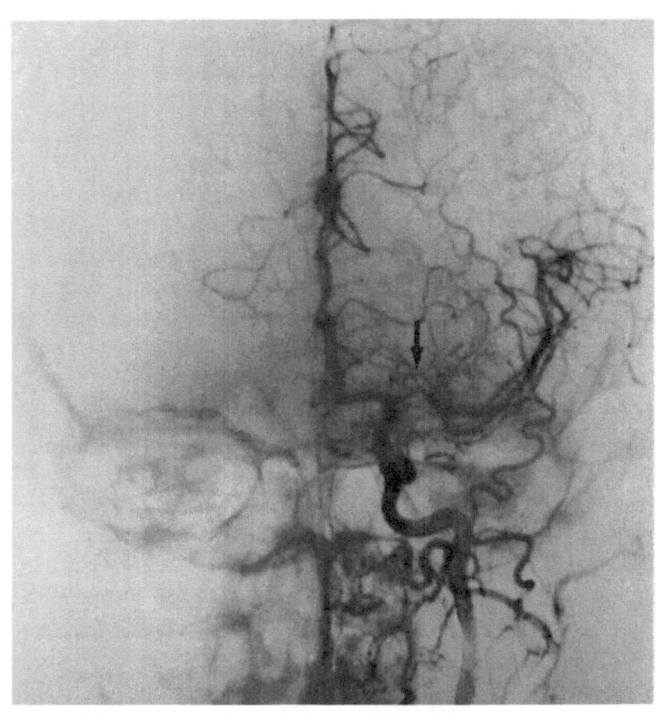

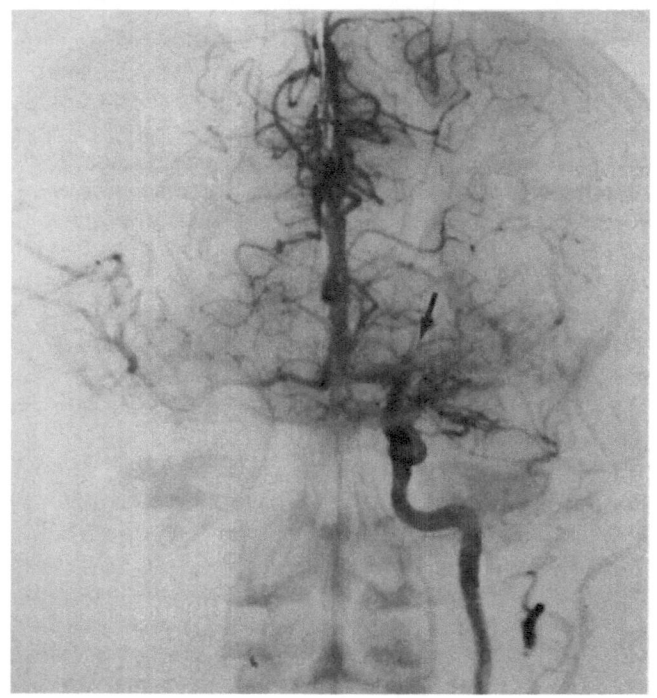

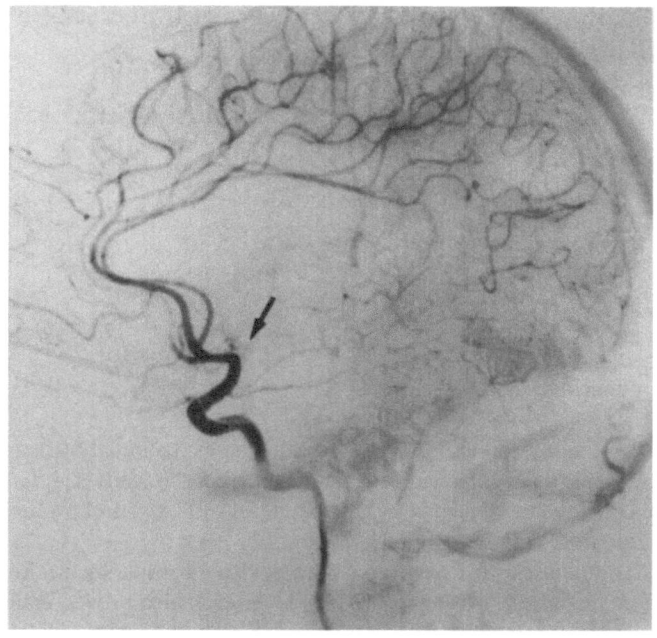

c

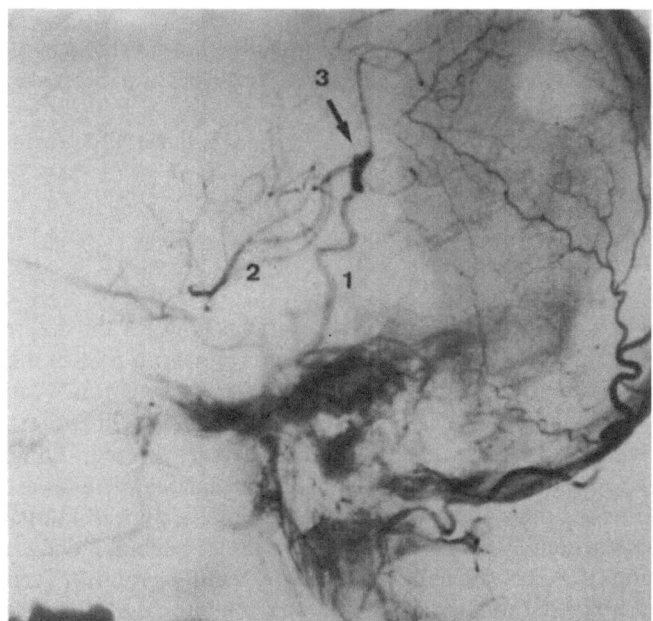

d

Fig. 2. a 46-year-old woman with a history of small CS. Pre-operative common carotid artery angiogram showing a severe stenosis of the MCA in its M1 area (*arrow*). **b, c** Same case 23 months after bypass operation. Postoperative clinical course remains free of new cerebral ischaemic episodes. Postoperative selective ICA angiogram demonstrate an occlusion of the MCA (*arrow*). **d** Same case. Postoperative selective external carotid artery angiogram showing patent bypass with retrograde filling of the MCA. 1= superficial temporal artery; 2= MCA; 3= site of EIAB

333

Indications and Results of Extracranial-Intracranial Bypass in Patients with Completed Stroke

W.Th. Koos, H. Schuster, G. Kletter, H. Ferraz, G.F. Gestring, and B. Richling

Introduction

Today it seems generally accepted that the extracranial-intracranial bypass procedure (EIAB) has a protective effect against further clinically significant cerebrovascular symptoms in cases of transient ischaemic attacks (TIA's) and prolonged reversible ischaemic neurological deficits (PRIND's).

The indications for treating patients with a completed stroke by an EIAB are different. Although there is evidence that this operation also proved beneficial in the treatment of selected patients with completed stroke (CS), the latter indication is unfortunately not yet widely accepted. This is mostly due to the relatively few published series of operated patients suffering from CS and to the difficulty, as stated by Chater et al. in 1977, in assessing the clinical value of any therapeutic measure directed at the treatment of cerebral ischaemia.

The following report reflects the current interest of our team in Vienna in the selection and treatment of patients with CS.

Material and Indications

The author's series consists of 181 patients in which the diagnosis of "completed stroke" was established. This number of patients represents 58% of the total of 310 operated cases. There were 125 men, and 56 women, ranging from 24 to 79 years of age, with a mean age of 55 years. There were 144 patients suffering from unilateral localized cerebrovascular occlusive disease and 37 patients presented with bilateral vascular lesions.

The patients were selected for an extracranial-intracranial arterial by-pass (EIAB) on the basis of their medical history, their present clinical status and angiographic findings, supplemented by such other tests as regional cerebral blood flow measurements with Xenon (rCBF) clearance, static cerebral scintigraphy with Technetium 99^m and computerized axial tomography (CT-scan). In most cases a "quantitative" dynamic serial scintigraphy was performed to compare the haemodynamics before and after operation.

The *clinical indications* for the EIAB in more than 310 patients operated on at the Department of Neurosurgery, University of Vienna, between 1975 and 1980 were as follows:

Transient ischaemic attacks (TIA)	in	23%	
Prolonged reversible neurological			37%
deficits (PRIND)	in	14%	
Progressive stroke (stroke in evolution)	in	5%	
Completed stroke	in	58%	

– the latter in the form of a single occurence or in the form of strokes with recurrent and/or intermittent attacks.

The neurological deficits in patients with completed stroke developed rapidly within several minutes and the patients recovered slowly during the following weeks: In 29 patients the completed stroke was preceded by TIA's. In all these patients we have to assume the presence of an area of low perfusion (marginal zone) around the infarcted area, in which neurons are still alive but do not function. Therefore neurological deficits can be improved in a certain number of patients with the restoration of normal perfusion pressure by revascularisation (EIAB).

The presentation of the *morphologic and functional correlates* to the above-mentioned clinical cases was the next step towards the selection of patients for an EIAB.

Four-vessel angiography of the cervical and cerebral vessels in addition to aortic arch angiography permitted localization of stenosing or occlusive vascular processes and revealed a possible multiplicity of the vascular lesions.

The transcutaneous measurement by *Doppler ultrasound* techniques over the supratrochlear and supraorbital arteries (terminal branch of the ophtalmic artery) detected a stenosis in the carotid artery with the probability of 90%. The procedure also proved useful for screening patients with possible extracranial occlusive disease before angiography.

For the selection of our patients with completed stroke for surgical revascularization procedures, *brain scan* and *computerized axial tomography (CT), and rCBF studies* provided, in addition to angiography, the most valuable information about the functional condition of the cerebral tissue in the infarct region (brain oedema, cerebral atrophy, cyst formation etc.). As a rule we found the Tc 99m brain scan positive from the 2nd to about the 6th week after the stroke, and this gave valuable functional information about the cerebral lesion.

The morphological information was obtained from CT scans which – even without enhancement – became positive six to eight weeks after the onset of symptoms.

An important diagnostic test to select completed stroke patients for surgery was measurements of rCBF with xenon clearance (by means of intra-arterial injection of Xe 133). Patients with general severe reduction of rCBF were poor candidates for operation, while patients with findings consisting of focal or relative focal ischaemic areas were considered suitable for EIAB. The focal ischaemic area, indicated by the rCBF measurements, probably represents an area of low cortical perfusion pressure, allowing a high flow through the surgically created anastomosis, which in turn diminishes the risk of occlusion.

The following *Vascular changes* in the cerebro-vascular system presented the most frequent indications for EIAB:

1. Occlusion of the cervical segment of the internal carotid artery (58%).

2. Stenosis of the siphon section of the internal carotid artery in its intracranial portion (6%), (on condition that the contralateral carotid artery is intact).
3. Occlusions of the main stem (15%) and the branches (10%) of the middle cerebral artery.

All patients with evidence of a *bilateral vascular lesion* such as a carotid stenosis on one side and a carotid occlusion on the contralateral side, were evaluated and managed according to the best clinical judgement. Our experience defends an old surgical principle. This states that direct reconstruction of the physiological cerebral blood supply has preference over an EIAB. Therefore, stenosis of the internal carotid artery in the neck was first treated by direct vascular surgery before an EIAB on the contralateral side was considered. In a number of cases, after endarterectomy of the cervical carotid, the EIAB proved to be unneccessary.

We would like particularly to emphasize that *advanced age* is not a contraindication, since this microsurgical procedure with adequate anaesthesia and careful pre-operative medication does not substantially burden the patients. Of the patients subjected to surgical treatment of cerebral infarction at our Neurosurgical Department 60% were older than 50 and 21% were even more than 60 years old.

The indication for an EIAB in stroke patients should be *carefully* evaluated if the *following vascular changes* are encountered angiographically:
1. *Occlusion of the Siphon Segment of the Internal Carotid Artery.* In the majority of these cases severe and irreparable neurological deficits are already present. No indication for operation!
2. *Stenosis of the Main Stem of the Middle Cerebral Artery.* Especially in younger patients the stenosing lesion is caused by a process other than arteriosclerosis and the stenosis is going to disappear spontanously after 2 to 6 months. In these patients it seems advisable to postpone operation and to follow the clinical course of the patient. Angiography should be repeated every 4 to 6 weeks. In the majority of patients complete recovery can be expected without any operation.

Methods

As the surgical procedure for revascularization, we performed an extracranial-intracranial arterial bypass (EIAB) in all 181 patients. In eight patients the bypass operation was done bilaterally and in two patients the procedure was repeated on the same side using another scalp artery. In 37 of these patients the EIAB had to be combined with a carotid artery endarterectomy in the neck because of multiple vessel involvement.

In cases of carotid artery stenosis in the neck and carotid artery occlusion on the other side, our present policy is to recanalize the stenosed artery first, following with the EIAB at a later date (in 6 to 8 weeks). In the meantime an optimal natural collateral circulation will establish. The timing for the contralateral EIAB depends on the clinical course and the results of repeated diagnostic studies (brain scans and CT) during this interval.

The operative procedure used for the EIAB is essentially unchanged since the first of our cases. The techniques used are described elsewhere.

Timing of Operation

The timing of an EIAB procedure proved to be of decisive importance in our patients with completed stroke.

Patients with clinical signs and symptoms of a completed stroke, providing they did not have impairment of consciousness, were operated on at the earliest four weeks after the onset of symptoms, while the optimal time for an EIAB operation proved to be between the 6th and 8th week after onset. For various reasons, however, operation was performed in about 60% of the patients between the third and the fifth month after the attack. In our experience an EIAB had been successful if performed after 8 months and later. In cases of completed stroke operation is inadvisable as long as the acute cerebral ischaemia persists. Our experience showed that patients operated on within a few hours of the onset of the clinical symptoms of cerebral infarction invariably succumbed to severe intractible cerebral oedema.

As regards the neurologists argument that the symptoms of cerebral infarction might spontaneously improve without surgical intervention, it may be maintained that our experience with the EIAB shows that the early additional blood supply ensured by the anastomosis may in many cases result in a restitution of neurological deficits immediately after operation. This phenomenon can be explained by the improved blood flow in the ischaemic marginal zone of the infarction. Without any doubt this approach can prevent an extension of the ischaemic tissue damage.

Operation offers the advantage of a shorter period of convalescence and a better prognosis for rehabilitation. At the same time the surgical procedure of an EIAB does not cause any strain to the patient. In fact, most patients are out of bed 2 to 3 days after the operation.

Results

The effects of the EIAB operation on the regional (and general) cerebral blood flow manifest themselves in a significant increase of cerebral perfusion. This newly established collateral circulation does not achieve its full effect on the cerebral blood flow until 6 to 8 months after the operation. The results of the EIAB operation in our patients with completed stroke are summarized as follows (Table 1).

We compared the *Neurological Condition* of the operated patients suffering from completed stroke at the end of observation periods from 6 months to 6 years postoperatively with their preoperative neurological symptoms. As the main symptoms we considered impairment of motor function, sensation, vision (visual field defects) and speech apart from the mental condition (impairment of memory and concentration, etc.). Improvement of pre-operative neurological deficits was achieved in 65% of patients.

The following neurological deficits improved or resolved completely (Table 2).

A significant phenomenon observed was the improvement of *intellectual functions (memory, concentration, attentiveness, emotional reactions,* etc.) in more than 70% of the patients in this group.

In patients with spastic paralysis of long standing which is frequently associated with aphasia, an improvement of the neurological status cannot be expected from a bypass operation. These patients should therefore not be subjected to operation!

337

Table 1. Results after EIAB (n= 310 cases, Department of Neurosurgery Vienna, 1965–1980)

Cerebral vascular insufficiency							Patency of anastomosis (angiographic control)	
Groups	Pre-operative status	Asympto-matic	Improved	Un-changed	Worse	Dead	Patent	Occluded
Transient ischaemic attacks (TIA)	70 (23%)	63 (90%)	2 (3%)	1 (2%)	– –	4 (5%)	(98%)	(2%)
Prolonged reversible neurologic deficits (PRIND)	43 (14%)	32 (75%)	–	11 (25%)	–	–	(97%)	(3%)
Progressive stroke	16 (5%)		10 (62%)	4 (22%)	1 (8%)	1 (8%)	(82%)	(10%)
Completed stroke	181 (58%)	6 (3%)	117 (65%)	43 (24%)	8 (4.5%)	7 (3.5%)	(90%)	(10%)
Total	310 (100%)	101 (33%)	129 (41.5%)	59 (19%)	9 (3%)	12 (3.5%)	(92%)	(8%)

Table 2. Improvement or complete regression of neurological deficits in 117 patients with completed stroke after EIAB (% of patients)

Motor deficits	67%
Sensory deficits	60%
Impairment of vision (visual field defects)	33%
Impairment of speech	53%
Impairment of intellectual functions	70%

Table 3. Surgical results after EIAB in patients with completed stroke (cerebral infarction) (n= 181)

Moderate to medium grade neurological deficits

Improved	72%
Unchanged	19%
Worse	3%
Dead (case mortality)	6%

Severe neurological deficits

Improved	44%
Unchanged	48%
Worse	6%
Dead	2%

The *results* of operations performed in patients with *completed stroke* (cerebral infarction) are displayed numerically as follows (Table 3).

The *Operative mortality* considering all surgical cases with completed stroke is 1%, the *mortality rate (case mortality)* up to 6 months after EIAB is 3.5%. The *late mortality* (3 to 6 years after operation) amounts to 12%, due to cardiac causes (6%), cerebrovascular causes (3.5%) and other causes (2.5%), such as pulmonary diseases, cancer, etc.

Postoperative follow-up angiographies showed *patent microanastomoses* in 92% of cases.

Of the patients with completed stroke who improved after EIAB procedures 117 were reviewed for longterm outcome, particularly their quality of life (Table 4).

Conclusion

The bypass operation yields absolutely satisfactory results even in patients with completed stroke, both those which present as single events or as recurrent or intermittent attacks.

All three studies, rCBF, brain scan and CT have to be regarded as complementary, and this combined diagnostic approach, in addition to the clinical status and course, and angiographic studies represent promising indications for a proper selection of patients presenting with completed stroke suitable for cranial revascularization procedures.

Table 4. Late results after EIAB in patients with completed stroke and improvement of neurological deficits (n= 117)

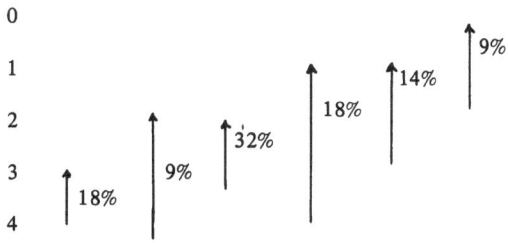

↑ = Improvement
0 = Patient full working, no neurological deficits
1 = Patient full working with slight neurological deficits
2 = Patient partially working with moderate neurological deficits
3 = Severe neurological deficits (at home)
4 = Severe neurological deficits (at hospital)

Summary

The extracranial-intracranial arterial bypass procedure (EIAB) proved beneficial in the treatment of patients with completed stroke. In 181 of a series of 310 operated patients with cerebrovascular insufficiency and occlusive disease the diagnosis of completed stroke was established. As a surgical revascularization procedure the EIAB was performed in all 181 patients; in 37 of them, because of multiple vessel involvement, the EIAB had to be combined with an extracranial carotid artery endarterectomy. In cases of carotid artery stenosis on one side and carotid artery occlusion on the other side the endarterectomy of the stenosed artery was carried out first, followed by the EIAB at a later date. The optimal time for operation in patients with completed stroke proved to be the 6th to 8th week after the stroke. Postoperative improvements in one or more neurological deficits were observed in 123 patients (68%) with completed stroke. The long term results (observation period up to 6 yrs after operation) proved to be satisfactory. The surgical mortality of 1% and the late mortality (case mortality) of 12% seem to be within reasonable limits.

References

1. Austin, G. (ed.): Microsurgical anastomoses for cerebral ischemia. Springfield, Ill.: C.C. Thomas 1976
2. Chater, N., Spetzler, R.F., Mani, J.: The spectrum of cerebro-vascular occlusive disease suitable for microvascular bypass surgery. Angiology 26, 235–251 (1975)
3. Gratzl, O., Schmiedek, P., Spetzler, R.F., Steinhofer, H., Marguth, F.: Clinical experience with extra-intracranial arterial anastomosis in 65 cases. J. Neurosurg. 44, 313–324 (1976)
4. Gratzl, O., Schmiedek, P., Steinhoff, H.: Five year follow-up of 65 patients treated with extra-intracranial bypass for cerebral ischemia. Advances in Neurosurgery 3, 115–117 (1976)
5. Fein, J.M., Reichmann, H.O.: Microvascular anastomoses for cerebral ischemia. New York, Heidelberg, Berlin: Springer 1978
6. Kletter, G.: The extra-intracranial bypass operation for prevention and treatment of stroke. Wien, New York: Springer 1979
7. Koos, W.T.: Die Bedeutung extra-intrakranieller Mikroanastomosen für die Hirndurchblutung. Akt. Gerontol. 10, 27–31 (1980)
8. Koos, W.T.: Die Behandlung zerebrovaskulärer Insulte mittels des extra-intrakraniellen arteriellen Bypasses. In: Die zerebrale Apoplexia. Barolin, G.S. (ed.), pp. 153–165. Stuttgart: Enke 1980
9. Koos, W.T., Kletter, G., Schuster, H.: Microsurgical extra-intracranial arterial bypass (EIAB) in patients with completed stroke. In: Cerebral vascular diaease 2. Meyer, J.S., Lechner, H., Reivich, M. (eds.), pp. 241–244. Amsterdam, Oxford: Excerpta Medica 1979
10. Spetzler, R.F., Chater, N.L.: Microvascular arterial bypass in cerebrovascular occlusive disease. In: Clinical neurosurgery. Koos, W.T., Böck, F., Spetzler, R.F. (eds.), pp. 242–247. Stuttgart: Thieme 1975
11. Tew, J.M., Jr.: Reconstrucitve intracranial vascular surgery for prevention of stroke. Clin. Neurosurg. 22, 264–280 (1975)
12. Yonekawa, Y., Yasargil, M.G.: Extra-intracranial arterial anastomosis: Clinical and technical aspects. Results. In: Advances and technical standards in neurosurgery, vol. 3. Krayenbühl, H. (ed.), pp. 47–78. Wien, New York: Springer 1976

The New Techniques of Vascular Reconstruction Applied to Cerebral Aneurysm Surgery

Z. Ito, H. Ohta, N. Yasui, and A. Suzuki

Introduction

Various kinds of extracranial-intracranial arterial bypasses (EIAB's) have been used to maintain the blood flow in the brain, when the elective obliteration of the main cerebral arteries was planned while treating aneurysms unsuitable for direct clipping.

However, when using these EIAB's, and mainly the superficial temporal artery (STA)-middle cerebral artery (MCA) bypass, some of the surgical problems could not be solved in certain cases: such as the following:

1. In treating anterior communicating artery aneurysms (Aco).
2. When the STA graft or the cortical MCA cannot be used in treating MCA or internal carotid artery (ICA) aneurysms.
3. When the shunt flow via the STA-MCA bypass channel may not be enough to maintain brain function.

To avoid these weak points, three new operative techniques have been created. In this paper, the indications, the operative techniques and the operative results are described.

Material and Method

In the surgical management of cerebral aneurysms, which were difficult and unsuitable for direct clipping and where the parent arteries were occluded by clipping, the intracranial interarterial anastomosis between the intra-sylvian M_2 branches (M_2–M_2 anastomosis) has been adapted for use in four cases with an MCA aneurysm, the interarterial anastomosis between distal ACA's (A_2–A_2 or A_3–A_3 anastomosis) in two cases with an Aco-aneurysm and the intrasylvian M_2 stem-cervical carotid bypass with an interposed radial artery (RA) graft (RA grafting) in three cases with an ICA aneurysm. In addition to these cases, the distal-inter-ACA anastomosis has been used in five cases with thrombotic occlusion of the unilateral A_1, A_2, or A_3, and the RA grafting was used in three cases with spontaneous occlusion of the ICA.

Operative Procedures

1. M_2–M_2 End-to-Side Anastomosis

An intrasylvian approach is used for operation on a MCA aneurysm. When the aneurysm has a complicated shape, such as when 2 or 3 branches of the M_2 Arise directly from the aneurysm itself or when an occlusion of one branch of the M_2 occurs at its origin during the operation, this anastomosis may be used.

After cutting off and reversing the branch of the M_2 which has become occluded, or which had to be sacrified to enable a precise clipping of the aneurysmal neck, the severed M_2 is anastomosed to the other patent M_2 in an end-to-side fashion (Fig. 1).

2. Interarterial Anastomosis Between Both Distal ACA's

In theory four kinds of interarterial anastomoses between distal ACA's may be performed for occlusions at the origin of a distal ACA or an A_1, as follows: an end-to-side, or a side-to-side, anastomosis between the A_2 and the contralateral A_2, at the origin of the distal ACA's; or an end-to-side, or side-to-side, anastomosis between both A_3's at the genu of the corpus callosum (Fig. 2).

The A_2–A_2 anastomosis is relatively difficult even when using a microsuturing technique, since the operating field is very narrow and deep, and an extremely skilful suturing technique is required. Either the A_3–A_3 end-to-side, or A_3–A_3 anastomosis, close to the corpus callosum, is the most feasible procedure. At present, the A_3–A_3 anastomosis is usually used to obtain a reflow in a distal ACA of the occluded side (1, 4).

a) A_2–A_2 End-to-Side Anastomosis. When the pericallosal artery (PrCA) on one side rises from the aneurysm itself or has already been occluded, the PrCA should be severed at its origin. Afterwards, an end-to-side anastomosis between the severed A_2 and the contralateral A_2 is carried out for the purpose of getting a new flow route called an "artificial" azygos anterior cerebral artery.

b) A_3–A_3 Side-to-Side Anastomosis. This anastomosis between both PrCA's is usually performed at the distal portion of the branching callosomarginal arteries. The interhemispheric fissure should be microsurgically dissected to expose both the PrCA's on the genu of the corpus callosum.

Both PrCA's should be pulled closely together for application of temporary clips. Each of the PrCA's is cut longitudinally for a length of about 2 mm on the slightly mesial parts of each artery.

At first, knot sutures are tied at both corners of the incised line on each PrCA. One end of the threads used for the cornering suture should be left sufficiently long to tie to both ends of the other threads used for the running sutures. After the running sutures between the inferior walls of the bilateral PrCA's, the single sutures on the superior walls of the bilateral PrCA's are inserted. The A_3–A_3 side-to-side anastomosis is then completed.

3. Intrasylvian MCA-Cervical Carotid Arterial Anastomosis with an Interposed Radial Arterial Graft

When a higher shunt flow is desired through the bypass channel than that provided by the STA-MCA bypass, a RA graft can be used to bridge the gap for an MCA-cervical carotid bypass. A RA graft 17 to 20 cm in length should be dissected from the forearm on the left side. To replace this portion of the radial artery, a reversed section of the radial vein from along side the artery is used. The free graft of the RA is then passed beneath the temporal muscle, the zygomatic arch and the mandible to the bifurcation of the common carotid artery. An end-to-side anastomosis between the peripheral end of the free RA graft and one branch of the M_2 at its origin in the Sylvian fissure is performed. Afterwards, an end-to-side anastomosis is completed between the proximal end of the radial arterial graft and the internal, external or common carotid artery. Systemic administration of heparin has never been needed either during or after the operation.

Results

1. Cases with M_2–M_2 End-to-Side Anastomosis

In four cases with MCA-aneurysms, in which the aneurysms operation resulted in occlusion of one or two branches of the M_2 portion of the MCA, this reconstructive procedure was performed.

One case was a 54-year-old female with a ruptured large aneurysm of the right MCA. The aneurysm, located at the trifurcation of the right MCA, was 2 cm in diameter and involved a posterior branch of the M_2.

After cutting off the posterior branch of the M_2, an end-to-side anastomosis between the posterior and the anterior branches of the M_2's was carried out (Fig. 1).

However, occlusion of the anterior branch of the M_2 occurred because atheroma plaque was dislodged from the vessel wall by the temporary clipping. The aneurysm was resected and a thrombo-endarterectomy of the anterior branch was also performed.

The postoperative angiogram after 40 days showed patency of the anastomotic channel (Fig. 3). She was left with a slight motor weakness of the left extremities.

In the other three cases, the anastomosis did not remain patent because all cases had significant sclerosis of both the donor and recipient vessels of the M_2's.

2. Cases with an Interarterial Anastomosis Between Both Distal ACA's

This anastomotic procedure has been used in two cases of aneurysm operations. One case was a 39-year-old man with an large unruptured aneurysm on an Aco, from which a left A_2 arose directly. To allow easy clipping of the aneurysmal neck, the left A_2 was cut off at its origin and was anastomosed to the right A_2 in the end-to-side position.

The postoperative angiogram showed normograde filling in the left distal A_2 through the patent anastomotic channel via the right A_2.

He was discharged on the eleventh postoperative day without any neurological deficit.

A second case was a 54-year-old man, in whom the postoperative angiogram demonstrated occlusion of the left A_2 after clipping of the Aco aneurysm. An A_3–A_3 side-to-side anastomosis was performed at four months and 13 days after the aneurysm operation. Although he suffered from slight mental disturbance, right hemiparesis, and motor aphasia in the pre-anastomotic period, only the motor aphasia disappeared after completing the patent anastomosis. In addition, in five cases with thrombotic occlusion of the unilateral A_1, A_2–A_3, or A_3, the A_3–A_3 anastomosis was carried out. In four of these cases, patency of the anastomotic channel was shown in the postoperative angiograms (Table 1).

3. Cases with MCA-Cervical Carotid Artery Anastomosis with an Interposed Radial Arterial Graft

In aneurysm operations, this procedure has been used for three cases.

Case 1 was a 25-year-old man, with a giant aneurysm of the right cervical ICA, who suffered from repeated TIA's. Immediately before ligation of a right cervical ICA and the RA bypass grafting, a right STA-MCA anastomosis was carried out in order to prevent cerebral ischaemia due to temporary occlusion of the M_2 during the anastomosis. In the postoperative angiogram 13 months later, good filling was seen in the right MCA territory, and also it was detected that the calibre of the RA graft had become larger and the patency of the STA-MCA bypass was still preserved (Fig. 4). During the two year follow-up period, he has never complained of a TIA or RIND.

Case 2 was a 64-year-old female, with a giant intracavernous aneurysms of the left ICA. After the STA-MCA anastomosis and trapping of the left ICA, this anastomotic procedure was performed. However, the STA-MCA bypass was not functioning and the shunt flow via the RA graft was insufficient to maintain brain function, because the calibre of the RA graft was very narrow, 1 mm in diameter, as was that of the STA graft. She was left with a severe right-sided hemiplegia and a disturbance of consciousness.

Case 3 was a 59-year-old man, in whom a left intracranial ICA occlusion resulted from a difficult operation on an ICA aneurysm. Severe ischaemic damage to the left hemisphere, especially the basal ganglia region, occurred postoperatively in spite of good collateral blood flow via the Aco from the right A_1.

On day 47 after the aneurysm operation, this anastomosis was performed on the left side. An angiogram on the 20th postoperative day showed a good reflow into the complete territories of the right MCA and the ACA through the RA graft. Up to 20 days after the anastomosis, the level of the consciousness gradually improved from a comatose to a somnolent state, but the right hemiplegia was not changed.

In addition, this reconstructive procedure was performed in three cases who had a thromboembolic occlusion of the ICA. In only one of these cases, the anastomotic channel became occluded by an embolus during the follow-up period.

Table 1. Operative results of the distal-inter-ACA anastomosis

Case No. (years, sex)	Diagnosis	Procedure	Occlusion → anastomosis	Patency	Outcome
1. 39, M	Cut off lt. A2 for clipping of a Big Aco–AN.	A2–A2 E · S	Immediately	+	Excellent 6 Y
2. 54, M	lt. A2 o after clipping of Aco–AN.	A3–A3 S · S	4 m 13 d	+	Good 3 Y
3. 54, M	Lt. A1 o + lt. IC s	A3–A3 S · S	38 d	+	worsened by postop. lt. IC o
4. 50, M	lt. A2–A3 o	A3–A3 S · S	5 m 21 d	–	–
5. 47, M	rt. A3 o + lt. IC o	A3–A3 S · S + lt. ST–MC	4 m	+	Excellent 2 Y
6. 59, M	lt. A1–A2 + lt. IC o	A3–A3 S · S + lt. ST–MC	2 m	+	Excellent 1 Y
7. 68, F	lt. A2–A3 o + lt. MC o	A3–A3 S · S + lt. ST–MC	1 m	+	Good 1 M

An= aneurysm; Aco= anterior communicating artery; MC= middle cerebral artery; ST= superficial temporal artery; ST–MC= ST–MC bypass; E · S= end-to-side anastomosis; S · S= side-to-side anastomosis; O= occlusion, S: stenosis

Discussion

Since Yasargil (1969) (12) first reported the use of an extracranial-intracranial arterial anastomosis (EIAB) in the management of an aneurysm by ligating a middle cerebral artery (MCA), several investigators (1, 2, 7–10) have discussed the idea that the superficial temporal artery (STA)–MCA anastomosis or the EIAB with a long saphenous vein graft could be employed to maintain blood flow in cases where elective occlusion of the parent arteries of aneurysms was required in treating aneurysms of the internal carotid artery (ICA) or MCA unsuitable for direct clipping, or where occlusion or damage to the parent arteries had occurred at the time of clipping the aneurysmal necks.

However, it was thought that these reconstructive procedures would be limited to use in the treatment of MCA or ICA aneurysms and not in other cases; as, for example, in cases of anterior communicating artery (Aco) aneurysms. For such cases, the following intracranial interarterial anastomoses, never before reported, should be used. In addition, the STA-MCA bypass could not be used in cases where the STA had already been damaged, where higher blood flow via the anastomotic channel than that provided by the STA graft would be desired. To solve these problems, the author has developed the new reconstructive procedures described in this report (for a summary of indications and advantages, see Table 2).

1. Interarterial Anastomosis Between the M Segments (M2–M2 Anastomosis). This procedure, useful for MCA aneurysm surgery, had not previously been reported. In each of four cases with MCA trifurcation aneurysms, one or two segments of the M_2 could not easily be dissected from the aneurysm, and the parent arteries of the aneurysm had severe atherosclerosis. Because of this, postanastomotic patency could be obtained in only one case after the thromboendarterectomy of the parent arteries.

However, this anastomotic procedure will result in the benefits of establishing normograde reflow, the anastomosis can be done in the same operating field as that of the aneurysm operation, and an aneurysm unsuitable for clipping may be easily obliterated by direct clipping after cutting off one or two segments of the M2. It should be decided on a case-by-case basis which is the more appropriate, this procedure or the STA-MCA anastomosis.

2. Distal-Inter-ACA Anastomosis (4). There had been no previous report of this procedure. It was found that clipping of the aneurysmal neck could be performed when there was a unilateral A1 with a hypoplastic Aco, or when an A2 segment had to be sacrificed to achieve occlusion of the aneurysmal neck. In these cases, only this anastomotic procedure could provide a reflow into the occluded ACA territory. Furthermore, this procedure can be also used for focal cerebral ischaemia, following thrombotic occlusion of the ACA on one side. The A3–A3 side-to-side anastomosis is the method most free from technical problems.

3. Intrasylvian MCA-Cervical Carotid Artery Anastomosis with a Radial Artery Graft (3): When a higher blood reflow than that provided in the STA-MCA anastomosis is desired, it is necessary that the inner calibre of both recipient and donor vessels should be larger than those of the STA graft and a MCA cortical branch. For this purpose, a free saphenous vein graft, developed by Lougheed (5), had been used.

346

However, Rhoton et al. (6), recommended that an arterial graft was superior to a venous graft for bypassing. In addition, the diameter and thickness of a vein graft is inadequate to MCA branches, and the use of a venous graft requires systemic administration of heparin. Accordingly, it was decided that a RA would be suitable for the bypass graft. A donor RA is approximately 2 to 3 mm in diameter, and the length available is usually 17 to 20 cm. In addition, the calibre of an intrasylvian M_2-stem selected as a recipient is 1.5 to 2.0 mm in diameter larger than that of a cortical MCA. Based on the mathematical analysis of the human arterial cast, Suwa et al. (11), extracted the experimental formula, Q= qr 2.7 (ml/sec.), for calculating the blood flow in a human artery with several branches. When the blood flows through the STA graft and the RA graft are compared by this formula, the blood flow via the RA graft in this procedure is 2 to 6.5 times that via the STA graft in the STA-MCA bypass.

In fact, the shunt flow through both grafts, actually measured by an electromagnetic flowmeter, was about 25—20 ml/min. in the STA graft, but is was approximately 100 ml/min. in the RA graft (2).

This procedure may be applied in the surgical treatment of inoperable giant aneurysms of the ICA, and in revascularization for treating cerebral ischaemia associated with, for example, an interhemispheric steal phenomenon caused by bilateral ICA lesions. Since the majority of giant aneurysms of the ICA produce their effect by behaving as an intracranial space-occupying mass, resection of the aneurysm, aneurysmorrhaphy or reduction of the aneurysm size would be the principal requirement. For these operations, the temporary occlusion of the parent artery would be needed for a relatively long time. During these manipulations, such a reconstructive procedure could prevent severe ischaemic damage of the brain.

Summary

The authors have developed three new vascular reconstructive procedures for the surgical treatment of cerebral aneurysms which are difficult or unsuitable for direct clipping.

Intracranial interarterial anastomoses, between two M2 branches in the Sylvian fissure and between distal anterior cerebral arteries (ACA), can be used in the surgical treatment of middle cerebral artery (MCA) aneurysms and anterior communicating artery (Aco) aneurysms, respectively. These procedures can result in normograde blood reflow through the anastomotic channel into the sacrificed arteries. When higher reflow than that obtained by a STA-MCA bypass is desired, a free long radial artery graft of the intrasylvian M_2 stem to a cervical carotid bypass can be used in treating internal carotid artery aneurysms unsuitable for direct clipping.

The operative procedures, indications and results are presented in this report.

Table 2. Operative indications and beneficial points of the intracranial interarterial anastomoses and the radial arterial grafting bypass

Procedure	Operative indication and beneficial points
Distal-inter-ACA anastomosis	1. In treating a big or giant Aco aneurysm difficult for direct clipping 2. In cases with: (a) unilateral A1 occlusion with a hypoplastic Aco (b) unilateral A2 or A3 occlusion
Inter-M2 anastomosis	1. Normograde reflow can be obtained 2. In treating a big MCA aneurysm not easy for direct clipping, including one or two of parent arteries 3. In cases with: (a) occlusion of one branch of M2 (b) the damaged STA
Intrasylvian M2 to cervical carotid bypass radial arterial graft	1. In treating inoperable giant ICA aneurysms 2. In cases with ICA occlusions, unilateral or bilateral 3. When a higher reflow is desired 4. Anastomotic technique is relatively easy and high patency rate is obtained 5. No necessity for systemic administration of heparin

References

1. Gelber, B.R., Sundt, T.M., Jr.: Treatment of intracavernous and giant carotid aneurysms by combined internal carotid ligation and extra- to intracranial bypass. J. Neurosurg. 52, 1–10 (1980)
2. Hopkins, L.N., Grad, W.: Extracranial-intracranial arterial bypass in the treatment of aneurysms of the carotid and middle cerebral artery. Neurosurgery 5, 21–31 (1979)
3. Ito, Z.: Extra-intracranial arterial bypass with long radial artery graft. In: 5th International Symp. on Microvascular Anastomosis for Cerebral Ischemia. Vienna 1980
4. Ito, Z.: A new technique of intracranial interarterial anastomosis between distal anterior cerebral arteries (ACA) for ACA occlusion and its indication. Neurol. Med. Chir. (Tokyo) 21 (1981) (in press)
5. Lougheed, W.M., Marshall, B.M., Hunter, M., Michel, E.R., Sandwith-Smyth, H.: Common carotid to intracranial internal carotid bypass venous graft. Technical note. J. Neurosurg. 34, 114–118 (1971)
6. Rhoton, A.L., Jr., Mozingo, J.R., Whang, C.J.: Comparison of blood flow and patency in arterial and vein grafts to the basilar artery. In: Microvascular anastomoses for cerebral ischemia. Reichman, O.H. (eds.), pp. 27–34. New York: Springer 1978
7. Sakaki, T., Kikuchi, H., Furuse, S., Karasawa, H., Yoshida, T., Onishi, H., Wakuda, S., Taki, K.: The usefullness of STA-MCA anastomosis in trapping vascular disorders. Neurol. Surg. 5, 253–260 (1977)
8. Spetzler, R.F.: Extracranial-intracranial arterial bypass to a single branch of the middle cerebral artery in the mangement of a traumatic aneurysm. Neurosurgery 4, 334–337 (1979)
9. Spetzler, R.F., Schuster, H., Roski, R.A.: Elective extracranial-intracranial arterial bypass in the treatment of inoperable giant aneurysms of the internal carotid artery. J. Neurosurg. 53, 22–27 (1980)
10. Spetzler, R.F., Rhodes, R.S., Roski, R.A., Likavec, M.J.: Subclavian to middle cerebral artery saphenous vein bypass graft. J. Neurosurg. 53, 465–469 (1980)
11. Suwa, N., Niwa, T., Fukasawa, H., Sasaki, Y.: Estimation of intravascular blood pressure gradient by mathematical analysis of arterial casts. Tohoku J. Exper. Med. 79, 168–198 (1963)
12. Yasargil, M.G.: Microsurgery applied to Neurosurgery. New York: Academic press 1969

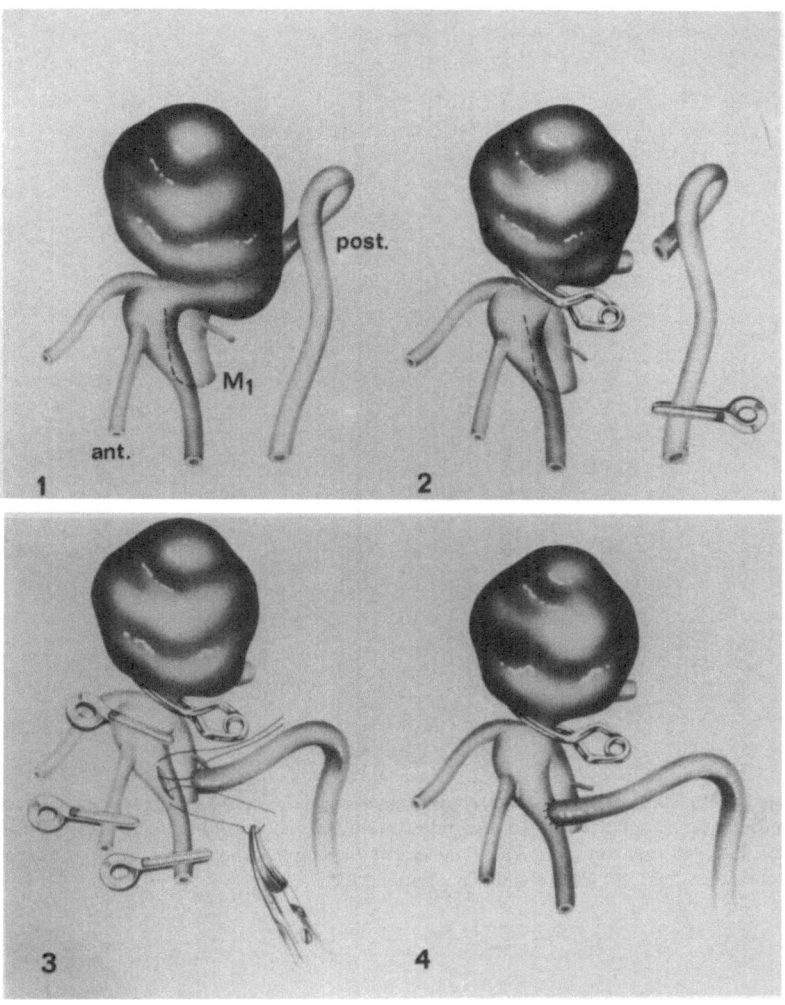

Fig. 1. Anastomotic technique of the M2—M2 end-to-side anastomosis. ant.= anterior branch of M2; post.= posterior branch of M2

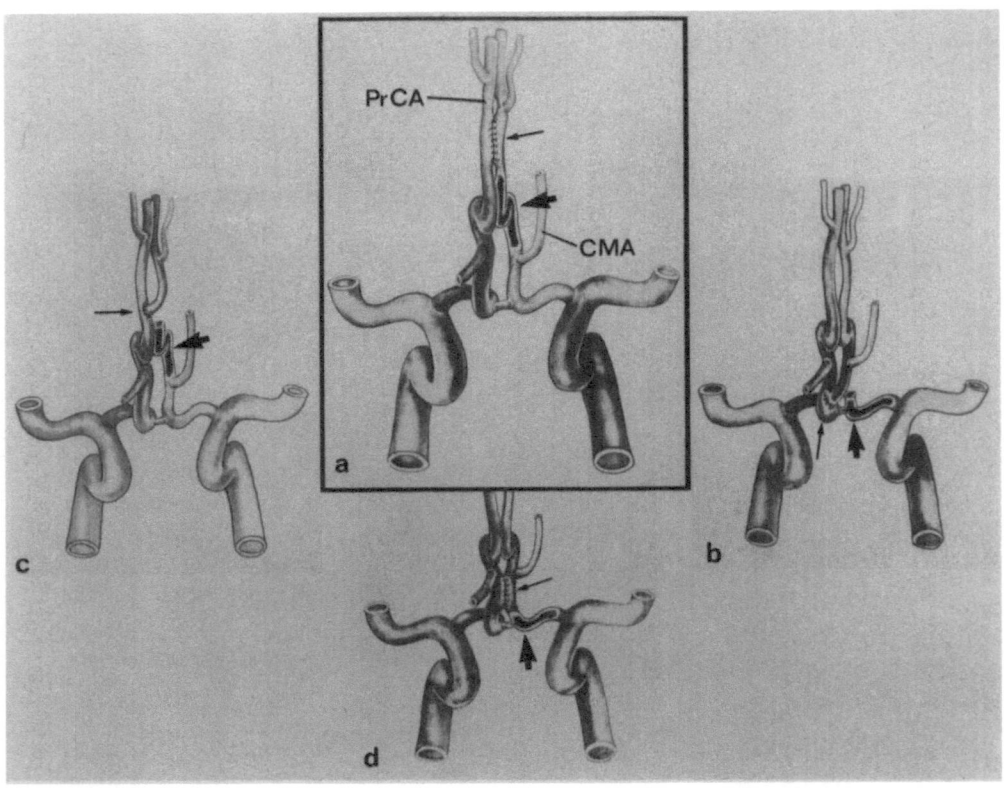

Fig. 2 a–d. Four kinds of the distal-inter-ACA anastomosis. The A3–A3 side-to-side anastomosis is the most suitable. **a, b, c** or **d**: A3–A3 side-to-side, A2–A2 end-to-side, A3–A3 end-to-side, or A2–A2 side-to-side anastomosis. Anastomotic site (*solid arrow*), occluded site (*open arrow*). PrCA= pericallosal artery; CMA= callosomarginal artery

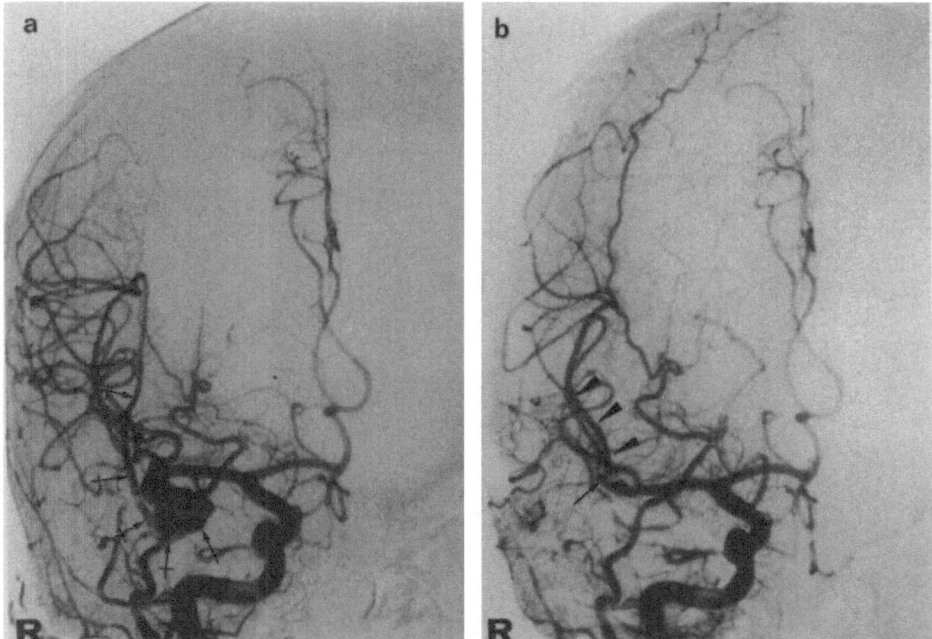

Fig. 3 a, b. A 54-year-old female with a M2–M2 end-to-side anastomosis used in treating an aneurysm of right middle cerebral artery (MCA). a Preoperative angiogram; note a large aneurysm of the right MCA trifurcation (→), including a posterior branch of MCA (↦). b Postoperative angiogram after 40 days. The aneurysm has disappeared. Note, no clip on the aneurysm site because of suturing the aneurysm neck after dissecting the aneurysm. The patent posterior branch of MCA rising from the anterior branch is revealed (▶). The anastomotic site (→)

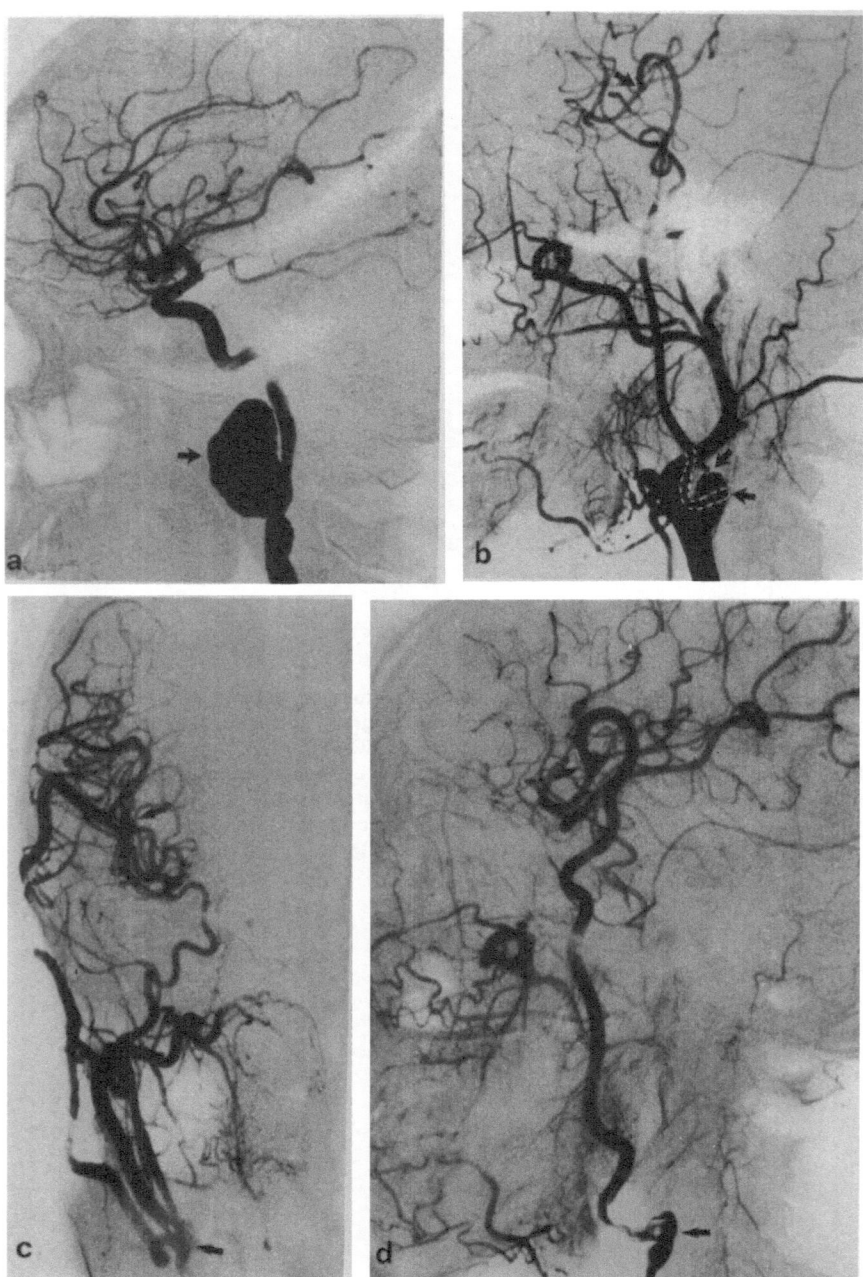

Fig. 4 a–c. A 25-year-old man with a radial arterial bypass graft between the right M2 and the cervical internal carotid artery (ICA) in treating a giant aneurysm of the right cervical ICA. **a** Preoperative angiogram. Note a giant aneurysm of right ICA cervical (→). **b** Postoperative angiogram after one week. The radial artery graft bypass (→) and the STA-MCA bypass are patent. **c** Antero-posterior and lateral views of postoperative angiograms after 13 months; the whole territory of MCA is filled via the RA graft. The RA graft bypass (→) is well functioning with a larger calibre than that in the angiogram one week postoperative. The STA-MCA bypass channel is also patent

Regional Cerebral Blood Flow in Transient Ischaemic Attacks, Effects of Reconstructive Vascular Surgery — A Study Using Xenon-133 Inhalation and Single-Photon Tomography

N.A. Lassen, L. Henriksen, R. Hemmingsen, and S. Vorstrup

Abstract

Regional cerebral blood flow (rCBF) was studied tomographically with 133-Xenon administered by inhalation over 1-min-period at a concentration of 10 mCi/l. A fast rotating ("dynamic") single-photon emission computed tomograph with four detector heads was used, an instrument that has been found to be well suited for detecting focal ischaemia.

In the present study the method was applied to a series of 12 patients with transient ischaemia attacks from the carotid territory which occurred days or weeks before the CBF study. Asymmetry of the CBF tomograms exceeding the normal limits was found in all 12 cases. In all but one severe stenosed or occluded internal carotid artery was found on the low flow side; the twelfth case had low grade stenosis and the flow asymmetry was probably accounted for by a CT-proven brain atrophy.

Tomographic CBF studies are considered essential in surgical management of TIA cases. The method presented is discussed relative to alternative approaches based on X-ray tomography and on positron tomography.

Introduction

Conventional single-photon detector systems, as multiple scintillation detectors or a gamma camera, have been widely used for measuring regional cerebral blood flow (rCBF) with Xenon-133. Administering the isotope by *intra-carotid injection* of Xenon-133 dissolved in saline, a fair degree of spatial resolution can be achieved in particular with respect to detecting areas of high blood flow in the cortex (1). The method is, however, quite insensitive for detecting areas of low flow, i.e. ischaemia. Indeed, if total ischaemia exists in an area, this will be completely overlooked. This phenomenon is accentuated in the atraumatic rCBF method based on a brief period of Xenon-133 *inhalation (or on i. v. administration),* as in this case a detector over a partially ischaemic area is recording counts from the opposite hemisphere as well as from scalp tissue.

These problems will be further commented on in the discussion. It may suffice here to state, that only by detecting the indicator *locally* — in the area of interest, avoiding superimposition of tissue layers — can ischaemia be studied adequately. Only by tomographic 3-dimensional detector systems can this be achieved. Our approach described below makes use of a fast rotating (dynamic) single-photon emission tomograph (2). Other tomographic techniques based on positron (dual-photon) emission tomography (CT scanning) will be considered.

Methods

The single-photon tomograph [1] we use was developed with the specific aim of allowing dynamic studies of the arrival and wash-out of Xenon-133 administered by inhalation (2). The instrument is similar to the one developed by Kuhl et al. some years ago (3). In essence it consists of 4 banks, each having 16 scintillation detectors. The instrument rotates at constant speed and collects data at short intervals (1/8 of a second). Thus, in each interval one "view" or "projection" of the isotope distribution in a slice of brain tissue is recorded. Conventional filtering and back-projection techniques are used for reconstructing the isotope distribution in the slice. Three slices of brain tissue are recorded simultaneously (Fig. 1a–c).

One half turn of the tomograph, allowing sampling of a complete set of projections, 40 in all, lasts 5 seconds. This rapid rotation is necessary because of the known speed of Xenon-133 arrival and wash-out from the brain: the tomograph must move so fast, that the Xenon-133 concentration is practically constant during collection of one complete set of projections. However, due to the low count rate a series of 5 second tomograms cannot be reconstructed with adequate resolution. Hence several sets of projections, usually 12, are added before reconstruction. As the raw data, the 12 sets added together, are the *average* count rates over one minute, the tomograms give the average isotope concentration in that minute. A series of four one-minute pictures is taken during and after the inhalation of Xenon-133 (10 millicuries/litre) for one minute.

Spatial Resolution. With the collimators used the resolution is approximately 1.7 cm in the plane and 2.0 cm vertical to the plane. Resolution is here given in the conventional terms of the full width of the bell shaped curve at half its maximal (peak) height (Full-Width-Half-Maximum, FWHM).

This rather coarse resolution is related to the basic problem of accomplishing dynamic tomograms, viz. the trade off between sensitivity (getting many counts in a short time for a given amount of isotope) and resolution (getting a small FWHM). In the system used here high sensitivity – of approx. 60,000 cps for a 20 cm diameter phantom with an isotope concentration of 1 μCi/ml – was necessitated by considerations of the radiation exposure: inhaling Xenon-133 10 mC/l for 1 minute gives an absorbed dose of ca. 0.4 rad in the critical organ – the lung (4). The gonadal dose is much lower, approx. 0.04 rad/study. While considerable below the exposure with most comparable positron emission tomographic studies, it was yet considered preferable not to exceed the dose mentioned in order to be free to perform repeated studies in normal volunteers without undue radiation exposure.

As mentioned, each slice is 2 cm thick. However, the distance between the midline of adjacent planes is 4 cm: each slice is seen by 4 cm of crystal length in order to achieve a high resolution. Thus a "non-seen" interval, 2 cm wide, exists between the slices. This

---

[1] Tomomatic 64, Medimatic Inc., Gersonsvej 7, 2900 Hellerup, Denmark

construction feature was considered necessary in order to achieve the sensitivity mentioned above. A series of contiguous slices can only be obtained by repeating the measurements after shifting the position 2 cm.

Calculation of rCBF. For each slice the raw data consists in the series of four one-minute -average-images-of Xenon-133 concentration. In addition the shape of the *input curve* to the brain is available as the concentration curve over the right lung is recorded. Based on these data rCBF is calculated using the *bolus distribution principle* on the "early picture", viz. the sum of the first and second one-minute pictures (5). This calculation is essentially the same as used by Kety in developing the autoradiographic method for calculating rCBF. However, as an individual scaling factor relating head counts to air curve is not available, the scaling is accomplished by using all four one-minute images.

This calculation has the advantage of exploiting the fair degree of isoefficiency in space and in time of the tomograph.

Results

Normal Man. With our routine positioning of the head the three slices are placed parallel to the orbito-meatal plane: OM + o cm, OM + 4 cm and OM + 8 cm. This means that the slice I (OM + 0) shows the cerebellum, the temporal lobe poles as well as an artifact anteriorly in the midline due to Xenon-133 in the nasal sinuses; slice II (OM + 4) cuts through the deep part of the hemispheres and displays the cortex of the juxtaposed mesial sides in the midline anteriorly and posteriorly as well as in both lateral (Sylvian) regions, as high flow regions — the basal ganglia are also represented as high flow regions but a clear resolution of the nuclei is not possible; slice III (OM + 8) gives a fairly uniform high flow map usually with evidence of the white matter — the centrum semiovale.

The flow level is normally about 60 ml/100g/min. The map is symmetrical with right and left side not deviating more than maximally 5% in mean CBF.

Apoplexy. The rCBF tomograms allow one to detect the ischaemic areas. In a series of 10 consecutive cases the flow maps showed low flow regions in the appropriate location in all cases (4). The defects tended to be larger than the hypodense areas on X-ray tomography. In one case studied several days after the onset of the stroke, the X-ray tomogram was still completely normal. Thus the CBF tomogram may reveal areas of *borderline* perfusion, a perfusion too low to sustain normal function and yet high enough to avoid frank tissue necrosis.

Transient Ischaemic Attacks, TIA. This preliminary report concerns a series of 12 patients with TIA arising from the carotid territory. The patients were studied days to weeks after the last TIA. All have stenosing arterial disease of the neck vessels. The X-ray tomograms ("CT-scans") showed possible small hypodense areas in two cases and a minor hypodense area in one case. Apart from moderate signs of cerebral atrophy in a few cases the other patients had normal X-ray tomograms. The X-ray tomograms were thus essentially negative with only one clearcut but small lesion, compatible with an old infarct in the hemisphere, corresponding to the TIA.

355

The CBF tomograms were asymmetrical in all 12 cases. In 11 of these the side with lower flow corresponded to the side with occluded or subtotally stenosed neck vessels. In 10 cases this was the side corresponding to the TIA (Fig. 1). The 11th case had occlusion of the internal carotid artery on the side with lower flow, but the TIA's stemmed from the opposite hemisphere supplied by a stenosed internal carotid artery.

In only one case, case 12, the CBF tomograms showed lower flow in a hemisphere supplied by normal neck arteries. This 71-year-old man – the oldest of the series – had signs of brain atrophy on the X-ray tomograms. His TIA arose one the side supplied by a moderately stenosed internal carotid artery, the opposite on appearing essentially normal. The fact that the CBF was lowest on the asymptomatic side (in the parietal lobe) indicates – correctly one might say – that between TIA's the symptomatic hemisphere had a normal arterial supply, viz. that the moderately stenosing lesion was of no haemodynamic importance. The asymmetry is probably due to side differences in the senile atrophy afflicting this patient.

Discussion

The patients studied in this series may not be representative of TIA cases in general. They were patients admitted to our vascular clinic for reconstructive surgery and had multiple and severe arterial occlusions. Thus we expect, that our finding – which surprised us – of clearcut asymmetry in all patients may not be confirmed in an unselected series of TIA cases.

However, for the type of patients here discussed having severe obstructions the positive result obtained is of considerable interest. Most of the patients had bilateral lesions and in almost all of them CBF tomography allowed us to identify the diseased side and thus to suggest a haemodynamic component perhaps repairable by surgery. Reconstructive surgery, including external-internal shunt in some, was in fact performed on most of our patients. Follow-up CBF tomograms are currently being made.

Concluding Comments

A three-dimensional method for studying regional blood flow must be considered essential for the study of cases of the type presented. Tomography allows one to eliminate the superimposition of tissue layers which invalidates methods only giving side views. Hence, using Xenon-133 inhalation our method is basically superior to the conventional methods, that are based on non-moving detector systems.

Can other tomographic methods be used to obtain CBF tomographically? Two other methods are currently being explored. The enhancement of routine X-ray tomograms by a freely diffusible X-ray absorbing indicator such as non-radioacitve ("cold") Xenon is used in several clinics (6). The signal-to-noise ratio is very unfavourable reducing the spatial resolution as integration over many pixels is necessary. Also, the anaesthetic properties of the Xenon gas constitute a limitation, as it means that the method cannot be considered completely atraumatic if applied to patients with intracranial space-occupying lesions. That only one slice is obtained per study is a technical problem, that could be overcome.

Positron emission tomography constitutes a technique very similar to ours. Limiting the discussion to the use of inert gases, the Krypton-77 inhalation studies by Yamamoto et al. must be emphasized (7). Being limited by a rather low counting rate their 10 second-integration-time pictures have a rather coarse resolution giving CBF maps quite similar to ours. The method is currently being applied to patients considered for reconstructive vascular surgery and the results obtained are of the same type as presented in this paper. The high cost of the positron emission technology and its cumbersomeness would seem to preclude its wider clinical use.

Single-photon emission tomography thus offers several advantages. It may be mentioned here, that CBF tomograms with improved resolution can be obtained with the same approach using more suitable radioactive tracers having a more ideal radiation energy such as Xenon-127, or Iodine-123 labelled isopropyl — amphetamine as recently proposed by Kuhl et al. (8).

References

1. Sveinsdottir, E., Larsen, B., Rommer, P., Lassen, N.A.: A multidetector scintillation camera with 254 channels. J. Nucl. Med. *18*, 168–174 (1977)
2. Stokely, E.M., Sveinsdottir, E., Lassen, N.A., Rommer, P.: A single photon dynamic computer-assisted tomograph (DCAT) for imaging brain function in multiple cross-sections. J. Comput. Assist. Tomogr. *4*, 230–240 (1980)
3. Kuhl, D.E., Edwards, R.Q., Ricci, A.R., Yacob, R.J., Mich, T.J., Alavi, A.: The Mark IV system for radionuclide computed tomography of the brain. Radiology *121*, 405–413 (1976)
4. Lassen, N.A., Henriksen, L., Paulson, O.B.: Regional cerebral blood flow in stroke by 133-Xenon inhalation using emission tomography. Stroke *12*, 284–288 (1981)
5. Celsis, P., Goldman, T., Henriksen, L., Lassen, N.A.: A method for calculating regional cerebral blood flow from emission computed tomography of inert gas concentrations; practical approach. J. Comput. Assist. Tomogr. *5*, 641–645 (1981)
6. Drayer, B.P., Wolfson, S.K., Reinmuth, O.W., Dujovny, M., Boenke, M., Cook, E.E.: Xenon enhanced CT for analysis of cerebral integrity, perfusion, and blood flow. Stroke *9*, 123–126 (1978)
7. Yamamoto, Y.L., Thompson, C., Meyer, E., Nukui, H., Matsunaga, M., Feindel, W.: Three dimensional tomographical regional cerebral blood flow in man, measured with high efficiency mini-BGO two ring positron device using Krypton-77. In: Cerebral blood flow and metabolism. Acta Neurol. Scand (Suppl. 72) *60*, 186–187 (1979)
8. Kuhl, D.E., Wu, J.L., Lin, T.H., Selin, C., Phelps, M.: Mapping local cerebral blood flow by means of emission computed tomography of N-Isopropyl-p (^{123}I) — Iodoamphetamine (IMP). J. CBF and Metab. (Suppl. 1) *1*, 25–27 (1981)

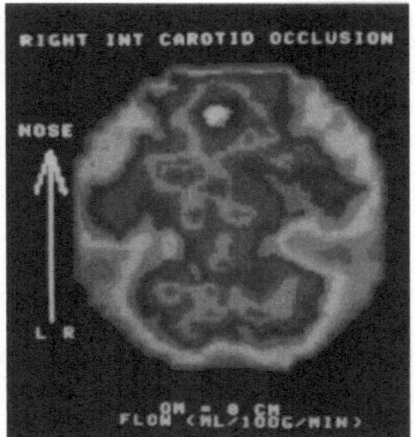

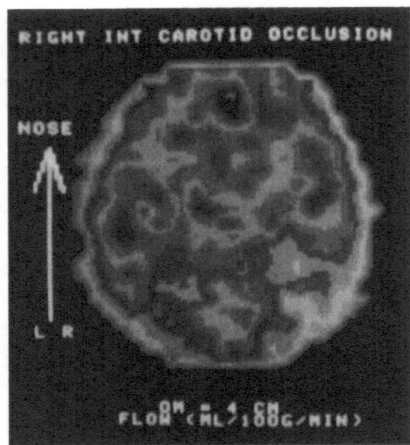

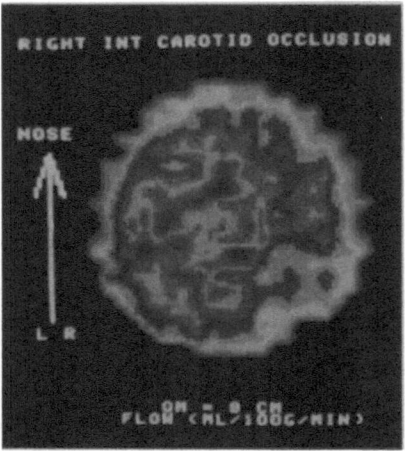

Fig. 1 a–c. CBF tomograms in a 50-years-old male with brief right-sided attacks of blindness and of contralateral hemiparesis, all arising in the upright posture. Right-sided common carotid artery occlusion, CT scan normal. Lower flow in right hemisphere showing insufficiency of collateral flow through circle of Willis. The study verifies the haemodynamic nature of the attacks. **a** OM + 0 cm: Lowest, one sees cerebellum, petrous bones, temporal poles and frontal lobe anteriorly with intense spot mesially (influenced by Compton scatter from nasal cavities?). Note that flow is lower in the right temporal pole than in the left. **b** OM + 4 cm: Middle, one sees, as high flow areas, the Sylvian cortex bilaterally and frontal and occipital cortex mesially. Note asymmetry with lowest flow in right centro-parietal cortex. **c** OM + 8 cm: Upper one sees the cortex. Note asymmetry of flow with right side much lower than left in particular posteriorly(watershed area between a. cer. med. and a. cer. post.)

358

Mechanism of Cerebral Vasospasm Induced by Oxyhaemoglobin

Y. Fujita, T. Shingu, H. Gi, O. Araki, M. Matsunaga, and H. Handa

Introduction

Vasocontractile responses to lytic products of erythrocytes have been well investigated (22, 23, 28, 29, 31) and these responses which are characteristically observed in the cerebral arteries are most strongly induced by oxyhaemoglobin (oxyHb), among other derivatives of haemoglobin (Hb) (9, 28, 29). However, the mechanism of the induction of oxyHb-induced contractile response on the vascular smooth muscle, especially in the cerebral arteries, remains unknown. Hb plays the physiological role of oxygen carrier in the biological system and Hb and its degradation products such as methaemoglobin (metHb), haematin, porphyrin and ferrous iron are important co-factors of enzymes which catalyze oxidation of polyunsaturated fatty acids (PUFAs), under experimental conditions (4, 20).

Recently, active oxygens have been detected in the biological system and their physiological and pathological roles have been postulated (8, 12). In the oxyHb, superoxide anions (O^-_2) are generated from human (3) and animal (19, 32) oxyHb (purified form) during auto-oxidation, but erythrocytes contain particular enzymes such as superoxide dismutase (SOD) (8, 12), catalase (5) and glutathione peroxidase (12) to prevent the deleterious effects of active oxygens. However, it is likely that haemolysate from disrupted erythrocytes may release acitve oxygens under conditions where these enzymes are dispersed in a hydrophilic state.

We now report the finding of radicals generated from oxyHb, the possible modality of oxygenation of PUFAs by these radicals and the inhibitory effects on the oxyHb-induced contraction in the cerebral arteries by scavengers and specific enzymes. The tentative mechanisms of vasocontractile response to oxyHb, are discussed, on the basis of our observations of different responses of cerebral arteries to agents such as sulhydryl reagent, local anaesthetics, and a cyclo-oxygenase inhibitor.

Materials and Methods

1. Generation of Active Oxygens from (Oxy) Hb of Human Red Blood Cells (RBCs)

It was of interest to determine whether SOD, catalase and glutathione peroxidase act normally and efficiently in diluted haemolysate, especially in the cerebrospinal fluid

(CSF) in the case of subarachnoid haemorrhage (SAH). We previously reported that SOD was sufficiently active to dismutate O^-_2 from RBCs incubated under sterile conditions at 37°C for 8 days, in the human CSF and in saline solution (9), yet hydrogen peroxide concentration increased under the same conditions (26).

Electron spin resonance (ESR) spectroscopy of active oxygen radicals was studied by the spin trapping method using a Joel FE1X spectrometer (Nihondenshi Co., Tokyo, Japan). The operating conditions were as follows: temperature: 23 ± 5°C, field modulation: 100 kHz, reference: 20 mW, field: 3550 ± 100 G, sweep time: 4 min, and response: 0.3. Materials; human Hb A was purified chromatographically according to the Huisman and Dozy method (13) and then frozen and dried. The weighed Hb which contained Tris-HCl was dissolved 10^{-6}M in 0.5 M phosphate buffer (pH 7.5). KO_2 (Research organic/inorganic chemical Co.), 5,5-dimethyl-l-pyrroline-N-oxide (DMPO, Sigma Co.) and α-tocopherol (Eisai Co.). DMPO was not further purified by using charcoal. The mixture of 50 μl of dissolved Hb and 50 μl of DMPO (10^{-2}M) was briefly shaken, sealed into a capillary glass tube and the ESR spectra were obtained. Figure 1 shows hyperfine structures (hfs) of adducted spin radicals from KO_2 (*1*), Hb (*2*), Hb plus α-tocopherol (*3*), also shows signals from DMPO only. On the right side of the figure are shown the molecular structures of adducted radicals postulated from an analysis of each hfs. An adducted OOH radical is obviously reduced by α-tocopherol treatment while the intensity of the carbon centred adduct (c) is not reduced. The carbon centred adduct signal may be an impurity of DMPO.

2. ESR Spectroscopy from the Mixture of PUFAs and (Oxy) Hb

Operating conditions were as follows; temperature: -196°C, reference: 8 mW, field: 3358 ± 2500 G, sweep time: 4 min, field modulation: 100 kHz, and response: 0.3. Figure 2 shows the ESR spectra of oxyHb (*1*), a mixture of linoleic acid and oxyHb (*2*) and a mixture of oleic acid and oxyHb (*3*). An abrupt increase in signals at 5.9, 4.3 and 2.0 in g values was observed immediately after the mixture of linoleic acid and oxyHb, but was not observed in the cases of a mixture of oleic acid and oxyHb. A signal at $g = 5.9$ indicates the high spin state of ferric iron, $g = 4.3$ signal coming from the non-haemiron, and $g = 2.0$ indicates free radical presence in the mixture. A characteristic increase in the signals at $g = 4.3$, 5.9 and 2.0 was reported in the case of the mixture of linoleic acid and lipoxygenase (soybean) (7) which has a high degree of specificity on substrates that have a pair of methylene groups interrupted by double bonds located between w6 and w10 (4). This increase indicated an interaction between Fe^{++} contained in the lipoxygenase and linoleic acid (7). Our findings suggest that the same interaction occurred in the mixture of oxyHb and linoleic acid and not in the mixture of oleic acid. This process seems important for initiation of oxygenation by iron containing compounds.

3. Vascular Contractile Responses

Mongrel dogs of both sexes and weighing 8 to 16 kg were anaesthetized with sodium pentobarbital (40 mg/kg i.v.) and exsanguinated from the femoral artery. The brain

360

and the distal portion of the superior mesenterium were removed. The basilar and middle cerebral arteries and the mesenteric artery were isolated. These vessels were cut helically at an angle of approximately $45°$ to the longitudinal axis into strips (approximately 20–25 mm in length, 1–2 mm in width). The strips were fixed vertically between hooks in a 20-ml bath containing the nutrient solution. The upper end of the strip was connected to the lever of forcedisplacement transducer (Nihonkoden Co. Tokyo, Japan). The resting tension was adjusted to 1.5 gram. The bathing solution was as follows (millimole concentration): Na^+ 162.1, K^+ 5.4, Ca^{++} 2.2, Cl^- 157.0, HCO_3^- 14.9, and dextrose 5.6. Before the start of experiments, the preparations were allowed to equilibrate for 90 to 120 minutes in the bathing medium and during this period, the solution was replaced every 20 minutes.

Drugs used were papaverine hydrochloride (Wako Co.), prostaglandin $F_{2\alpha}$(Ono Co.), Catalase (Aldrich Co.), dibucaine (Teikokukagaku Co.), superoxide dismutase and indomethacin (Sigma Co.), α-tocopherol, 1,4,–diazabicyclo–2,2,2–octane (DABCO, Sigma Co.), N-ethylmaleimide (NEM, Wako Co.), and dithiothreitol (DTT, Wako Co.). The Hb was spectrophotographically identified as oxyHb when it was added to the bathing medium and this medium was bubbled with a mixture 95% O_2 and 5% CO_2 and maintained at $37 \pm 0.5°C$.

a) Vascular Contractile Responses to KO$_2$ (Fig. 3)

The KO_2 which generates O^-_2 was dissolved in distilled water and immediately added cumulatively to the bathing solution. The solution was freshly prepared at each time of addition. The vascular contractile responses were dose-dependently obtained within a ranged of concentrations (0.25 – 2 mM/ml) of KO_2, but when the concentration was over 2 mM, contraction was sustained and the contracted artery was not relaxed by papaverine (PA, $10^{-4}M$) and 5 mM K^+. The maximum contraction obtained by the cumulative addition method (2 mM) was smaller than the one administration method of the total concentration of the cumulatively added KO_2 while 2 mM K^+ produced no contraction in the cerebral artery. In Ca^{++} free medium, KO_2 induced strong and sustained contractions.

Relaxation of the cerebral arteries induced by 5 mM K^+ in normal K^+ solution is due to stimulation of the electrogenic sodium pump (6, 16, 30) which is inhibited by ouabain, and relaxation by papaverine is due to stimulation of cyclic nucleotide synthesis (30). Ineffectiveness of a small amount of K^+ and papaverine treatment on relaxation of the sustained contraction by KO_2 may indicate that KO_2 damages the $Na^+ -K^+$ activated ATPase system and also impairs the ATP production mechanism in the smooth muscle cells of the artery.

b) Relaxation by 5 mM K$^+$ in OxyHb-Induced Contractile Response

When inhibitory effects of agents such as DTT and scavengers on the oxyHb-induced contraction were estimated, the measurements of the responses were made at three steps. At the first step, a response to oxyHb was measured. At the second step, agents to be estimated for their inhibitory effect were added, the incubation carried out for 20 to 30 minutes in the bathing medium and the response to the same dosage of oxyHb was measured. The third step was to measure recovery from the inhibitory effects. The first step is expressed as 'pre' and the third step is expressed as 'post' in the figures.

5 mM K^+—induced relaxation was estimated in a series of experiments to determine the DTT effects on the oxyHb-induced vasoconstriction. Five mM K^+ was added to the bathing medium when the oxyHb-induced contraction reached a maximum plateau. A transient relaxation was observed. Figure 4 illustrates percentage of relaxation by 5 mM K^+ calculated as shown in the lower fugure. These data indicate that oxyHb does not completely inactivate the ouabin sensitive sodium pump. Enhancement of the relaxing response after treatment of DTT may indicate that the sodium pump is partially inhibited by oxyHb. We found that high concentrations and long applications of haemolysate induced a prolonged vasoconstriction which was not altered by 5 mM K^+ and papaverine hydrochloride (10^{-4}M) (unpublished data). Thus, the initiation of vasocontraction may be brought about by inactivation of Na^+-K^+-activated ATPase in the artery exposed to oxyHb.

c) Vascular Responses to Scavengers and Enzymes

Experimental procedures involved the three steps described in b). The concentrations used were: Catalase 15 μg/ml, SOD 50 μg/ml, catalase and SOD 15 μg + 50 μg/ml, α-to-copherol 1.2 x 10^{-4}M, and DABCO 10^{-4}M. The concentrations of the two enzymes were the same respective concentrations which inhibited oxygenation of linoleic acid by fusarium lipoxygenase (18). Incubation time was 30 minutes and catalase and α-to-copherol slightly relaxed the basal tonus of the vessels, but not for longer than 20 min. Figure 5 indicates that catalase, α-tocopherol, and DABCO significantly inhibited the contractile responses induced by oxyHb, compared to pre and post the response. Unexpected, SOD increased the basal tonus and after catalase treatment did not relax the tonus. On the contrary, SOD following the catalase treatment showed a greater potency of inhibition than did the catalase alone.

Catalase and α-tocopherol are substances which removed hydroxy radicals and DABCO is a scavenger of singlet oxygen (2, 12). Inhibition of contraction induced by oxyHb indicates that this contraction might be induced by hydroxy or singlet oxygen derived from oxyHb. The reason why SOD, dismutates O^-_2 to H_2O_2, and dose not reduce but rather increases the vasotonus is unknown. However, we speculated that SOD can dismutate O^-_2, subsequently increasing H_2O_2 the amount of which generates the hydroxy radical (Haber-Weiss reaction) in the presence of Fe ions.

d) Vasoconstrictive Responses to Prostaglandin (PG) $F_{2\alpha}$ and Modification of These Responses by DTT and NEM

Asano and Hidaka (1) reported that lipoperoxide formed by lipoxygenase induced contractions in the rabbit aortic strips and that these contractions were attenuated by NEM, 2-mercaptoethanol and dithioerythrotol. Johnson and Colleagues (15) and Greenberg

362

et al. (10) postulated that membrane disulphide groups might be integral components of vascular smooth muscle receptors for PGs. For this reason we attempted to determine why the cerebral arteries have a characteristic strong contractibility to oxyHb.

Figure 6 shows the inhibitory effects of DTT on the oxyHb-induced constriction in the cerebral artery. The contractile responses by PG $F_{2\alpha}$ although not reduced in the cerebral arteries were reduced significantly in the mesenteric arteries (Fig. 7). NEM induced sustained contraction in the cerebral arteries (Fig. 6b). These findings suggest that oxyHb-induced contraction may be brought about through a disulphide-containing structure such as PG receptors but the process is not the same as in the case of PG $F_{2\alpha}$ in the cerebral artery. The blocking of sulphydryl groups of components in the vascular smooth muscle cells may induce the contractile response.

e) Inhibitory Effects of Dibucaine and Indomethacin on the Contraction by OxyHb

There is also the possibility that the oxygenative action of oxyHb may be a trigger which releases vasoconstricting substances or stimulates synthesis of intrinsic vasoconstricting substances such as PGs and thromboxanes in the vessels. Local anaesthetics such as dibucaine, tetracine, and procaine inhibit platelet aggregation by decreasing the phospholipase activity and competitively inhibit C kinase activity against phospholipids. Indomethacin is an inhibitor of cyclo-oxygenase which catalyzes PG synthesis. Figure 8 a demonstrates that dibucaine does not inhibit the oxyHb-induced contraction while the 30 mM K^+ -induced contraction is completely blocked. Figure 8 b shows that indomethacin does not inhibit the oxyHb-induced contraction. The same dosage of indomethacin increased the basal tonus in the mesenteric arteries. These findings suggest that it is unlikely that oxyHb is a trigger releasing or synthesizing vasoconstriction PGs.

Discussion

From our results with the ESR spin trapping method, two radicals generated from oxyHb were analysed. One is a hydroperoxy radical ($\cdot$OOH) and the other is an isomer of the former. The latter has a intramolecular hydrogen bonding between hydrogen in the hydroperoxy group and the oxygen bound to nitrogen in DMPO. Superoxide is 4.88 in pKa, thus almost all of these radicals exist in the form of O^-_2 in the neutral aqueous solution and HO_2 in the acidic solution. Although we could detect O^-_2 adduct in KO_2 solution in 0.5 M phosphate buffer (pH 7.5), we did not detect the same hfs in oxyHb in the same buffer solution. Adducted O^-_2 is easily protonated and forms $\cdot$ OOH (14). Thus, it is clear that oxyHb does generate O^-_2 radicals. We found no evidence for hydroxy radical ($\cdot$OH) generation in the oxyHb hfs. The Hb used for the chromatographical elution solution contained Tris buffer and this buffer is able to trap hydroxy radicals (14). Perhaps this is why the hydroxy radicals were not detected in our Hb.

The target compound which is directly oxidized by superoxide has not been detected, but quinone and thiol compounds are candidates for target compounds. Although PUFAs are not directly oxidized by superoxide, hydroxy and hydroperoxy radicals react well with PUFAs. Vasoncontrictive responses to KO_2 were enhanced by the addition of Fe^{++}

to the bathing medium (Fig. 3). Vasoconstriction induced by KO_2 may be due to inactivation of Na^+-K^+-activated ATPase. Because this enzyme has SH groups as the active centre and it is a membrane bounded enzyme, it is likely that this enzyme is oxidized by hydroxy, hydroperoxy radicals and by oxidized PUFAs and even directly by O^-_2. NEM, SH blocking agent, induced sustained contractions in the cerebral arteries and these contractions were not relaxed by papaverine and 5 mM K^+ (Fig. 6b). Ouabain induces vasocontraction by inhibition of Na^+-K^+ – activated ATPase. This Na pump enzyme was partially inhibited in the contracted cerebral arteries by oxyHb (Fig. 4). This inhibition may be due to a direct oxidation of SH groups by O^-_2 derived from oxyHb, however, the inhibitory effects of scavengers and catalase on the oxyHb-induced contractions indicate that these contractions may be due to hydroxy, hydroperoxy radicals and singlet oxygen from oxyHb (Fig. 5). With DTT, oxyHb-induced contractions were reduced (Fig. 6) and the relaxation seen with 5 mM K^+ of these contractions was slightly but significantly enhanced by DTT treatment (Fig. 4). These findings indicate that oxidation of SH groups may contribute to the oxyHb-induced vasoconstriction or vasocontraction may be mediated via disulphide bonds by the oxidized substances, as the result of active oxygens. Vasocontrictions are actually induced by oxidized lipids (1).

Many Fe containing compounds and iron itself are co-factors of oxygenative enzymes. Chan et al. (4) reported that haem-proteins regioselectively catalyze the oxygenation of linoleic acid, similarly to those of lipoxygenase. We confirmed the similarity of oxyHb to lipoxygenase by ESR spectroscopy (Fig. 2). Lipoxygenase is a non-haem enzyme, thus it has a signal at $g= 4.3$ without substrates (7). Although oxyHb has no signal at the same g value, this signal appeared immediately after mixing with linoleic acid. This finding indicates that conformational changes of oxyHb occurred with PUFAs. Fe of oxyHb is located in a haem-pocket (24) which is surrounded by hydrophobic molecules, therefore, it is unlikely that Fe in the oxyHb is easily contiguous to the target compound for oxygenation, if conformational changes do not occur. OxyHb has mechanisms of oxygenation different from soybean lipoxygenase. A characteristic signal appearance, high spin signals of ferric Fe in proto-haem, signal at $g= 4.3$, and $g= 2.00$ (free radical signal), was also reported in the mixture of linoleic acid and fusarium lipoxygenase which has a proto-haem, and does not demand active oxygen as activator for enzyme activity (16). The method of oxygenation of PUFAs by oxyHb is similar to that of fusarium lipoxygenase. It is concluded that this specific modality of oxygenation may explain why oxyHb has the most potent vasocontractile response among all Hb derivatives.

Hydroperoxides formed by enzymatic oxygenation by lipoxygenase from arachidonic acid and linoleic acid are hydroperoxy-eicosatetraenoic acid (HPETE) and hydroperoxy-octadecadienoic acid, respectively. They are not true prostanoids but do have diverse biological activities (11, 25, 27). Toda (31) postulated that Hb-elicited vasocontraction mainly by release of vasoconstricting prostaglandins from the arterial wall. We demonstrated that blocking of releasing and synthesis of prostaglandins could not reduce the contraction by oxyHb (Fig. 8). The oxyHb-induced contraction may be mediated through a prostaglandin-like receptor because it has disulphide bonds but probably not through prostaglandin receptors in the cerebral artery (Figs. 6, 7).

HPETE inhibits PGI_2 synthesis which dilates vessels (11, 21). Prolongation of vasospasm might be due to inhibition of PGI_2 synthesis by the HPETEs that were derived from regioselective oxygenation of arachidonic acids by oxyHb.

Conclusion

OxyHb-induced contractile response may be mainly due to regioselectively oxygenated PUFAs, such as HPETEs and not to prostaglandins, as the result of hydroxy, hydroperoxy radicals and of singlet oxygen derived from oxyHb. Such would explain why oxyHb induced the strongest contractions, among all the Hb derivatives used. The regioselectively oxygenated PUFAs induced contraction through disulphide containing structures such as prostaglandin receptors. This structure differs with the organs.

References

1. Asano, M., Hidaka, H.: Contractile response of isolated rabbit aortic strips to unsaturated fatty acid peroxides. Pharmacol. Exp. Ther. 3, 347−353 (1979)
2. Brabham, D.E., Lee, J.: Excited state interaction α-tocopherol and molecular oxygen. J. Phys. Chem. 80, 2292−2296 (1976)
3. Brunori, M., Falcioni, G., Fioretti, E. et al.: Formation of superoxide in the autoxidation of the isolated and chains of human hemoglobin and its involvement in hemichrome precipitation. Eur. J. Biochem. 53, 99−104 (1975)
4. Chan, H.W.-S., Newby, V.K., Levett, G.: Metal ion-catalysed oxidation of linoleic acid. Lipoxygenase-like regioselectivity of oxygenation. J.C.S. Chem. Comm. 82−83 (1978)
5. Chance, B., Sies, H., Boveris, A.: Hydroperoxide metabolism in mammalian organs. Physiol. Rev. 59, 527−605 (1979)
6. Chen, W.T., Brace, R.A., Scott, J.B. et al.: The mechanism of the vasodilator action of potassium. Proc. Soc. Exptl. Biol. Med. 140, 820−824 (1972)
7. De Groot, J.J., Veldink, G.A., Vliegenthart, J.F.G., et al.: Demonstration by EPR spectroscopy of the functional role of iron in soybean lipoxygenase-1. Biochim. Biophys. Acta 377, 71−79 (1975)
8. Fridovich, I.: The biology of oxygen radicals. Science 201, 875−880 (1978)
9. Fujita, Y., Shingu, T., Yamada, K. et al.: Noxious free radicals derived from oxyhemoglobin as a cause of prolonged vasospasm. Neurologia. Med. Chir. 20, 137−144 (1980)
10. Greenberg, S., Kadowitz, P.J., Long, J.P. et al.: Studies on the nature of a prostaglandin receptor in canine and rabbit vascular smooth muscle. Cir. Res. 39, 66−76 (1976)
11. Ham, E.A., Egan, R.W., Soderman, D.D. et al.: Peroxidase-dependent deactivation of prostacyclin synthetase. J. Biol. Chem. 254, 2191−2194 (1979)
12. Hayaishi, O., Asada, K.: Biochemical and medical aspects of active oxygen. Tokyo: University Tokyo Press 1979
13. Huisman, P.H.J., Dozy, A.M.: Studies of the heterogeneity of hemoglobin. IX. J. Chromatogr. 19, 160−169 (1965)
14. Janzen, E.G.: A critical review of spin trapping in biological system. In: Free radicals in biology. Pryor, W.A. (ed.) pp. 115−154. New York: Academic Press 1980
15. Johnson, M., Jessup, R., Ramwell, P.W.: The significance of protein disulfide and sulfhydryl groups in prostaglandin action. Prostaglandin 5, 125−136 (1974)
16. Lockette, W.E., Webb, R.C., Bohr, D.F.: Prostaglandins and potassium relaxation in vascular smooth muscle of the rat. The role of Na-K-ATPase. Cir. Res. 46, 714−720 (1980)
17. Matsuda, Y., Beppu, Y., Arima, K. et al.: Spin-state exchanges in fusarium lipoxygenase on binding of linoleic acid. Biochem. Biophys. Res. Commun. 86, 319−324 (1979)

18, Matsuda, Y., Beppu, T., Arima, K.: Possible mechanism of oxygen activation in linoleate per-oxidation by fusarium lipoxygenase. Agric. Biol. Chem. *43*, 1179–1186 (1979)

19. Misra, M.P., Fridovich, I.: The generation of superoxide radical during the oxidation of hemo-globin. J. Biol. Chem. *247*, 6960–6962 (1972)

20. Miyamoto, T., Ogino, N., Yamamoto, S. et al.: Purification of prostaglanding endoperoxide synthetase from bovine vesicular gland microsomes. J. Biol. Chem. *251*, 2629–2636 (1976)

21. Moncada, S., Grygleski, R.J., Bunting, S.: A lipid peroxide inhibits the enzyme in blood vessel microsomes that generate from prostaglandin endoperoxides the substance (PGX) which pre-vents platelet aggregation. Prostaglandins *12*, 715–737 (1979)

22. Osaka, K.: Prolonged vasospasm produced by the breakdown products of erythrocytes. J. Neu-rosurg. *47*, 403–411 (1977)

23. Ozaki, N., Mullan, S.: Possible role of the erythrocyte in causing prolonged cerebral vasospasm. J. Neurosurg. *51*, 775–778 (1979)

24. Perutz, M.F.: Stereochemistry of cooperative effects in hemoglobin. Nature *228*, 726–734 (1970)

25. Rome, L.H., Lands, W.E.M.: Properties of a partially-purified preparation of the prostaglandin-forming oxygenase from sheep vesicular gland. Prostaglandins *10*, 813–824 (1975)

26. Shingu, T., Fujita, Y., Handa, H. et al.: Intracranial hematomas and deleterious radicals derived from oxyhemoglobin. In: Ischemia and cell damage. Asano, T. (ed.), pp. 109–114. Tokyo: Nyuron Shya 1980

27. Siegel, M.E., McConnell, R.T., Abrahams, S.L., et al.: Regulation of arachidonate metabolism via lipoxygenase and cyclooxygenase by 12-HPETE. Biochm. Biophys. Res. Commun. *89*, 1273-1280 (1979)

28. Sonobe, M., Suzuki, J.: Vasospasmogenic substance produced following subarachnoid haemorr-hage, and its fate. Acta Neurochir. *44*, 97–106 (1978)

29. Tanishima, T.: Cerebral vasospasm: Contractile activity of hemoglobin in isolated canine basilar arteries. J. Neurosurg. *53*, 787–793 (1980)

30. Toda, N.: Responsiveness to potassium and calcium ions of isolated cerebral arteries. J. Physiol. *277*, 1206–1211 (1974)

31. Toda, N., Shimizu, K., Ohta, T.: Mechanism of cerebral arterial contraction induced by blood constituents. J. Neurosurg. *53*, 312–322 (1980)

32. Weber, B., Oudega, B., Van Gelder, B.F.: Generation of superoxide radicals during the autoxi-dation of mammalian oxyhemoglobin. Biochim. Biophys. Acta *302*, 475–478 (1973)

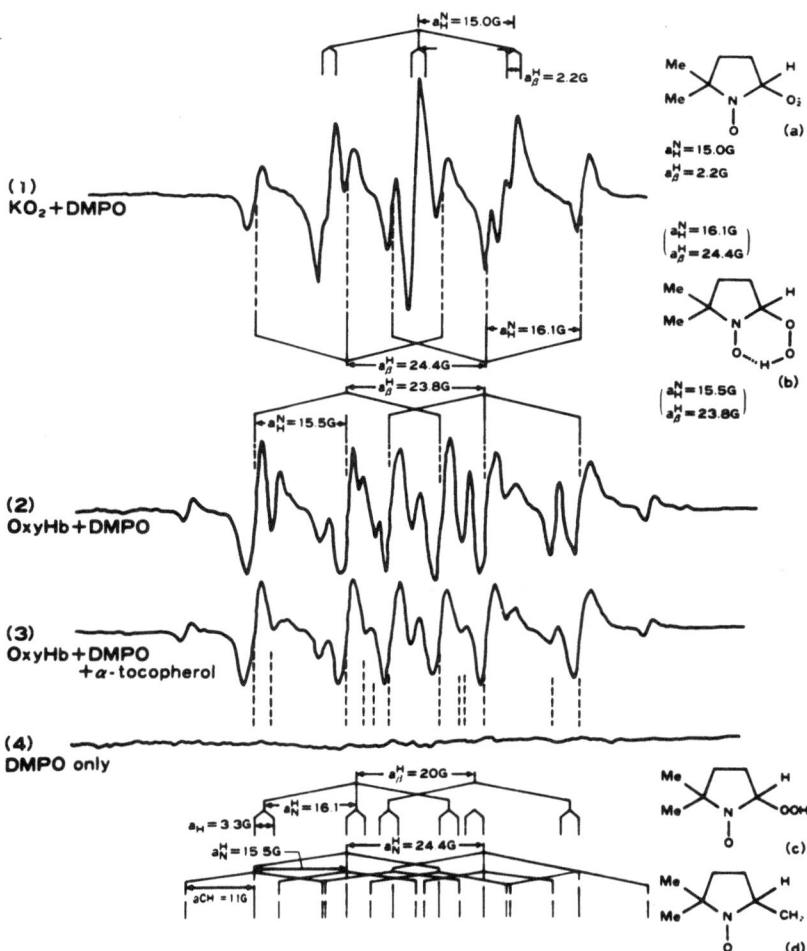

Fig. 1. ESR spectra of adducted spin radicals from KO_2 and oxyHb, hyperfine structures (hfs) and their molecular structures. (1)= signals from mixture of KO_2 and DMPO; (2)= mixture of oxyHb and DMPO;(3), (2)= + α-tocopherol; (4)= DMPO only. Used concentration: KO_2 10^{-4}M, oxyHb 10^{-5}M, α-tocopherol 1.2×10^{-4}M and DMPO 10^{-2}M. In the right side of the fugure molecular structures [(a) to (d)] are shown by analysis of hfs from spectra

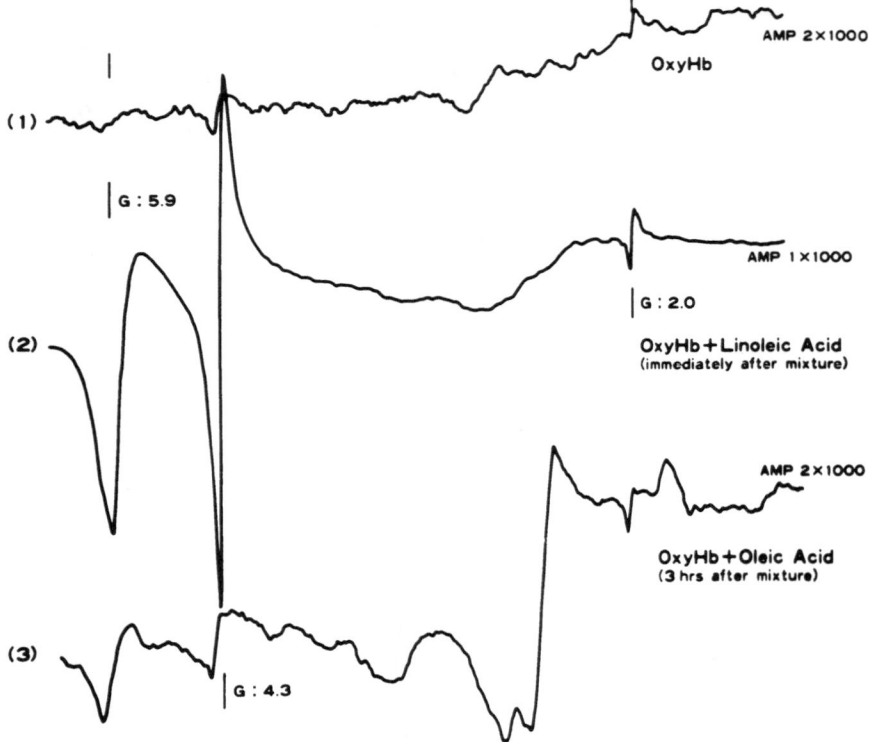

AMP 2×1000

OxyHb

(1)

G : 5.9

AMP 1×1000

G : 2.0

OxyHb+Linoleic Acid
(immediately after mixture)

(2)

AMP 2×1000

OxyHb+Oleic Acid
(3 hrs after mixture)

(3)

G : 4.3

Fig. 2. ESR spectra of oxyHb alone (1), oxyHb and linoleic acid (2), and oxyHb and oleic acid (3). The mixtures were made under aerobic condition. Originally oxyHb did not have a paramagnetic species, but the Hb produced a weak signal at g= 4.3, thereby suggesting that some portion of oxyHb was degraded to the non-haem form

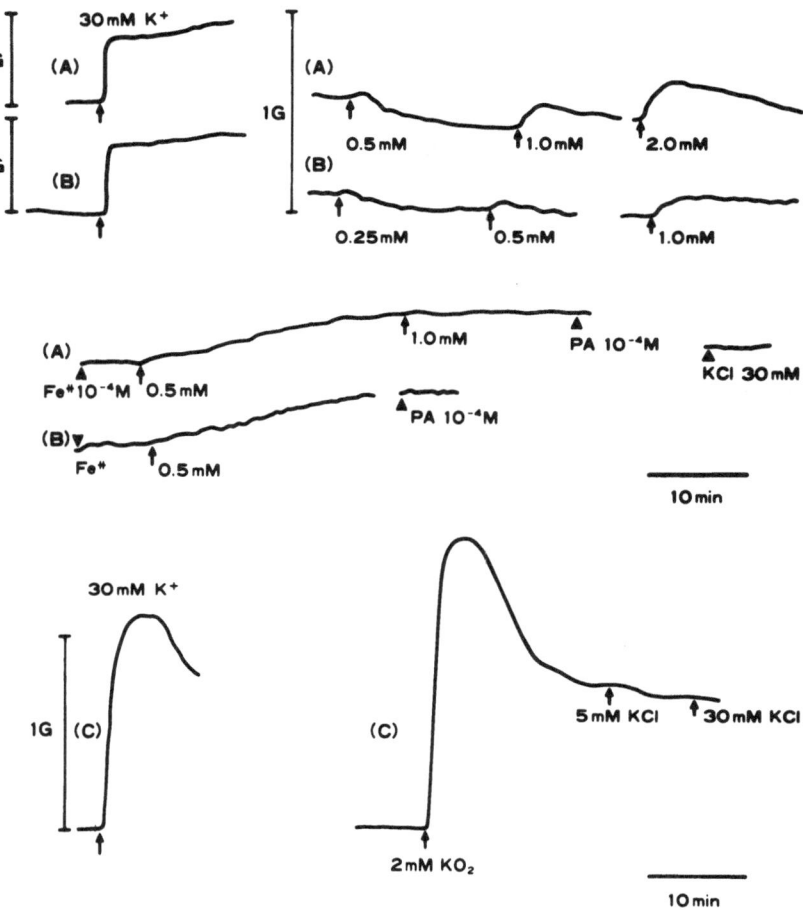

Fig. 3. Vasocontractile responses of the canine cerebral arterial strips to KO_2. Cumulatively added KO_2 (0.25 to 2 mM) dose-dependently induced vasoconstriction of the cerebral arterial strips (upper *A*, *B*). After application of $FeCl_2$ (10^{-4}M) to the same arterial strips, sustained contraction was induced by additional 0.5 mM KO_2 (total dosage was 2.5 mM in A, 1.5 mM in B strip). These sustained contractions did not relax with papaverine (10^{-4}M) and were not further constricted by 30 mM K^+. A strip (c) showed a strong constriction with one administration of 2 mM KO_2

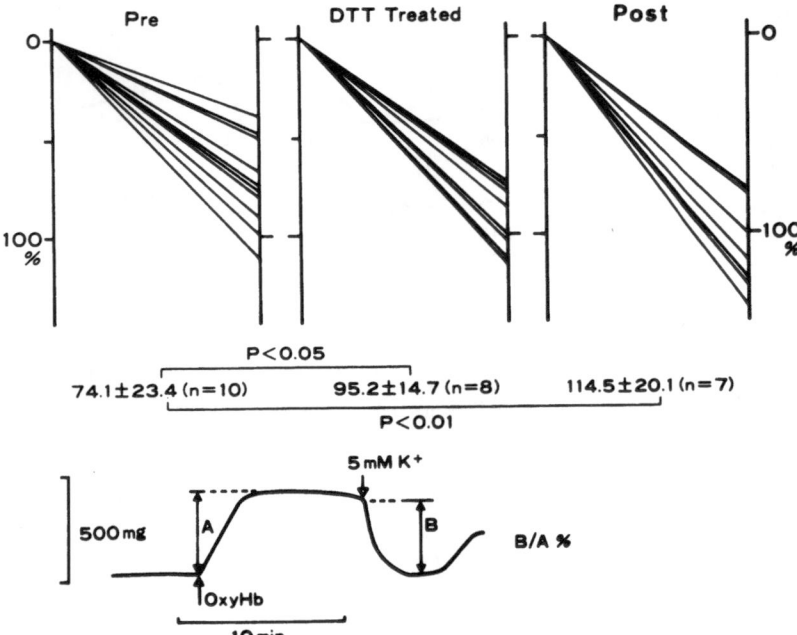

Fig. 4. Percentage relaxation by 5 mM K$^+$ of the oxyHb-induced contraction in the dog cerebral artery. Pre and post responses to oxyHb were compared with the responses after treatment of DTT. DTT was treated for 20 min before oxyHb addition. Percentage of relaxation by 5 mM K$^+$ was calculated according to the lower figure and formula

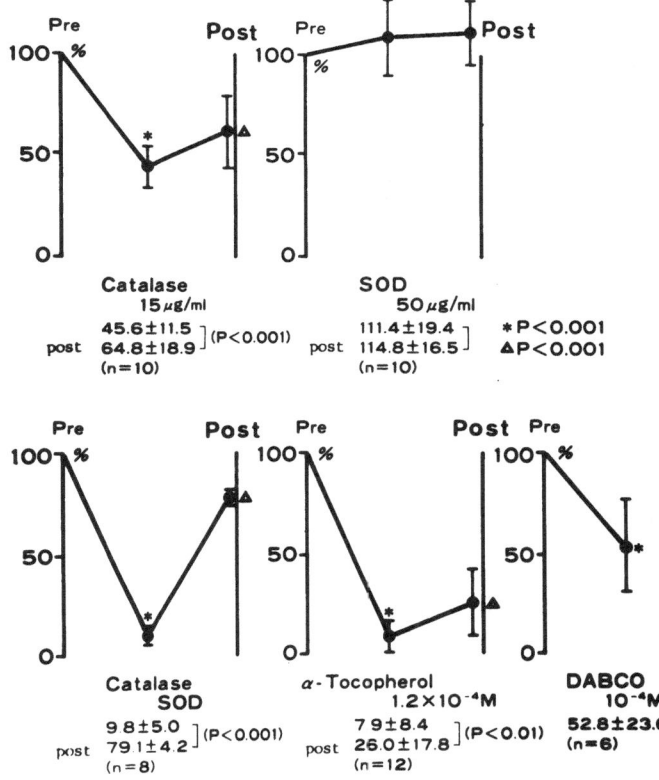

Fig. 5. Inhibitory effects on the oxyHb-induced contraction by scavengers and enzymes which remove active oxygens. OxyHb concentration was 10^{-6}M. Thirty minutes were allowed for incubation after treatment with scavengers and enzymes and then oxyHb was added to the medium. Statistical significance between pre (first step) and the response after treatment of scavengers and enzymes (second step) (p ⟨ 0.001), statistical significance between response after treatment (second step) and post response (third step) is shown in the figure, and the hollow triangles show the significance between pre (first step) and post (third step) (p ⟨ 0.001). DTT= dithiothreitol 10^{-4}M. SOD= superoxide dismutase; DABCO= diazabicyclo-2.2.2.-octane

371

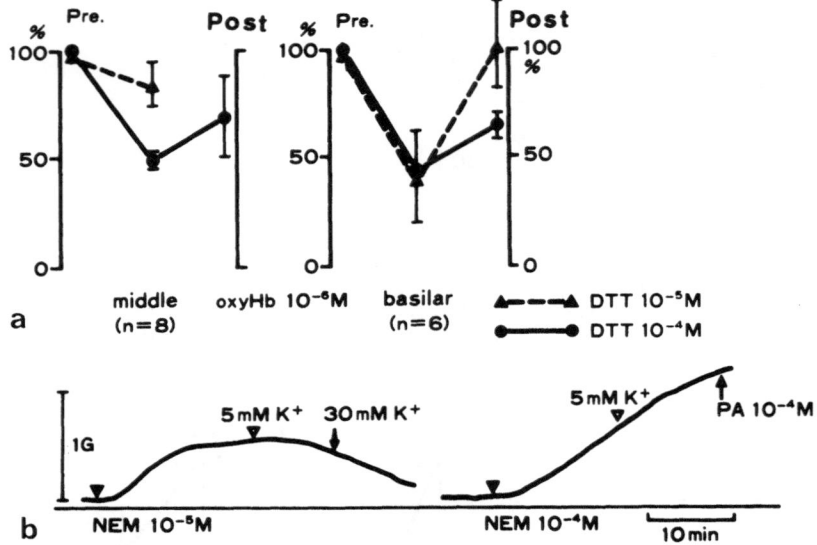

Fig. 6 a,b. Inhibitory effects of DTT on the oxyHb-induced contraction in the dog cerebral artery (a) and contractile response to NEM. Sustained contraction induced by NEM was not relaxed by 5 mM K^+, and papverine hydrochloride ($10^{-4}M$) and not further constricted by 30 mM K^+ (b). NEM= N-methyl-maleimide

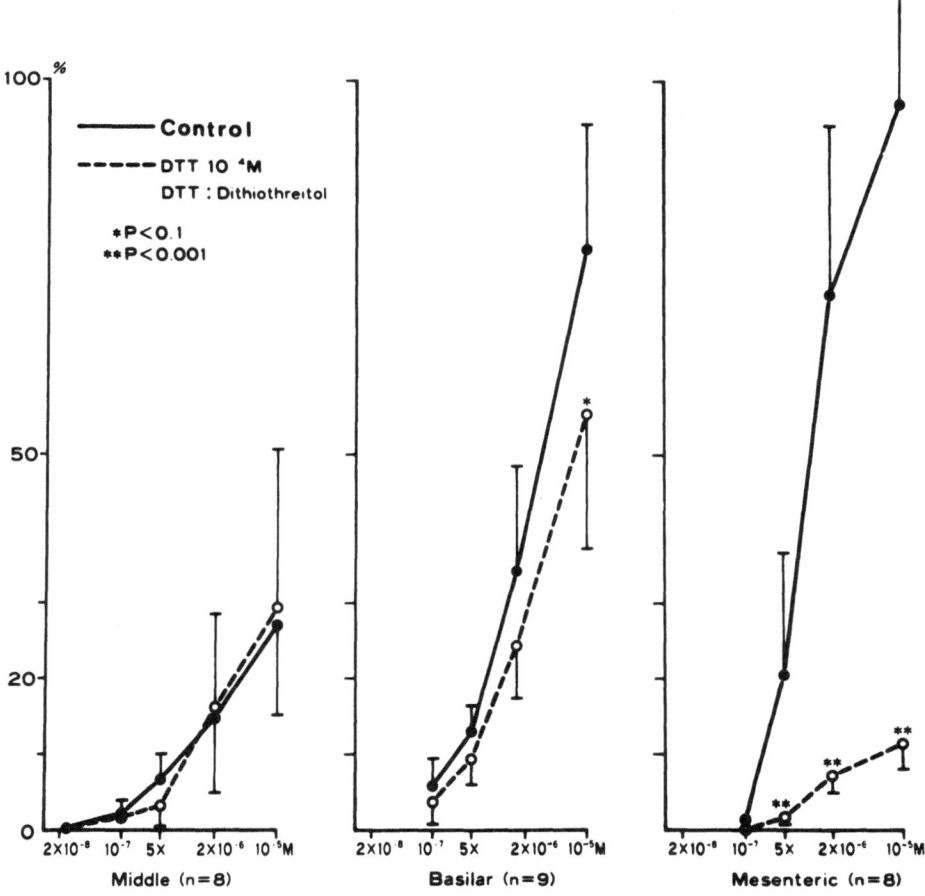

Fig. 7. Inhibitory effects by DTT on the PG F$_{2\alpha}$-induced contraction in the middle cerebral, basilar and mesenteric arteries. Inhibitory effects by DTT on the cerebral arteries were not statistically significant, while the mesenteric artery was markedly inhibited by the same dosage of DTT applied to the cerebral artery

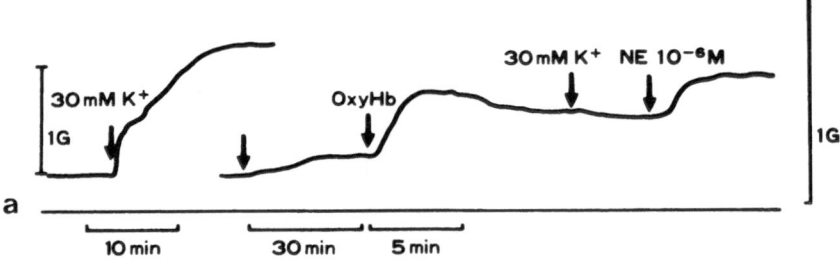

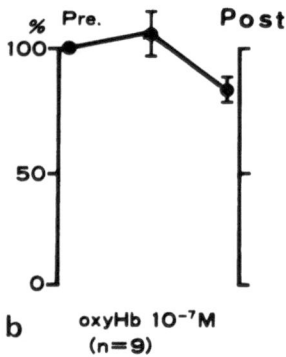

Fig. 8 a,b. The effects of dibucaine on the oxyHb-induced contraction is shown in **a**. Dibucaine did not block the contraction induced by oxyHb but did completely block the 30 mM K$^+$-induced contraction. Indomethacin (10^{-5}M) was added and the preparation was incubated for 20 min. Application of indomethacin enhanced the vasotonus in the cerebral artery (**b**). OxyHb was added after the contraction induced by indomethacin had reached a plateau. Indomethacin did not inhibit the oxyHb-induced contraction

Vasospastic Activity of Haemorrhaghic CSF – Its Effects "in Vitro"

M. Costal, A. Campero, and R. Rodriguez Rey

Introduction

Cerebral vasospasm (CVS) is the result of an active contraction, excessive in its intensity and duration, of the muscular layer of an intracranial artery (1, 16, 28).

This contraction (accompanied by the reaction of other components of the arterial wall) *can be observed and even measured only in extracerebral vessels;* it seems to be self perpetuating, and initiated by mechanical as well as biochemical factors. Thus, the original stimulus might generate a "cascade" phenomenon which, eventually, leads to a loss of the brain's blood flow autoregulation.

The study of CVS is conveniently divided into the three following parts:
1. The artery, with the neuroreceptors and its arachnoid strands.
2. The intra-arterial blood and its content.
3. The cerebrospinal fluid (CSF), in contact with neural tissue (producer of neurotransmitters ?), and surrounding the artery.

If we think in terms of *integrative concepts*, the artery would be inside a "black box", in which the Input (e) would be the subarachnoid haemorrhage (SAH), the Output (s) would be the loss of blood flow self regulation, and the Function of Transference (f) would be the *arterial spasm* (7, 18):

$$S = e \times F.$$

Material and Methods

Since the early works by Florey, Bagley, Riser, Echlin and Rimmenschneider (8, 9, 11, 17, 31), many investigators have tried to find an answer to the pathophysiology of CVS with *experimental models.*

In the present experience, the vasospastic activity (VSA) "in vitro" of haemorrhagic CSF has been studied, correlating the findings with the percentage of angiographic CVS. The clinical history of 200 patients with SAH of different aetiology was used: 83 aneurysms, 12 arterio-venous malformations (AVM), 15 intracerebral haematomas, and 90 due to other causes (SAH plus severe arterial hypertension).

No CVS has been recorded either in AVM, or in SAH due to intracerebral haematomas. However, a 33% of CVS in SAH due to head injuries has been found.

From the total number of patients, we used 108 samples of haemorrhagic CSF, taken *at random,* from lumbar punctures carried out according to the medical indications in each donor.

The CSF was used within the first two hours after removal and put in a chamber where it "bathed" a segment of artery extracted surgically from healthy dogs and rabbits. The system was kept at $37^{\circ}C-37.6^{\circ}C$ at an alkaline p^H of 7.3–8.3. In order to estimate the contraction, the artery was connected to a force transducer which works with 10 volts excitation at a square wave of 5000 cps, using a full range of $-5g$ to $+5g$, with deflections of 0.1 mm; the instrument included a connector for simultaneous recording with a two channel polygraph; the artery was stretched previously with a tension of 0.05 to 0.10 g. For calibration, we used normal CSF with autologous or heterologous peripheral blood; this mixture resulted in a weak and less frequent contraction.

Results

We observed that the contraction develops slowly, in a matter of hours. Occasionally, it was possible to see some oscillations in the dynamometer, that might be due to spontaneous activity of the artery. When present, the contraction achieved a force of at least 1.6 g and lasted 4 to 6 hours.

The maximum of *in vitro* contraction takes place at the end of the second week post SAH (Table 1). Comparatively, we have observed a lesser proportion of angiography CVS (309 angiographies) (Table 2).

Table 1. Percentage of *in vitro* contraction in relation to the time after SAH

Days after SAH	Contraction (%)
0– 4	33.33
5– 8	68.75
9–12	75.00
13–16	57.00

Table 2. Percentage of angiographic vasospasm in relation to the time after SAH

Days after SAH	Vasospasm (%)
0– 4	16.62
5– 8	44.68
9–12	66.41
13–16	57.14

Discussion

The biochemical factors that participate in CVS, which is a *local, intracranial pheno-menon*, "arrive" at the site of the ultimate effector, that is, the muscle fibre, either through the intra-arterial circulation, or the synaptic neuroreceptors (26), or rather poured into the CSF. Some 25 to 30 biochemical agents in a probably blocked suba-rachnoid space, allow this space to act as a true factory of vasospastic substances (34). These agents (norepinephrine, serotonin, histamine, thromboxane, dopamine, prostag-landins, breakdown products of erythrocytes, oxyhaemoglobin and methaemoglobin and their peroxides, fibrinogen-degradation products etc.) (5, 19, 20), liberated from platelets, erythrocytes, or from the brain tissue itself, plus the extravasated blood as a whole, and, perhaps, other neurotransmitters (endorphins ?) might act synergistically upon a sensitized artery. (Eg. ruptured aneurysm, haemorrhage-clot formation, dislo-cation-ruptured arachnoid) (6, 10, 12, 13, 22–25, 32, 33).

In the present series, the working hypothesis was based on the action of the CSF with all the agents within it, after a SAH. One can understand the fact that no experimental model corresponds exactly with the humane situation (difference in onset, environment, species etc.) (2–4, 27, 29, 30). Besides, we have not distinguished the action of each vasospastic agent.

Conclusion

There is certain correlation between the frequency of angiographic CVS and the vaso-spastic activity of haemorrhagic CSF "in vitro". Apparently, both involve a time factor, which gives the process a sort of *temporal profile* (Fig. 1).

There seems to be greater vasospastic activity of post SAH CSF when acting "in vitro"; marked activity has been found even later than two weeks after a SAH. This exprimental contraction (immediate contraction) does not depend on age, sex, type or site of the lesion.

References

1. Alksne, J.F., Smith, F.W.: Experimental models of spasm. Clinical Neurosurg. *24*, 216–227 (1978)
2. Allen, G.S., Henderson, L.M., Chou, S.N., French, L.A.: Cerebral arterial spasm. J. Neurosurg. *40*, 433–441 (1974)
3. Allen, G.S.: Cerebral arterial spasm. J. Neurosurg. *40*, 442–450 (1974)
4. Allen, G.S.: Cerebral arterial spasm. Surg. Neurol. *6*, 71–80 (1976)
5. Asano, T., Tanishima, T., Sano, K.: Possible participation of the free radical reaction initiated by clot lysis in the pathogenesis of vasospasm following subarachnoid hemorrhage. Second Inter-national Workshop on Cerebral Vasospasm (Abstracts) Amsterdam, July 1979
6. Arutiunov, A.I., Baron, M.A., Majorova, N.A.: The role of mechanical factors in the pathogenesis of short-term and prolonged spasm of the cerebral arteries. J. Neurosurg. *40*, 459–472 (1974)
7. Betti, O.: La circulación cerebral. Eudeba 1976
8. Ecker, A., Riemenschneider, P.A.: Arteriographic demostration of spasm of the intracranial ar-teries, with special reference to saccular aneurysms. J. Neurosurg. *8*, 660–667 (1951)
9. Echlin, F.A.: Vasospasm and focal cerebral ischemia: an experimental study. Arch. Neurol. Psy-chiat (Chicago) *47*, 77–96 (1942)

10. Echlin, F.A.: Spasm of basilar and vertebral arteries caused by experimental subarachnoid hemorrhemorrhage. J. Neurosurg. *23*, 1–11 (1965)
11. Echlin, F.A.: Current concepts in the etiology and treatment of vasospasm. Clinical Neurosurg. *15*, 133–160 (1968)
12. Echlin, F.A.: Experimental vasospasm, acute and chronic, due to blood in the subarachnoid space. J. Neurosurg. *35*, 646–656 (1971)
13. Echlin, F.A. , Smith E. Robertson (eds.): Subarachnoid hematology. pp. 112–113. Springfield 1975
14. Fein, J.M., Boulos, R.: Local cerebral blood in experimental middle cerebral artery vasospasm. J. Neurosurg. *39*, 337–347 (1973)
15. Fein, J.M.: Brain energetics and circulatory control after subarachnoid hemorrhage. J. Neurosurg. *45*, 498–507 (1976)
16. Fleischer, A.S., Rudman, D.R., Fresh, C.B., Tindall, G.T.: Concentration of 3', 5' cyclic adenosine monophosphate in ventricular CSF of patients following severe head trauma. J. Neurosurg. *47*, 517–524 (1977)
17. Florey, M.: Macroscopic observations on the circulation of the blood in the cerebral cortex. Brain *48*, 43–64 (1925)
18. Gunther, B., Hodgson, G. (eds.): Fisiologia Integrativa. Ediciones de la Universidad de Chile 1979
19. Handa, J., Yoneda, S., Matsida, M., Handa, H.: Effects of prostaglandins A_1, E_1 and F_2 on the basilar artery of cats. Surg. Neurol. *2*, 251–255 (1974)
20. Ishii, S., Ito, M., Miyaoka, M., Nonaka, T.: The causative factors of vasospasm and its treatment. Second International Workshop on Cerebral Vosospasm. (Abstracts) Amsterdam, July 1979
21. Kapp, J.P., Odom, G.L.: Cerebral arterial spasm, Part 1: Evaluation of experimental variables affecting the diameter of the exposed artery. Neurosurg. *29*, 331–338 (1968)
22. Nagai, H., Susuki, Y., Sugiura, M., Noda, S., Mabe, H.: Experimental cerebral vasospasm. J. Neurosurg. *41*, 285–292 (1974)
23. Nagai, H., Noda, S., Mabe, H.: Experimental cerebral vasospasm. J. Neurosurg. *42*, 420–428 (1975)
24. Nagai, H., Noda, S., Mabe, H.: Experimental cerebral vasospasm (Part 2). J. Neurosurg. *42*, 420–428 (1975)
25. Pardal, E., Zamboni, O., Fernandez Pardal, M.: Hemorragia subaracnoidea y vasoespasmo cerebral. p. 33. Sociedad Neurológica Argentina (Tucumán) 1977
26. Peerless, S.J., Yasargyl, M.G.: Adrenergic innervation of the cerebral blood vessels in the rabbit. J. Neurosurg. *35*, 148–154 (1971)
27. Petruck, K.C., Weir, B.K.A., Overton, T.R.: The effect of graded hypocapnia and hypercapnia on regional cerebral blood flow and cerebral vessel caliber in the rhesus monkey of cerebral hemodynamics subarachnoid hemorrhage and internal carotid spasm. Stroke *5*, 230–246 (1974)
28. Rosenblum, W.I., Zweifach, B.W.: Cerebral microcirculation in the mouse brain. Arch. of Neurology *9*, 102–423 (1963)
29. Rosenblum, W.I.: Cerebral arteriolar spasm inhibited by adrenergic blocking agents. Arch. Neurology *21*, 196–302 (1969)
30. Simeone, F.A., Vinall, P.: Mechanisms of contractile response of cerebral artery to externally applied fresh blood. J. Neurosurg. *43*, 37–47 (1975)
31. Stolarza, I., Benain, J.: Consideraciones sobre las hemorragias subaracnoideas. p. 32. Sociedad Neurológica Argentina (Tucumán) 1977
32. Sundt, T.M., Jr., Szurzewski, J., Sharbrough, F.W.: Physiological considerations, important for the management of vasospasm. Surg. Neurology *7*, 259–267 (1977)
33. Sundt, T.M., Jr.: Cerebral vasospasm following subarachnoid hemorrhage: Evolution, management and relationship to timing of surgery. Clinical Neurosurg. *24*, 228–239 (1978)
34. White, R.P.: Overview of the pharmacology of vasospasm. Second International Workshop on Cerebral Vasospasm (Abstracts) Amsterdam, July 1979

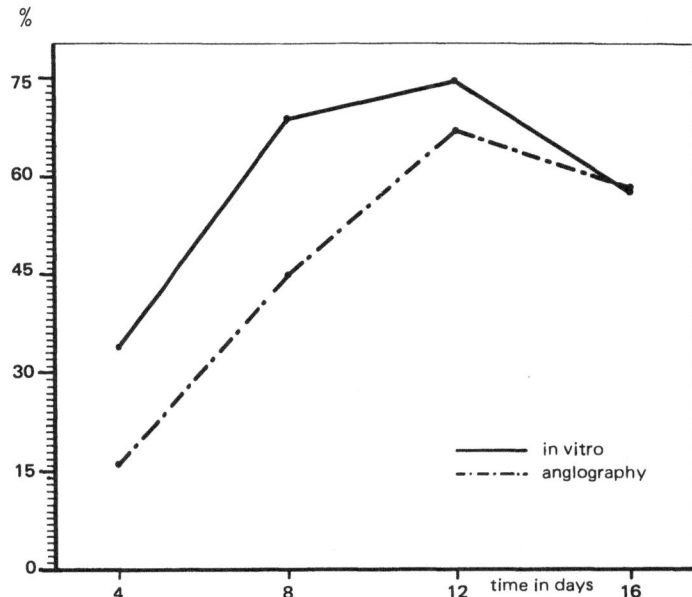

Fig. 1. Correlation of the temporal profile between antiographic vasospasm and *in vitro* contraction

Anutensin — A New Factor in Delayed Cerebral Vasospasm

R.L.G. Newcombe and W.J. Cliff

In cerebral vasospasm there appears to be an initial brief phase of spasm followed by no spasm for some days and then prolonged contraction of often two or three weeks duration. Such a time course is very similar to that of granulation tissue in healing wounds (1).

A natural agonist in blood and lymph producing wound contraction has been described (2). This substance has a molecular weight of approximately 1,000 and has been provisionally named anutensin. It is also found in urine, saliva and cerebrospinal fluid.

We have investigated Anutensin as a possible plasma factor in the production of cerebral vasospasm after subarachnoid haemorrhage. In the course of this work we have demonstrated in human arteries of the circle of Willis spontaneous rhythmic activity which may be of importance in the mechanisms of cerebral autoregulation.

Methods

Segments of the basal anterior cerebral, middle cerebral or posterior cerebral arteries each 6 mm long have been dissected fresh as soon as possible after autopsy and suspended in a small volume (1 ml) tissue bath containing Tyrode solution. By a light beam and photo-electric cell recording solution the changes of vessel diameter have been displayed. A mixture of 95% oxygen and 5% carbon dioxide was bubbled through the chamber and the temperature maintained at 37°C. Responses have been obtained up to 72 hours after death.

Vasoactive test solutions have included Prostaglandin $F2a$, nor-Epinephrine, Vasopressin, Angiotensin and the newly discovered substance Anutensin.

Results

In the vessels of five subjects, all male, aged 18—66 years, we have noted rhythmic activity. It was spontaneous at a rate of 1—1.5 beats per minute in two subjects. In other subjects it was provoked by a moderate contraction after the application of a vasoactive agent. Rhythmic activity has been noted in the anterior cerebral artery, the anterior communicating artery, middle cerebral artery, posterior cerebral artery and basilar artery. In Fig. 1 the dose response curve to Prostaglandin F2 is demonstrated. Rhythmic

Modern Neurosurgery 1. Edited by M. Brock
© Springer-Verlag Berlin · Heidelberg 1982

activity was abolished in strong tonic contraction, but after washing phasic activity of large amplitude (50% of maximal contraction) is seen.

Anutensin produces a strong and prolonged tonic contraction (Fig. 2). It also stimulates phasic activity.

Discussion

An unidentified contractile substance in normal human serum was found by Starling et al. (3) to produce tonic contractions of human basilar artery. At least some of this contractile effect may be due to Anutensin.

This new substance which strongly contracts granulation tissue is of particular interest because of the prolonged contractile effect and the apparent stability of the substance. We are hoping to establish the molecular composition, proceed to synthesis and then to develop a radio immune assay. Preliminary studies of various chromatographic fractions suggest that there may also be a naturally occurring antagonist. It is probably a peptide but at least in granulation tissue is quite unlike other known contractile agents in that is it produces very strong and prolonged contractions.

Phasic contractility of the cerebral arteries, also found by Miller (5), suggests that a pacemaker type of activity may be present with one smooth muscle cell inducing synchronous activity in others, similar to propagation in visceral smooth muscle. The finding supports the hypothesis of Falkow (4) that rhythmic contractility is essential to a myogenic mechanism in autoregulation, and suggests that such a mechanism exists in addition to neural factors and to changes in the chemical environment.

Conclusion

A peptide like substance which causes prolonged contraction of granulation tissue and which is present in blood may be a factor in cerebral vasospasm after subarachnoid haemorrhage.

Phasic activity of arteries of the human circle of Willis have been demonstrated and this suggests that a myogenic mechanism of autoregulation exists.

References

1. Kennedy, D.F., Cliff, W.J.: A systematic study of wound contraction in mammalian skin. Pathology *11*, 207–222 (1979)
2. Kennedy, D.F., Cliff, W.J.: A Natural agonist in blood and lymph producing wound contraction. Proceedings of the Australian Physiological and Pharmacological Society *9*, 47 (1978)
3. Starling, L.M., Boullin, D.J., Grahame-Smith, D.G., Adams, C.B.T., Gye, R.S.: Responses of isolated human basilar arteries to 5 – hydroxytryptamine, noradrenaline, serum, platelets, and erythrocytes. Journal of Neurology, Neorosurgery and Psychiatry *38*, 650–656 (1975)
4. Folkow, B.: Description of the myogenic hypothesis. Circulation Res. *15* (Suppl), 279–87 (1974)
5. Miller, C.A., Yason, D., Locke, G., Hunt, W.E.: Autonomous activity in human basilar artery: Relationship to derebral vascular spasm. Neurology (Minneap.) *21*, 1249–1254 (1971)

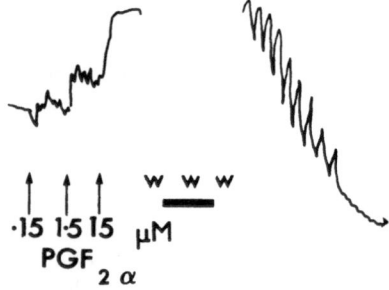

Fig. 1. Response of basilar artery to prostaglandin F2a (PGF2α). Good phasic contractions at lower doses. After wash (w) strong phasic regular contractions at the rate of 1 per min. Time bar, 4 min

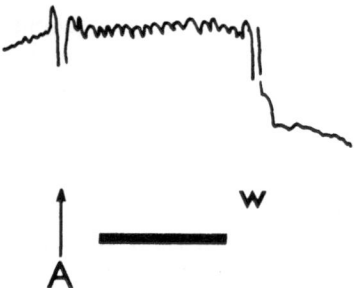

Fig. 2. Phasic activity induced by anutensin (A). Tonic contraction brought to an end by wash (W). Right middle cerebral artery from male, 20 years, death due to subarachnoid haemorrhage. Time bar, 8 min

Studies on Cerebral Vasospasm

L. Brandt, B. Ljunggren, K.-E. Andersson, and B. Hindfelt*

"It is with a considerable degree of genuine humility that we broach the topic of cerebral vasospasm. This humility is the result of 20 years of disappointment, frustration, and bewilderment. The feeling of helplessness related to the relentness deterioration of a patient with this entity is matched only by that associated with the care of the victims of spinal cord injury. This is a feeling we have all shared and this has been the primary force driving all of us. It has literally compelled us to turn to the laboratory for answers, and there, in spite of heroic efforts, few revelations and no miracles have emerged."

(Thoralf Sundt & Dudley Davis, The Mayo Clinic, 1979)

In 1893 William Gowers concluded that "If the diagnosis of an intracranial aneurysm is certain, the prognosis is extremely grave" (1). This statement is unfortunately still valid.

When in 1920 the British neurologist, Sir Charles Symonds, for some months worked as a voluntary assistant with Harvey Cushing at the Peter Bent Brigham Hospital in Boston, he suggested the diagnosis of a suprasellar aneurysm in a patient whom Cushing was about to operate on. Cushing scoffed at the suggestion. An uncontrollable haemorrhage terminated the operation (2).

It happened that the only time Cushing could attend the autopsy was the following afternoon, on which Symonds and the resident, and, as it turned out later, Cushing himself, had tickets for a critical world series baseball game. Cushing decided that the autopsy should be held at that time anyway, and that they all must be present, which they were. When the aneurysm was disclosed Cushing turned to Symonds: "Symonds, you made the correct diagnosis; either it was a fluke, or there was a reason for it. If so, you will prove it. You will cease your ward duties as from now and spend all your time in the library". The resulting paper, giving the first account of the significance of subarachnoid haemorrhage in the diagnosis of aneurysm, appeared in 1923 (3). Symond's correct conclusion and Cushing's initiative involved a break-through for clinical diagnosis of intracranial aneurysms.

The first deliberate intracranial attack on a ruptured intracranial aneurysm was carried out by Dott in 1931 (4). On March 23rd 1937 Walter Dandy performed the first successful clipping of an intracranial aneurysm (5). He subsequently first reported on a series of operated aneurysm patients in 1944 (6). During the next decades, however, little evidence arose favouring surgical treatment as compared to the natural history of the disease.

* Part of this study was supported by grants from Greta and Johan Kocks Foundation and Thorsten and Elsa Segerfalks Foundation

It gradually became clear that many patients did not die from rebleeding but from ischaemic complications related to the haemorrhage and the frequent occurrence of co-existing intracranial arterial spasm became recognized. Even although the pathophysiological significance of cerebral arterial spasm has been questioned as recently as 1975 (7), most investigators agree with the concept that the presence of spasm to such an extent that cerebral perfusion is affected is important in determining the clinical outcome.

The swedish pioneers, Herbert Olivecrona and Gösta Norlén, in 1953 concluded that no operation should be performed until the third week after the aneurysm rupture (8). However, by that time approximately half of the patients have died or become severely disabled by recurrent haemorrhages and complicating cerebral ischaemic dysfunction. Towards the end of the 1950's the aneurysm surgeon, Wylie McKissock in London even stopped operating on ruptured intracranial aneurysms supporting the idea that surgery at any time was not superior to the natural course of the disease (9).

In 1969 Hamby reviewed the technical aspects of improvements in aneurysm exposure as they had evolved in the previous half century (10). Pool in 1965 first wrote on the use of the operating microscope in intracranial aneurysm surgery (11). Yasargil advanced the state of the art of microtechnique for aneurysm surgery, reporting a remarkable drop in mortality rates (12, 13). Use of the operating microscope or its equivalent subsequently has become standard technique in the surgery of intracranial aneurysms (14).

Despite the common occurrence of cerebral vasospasm in conjunction with aneurysmal subarachnoid haemorrhage it was not until 1965 that the time-course of this phenomenon was elucidated by Kagström et al. (15) who demonstrated that vasospasm shown by angiography does not occur until some days after the bleed. This was a further support for a relationship between angiographic vasospasm and delayed cerebral ischaemic dysfunction. However, several reports on this subject have not been able to establish an absolute correlation between delayed ischaemic dysfunction (DID) and angiographic spasm. As angiography does not demonstrate calibre changes in the resistance vessels it has been suggested that delayed ischaemic dysfunction without an angiographic correlate is due to arteriolar narrowing. The fact that even pronounced angiographic vasospasm may occur without concomitant ischaemic deficits has been explained by Simeone et al. (16) who showed that in experimental subarachnoid haemorrhage the cerebral blood flow is not consistently reduced until the arteries have become constricted to about one half of their control lumen. According to these findings, reduction in cerebral arterial lumen by vascular spasm does not cause ischaemia, unless the arterial diameter is critically reduced, provided that other compensatory mechanisms are present.

What is the cause of cerebral vasospasm? Already in 1839, John Hunter considered constriction of arteries to be one of the physiological mechanisms responsible for the control of haemorrhage. From later work it is well known that mechanical, chemical and electrical stimulation may induce arterial constriction. Even such nonspecific agents as room air or distilled water are known to induce cerebral vasoconstriction (17).

During the last two decades an immense number of studies have been undertaken to elucidate the pathophysiology of cerebral vasospasm and delayed ischaemic dysfunction after aneurysmal subarachnoid haemorrhage, but they "have produced more questions than answers" (Sundt and Davis, 1979) (18).

384

The significance of the various mechanisms possibly involved in the phenomenon remains controversial. A large number of different substances has been suggested to account for the pathogenesis of delayed cerebral hypoperfusion and the list has grown as new vasoactive agents have been discovered. The fact, that vasospasm is not a constant consequence of aneurysmal subarachnoid haemorrhage, may indicate that variations exist between individuals as regards cerebrovascular responses to chronic exposure to blood-contaminated cerebrospinal fluid.

When shall the sword of Damocles, hanging over the head of the patient with a ruptured intracranial aneurysm, be removed? The great improvements in surgical techniques and the refinement of neuroanaesthesia in the last decade have markedly improved the results of operation (19–25). However, the timing of the operation remains controversial (26), although it appears that most neurosurgeons still favour delayed operation as the best method of reducing postoperative ischaemic complications. Very early operation is, however, increasingly proposed with a view to improving the overall outcome and preventing delayed ischaemic dysfunction not only by preventing rebleeding but also by operative removal of perivascular blood collections (19, 21, 27).

Several studies have confirmed the presence of vasoconstrictor substances in post-haemorrhagic cerebrospinal fluid (CSF) from patients suffering from aneurysmal subarachnoid haemorrhage (SAH). So far no complete information about the identities of the vasoconstrictor substances in the CSF is available. It has been proposed in some earlier studies that the development of vasospasm and delayed cerebral ischaemic dysfunction is paralleled by an increase in the concentration of vasoconstrictor agents in the CSF (28, 29).

The presence or absence of cerebral vasoconstriction after aneurysmal SAH implies an interaction between vasoconstrictor substances in the post-haemorrhagic CSF and protective mechanisms in the cerebral arterial wall to maintain normal vascular tone. Most experimental results on vasospasm have been obtained in studies on inbreed animals with relatively homogeneous vascular responses. The capricious appearance of vasospasm in some but not all patients with an aneurysmal SAH may be due to variations in the vascular responsiveness. This is supported by clinical experience from early aneurysm surgery: some patients with heavily blood-contaminated subarachnoid spaces in whom a wash-out was not technically feasible, did not however develop any indication of cerebral arterial spasm or delayed ischaemic dysfunction. This may imply marked individual characteristics in human cerebral arteries and arterioles.

Because of the numerous substances incriminated in vasospasm, a variety of drugs have been tried in an effort to prevent or treat intracranial spasm following SAH. Despite many promising preliminary investigations, the final results have been disappointing. Some of the failures may be ascribed to the fact that the basis for the trials has been derived entirely from experimental animals. However, there is no pattern of delayed ischemic events in animals that parallels the syndrome of cerebral vasospasm seen in humans. This brings Pope's dictum to the fore: "The proper study of mankind is man".

Lately, evidence has been accumulating suggesting that other mechanisms may be involved in the pathogenesis of cerebral ischaemic dysfunction in SAH patients. Among these are lesions in the wall of the spastic artery, including endothelial damage with associated thrombus formation (30, 31). Based upon the knowledge that vasoactive prostaglandins are synthesized in the endothelium, it has been suggested that cerebral vasospasm may represent insufficient synthesis of dilatatory arachidonic acid metabolites. Experimental studies and studies of cerebral arteries from patients who have died from delayed cerebral dysfunction after SAH have demonstrated marked morphological changes within the vessel wall paralleling the onset of vasospasm. Elevated levels of lipid peroxides have also been implicated in vasospasm, and it has been speculated that vasospasm may be the result of an interaction between accumulated hydroperoxides, derived from the lysed blood clot, and a modified synthesis of prostaglandins. This should provide the predominance of vasoconstrictor metabolites (32–35) (Fig. 1).

The failure of prior attempts to treat cerebral vasospasm with various agents, utilizing different mechanisms, suggests that a reasonable approach to the problem would be interfering with the final step in the smooth muscle contraction mechanism. It is generally accepted that changes in the concentration of calcium ions within the smooth muscle cell regulate several cellular processes, including the final step in the excitation-contraction coupling. Several studies have shown that smooth muscle is dependent on an extracellular source of calcium to initiate and maintain contraction. Intracellularly stored calcium is also involved, but is of less importance.

Many pharmacological agents blocking transmembrane calcium-flux are used clinically, especially in cardiovascular disorders. Many substances are classified as "calcium antagonists", but only a few of them are considered selective influx-blockers. However, contradictory information about the exact site of action has been presented even for these drugs as well as indications of regional and species differences. Most information on the effects of calcium-inhibiting drugs have been obtained from animal studies on the systemic circulation. There is little information about the cerebrovascular effects, especially in humans.

Current Studies

Vasospasm in Early Aneurysm Surgery

In a consecutive series of patients with a ruptured aneurysm of the anterior part of the circle of Willis, referred to the neurosurgical clinic in Lund, early intracranial operation (within 2.5 days post-SAH) was performed in 81 patients (36). Fifty-five patients had their operation eight days or more after aneurysm rupture. No operation was performed in the interval 2.5–8 days post-SAH, and early operation was only performed in patients in neurological Grade I to III according to the classification of Hunt and Hess (37). A comparison was made between the outcome in patients receiving early operation and the outcome in those patients who would have fulfilled our criteria for such an operation (Grade I–III within 48 hours post-SAH), but who were not operated on early. The comparison indicates that early operation resulting in 74% good recoveries, 10% morbidity and 16% mortality is superior to delayed treatment, which resulted in 56% good recoveries, 18% morbidity and 26% mortality. In fact, when considering good recoveries only, the results of early operation were fully comparable to the results in the selected group of patients subjected to conventional delayed operation (74% versus 76% good recoveries).

It has been proposed that early and extensive peroperative removal of perivascular blood collections should be effective in minimizing the occurrence of vasospasm and delayed ischaemic dysfunction (21, 27, 38—40). In previous literature the incidence of delayed ischaemic dysfunction after aneurysmal subarachnoid haemorrhage ranges from 1/4 to 1/3 (38, 41). The 21 per cent incidence of delayed ischaemic dysfunction in the current series of early operated patients indicates that our present operative procedures do not eliminate but may reduce the incidence of delayed ischaemic dysfunction. If three patients are excluded, in whom intraoperative cistern cleaning could not be performed for various reasons (36), the incidence of delayed ischaemic dysfunction was 18% (14 out of 78 patients).

Some patients developed severe angiographic vasospasm but remained symtomfree whilst other patients with severe ischaemic deficits of delayed onset only showed a moderate narrowing of the larger cerebral arteries on angiography. The observations not only stress the importance of the distribution of vasospasm but also that spasm in the conducting arteries is only one factor determining brain perfusion after aneurysmal SAH (36).

CSF Effects on Resistance Vessels

In an *in vivo* study on cat pial arterioles periarteriolar microinjections of CSF from SAH patients induced pronounced vasoconstriction (42). These results support the concept that the sometimes obvious discrepancy between arterial spasm visualized by angiography and delayed cerebral ischaemic dysfunction may represent regional differences in vascular response to post-hemorrhagic CSF. One of the CSF specimens used in the present study was obtained from a patient without delayed ischaemic deficits. When compared with the effects of CSF from patients with ischaemic deficits, no obvious differences in vasoconstrictor activity was observed. These observations may indirectly imply variations in vascular responsiveness between patients. This stimulated us to make an *in vitro* study of the responsiveness of human pial arteries.

Variations in Cerebrovascular Responsiveness Between Individuals

Small cortical arteries were removed from macroscopically normal parts of the brain before decompressive lobectomy in patients suffering from cerebral gliomas not infiltrating the cortex (43). The reactivity of the vessel segments was tested to various vasoactive substances (prostaglandin F_{2a}, noradrenaline, serotonin, human plasma and CSF from patients with aneurysmal SAH). There was a marked variability between arteries from different individuals. The finding of a markedly individual profile in terms of reactivity toward vasoactive substances emphasizes the importance of a human cerebral vessel wall factor in the pathogenesis of cerebral vasospasm. These observations may account for the fact that delayed arterial/arteriolar narrowing does not always occur after aneurysmal SAH despite the presence of heavily blood-contaminated CSF spaces as indicated by computer tomography or observed at early operation. However, the pattern of individual vascular response to different CSF specimens was rather consistent. These findings, as well as the observations of CSF effects on resistance vessels where CSF specimens from different donors had a consistent vasoconstrictor effect, prompted an investigation of vasoconstrictor activity in serial CSF samples from SAH patients.

Vasoconstrictor Activity in Post-SAH CSF

CSF vasoconstrictor activity was examined in serial samples obtained from patients undergoing early operations for a ruptured aneurysm (44). Five patients remained symtom-free and five developed delayed neurological deficits. There was no relationship between vasoconstrictor activity in postoperative CSF samples and clinical condition or angiographic vasospasm (44). The highest activities were seen in three patients very soon after SAH and were associated with neither angiographic spasm or cerebral ischaemic dysfunction nor with later development of delayed ischaemic deficits. The generally low values for vasoconstrictor activity could probably be ascribed to the operative procedures with early drainage of blood-contaminated CSF from the basal cisterns. The study (44) confirmed that there are no major differences in CSF vasoconstrictor activity between patients with and without cerebral ischaemic dysfunction after aneurysmal SAH, and clinical deterioration is *not* paralleled by an increased vasoconstrictor activity in CSF.

Prostaglandin Metabolism and Vasospasm

Previous studies have demonstrated that an intact prostaglandin synthesis may be necessary for the maintenance of normal cerebrovascular tone, but also that disturbances of the prostaglandin synthesis seem to be involved in the pathogenesis of delayed cerebral vasospasm (45). Based on the knowledge that on one hand prostacyclin (PGI_2), a main arachidonic acid metabolite with vasodilating properties, is mainly formed by the endothelial layer, and that on the other hand experimental SAH results in progressive ultrastructural endothelial lesions (30, 31), it has been proposed that vasoconstriction after SAH may be due to impaired PGI_2 synthesis (46). Based on this assumption, it was suggested that inhibition of prostaglandin synthesis may effect CSF-induced contractions.

To that end, the vascular responses to post-haemorrhagic CSF were studied before and after pretreatment of human pial vessel segments with the cyclo-oxygenase inhibitor indomethacin (47). There was a marked augmentation of the CSF-induced contractions, in some experiments more than ten-fold, after indomethacin incubation of the arteries. The results suggest that the development of delayed cerebral vasospasm might be due to local disturbance of the synthesis of PGI_2 and/or other vasodilatatory arachidonic acid metabolites. This concept is further supported by the observations that PGI_2 had a very marked relaxant effect on contractions induced by post-haemorrhagic CSF. One might speculate whether the observations of marked individual variations in vascular responsiveness to post-haemorrhagic CSF represent vascular differences in arachidonic acid metabolism between individuals.

Since the mechanisms responsible for delayed cerebral vasospasm after aneurysmal SAH are unknown, it is not surprising that no specific blocking agents have emerged. Theoretically, it should be possible to counteract cerebral vasoconstriction irrespective of what agents are responsible, if all mechanical activation occurred through a final common step that could be blocked. There is abundant evidence that the cytoplasmic concentration of free Ca^{2+} available to the contractile proteins determines the mechanical activity of the smooth muscle cell. Control of this calcium concentration thus means control of the mechanical activity, However, the intracellular concentration of calcium is regulated by a complex system of ion fluxes between the extracellular and intracellular spaces, and by translocations of calcium within the cell.

Two types of calcium-dependent activation mechanisms in smooth muscle have been suggested. One of these is correlated to spike discharges and is responsible for phasic activation (P-mechanism) (48). This type of activation corresponds to "electro-mechanical coupling" (49) (Fig. 2). The other activation mechanism is correlated to spike-free depolarization and is responsible for tonic activation (T-mechanism) (48), mainly corresponding to "pharmaco-mechanical coupling" (49) (Fig. 2). It has been suggested (50) that in electro-mechanical coupling calcium influx occurs through specific channels in the membrane (membrane potential sensitive calcium channels, MPS-C). These channels can be effectively blocked by calcium "antagonists" or "blockers", e.g., nifedipine (51). On the other hand pharmaco-mechanical coupling may involve another type of calcium channel (the receptor-operated calcium channel, RO-C) (50), which is not affected by changes in membrane potential and can not be effectively blocked by calcium antagonists. However, calcium antagonists, e.g., nifedipine may also affect later steps in the excitation-contraction process. including inhibition of release of intracellularly stored calcium (52).

If the assumption is correct that calcium antagonists selectively block the MPS-C, and not the RO-C, one would expect that the relaxant effect of nifedipine on contractions induced by amines was less than that produced by potassium, as contractions induced by potassium are mainly mediated via MPS-C (50). This was shown in an *in vitro* study of human pial arteries (53). Vessels contracted by potassium were almost completely relaxed by nifedipine and nimodipine, whereas the calcium antagonists in the same concentrations only reduced contractions induced by noradrenaline by 70%, those by 5-hydroxytryptamine by 60%, and those by prostaglandin F_{2a} even less (53). The observations are in agreement with the assumption that these agents cause contraction of the vessels by stimulating calcium influx through RO-C:s, or by mobilizing intracellularly stored calcium, possibly in addition to causing an increased calcium influx through MPS-C:s. When compared to the observations in our study with indomethacin (47), where it was found that prostacyclin only partly counteracted potassium-induced contraction, whereas contractions induced by noradrenaline, 5-hydroxytryptamine and prostaglandin F_{2a} were completely relaxed, one might speculate whether prostacyclin, in contrast to nifedipine, interferes with the RO-C:s in the vascular smooth muscle cell. It was shown that the relaxant effect of nifedipine occurred at lower concentration in cerebral than in mesenteric arteries (53). It was also found that the threshold for potassium-induced contraction of human pial arteries was lower than that of mesenteric arteries (53). If an elevated potassium concentration in the CSF contributes to the syndrome of cerebral vasospasm, then calcium antagonists might be of therapeutical value.

Studies of the effects of topical microapplication of nifedipine on cat cortical pial microvasculature under normal conditions revealed that nifedipine induced very marked concentration-dependent arteriolar dilatations (54). The similar though less pronounced effect on the venules confirms the existence of contractile properties in the wall of human cerebral venules. Considering that about 80% of the total intracranial blood volume is distributed in the venous part of the cerebral vasculature, the finding of venular dilatation must be taken into account when calcium blockers of the nifedipine type are considered as treatment alternatives in cerebrovascular disorders. After occlusion of the middle cerebral artery, all pial arterioles in the antero-lateral, suprasylvian and ectosylvian gyruses dilated. The dilatations in the antero-lateral gyrus were sustained whereas constriction occurred in the suprasylvian gyrus and most frequently in the ectosylvian gyrus 2–9 minutes after occlusion. Also in arterioles constricted after occlusion of the middle cerebral artery, nifedipine induced concentration-dependent dilatations (54).

So far no explanation has been put forward to explain the biphasic sequence of arteriolar calibre changes in focal ischaemia (G. Teasdale: personal communication, 1981). The nifedipine-induced relaxation of constricted 'ischaemic' arterioles suggests that the mechanisms behind the delayed ischaemic arteriolar constriction is dependent on extracellular calcium. The occurrence of pronounced cortical vasoconstriction in focal ischaemia may be of relevance not only in the pathogenesis of stroke, but also in cerebral vasospasm after SAH. Provided that proximal vasospasm in the conducting arteries is sufficient to produce distal ischaemia, and that the observed phenomenon is not only a phenomenon in the cat, one might speculate whether a similar 'ischaemic' vasoconstriction in cortical areas may contribute to delayed ischaemic dysfunction after SAH. If the observed delayed cortical vasoconstriction is due to an increased concentration of potassium in the perivascular space, then the lower threshold observed for potassium-induced contractions on human cerebral arteries might lead to an aggravation of this phenomenon in humans.

General Conclusions of Current Studies

Early aneurysm surgery (within approximately 60 hours post-SAH) is superior to conventional delayed treatment. This form of management eliminates repeat SAH:s but does not dramatically reduce the incidence of delayed cerebral ischaemic dysfunction.

In vivo, post-haemorrhagic CSF induces pronounced constriction of cat pial arterioles, i.e. resistance vessels not discernible on arteriograms. These constrictions are effectively blocked by nifedipine.

In vitro, human pial arteries show marked individual variations in the response to post-haemorrhagic CSF, plasma, and amines. These findings may be relevant for the capricious appearance of cerebral vasospasm in only some patients, whereas other patients with severely blood-contaminated CSF spaces completely escape this dreaded complication. There is no close relationship between vasoconstrictor activity in post-haemorrhagic CSF and clinical condition or angiographic evidence of vasospasm, i.e. delayed deterioration or development of angiographic vasospasm is not paralleled by an increase in CSF vasoconstrictor activity. Removal of subarachnoid blood clots and blood-contaminated cisternal CSF in early aneurysm operations results in generally low CSF vaso-constrictor activity.

In vitro, contractions of human pial arteries induced by acute exposure to CSF from SAH patients are markedly increased after interference with the arachidonic acid metabolism by the use of indomethacin. These results suggest that the development of delayed cerebral vasospasm may be due to a local disturbance of the synthesis of vasodilatatory arachidonic acid metabolites. This suggestion is further supported by the observation that prostacyclin has a pronounced relaxant effect on contractions induced by post-haemorrhagic CSF.

Potassium, amines and prostaglandin F_{2a} activate isolated human pial and mesenteric arteries by partly different calcium-dependent mechanisms. The threshold for potassium-induced contractions is lower in human pial as compared to human mesenteric arteries. The calcium antagonists nifedipine and nimodipine have pronounced relaxant effects on human pial arteries contracted by potassium, amines and prostaglandin F_{2a}, being most potent on potassium-induced contractions.

In vivo, topical application of nifedipine causes marked concentration-dependent pial arteriolar dilatation, increasing with decreasing vessel size. Nifedipine induces venular dilatations as well, which however are less pronounced but more long-lasting than the nifedipine-induced arteriolar dilatations. Nifedipine also dilates arterioles in ischaemic cortex, which have constricted after occlusion of the middle cerebral artery.

The fact that calcium antagonists are effective dilatators of human cerebral arterial segments *in vitro* as well as cat pial arteries *in vivo* under normal conditions as well as when contracted by exposure to post-haemorrhagic CSF and other vasoactive substances does not imply that such agents are effective clinically once the process of cerebral vasospasm is established.

References

1. Gowers, W.R.: Intra-cranial aneurism. In: A manual of diseases of the nervous system. Vol. II, pp. 529–540. London: J. & A. Churchill 1893
2. Denny-Brown, D., Harvey Cushing: The man. J. Neurosurg. *50*, 17–19 (1979)
3. Symonds, C.: Contributions to the clinical study of intracranial aneurysms. With Harvey Cushing. (Reprinted from Guy's Hospital Reports, 1923) In: Studies in Neurology. pp. 27–47. London: Oxford University Press 1970
4. Dott, N.M.: Intracranial aneurysms: cerebral arterio-radiography: surgical treatment: Edinburgh Med. J. *40* (Section on Trans. Med-Chir. Soc. Edinburgh), 219–234 (1933)
5. Dandy, W.E.: Intracranial aneurysm of the internal carotid artery. Cured by operation. Annals of Surgery *107*, 654–659 (1938)
6. Dandy, W.E.: Intracranial arterial aneurysms. New York and London: Hafner; Ithica, New York: Comstock Publishing Co. 1944 (reprinted 1969)
7. Millikan, C.H.: Cerebral vasospasm and ruptured intracranial aneurysm. Arch. Neurol. *32*, 433–449 (1975)
8. Norlén, G., Olivecrona, H.: The treatment of aneurysms of the circle of Willis. J. Neurosurg. *10*, 404–415 (1953)
9. Bucy, P.C.: Editorial reply in Surg. Neurol. *14*, 386 (1980)
10. Hamby, W.B.: Intracranial surgery for aneurysms. Progr. Neurol. Surg. *3*, 1–65 (1969)
11. Pool, J.L.: New dimension in aneurysm surgery. Columbia Univ. Phys. Surg. Q *10*, 18–20 (1965)

12. Yasargil, M.G., Fox, J.L.: The microsurgical approach to intracranial aneurysms. Surg. Neurol. *3*, 7–14 (1975)
13. Yasargil, M.G., Fox, J.L., Ray, M.W.: The operative approach to aneurysms of the anterior communicating artery. In: Advances and technical standards in neurosurgery. Vol. 2. Krayenbühl, H. (ed), pp. 113–170, New York, Wien: Springer 1974
14. Fox, J.L., Ablin, M.S., Bader, D.C.H. et al.: Microsurgical treatment of neurovascular disease. Neurosurgery *3*, 285–337 (1978)
15. Kågström,E., Greitz, T., Hanson, J. et al.: Changes in cerebral blood flow after subarachnoid hemorrhages. In: Proceedings of the Third International Congress of Neurological Surgery, 1965. Excerpta Med. Int. Cong. Series *110*, 629–633, Amsterdam 1966
16. Simeone, F.A., Trepper, P., Brown, D.: Cerebral blood flow evaluation of prolonged experimental cerebral vasospasm. J. Neurosurg. *37*, 302–311 (1972)
17. Kapp, J., Mahaley, M.S. Jr., Odom, G.L.: Cerebral arterial spasm. Part 1: Evaluation of experimental variables affecting the diameter of the exposed basilar artery. J. Neurosurg. *29*, 331–338 (1968)
18. Sundt, I.M., Davis, D.H.: Reactions of cerebrovascular smooth muscle to blood and ischemia: primary versus secondary vasospasm. In: Cerebral arterial spasm: Proceedings of the Second International Workshop. Wilkins, R.H. (ed), pp. 244–250. Baltimore: Williams & Wilkins Co. 1980
19. Mizukami, M., Kawase, T., Tazawa, T. et al.: Hypothesis and clinical evidence for the mechanism of chronic cerebral vasospasm after subarachnoid hemorrhage. In: Cerebral arterial spasm: Proceedings of the Second International Workshop. Wilkins, R.H. (ed.), pp. 97–106. Baltimore: Williams & Wilkins Co. 1980
20. Samson, D.S., Hodosh, R.M., Reid, W.R. et al.: Risk of intracranial aneurysm surgery in the good grade patient: early versus late operation. Neurosurgery *5*, 442–426 (1979)
21. Sano, K., Saito, I.: Timing and indication for surgery for ruptured intracranial aneurysms with regard to cerebral vasospasm. Acta Neurochir. *41*, 49–60 (1978)
22. Sundt, M., Jr.: Cerebral vasospasm following subarachnoid hemorrhage: evolution, management, and relationship to timing of surgery. Clin. Neurosurg. *24*, 228–239 (1977)
23. Weir, B., Aronyk, K.: Management mortality and the timing of surgery for supratentorial aneurysms. J. Neurosurg. *54*, 146–150 (1981)
24. Yasargil, M.G., Smith, R.D.: Surgery on the carotid system in the treatment of hemorrhagic stroke. In: Stroke. Advances in Neurology, Vol. 16. Thompson RA, Green JR (eds.), pp. 181–209. New York: Raven Press 1977
25. Yoshimoto, T., Uchida, K., Kaneko, T. et al.: An analysis of follow-up results of 1000 intracranial saccular aneurysms with definitive surgical treatment. J. Neurosurg. *50*, 152–157 (1979)
26. Adams, H.P., Kassel, N.F., Torner, J.C. et al.: Early management of aneurysmal subarachnoid hemorrhage. A report of the Cooperative Aneurysm Study. J. Neurosurg. *54*, 141–145 (1981)
27. Suzuki, J., Onuma, T., Yoshimoto, T.: Results of early operations on cerebral aneurysms. Surg. Neurol. *11*, 407–412 (1979)
28. Boullin, D.J., Mohan, J., Grahame-Smith, D.G.: Evidence for the presence of a vasoactive substance (possibly involved in the aetiology of cerebral arterial spasm) in cerebrospinal fluid from patients with subarachnoid haemorrhage. J. Neurol. Neurosurg. Psychiat. *39*, 756–766 (1976)
29. Sano, K., Saito, I.: Timing of microsurgical treatment of ruptured intracranial aneurysms. In: Cerebral arterial spasm. Proceedings of the Second International Workshop. Wilkins, R.H. (ed.), pp. 447–454. Baltimore: Williams & Wilkins Co.1980
30. Alksne, J.F., Branson, P.J.: Pathogenesis of cerebral vasospasm. Neurol. Res. *2*, 274–282 (1980)
31. Tanabe, Y., Sakata, K., Yamada, H. et al.: Cerebral vasospasm and ultrastructural changes in cerebral arterial wall. An experimental study. J. Neurosurg. *49*, 229–238 (1978)
32. Asano, T., Tanishima, T., Sasaki, T. et al.: Possible participation of free radical reactions initiated by clot lysis in the pathogenesis of vasospasm after subarachnoid hemorrhage. In: Cerebral arterial spasm:Proceedings of the Second International Workshop. Wilkins, R.H. (ed.), pp. 190–201. Baltimore: Williams & Wilkins Co. 1980
33. Sano, K., Asano, T., Tanishima, T. et al.: Lipid peroxidation as a cause of cerebral vasospasm. Neurol. Res. *2*, 253–271 (1980)

34. Sano, K., Sasaki, T., Asano, I.: Cerebral Vasospasm: The result of lipid peroxidation leading to inhibition of prostacyclin biosynthesis in the cerebral artery. Presented at the 50th Anniversary Meeting of the American Association of Neurological Surgeons in Boston 5/4–9/4 1981. In: Congress Scientific Manuscripts. (Paper 52)

35. Sasaki, T., Wakai, S., Asano, T. et al.: The effect of a lipid hydroperoxide of arachidonic acid on the canine basilar artery. An experimental study on cerebral vasospasm. J. Neurosurg. 54, 357–365 (1981)

36. Ljunggren, B., Brandt, L., Kågström, E., Sundbärg, G.: Results of early operations for ruptured aneurysms. J. Neurosurg. 54, 473–479 (1981)

37. Hunt, W.E., Hess, R.M.: Surgical risk as related to time of intervention in the repair of intracranial aneurysms. J. Neurosurg. 28, 14–19 (1968)

38. Saito, I., Ueda, Y., Sano, K.: Significance of vasospasm in the treatment of ruptured intracranial aneurysms. J. Neurosurg. 47, 412–429 (1977)

39. White, R.P.: Multiplex origins of cerebral vasospasm. In: Cerebrovascular diseases. Eleventh Princeton Conference. Price, T.R., Nelson, E. (eds.), pp. 307–319. New York: Raven Press 1979

40. Wilkins, R.H.: The role of intracranial arterial spasm in the timing of operations for aneurysm. Clin. Neurosurg. 29, 121–134 (1968)

41. Post, K.D., Flamm, E.S., Goodgold, A. et al.: Ruptured intracranial aneurysms. Case morbidity and mortality. J. Neurosurg. 46, 290–295 (1977)

42. Brandt, L., Ljunggren, B., Andersson, K.-E., Hindfelt, B., Teasdale, G.: Vasoconstrictive effects of human post-hemorrhagic cerebrospinal fluid on cat pial arterioles in situ. J. Neurosurg. 54, 351–356 (1981)

43. Brandt, L., Ljunggren, B., Andersson, K.-E., Hindfelt, B.: Individual variations in response of human cerebral arterioles to vasoactive substances, human plasma, and cerebrospinal fluid from patients with aneurysmal subarachnoid hemorrhage. J. Neurosurg. 55, 431–437 (1981)

44. Boullin, D.J., Brandt, L., Ljunggren, B., Tagari, P.: Vasoconstrictor activity in cerebrospinal fluid from patients subjected to early surgery for ruptured intracranial aneurysms. J. Neurosurg. 55, 237–245 (1981)

45. Pickard, J.D., Tamura, A., Stewart, M. et al.: Prostacyclin, indomethacin and the cerebral circulation. Brain Res. 197, 425–431 (1980)

46. Boullin, D.J., Bunting, S., Blaso, W.P. et al.: Responses of human and baboon arteries to prostaglandin endoperoxides and biologically generated and synthetic prostacyclin: their relevance to cerebral arterial spasm in man. Br. J. Clin. Pharmacol. 7, 139–147 (1979)

47. Brandt, L., Ljunggren, B., Andersson, K.-E., Hindfelt, B., Uski, T.: Effects of indomethacin and prostacyclin on isolated human pial arteries contracted by cerebrospinal fluid from patients with aneurysmal subarachnoid hemorrhage. J. Neurosurg. 55:877–883 (1981)

48. Golenhofen, K., Hermstein, N.: Differentiation of calcium activation mechanisms in vascular smooth muscle by selective suppression with verapamil and D600. Blood vessels 12, 21–37 (1975)

49. Somlyo, A.V., Somlyo, A.P.: Electromechanical and pharmacomechanical coupling in vascular smooth muscle. J. Pharmacol. Exp. Ther. 159, 129–145 (1968)

50. Bolton, T.B.: Mechanisms of action of transmitters and other substances on smooth muscle. Physiol. Rev. 59, 606–718 (1979)

51. Fleckenstein, H.: Specific pharmacology of calcium in myocardium, cardiac pacemakers, and vascular smooth muscle. Ann. Rev. Pharmacol. Toxicol. 17, 149–166 (1977)

52. Church, J., Zsoter, T.: Calcium antagonistic drugs. Mechanisms of action. Can. J. Physiol. Pharmacol. 58, 254–264 (1980)

53. Brandt, L., Andersson, K.-E., Edvinsson, L., Ljunggren, B.: Effects of extracellular calcium and calcium antagonists on contractile responses of human and mesenteric arteries. J. CBF and Metabolism 1, 339–347 (1981)

54. Brandt, L., Ljunggren, B., Andersson, K.-E., MacKenzie, E.T., Tamura, A., Teasdale, G.: Effects on feline cortical pial microvasculature of topical application of a calcium antagonist (Nifedipine) under normal conditions and in focal ischemia. J. CBF and Metabolism (in press)

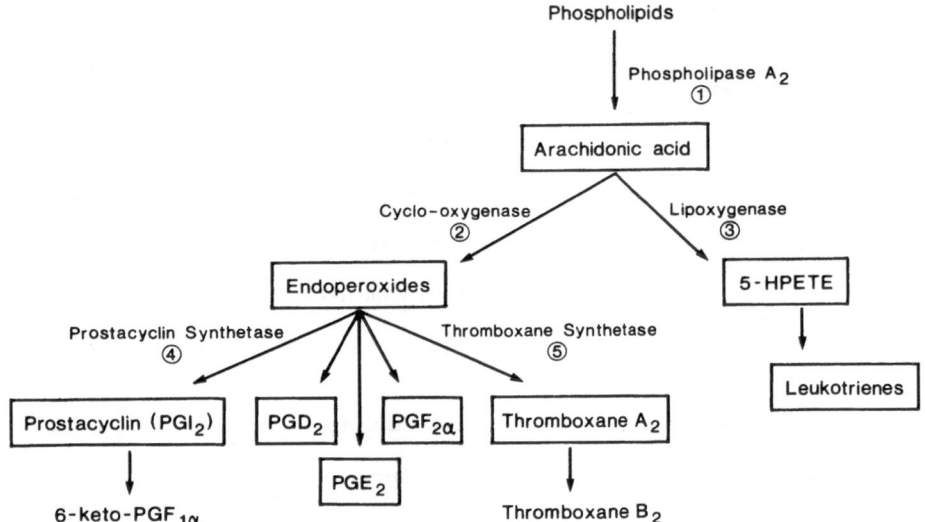

Fig. 1. Metabolism of arachidonic acid

(1) = can be inhibited by e.g., mepacrine, glucocorticosteroids

(2) = can be inhibited by anti-inflammatory drugs, e.g., indomethacin

(3) = can be inhibited by e.g., eicosatetraynoic acid (ETYA)

(4) = can be inhibited by e.g., tranylcypromine

(5) = can be inhibited by e.g., butylimidazole

394

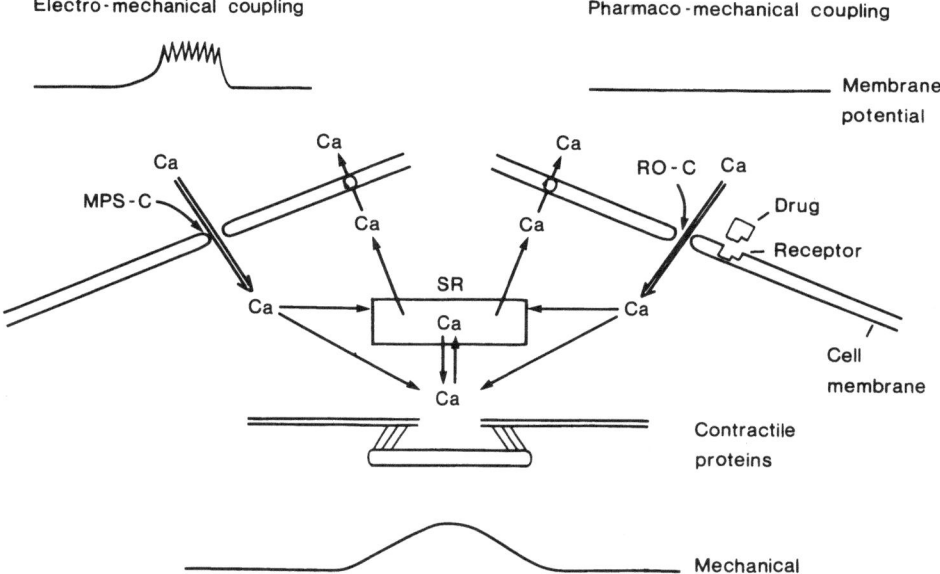

Electro-mechanical coupling

Pharmaco-mechanical coupling

Membrane potential

Ca

Ca

MPS-C

Ca

Ca

RO-C Ca

Ca

Ca

Drug

Receptor

SR

Ca

Ca

Ca

Cell membrane

Ca

Contractile proteins

Mechanical activity

Fig. 2. Electro-mechanical and pharmaco-mechanical coupling in vascular smooth muscle. MPS-C = membrane potential sensitive Ca channel; RO-C = receptor operated Ca channel; SR = sarcoplasmic reticulum

Cerebral Oedema Following Experimental Subarachnoid Haemorrhage

T. Shigeno, E. Fritschka, J. Schramm, and M. Brock

Introduction

Despite the fact that cerebral oedema appears to be a common complication of subarachnoid haemorrhage (SAH) due to a ruptured cerebral aneurysm, measurements of brain tissue water content have not been carried out in this condition (6). For this reason, we have analysed the development of cerebral oedema in experimental SAH in cats.

Material and Methods

To simulate human SAH the following three conditions are required; 1: arterial wall injury: 2: acute increase of intracranial pressure (ICP); 3: a sufficient amount of subarachnoid blood clot. To achieve this purpose, SAH was induced in cats under controlled ventilation by withdrawing needles previously pierced into one or both infraclinoid internal carotid arteries through a unilateral transorbital approach (Fig. 1). Anaesthesia was induced with Nembutal and maintained by a nitrous oxide-oxygen mixture.

The following vital signs were monitored: blood pressure, blood gases, body temperature. ICP in the cisterna magna and in the chiasmatic cistern, cortical EEG and somatosensory evoked potentials (SEP) to sciatic nerve stimulation. Ten animals were observed for 3 to 24 hours.

Using labelled microspheres of 15μ diameter, four serial determinations of regional cerebral blood flow (rCBF) were performed in one group of five animals before and immediately after the SAH as well as 10 to 20 minutes, and 3 to 6 hours after the SAH. RCBF was obtained in 60 areas of the brain from tissue samples weighing less than 200 mg. In these animals, brain tissue water content was determined as a percentage by the vacuum freeze-drying and weighing procedure in the same samples of brain tissue used for rCBF measurement. In another group of five animals, specific gravity of brain tissue was measured by microgravimetry (11) in samples of brain tissue weighing 30 to 50 mg. Normal values of regional specific gravity and water content of brain tissue had been determined previously and these are to be reported (Shigeno, Brock et al). Disturbances of blood-brain barrier were demonstrated by systemic injection of Evans blue.

Modern Neurosurgery 1. Edited by M. Brock

Results

Three patterns of ICP changes were observed, depending on the severity of the SAH (Fig. 2). In grade I (n= 4), after an acute rise of ICP to about 50 mm Hg, control values were reached again within ten minutes. Blood pressure did not change significantly. In grade II (n= 4), ICP increased up to 200 mm Hg with a concomitant rise of blood pressure and a total supression of EEG and SEP. Ten to 20 minutes later, ICP nearly returned to control values, accompanied by a partial recovery of electrical activities. In contrast, in grade III, the ICP increase above 100 mm Hg was sustained for more than one hour, and systemic hypotension and death followed. Necropsy revealed a close relationship between the above-mentioned grading and the amount of subarachnoid blood clot spreads over the cerebral hemisphere (Fig. 3). Extravasation of Evans blue was observed only in grade II animals, and was located mainly in the parasagittal water-shed areas and in the basal ganglia.

There were also three grades of patterns of rCBF changes (Fig. 4). RCBF changes were estimated as percentages in the parasagittal area, in the sylvian region and in the brain stem. Grade I corresponded to a slight decrease in rCBF. In grade II, rCBF decreased markedly in the cerebral hemisphere, while brain stem circulation was relatively preserved. In these animals, 10 to 20 minutes after haemorrhage, hemispheric rCBF increased even above control values, running parallel with the decrease in ICP and indicating reactive hyperaemia. Three to six hours later, a marked reduction of rCBF was again observed. In grade III, rCBF remained nearly zero after SAH. There was a tendency towards a greater rCBF reduction in the parasagittal area as compared to the sylvian region. However, when including those tissues without significant rCBF reduction the distribution of rCBF decrease was not homogeneous.

The difference in specific gravity from control values in each corresponding area was estimated in the parasagittal cortex and subjacent white matter, as well as in the sylvian cortex and subjacent white matter (Fig. 5). A marked decrease in specific gravity was observed only in grade II animals, particularly in the parasagittal area. These animals had a moderate arterial hypertension up to 160 mm Hg. In grade I or III, there was even a tendency for the specific gravity to increase. This may be a result of increased cerebral blood volume, since the specific gravity of blood is higher than that of brain tissue (11). The percentage increase in brain tissue water content was also estimated in the same manner. A marked increase was observed only in grade II animals (Fig. 6).

When rCBF and percentage brain tissue water content were measured simultaneously, rCBF values immediately after SAH were plotted against brain water content (Fig. 7). In animals of grade II, with reactive hyperaemia, a significant increase of water content was observed only in areas in which rCBF had decreased below 20 ml/100g/min both in grey and white matter. In contrast, in grade III animals, with a permanent decrease of rCBF below 10 mg/100g/min, there was no significant increased in water content.

Discussion

The occurrence of cerebral oedema after experimental SAH is documented for the first time in this study, using a newly developed surgical approach and a microdetermination of brain tissue water content. The validity of the present experiments is corroborated by the acute increase in ICP above 200 mm Hg leading to global cerebral ischaemia, as well as by the presence of subarachnoid blood clots over the cerebral hemisphere. In the previous report by Hayakawa et al. (4), the increase of ICP was up to 50 mm Hg after puncture of the middle cerebral artery of the cat. With this ICP increase however, we were unable in this study to produce either significant cerebral ischaemia or oedema, as was demonstrated in the grade I animals.

It has been clearly shown that cerebral oedema complicating SAH is caused by the combination of an initial cerebral ischaemia with subsequent recovery of cerebral circulation. An acute increase in ICP as a result of cerebral tamponade appears to be a primary factor causing global cerebral ischaemia, as was also reported by Asano et al. (1). This may be aggravated by impairment of pressure-buffering capacity due to acute hydrocephalus, as frequently observed in patients with acute SAH (9). Since rCBF decreased in a patchy and unhomogeneous distribution, constriction of pial vessels in contact with subarachnoid blood clots might be another factor causing microcirculatory disturbances (3, 5). The parasagittal water-shed areas tend to be more affected by ischaemia and subsequent cerebral oedema, particularly in cases of arterial hypertension following SAH. Asano et al. (1) also showed such a preferential distribution for so-called no-reflow areas after experimental SAH. Even hypertension alone has been reported to cause alterations in the cerebral circulation and extravasation of protein-bound tracers in these boundary areas (8). Increased sympathetic activity and hypertension have been reported in patients with SAH (2, 10). In contrast to grade II animals, which showed a marked decrease in brain tissue specific gravity, corresponding to an increase of brain tissue water content, cerebral oedema could not be detected in the grade III animals with severe SAH, indicating that there is no water increase in no-flow areas.

Since hypervolaemic hypertension has recently been proposed for the treatment of ischaemia following SAH (7), it should be born in mind that post-ischaemic overperfusion might accelerate the development of cerebral oedema as demonstrated by our results.

References

1. Asano, T., Sano, K.: Pathogenetic role of no-reflow phenomenon in experimental subarachnoid hemorrhage in dogs. J. Neurosurg. 46, 454–466 (1977)
2. Benedict, C.R., Loach, A.B.: Sympathetic nervous system activity in patients with subarachnoid hemorrage. Stroke 9, 237–244 (1978)
3. Hart, M.N.: Morphometry of brain parenchymal vessels following subarachnoid hemorrage. Stroke 11, 653–655 (1980)
4. Hayakawa, T., Walts, A.G.: Experimental subarachnoid hemorrage from a middle cerebral artery. Neurologic deficits, intracranial pressures, and pulse rates. Stroke 8, 421–426 (1977)
5. Herz, D.A., Baez, S., Shulman, K.: Pial microcirculation in subarachnoid hemorrage. Stroke 6, 417–424 (1975)
6. Katzman, R., Clasen, R., Klatzo, I., Meyer, J.S., Pappius, H.M., Waltz, A.G.: Report of joint committee for stroke responses. IV. Brain edema in stroke. Stroke 8, 510–540 (1977)
7. Kosnik, E.J., Hunt, W.E.: Postoperative hypertension in the management of patients with intracranial arterial aneurysms. J. Neurosurg. 45, 148–154 (1976)

8. MacKenzie, E.T., Strandgaard, S., Graham, D.I., Jones, J.V., Harper, A.M., Farrar, J.K.: Effects of acutely induced hypertension in cats on pial arteriolar caliber, local cerebral blood flow, and the blood-brain barrier. Stroke *39*, 33–41 (1976)
9. Shigeno, T., Aritake, K., Saito, I., Sano, K.: Hydrocephalus following early operation on ruptured cerebral aneurysms: significance of long-term monitoring of intracranial pressure. In: Intracranial pressure IV: Shulman, K., Marmarou, A., Miller. J.D., Becker, D.P., Hochwald, G.H., Brock, M. (eds.), pp. 235–240. Berlin, Heidelberg, New York: Springer 1980
10. Shigeno, T., Mori, K., Saito, I., Sano, K., Brock, M.: Early operation of ruptured cerebral aneurysms: The role of norepinephrine in subarachnoid hemorrhage and in experimental vasospasm. In: Advances in neurosurgery, Vol. 9. Schiefer, W., Klinger, M., Brock, M. (eds.), pp. 189–196. Berlin, Heidelberg, New York: Springer 1981
11. Shigeno, T., Shigeno, S., Fritschka, E., Cervos-Navarro, J., Brock, M.: Fundamental problems and improved methods in the measurement of specific gravity of brain tissue. J. CBF Metabol. *1* (Suppl. 1) 158–159 (1981)
12. Shigeno, T., Brock, M., Shigeno, S., Fritschka, E., Cervos-Navarro, J.: The determination of brain water content: Microgravinetry versus drying-weighing. J. Neurosurg. (in press)

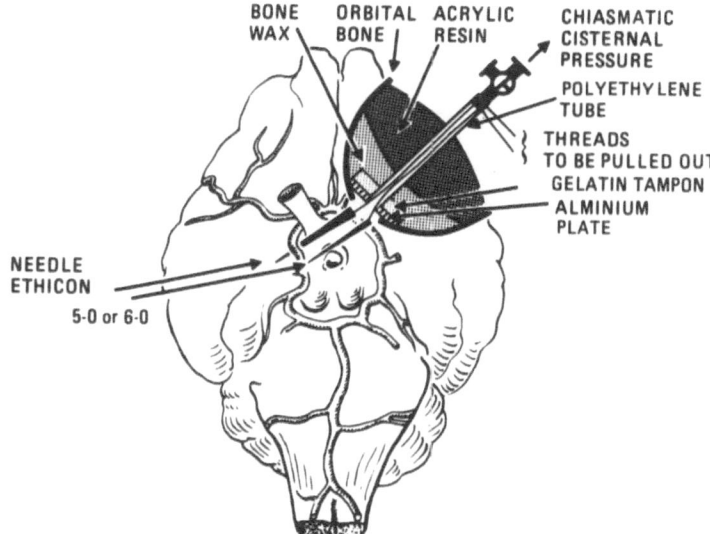

Fig. 1. Operative procedure for the production of experimental SAH

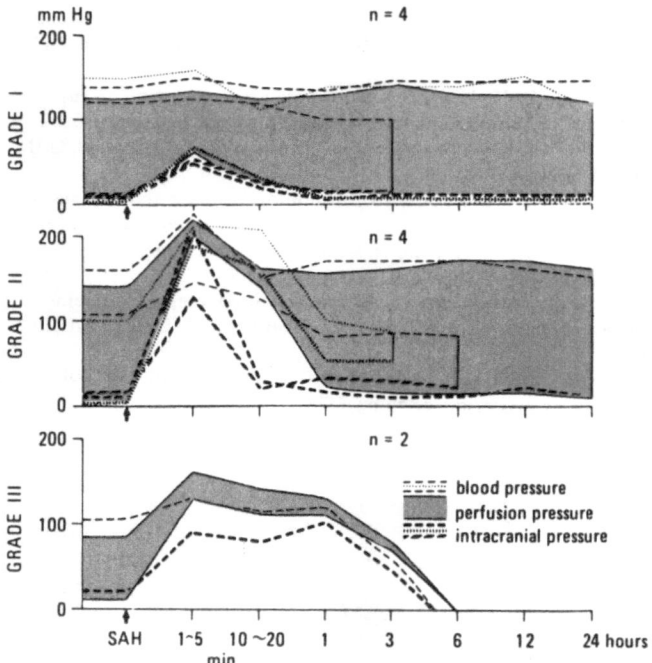

Fig. 2. Changes of blood pressure and ICP after SAH, classified into three grades. Shaded area shows perfusion pressure in a representative case

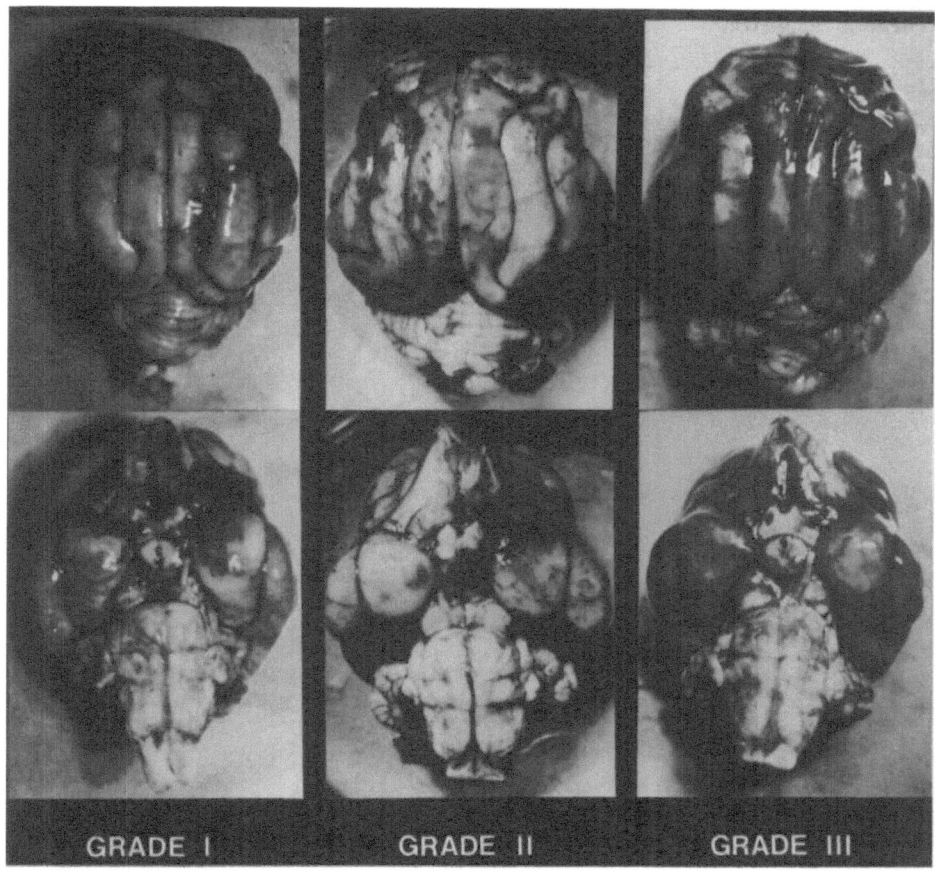

Fig. 3. Gross appearance of the brain with SAH in each grade. There is a close relationship between the severity of SAH and the grading. Extravasation of Evans blue is present in the parasagittal watershed area of the grade II animal

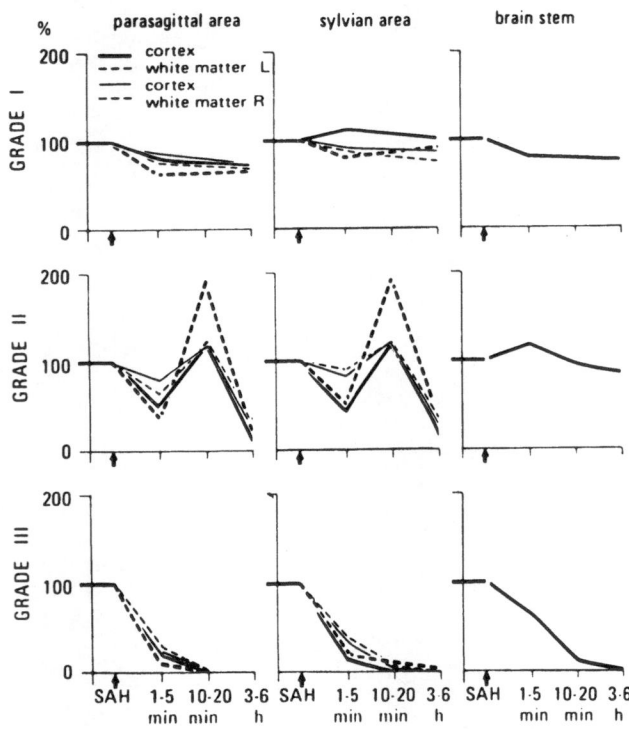

Fig. 4. Changes of rCBF after SAH in a representative case belonging to each grade. Marked reactive hyperaemia was only observed in grade II

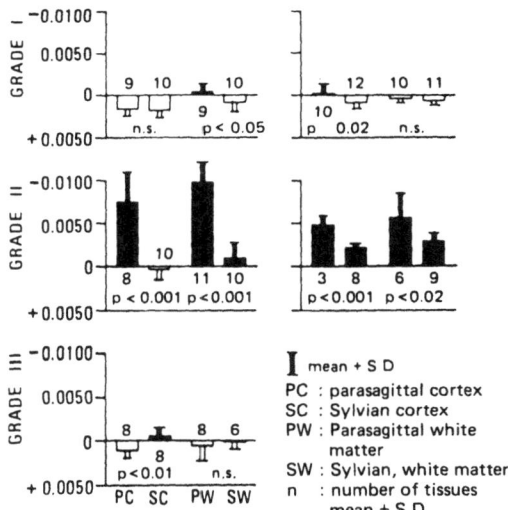

Fig. 5. Changes of specific gravity of brain tissue from five animals classified into three grades. A marked decrease in specific gravity was only observed particularly in the parasagittal areas of grade II animals

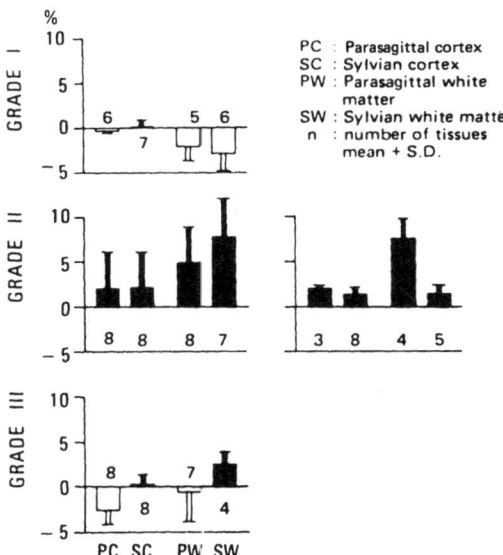

Fig. 6. Percentage changes of water content of brain tissue from four animals. A marked increase in water content was only observed in grade II animals

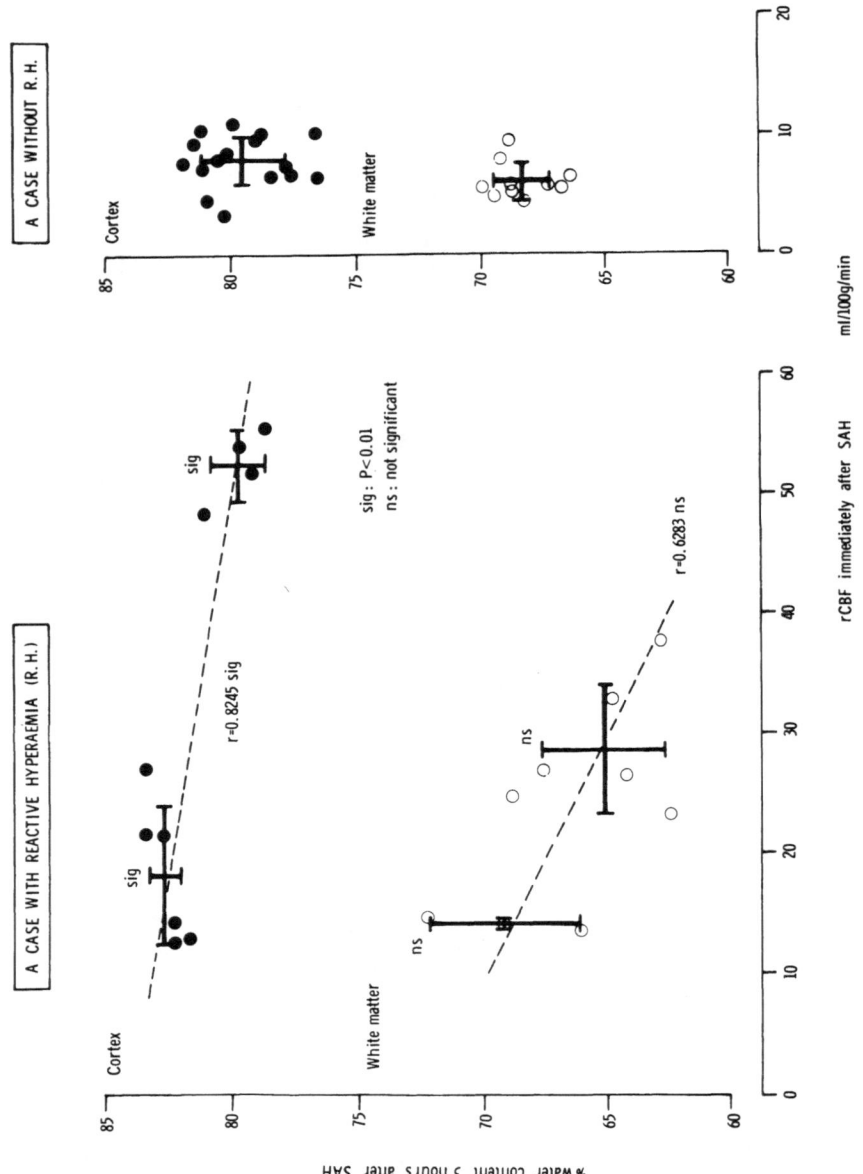

Fig. 7. Relationship between the water content and the value of rCBF immediately after SAH in a representative case from grade II and grade III. Each point represents a value from one sample of brain tissue. In a grade II animal with reactive hyperaemia, a marked increase in water content was ob observed in those areas where rCBF decreased below 20 ml/100g/min, particularly in the grey matter. In a grade III animal with sustained no flow, no increase in water content was evident

The Effect of Carotid Ligation on Cerebral Aneurysmal Size and on Aneurysmal Production in Man

B. Vlahovitch, J.M. Fuentes, and Y. Choucair

Introduction

Carotid ligation is still sometimes performed in the treatment of particular intracranial aneurysms, most often of the giant type. Naturally this method is employed when direct surgical approach is considered to be too risky.

Generally, carotid ligation must be preceded by the usual different tests of good tolerance with even progressive clamping (Selverstone), and as in one of our cases, by protection with an intracranial-extracranial by-pass. It also seems useful during the first week which immediately follows the ligation, to add to the treatment a small dose of heparin, by infusion.

Five representative cases were chosen out of the twenty carotid ligations done for cerebral vascular malformations.

In three of our cases of giant aneurysms, the active size of the vascular anomaly has greatly diminished and, in one case, completely disappeared 17 years later. While the active size improved (angiographic picture) in an enormous aneurysm measuring 4 x 2.5 cm there was a persisting pseudo-tumoural effect due to the clotted part of the malformation (CT scan picture) which, even three years later, gave rise to some slight neurological symptoms. A giant serpiginous aneurysm also had a complete lack of opacification after treatment.

Carotid ligation, was followed in one case, by a growth of the aneurysm located on the carotid bifurcation. In the last case a new anterior communicating artery aneurysm developed, which can be compared with the experimental description of Hashimoto and Hassler.

Summary of Cases

Case 1: S.R. (Fig. 1)

This 45-year-old father of four children, a hard worker and right-handed was seen for the first time in April 1978. In November 1977, he had sudenly complained of acute headache and of a slight right-sided facio-brachial paresis without aphasic symptoms. He was examined by a neurosurgical team and then had a left carotid angiogram which showed a giant carotid bifurcation aneurysm, about 4 x 2.5 cm and two smaller aneurysms, one on the left Sylvian artery and the other on the right carotid bifurcation. No neurosurgical treatment was advised for him at that time.

When we had the opportunity to see the patient, he had severe headache and a variable right facio-brachial paresis. Four-vessel angiography showed that the left hemisphere was well irrigated by the right carotid and also by the left vertebral artery. His arterial blood pressure was 140/80 mm Hg and his pulse 75. We carried out all the different clinical and EEG arterial compression tests, and we came to the conclusion that the patient tolerated left carotid compression very well for ten minutes. Common carotid ligation was performed on 11th May 1978. The internal carotid artery was occluded first of all and this showed that the residual intravascular carotid pressure fell from 140 mm Hg to 100 mm Hg. When the common carotid artery was occluded the residual internal carotid pressure fell to 80 mm Hg. Finally the common carotid was ligated.

This operation was done under local anaesthesia and was well tolerated. Immediately afterwards the patient was given post-operative treatment with vasodilator drugs and also an intravenous infusion of heparin, 150 mg/day for one week (3).

A post-operative right carotid angiogram showed that the aneurysm had diminished by more than 50%. The CT scan showed a large opto-striate lesion with enhancement by contrast injection giving a characteristic rosette appearance (18) of the aneurysm. The aneurysmal wall was calcified, which gave a ring-like hyperdense picture on the scan.

The patient went home to convalesce and was well for two years. Then again he suddenly had headache with a slight right-sided paresis.

He was readmitted to the neurosurgical department where treatment by Decandron produced a general remission of all the symptoms, probably in relation with an oedematous and ischaemic effect. At this moment, the new CT scan analysis showed that the giant aneurysm was still incompletely thrombosed.

During the early part of 1981, the patient was again very well with episodic headache and practically no residual right motor deficit. The CT scan demonstrated a completely clotted left carotid bifurcation giant aneurysm, but with a ring-like enhancement on the lateral superior border of the lesion (5). Also, the frontal hypodensity at the periphery of the lesion was still present without significant change.

Finally, four-vessel angiography showed that the size of the active giant aneurysm had diminished by 95% with no change in the two other small aneurysms. Three years after treatment of this left bifurcation giant aneurysm by carotid ligation this patient was practically independent without any obvious neurological deficit, but he was having some headache and was still unable to work.

Comment

In this case of giant aneurysm of the left carotid bifurcation, situated at the internal part of the perforating hemisphere branches, direct operation was not undertaken, but common carotid ligation was well tolerated. Two years later, the patient had a recurrence of symptoms with a right hemiparesis which was accompanied by cerebral swelling and frontal hypodensity in the CT scan.

As regards this patient, we must stress the remarkable reduction in the size of the aneurysm, 50% in the first year and 95% three years later.

We then noticed that a progressive thrombosis of the aneurysmal mass gave a CT scan image two years later with a rosette appearance and three years later a completely thrombosed lesion with, nevertheless, a small capsular ring sign on enhancement. This last image proves that there is in the capsule of the clotted aneurysm a vascularization which must not be mistaken for the residue of an active malformation (5, 18).

This patient did not have any extracranial-intracranial by-pass which might possibly have offered more protection to his left hemisphere from ischaemia with CT scan hypodensity. He may also need in the near future to have the clot excised to diminish the still persisting tumoral effect.

Case 2: T.L. (Fig. 2)

In May 1974, this 28-year-old woman with usual menstrual headache began to suffer progressively from neck pain with some vomiting, of one week duration. This condition was accompanied by unsteadiness of gait and pailloedema, but without obvious neurological deficit or neck stiffness. Ventriculography was normal without raised CSF pressure or haemorrhage.

In June 1974, a comatose state suddenly developed with a left hemiplegia. A right carotid angiogram revealed a saccular aneurysm at the carotid bifurcation without any haematoma. She slowly recovered consciousness and the hemiplegia improved. After successful compression tests had been carried out, the right common carotid was ligated under local anaesthesia. The patient recovered very rapidly and was discharged to a convalescent home.

In May 1975, she again suffered from severe headache with vomiting, slight neck stiffness and increasing left hemiparesis, without any disorder of consciousness. A left carotid angiogram showed that the right internal carotid bifurcation aneurysm had increased in size by about 20%.

After this possible attack of rebleeding the patient again resumed her normal life, but with episodic occipital headache.

In 1980, a CT scan analysis conformed, after enhancement, a hyperdense image on the right internal carotid, with a hydrocephalic right lateral ventricle.

A complete angiographic examination showed that the right carotid bifurcation aneurysm which filled from the left side, had grown by about 100% and was surrounded by an incomplete circular calcification. In fact, the vessels of the anterior part of the circle of Willis were greatly enlarged in this case, but without any new 'iatrogenic' aneurysm on the other cerebral arteries.

Comment

This patient had a ruptured internal carotid bifurcation aneurysm which responded very well to the treatment by common carotid ligation, but she almost had another episode of aneurysmal rupture one year later. The arteriographic control at this time showed that her aneurysm had increased in size by about 20%. At a second angiographic follow-up made six years later, this aneurysm had increased in size by 100%.

Such evolution of a cerebral aneurysm has already been described by Odom (17) in 1962, Cuatico et al. in 1967 (2) and Shiobara et al. in 1980 (20). It seems likely that the hydrodynamic force theory (4) cannot be the only explanation of the growth of the aneurysm, and one should also consider the post-rupture repair mechanism (24) which is what probably happened in our case.

The positive and negative changes in aneurysmal size after carotid ligation are, in general, not rapid but may take several years.

Case 3: A.M.

A 32-year-old female who, from 1975 onwards after the birth of her son, was treated for headache and for diminishing vision in the left eye and transient paresis of the right upper limb.

In 1977, a left carotic angiogram showed a giant serpiginous carotid aneurysm but the patient would not agree to any surgical treatment.

In 1980, she began to have generalized epilepitc attacks and was admitted to the neurosurgical department for treatment of this vascular malformation. The four-vessel angiography showed that the giant, serpiginous left carotid aneurysm was situated under a well-developed circle of Willis.

The lesion was also apparent on CT scan, with a calcified wall and it showed good enhancement after contrast injection. It was decided to perform a trapping operation. Although the patient tolerated the left carotid compression test she was first given an extracranial-intracranial arterial by-pass. Three weeks later she underwent a progressive surgical occlusion of her left internal carotid artery with a Selverstone clamp. At this time she had a left regional carotid blood-flow estimation, by the Xenon clearance method. This study clearly proved that the complete occlusion of the left internal carotid had reduced the flow to 10 cc/100g/min in the frontal region, leaving it at 35 cc/100g/min in the temporal region with the extracranial-intracranial by-pass. After the operation the vision in the left eye recovered well and she had no more transient right arm paresis. She continued to have fits which were controlled by phenobarbitone.

A complete angiographic control showed only a minimal filling of the aneurysm by the left ophtalmic artery via the external carotid.

CT scan control, with and without enhancement, was practically unchanged so that entrapment of the aneurysm was judged to have been useless.

Comment

The technique used to ensure the good tolerance of internal carotid artery occlusion, by extracranial-intracranial by-pass and progressive Selverstone clamping is now commonly accepted. While clamping the carotid artery the regional blood-flow study gives a precise idea of the function of the arterial by-pass as in our case, so this can indicated that the blood flow will be sufficient to ensure satisfactory function in the hemisphere.

In many recent works (6, 21–23) the usefulness and security achieved by the arterial by-pass has been stressed. The cerebral blood-flow measurements with carotid occlusion must also be regarded as very helpful (7, 23).

Case 4: R.J.

In July 1965, a healthy 41-year-old man suffered an acute headache after a severe boat of coughing. He also had neck stiffness and vomiting but no other neurological symptoms. Lumbar puncture confirmed a subarachnoid haemorrhage.

After three weeks bed rest the patient underwent a four-vessel angiographic study, which showed a small aneurysm on the right internal carotid at the level of the anterior clinoid process, with a good functional circle of Willis.

On 28th August 1965 the blood pressure was 140/80 mm Hg and after a well-tolerated carotid compression test a right common carotid ligation was performed under local anaesthesia. The immediate follow-up was very good and the patient was discharged home ten days later. He resumed his former work without trouble, two months later.

In 1971 he again suffered a sudden acute headache with neck stiffness but without vomiting or neurological deficit. Lumbar puncture was normal. In spite of this, the patient was admitted to the neurosurgical department and again had a complete cerebral angiography. On the left side, the vertebral artery was normal and the left carotid showed the two anterior cerebral and the two middle cerebral arteries without any new aneurysm or displacement, but only slight atherosclerosis of the main trunks. On the right side it was possible to puncture the internal carotid artery above the previous ligature and to do an angiogram. This one showed a filling of the internal carotid artery, its cavernous portion, the right external carotid and the right middle cerebral artery but with poor contrast in the anterior cerebral artery. The right internal carotid artery was thin and the old aneurysm was no longer visible. The patient was discharged on medical treatment and he rapidly returned to work.

In January 1980, fifteen years after the first attack, this patient was seen again in very good condition. He continues to work hard, quite normally and he did not complain of any headache or vertigo. His blood pressure was 150/100 mm Hg and he only has a slight hearing and visual defect.

Comment

In this case of a simple internal carotid aneurysm, common carotid ligation gave a good result with disappearance of the lesion, but two things are important to notice: firstly that he had a clinical episode suggestive of rebleeding, but without subarachnoid haemorrhage and secondly the right internal carotid beyond the ligature was not thrombosed six years after. It may be that this phenomenon has not given the opportunity for the formation of a new iatrogenic aneurysm of the Hassler-Hashimoto type in this patient.

Case 5: G.M. (Fig. 3)

This patient, a 33-year-old farmer, was seen for the first time in 1962 on account of a subarachnoid haemorrhage. Bilateral carotid angiography showed a giant aneurysm (2.5 x 1.5 cm) of the right posterior communicating artery. This was treated by ligation of the right common carotid artery.

The patient recovered completely and returned to a normal working life for seventeen years. Then, suddenly he had another attack of subarachnoid haemorrhage. Angiography of all the cerebral arteries showed a new saccular aneurysm on the anterior communicating artery, which was not there on the first occassion. The aneurysm was also clearly visible on the CT scan, although the old giant aneurysm on the right posterior communicating artery had completely disappeared and was probably cured.

As a preliminary to a direct surgical attack on this new aneurysm we tried, with the help of the vascular surgeons to perform a right subclavian – right external carotid by-pass, but this unforunately failed. Nevertheless this patient was successfully operated on by direct clipping of this new aneurysm.

Comment

This case is a good illustration of two important things. First of all the giant aneurysm of the psoterior communicating artery was completely cured by the common carotid ligation and could no longer be seen on the scan picture. Secondly this case proves that the second subarachnoid haemorrhage was caused seventeen years later by a new iatrogenic anterior communicating artery aneurysm not previously seen on the old angiogram.

This sort of complication after carotid ligation is similar to the results of Hassler's experimental work on the rabbit (14) and also, more recently, of Hashimoto et al. on the rat (9–13). The development of the aneurysm is probably provoked by the haemodynamic modifications in the anterior part of the circle of Willis.

Hassler and Hashimoto have also pointed out the strong probability of these aneurysms developing (14% and 50%) (13, 14). We think that these figures are too high and, in any case, are difficult to prove in man.

In cases of carotid ligation one is not allowed to use invasive methods such as arteriography to look for new aneurysms (17), and at present CT scan is still unable to show accurately a small non-ruptured aneurysm.

Discussion

In the neurosurgical treatment of cerebral aneurysms the place of the old Hunterian principle consisting of carotid ligation still survives almost exclusively for the management of giant sized malformations.

In fact, in some recent large series of cases of intracranial carotid artery giant aneurysms, it appears that carotid ligation or trapping were still used in 43% of 51 cases (23), in 40% of 25 cases (15) and 33% of 66 cases (3). For the remaining distally located giant aneurysms of the cerebral vessels direct neurosurgical approach prevails but, of course, with a higher operative risk.

One must bear in mind that even with the most sophisticated security methods used before occlusion some unforseeable dangers still persist. Among these security methods, extracranial-intracranial arterial by-pass (1, 15, 19, 21–23, 26) and blood-flow measurements are the most useful.

The result of carotid ligation, as in our first case, was a striking reduction in the active volume of the malformation over a three year follow-up period, probably produced by deviation of the blood jet stream effect (5). Even if a CT scan still shows a huge pseudotumoural lesion, it is nevertheless completely clotted and is acting only like a space-occupying lesion. In this case also, at the end of the period of complete thrombosis of the aneurysm, the CT scan showed a ring sign enhancement of the capsule which confirmed a thickened vascular wall (5).

Even if in case 5, the giant right posterior communicating artery aneurysm appears definitely cured seventeen years after carotid ligation, in case 2 the carotid bifurcation aneurysm became progressively larger over a seven year period, similar to the cases of Cuatico and others (2, 20, 25).

The occurence of a iatrogenic aneurysm of the anterior communicating artery in case 5, seventeen years after the carotid ligation must be referred to the pioneer experimental work of Hassler and Hashimoto (9, 14). Hashimoto et al. (9) showed that carotid occlusion with the addition of arterial hypertension and the use of 'lathyrogens', started aneurysmal formation absolutely similar to the human cases especially in two principal spots on the circle of Willis, namely, the anterior and posterior communicating arteries. The major haemodynamic change in flow occuring in these regions probably explains the development of new aneurysms after carotid ligation, demonstrated since 1965 by Gurdjian et al. (8) for the anterior communicating artery and by the works of Klemme et al. (16) and of Winn et al. (25) in 1977 for the posterior communicating artery.

The changes in size of an aneurysm after carotid ligation depend on this factor (4) and possibly also on the post-aneurysmal rupture repair mechanisms (24). It looks important to be aware that many different changes in aneurysmal pathology may be brough about by carotid occlusion and sometimes, as in our cases 1, 2 and 5, only after a long delay.

Conclusion

These few cases of aneurysms treated by carotid ligation may have no statistical value, but they are sufficient to draw attention to some particular long-term results and also to the complications of rebleeding. Among the results there are not only the already known positive and negative effects on the size of the aneurysm after carotid ligation, but also the complications of subarachnoid rebleeding caused by other aneurysms not previously demonstrated by a total cerebral angiography.

These iatrogenic aneurysms give a particular importance to the experimental work of Hassler and Hashimoto. They also indicate the necessity when treating aneurysms of having a complete arteriographic investigation and a long-term follow-up.

Summary

In the past history of neurosurgery carotid ligation has been the main treatment of intracranial aneurysms and even nowadays it still remains a useful measure in some particular cases. It was specially performed in three patients with *giant aneurysms,* which were deemed unsuitable for direct clipping, with quite a good reduction in size, or even disappearance of the lesion. In these cases among the methods used to avoid the risks of carotid ligation, one patient had an anastomosis of the superficial temporal to the middle cerebral artery performed beforehand.

However, carotid ligation may sometimes have a contradictory effect on the growth of the aneurysm, as in one of our cases, or may even produce a *new iatrogenic anterior communicating artery aneurysm* of the Hassler-Hashimoto type. This last occurence happened 17 years after common carotid ligation for a giant aneurysm of the posterior communicating artery, which itself was completely cured.

It seems that interfering with carotid blood flow by ligation induces in man, as in the experimental animal, a haemodynamic aneurysm-producing effect.

References

1. Ammerman, B.J., Donald, R., Smith: Giant fusiform middle cerebral aneurysm: successful treatment utilizing microvascular by-pass. Sug. Neurol. 7, 5, 255–257 (1977)
2. Cuatico, W., Cook, A.W., Tyshchenko, V., et al.: Massive enlargement of intracranial aneurysms following carotid ligation. Arch. Neurol. 17, 609–613 (1967)
3. Drake, G.C.: Giant intracranial aneurysms: experiences with surgical treatment in 174 patients. Clinical neurosurgery 26, 12–95 (1979)
4. Ferguson, G.G.: Physical factors in the initiation, growth and rupture of human intracranial saccular aneurysms. J. Neurosurg. 37, 666–677 (1972)
5. Fodstad, H., Liliequist, B., Wirell, S., Nilsson, P.-E., Boquist, L., Rahman, A.A.: Giant serpentine intracranial aneurysm after carotid ligation. J. Neurosurg. 49, 903–909 (1978)
6. Gelber, B.R., Sundt, T.M.: Treatment of intracavernous and giant carotid aneurysms by combined internal carotid ligation and extra to intracranial by-pass. J. Neurosurg. 52, 1–10 (1980)
7. George, R., Leibrock, L., Epstein, M.: Long term analysis of cerebrospinal fluid shunt infections. J. Neurosurg. 51, 6. 804–811 (1979)
8. Gurdjian, E.S., Lindner, D.W., Thomas, L.M.: Experiences with ligation of the common carotid artery for treatment of aneurysms of the internal carotid artery. With particular reference to complications. J. Neurosurg. 23, 3, 311–318 (1965)
9. Hashimoto, N., Hazama, F., Handa, H.: Experimentally induced cerebral aneurysms in rats. Surg. Neurol. 10, 3–8 (1978)
10. Hashimoto, N., Handa, H., Hazama, F.: Experimentally induced cerebral aneurysms in rats. Surg. Neurol. 11, 243–246 (1979)
11. Hashimoto, N., Handa, H., Hazama, F.: Experimentally induced cerebral aneurysms in rats: Pathology. Surg. Neurol. 11, (4), 299–304 (1979)
12. Hashimoto, N., Nagata, I., Handa, H.: Experimentally induced cerebral aneurysms in rats: Cerebral angiography. Surg. Neurol. 12, (5), 419–424 (1979)
13. Hashimoto, N., Handa, H., Nagata, I., Hazama, F.: Experimentally induced cerebral aneurysms in rats: Relation of hemodynamics in the circle of Willis to formation of aneurysms. Surg. Neurol. 13, (1), 41–45 (1980)
14. Hassler, O.: Experimentally carotid ligation followed by aneurysmal formation and other morphological changes in the circle of Willis. J. Neurosurg. 20, 1–7 (1963)
15. Hosobuchi, Y.: Direct surgical treatment of giant intracranial aneurysms. J. Neurosurg. 51, 743–756 (1979)
16. Klemme, M.W.: Hemorrhage from a previously undemonstrated intracranial aneurysm as a late complication of carotid artery ligation. J. Neurosurg. 46, 654–658 (1977)
17. Odom, G.L., Woodhall, B., Tindall, G.T. et al.: Changes in distal intravascular pressure and size of intracranial aneurysm following common carotid ligation. J. Neurosurg. 19, 41–50 (1962)
18. Petit Perrin, D., Aubin, M.L., Vignaud, J.: Apport de la scanographie au diagnostic des anévrysmes géants intra-crâniens. C.T. Findings in giant intracranial aneurysms. Neuroradiology. 6, 317–326 (1979)
19. Pia, H.W.: Large and giant aneurysms. Neurosurg. Rev. 3, 7–16 (1980)
20. Shiobara, R., Shigeo, T., Shigemaru, M., Ziro, T.: Surgery of posterior communicating artery aneurysms that enlarge after common carotid ligation. J. Neurosurg. 52, 116–119 (1980)
21. Sindou, M., Brunon, J., Fischer, G., Goutelle, A., Mansuy, L.: L'anastomose extra intra cranienne préalable à la ligature de la carotide. Intérêt à propos d'un cas d'anévrysme traumatique de la carotide interne cervicale. Neurochirurgie 23, (3), 205–213 (1977)

22. Spetzler, F.R., Schuster, H., Roski, R.A.: Elective extracranial intracranial arterial by-pass in the treatment of inoperable giant aneurysms of the internal carotid artery. J. Neurosurg. *53*, 22−27 (1980)
23. Sundt, T.M., Piepgras, D.G.: Surgical approach to giant intracranial aneurysms. Operative experience with 80 cases. J. Neurosurg. *51*, 731−742 (1979)
24. Suzuki, J., Ohara, H.: Clinicopathological study of cerebral aneurysms. Origin rupture, repair and growth. J. Neurosurg. *48*, 505−514 (1978)
25. Winn, H.R., Richarson, A.E., Jane, J.A.: Late morbidity and mortality of common carotid ligation for posterior communicating aneurysms. A comparison of conservative treatment. J. Neurosurg. *47*, 727−736 (1977)
26. Yasargil, M.G.: Microsurgery applied to neurosurgery. New York: Academic Press 1969

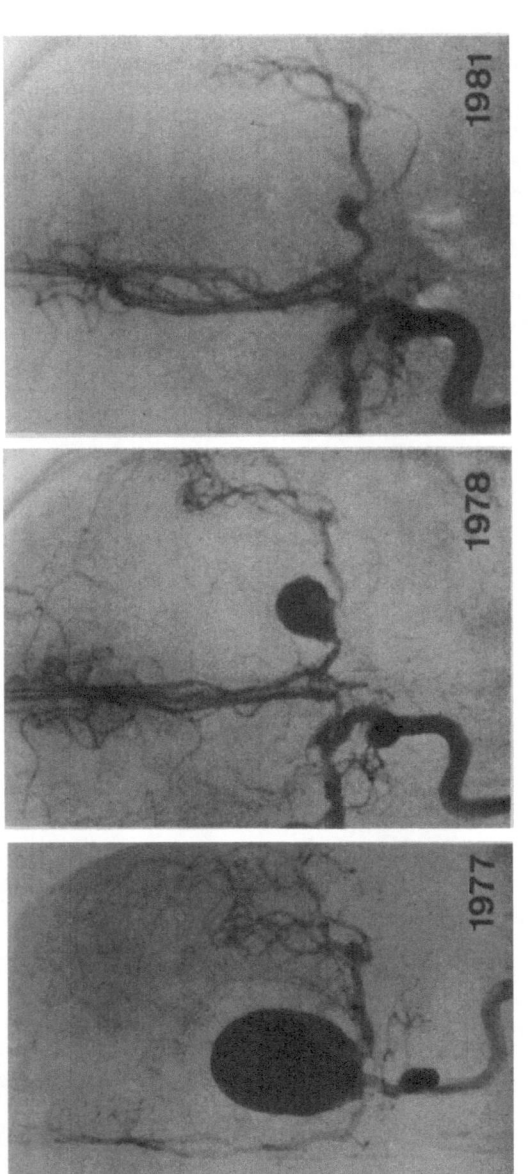

Fig. 1. Three years follow-up of a left carotid bifurcation giant aneurysm (case 1) treated by carotid occlusion

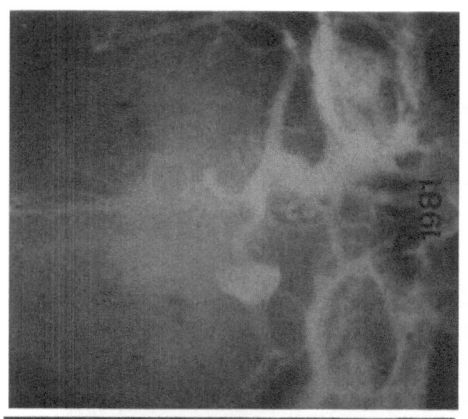
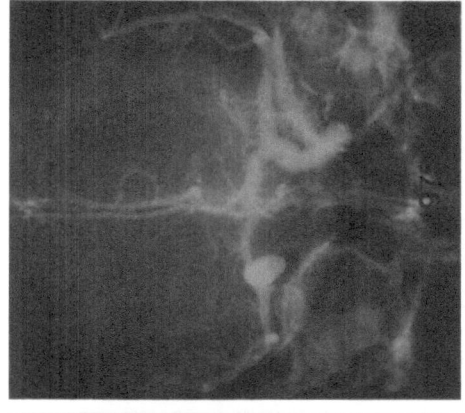
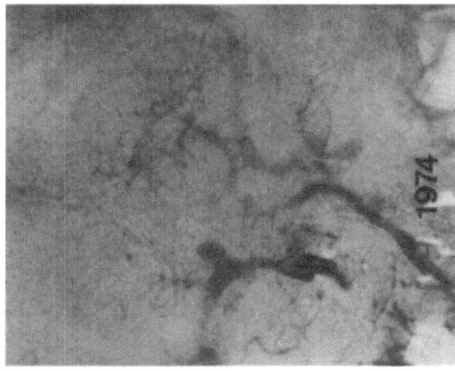

Fig. 2. Right carotid bifurcation aneurysm who enlarges after carotid occlusion (case 2)

415

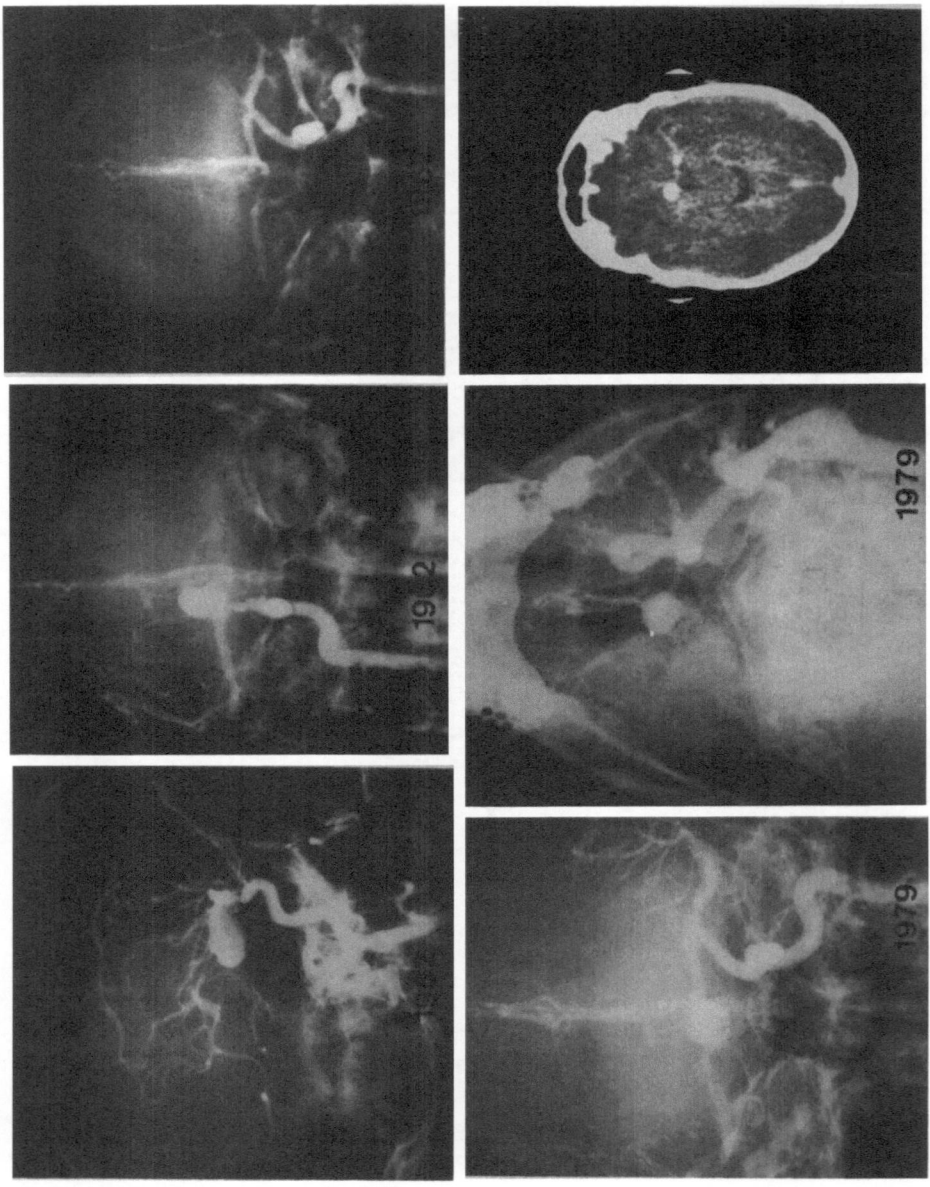

Fig. 3. *Above:* right posterior communicating giant aneurysm with normal anterior communicating artery (case 5). *Below:* iatrogenic anterior communicating aneurysm 17 years after right carotid occlusion (case 5)

The Natural History of Cerebral Aneurysms:
The Rate of Late Rebleeding

H.R. Winn, A.E. Richardson, and J.A. Jane

Introduction

Previous studies attempting to define the natural history of ruptured cerebral aneurysms have, in general, concentrated on the short-term outcome and have concluded that the risk of further haemorrhage and death was greatest in the first few weeks after the initial haemorrhage. Subsequent to this acute time period, the rate of rebleeding and death was assumed to be minimal, thus leaving the patient who survived the initial hemorrhage at low risk.

However, recent (10–15) long-term evaluations of aneurysm patients treated by conservative means have indicated that the survivors continue to remain at risk of suffering a further haemorrhage even years after their initial haemorrhage. Thus, cerebral aneurysms should not be considered an acute phenomenon, but a chronic disease. The present chapter will review these studies, and stress the late rebleeding rate during the first decade after the initial haemorrhage.

Material and Approach

Patients

Six hundred and eighty-five patients from the Atkinson Morley's Hospital and the National Hospital at Queen Square, described in previous publications (3–9), provided data for the assessment of the long-term prognosis of ruptured intracranial aneurysms. All patients suffered a subarachnoid haemorrhage (SAH), as documented by lumbar puncture, and the aetiology was confirmed by arteriography. All patients were treated by bed rest. Many of the patients were assigned to conservative therapy as part of a randomized treatment trial (3–6). After six months, 383 patients remained alive (Table 1). These 383 patients were then followed at yearly intervals to determine the rate of late haemorrhage. We have (12, 13) defined late haemorrhage as a SAH which occurs more than six months after the initial bleeding episode. In general, late rebleeding occurred at a rate of at least 3% per year, irrespective of site or multiplicity. Each site will be considered, but because the anterior circulation has been more extensively studied, anterior cerebral artery (ACA) and posterior cerebral artery (PCA) aneurysms will be stressed.

Table 1. Late rebleeding in patients treated for initial SAH with 6 weeks of bedrest

Aneurysm location	No. of patients alive at 6 months	Patients suffering late haemorrhage
ACA/PCA	213	61 (29%)
MCA	75	23 (31%)
VBA	25	9 (36%)
Multiple	70	21 (30%)

ACA= anterior communicating artery aneurysms; PCA= posterior communicating artery aneurysms; PCA= posterior communicating artery aneurysms; MCA= middle cerebral artery aneurysms; VBA= vertebral/basilar artery aneurysms

Results

Anterior Circulation

At six months, a total of 213 patients with ACA and PCA aneurysms were available for study. Some of the patients were followed for up to 21 years (11, 12, 14, 15). Initially, we analyzed only the first 10 years in detail (14). The number of ACA and PCA patients lost to follow-up over the first ten years was 26 out of 213 (12%).

Of the 213 survivors at six months, 54 patients rebled during the first ten years and 61 (29%) patients rebled over the entire duration of the follow-up period (average duration= 8.4 years). Figure 1 [1] illustrates that the peak incidence of rebleeding centred around year 3. The peak was noted for both ACA and PCA aneurysms. Symptom-free intervals of more than ten years were noted in seven cases.

Figure 2 illustrates the late rebleed rates for ACA and PCA patients between one and ten years after the initial haemorrhage. In an attempt to develop maximal and minimal yearly rebleed rates, patients lost to follow-up were assumed either to have rebled in the year lost or to be alive and free from subsequent subarachnoid hemorrhage. Obviously, the former assumption (that those patients lost to follow-up have rebled in the year in which they were lost) accounts for the highest rate of rebleeding, whereas the latter assumption (that those patients lost to follow-up were alive and did not rebleed) accounts for the lowest rate of rebleeding. The actual rate of rebleeding will fall between the two extremes and, in general, averages 3% per year.

In Fig. 3, the rate of rebleeding during the acute phase for ACA and PCA patients, as measured in days, is contrasted with the rate of rebleeding during the long-term follow-up, as measured in years. ACA and PCA aneurysms had similar late rebleeding rates. Subsequent analysis of ACA patients revealed that the rebleeding rate persisted unchanged into the second decade (14).

Of 61 patients suffering a late haemorrhage, 37 died as a result of their initial late rebleed. Thus, late rebleeding was fatal in 67% of all cases, and the yearly fatal late rebleed rate averaged 2% per year. Second and third late rebleeding episodes in four ACA and PCA patients were uniformly fatal.

[1] Figs. 1–4 with permission of the *Annals of Neurology*

An additional 25 patients died of causes not associated with late rebleeding. The overall death rate (late rebleed deaths, plus non-late rebleed deaths) was then calculated and compared to expected mortality for a similar population matched with regard to age and sex. A statistical difference at five and ten years was evident (Fig. 4).

Late Rebleeding Rates at Other Aneurysm Sites

Table 1 documents the total percentages of late rebleeding at all sites. The rates did not differ with respect to location of the original ruptured aneurysm. Moreover, fatal late re rebleeding occurs at a similar rate (60–70%) with all aneurysm sites.

The reader should note that the presence of multiple aneurysms in non-surgically treated patients did not increase the risk of a late haemorrhage. In the 21 patients with multiple aneurysms suffering a late haemorrhage, there was no evidence that an intact aneurysm had ruptured. Therefore, late haemorrhage in patients with multiple aneurysms is, in fact, a late rebleed. The aneurysms which originally ruptured can be thought of as the weakest link in a chain and destined to be the site of future rupture in untreated patients. In patients with multiple aneurysms in whom the ruptured aneurysm is treated by direct operation, intact aneurysms rupture at approximately a third (1%) of the yearly late rebleed rate associated with single ruptured aneurysms treated by bed rest (11).

Characteristics of Late Rebleeding Patients

Having defined the rate of late haemorrhage, we then attempted to determine if there were any distinguishing characteristics which would predict which patients would suffer a late rebleed.

Factors such as age, sex, blood pressure on admission and during subsequent examination, neurological state and size of the aneurysm were examined. Hypertension increased the risk of a late haemorrhage in patients with PCA and multiple aneurysms. In addition, PCA females were at additional risk.

There was no relationship between the patients' age and the occurrence of either non-fatal or fatal late haemorrhage. This is illustrated in Table 2 which considers only ACA and PCA patients, but is true for all other locations and presence of multiplicity. Thus, youth does not confer any immunity to late rebleeding if the follow-up is long enough. However, a highly significant relationship was found by plotting patients' age against the time to late rebleed (Table 3). The average time to rebleed for patients less than 40 years old was found to be almost ten years, whereas that of patients older than 40 years was 4.4 years.

The size of the aneurysm found by arteriography at the time of the original SAH did not correlate with subsequent late rebleeding. In order to answer the question whether change in size of the aneurysm would predict subsequent late haemorrhage, 60 patients, all with ACA aneurysms, routinely had arteriography performed six months after the original haemorrhage. No statistical correlation could be found between the subsequent late haemorrhage and changes in the size of the aneurysm in these 60 patients (Table 4). However, an additional 17 patients had arteriography at the time of their subsequent

Table 2. Relationship of patient age to occurrence of late haemorrhage (ACA and PCA patients)

0–30 years	31–40 years	41–50 years	51–60 years	61–73 years	Total
5/10	9/34	16/52	23/76	8/33	61/213
(28%)	(26%)	(30%)	(30%)	(24%)	(29%)

Table 3

Age of patient (n)	Average time to late rebleed (years)
⟨ 40 years (17)	9.8
⟩ 40 years (44)	4.4 [a]

[a] $p < 0.001$ by t-test

Table 4. Change in aneurysm (ACA) size as judged by arteriography 6 months after initial haemorrhage

Arteriographic finding	No. of patients	No. with subsequent late haemorrhage
Increase in size	21	6 (29%)
No change	28	11 (39%)
Decrease in size	11	1 (9%)
Total	60	18

late haemorrhage (1–9 years after initial haemorrhage). All 17 of these patients, in contrast to the patients arteriogrammed routinely at six months, showed an increase in aneurysm size compared with the size in the original arteriography.

Conclusion

The data we have analyzed indicate that the late rebleeding rate in conservatively treated patients averages 3% per year, with a fatal rebleed rate of 2% annually during the first decade. Late rebleeding is defined as subarachnoid haemorrhage occurring more than six months after the initial bleeding episode. Such an event was thought to be rare, but additional reports (1, 2) support our earlier findings.

Studies of the natural history of cerebral aneurysms have been confined in large part to the acute period after subarachnoid haemorrhage and have had varied success in defining factors related to rebleeding. In a similar fashion, surgical series have, in general, dealt with the short-term prognosis. Although a ruptured cerebral aneurysm has previously been considered an acute entity, the evidence of a constant yearly rebleed rate of 3% in conservatively managed patients emphasizes the chronicity of this disease process. Therefore assessment of treatment for cerebral aneurysms must no longer deal merely with the short-term prognosis.

References

1. Henderson, W.G., Torner, J.C., Nibbelink, D.W.: Intracranial aneurysms and subarachnoid hemorrhage. Report on a randomized treatment study. Stroke 8, 579–589 (1977)
2. Kaste, M., Troupp, H.: Subarachnoid haemorrhage: Long-term follow-up results of late surgical versus conservative treatment. Brit. Med. J. 1, 1310–1311 (1978)
3. McKissock, W., Richardson, A., Walsh, L.: "Posterior communicating" aneurysms: a controlled trial of the conservative and surgical treatment of ruptured aneurysms of the internal carotid artery at or near the point of origin of the posterior communicating artery. Lancet 1, 1203–1206 (1960)
4. McKissock, W., Richardson, A., Walsh, L.: Middle cerebral aneurysms. Further results in the controlled trial of conservative and surgical treatment of ruptured intracranial aneurysms. Lancet 2, 417–421 (1962)
5. McKissock, W., Richardson, A., Walsh, L.: Anterior communicating aneurysms: trial of conservative and surgical treatment. Lancet 1, 873–876 (1965)
6. McKissock, W., Richardson, A., Walsh, L., Owens, E.: Multiple intracranial aneurysms. Lancet 1, 623–626 (1964)
7. Richardson, A.E.: Surgery of basilar aneurysms. Psychiatria, Neurologia, Neurochirurgia 75, 441–443 (1972)
8. Richardson, A.E., Jane, J.A., Payne, P.M.: Assessment of the natural history of anterior communicating aneurysms. J. Neurosurg. 21, 266–274 (1964)
9. Richardson, A.E., Jane, J.A., Yashon, D.: Prognostic factors in the untreated course of posterior communicating aneurysms. Arch. Neurol. 14, 172–176 (1966)
10. Winn, H.R., Berga, S.L., Richardson, A.E., Jane, J.A., Waldman, M.T., O'Brien, W.M.: The natural history of vertebral basilar (VBA) aneurysms. (Abstract) Stroke 12, 120 (1981)
11. Winn, H.R., Berga, S.L., Richardson, A.E., Waldman, M.T., O'Brien, W.M., Jane, J.A.: Long-term evaluation of patients with multiple cerebral aneurysms. (Abstract) Annals of Neurol. 10, 106 (1981)
12. Winn, H.R., Richardson, A.E., Jane, J.A.: Late morbidity and mortality in cerebral aneurysms: a ten year follow-up of 364 conservatively treated patients with a single cerebral aneurysm. Trans. Amer. Neurol. Assn. 98, 23–24 (1973)
13. Winn, H.R., Richardson, A.E., Jane, J.A.: The long-term prognosis in untreated cerebral aneurysms: I. The incidence of late hemorrhage in cerebral aneurysm: A 10-year evaluation of 364 patients. Annals of Neurol. 1, 358–370 (1977)
14. Winn, H.R., Richardson, A.E., Jane, J.A.: Fifteen-year rebleed rate in 258 nonsurgically treated patients with a single anterior communicating artery aneurysm. (Abstract) Neurosurg. 2, 165 (1978)
15. Winn, H.R., Richardson, A.E., O'Brien, W., Jane, J.A.: The long-term prognosis in untreated cerebral aneurysms: II. Late morbidity and mortality. Annals of Neurol. 4, 418–426 (1978)

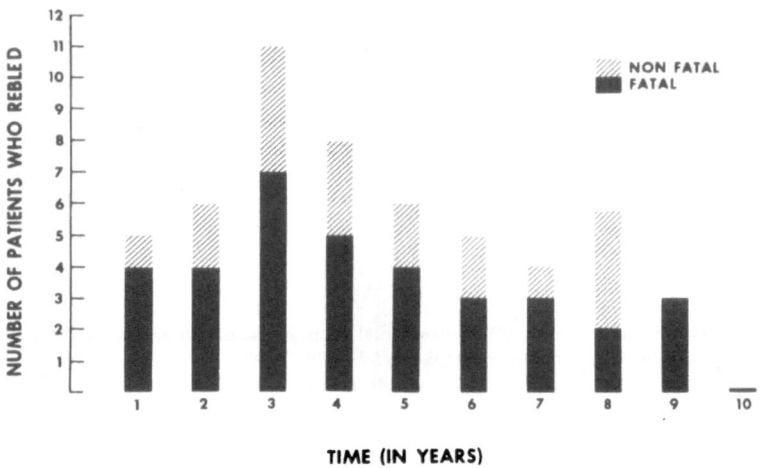

Fig. 1. Number of patients with ACA or PCA aneurysms who rebled within each year during the first decade. Seven rebleeds were noted during the second decade (13)

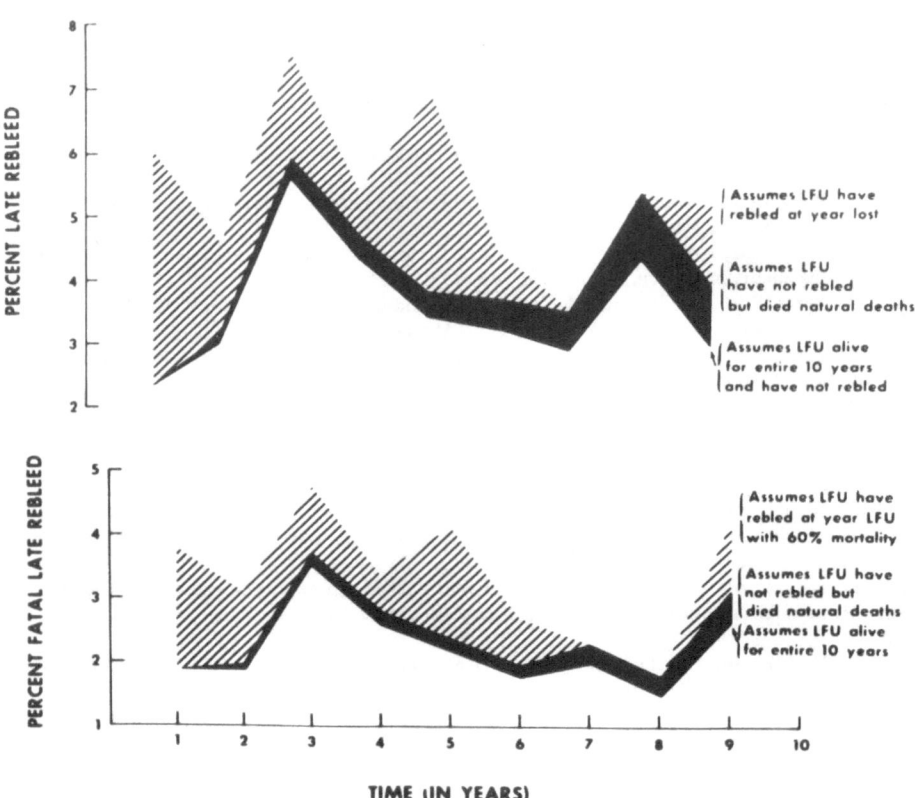

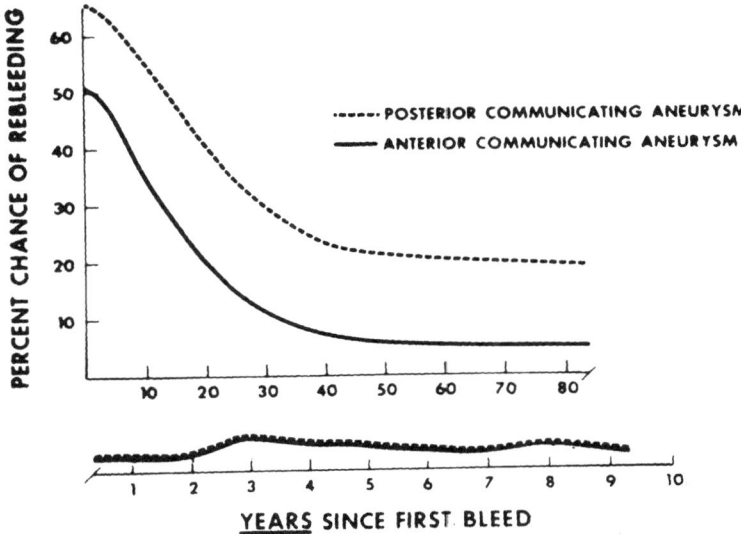

Fig. 3. Rate of rebleeding during the acute period measured in days contrasted with the long-term course measured in years (13)

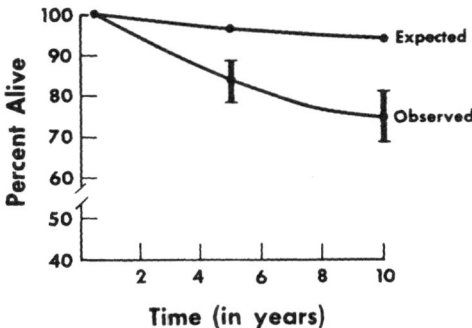

Fig. 4. Expected vs. observed mortality for ACA and PCA patients. Expected survival was based on a life insurance table for a similar population by age and sex (15)

Fig. 2. Percentage of ACA and PCA patients rebleeding in each year. Upper graph represents total late rebleeds; lower graph represents fatal late rebleeds. The lower limit on each graph assumes that the patients lost to follow-up (LFU) are alive. The intermediate limit assumes that the patients LFU have died natural deaths (i.e., not related to subarachnoid hemorrhage); upper limit assumes that patients LFU have bled in the year lost (13)

Early Operation on Ruptured Cerebral Aneurysms –
Results of 120 Cases Operated on Within One Week After SAH

I. Saito, K. Aritake, and K. Sano

Introduction

For cases with ruptured cerebral aneurysms in the acute stage, or still suffering the effects of subarachnoid haemorrhage (SAH), the question of whether to operate or not is a controversial problem.

The most important purpose of operating on ruptured cerebral aneurysms is to prevent their rebleeding. The Cooperative study (7) in the United States showed that the rate of rebleeding was highest at around 7 days after the onset of SAH. Therefore, theoretically, operation on ruptured aneurysms should be done as early as possible after SAH. Since the beginning of 1970, microsurgery was introduced in our operations on cerebral aneurysms and we actively performed early operations on ruptured aneurysms. In May, 1972, at the first Conference of Surgical Treatment of Stroke in Japan, we reported our experiences of early operations on ruptured aneurysms and the following was the conclusion: In the early stage, the operative results, did not always depend upon the grade of patients. Four out of six operative deaths among 22 cases operated on within two weeks after SAH was due to postoperative vasospasm and these four cases were all submitted to surgery for aneurysm between day 3 and day 7 (the day of SAH was counted as day 0). In contrast, in cases operated on on day 0, 1 and 2, the intervention was well tolerated except patients in Grade 5 according to Hunt's system. These results were explained as follows (16): Vasospasm in the natural course of SAH appeared frequently after day 5 and was never found earlier than day 4. The substances causing vasospasm are probably produced in the latter half of the first week after SAH and the cerebral arteries are inclined to vasospasm in this period. Therefore, operations between day 3 and 7 after SAH may enhance the anticipated vasospasm. In operations performed within 3 days of the SAH, on the other hand, extravasated blood clots could be easily removed from the area of the cerebral arteries, and the postoperative vasospasm tends not to develop and, if present, is mild.

Since those days, our policy of treatment for ruptured aneurysms in the acute stage is as follows:

1. In the first 3 days after SAH, all cases are indicated for direct surgical intervention on the aneurysm except cases in neurological Grade 5.
2. Between day 3 and day 7 after SAH, the period of incipient vasospasm, cases in Grade 3 or 4 are treated with administration of antifibrinolytic agents and direct operation is postponed until they show improvement in their neurological condition.

    Modern Neurosurgery 1. Edited by M. Brock

3. In the second week, that is to say, the period of the vasospasm, any patient who demonstrates neurological deterioration is submitted to angiography in order to detect vasospasm. If vasospasm is shown in the angiogram, aneurysm surgery is postponed until the patient begins to show an improved state of consciousness. Direct operation should not be delayed more than two weeks after the onset of the vasospasm because of the danger of rebleeding when vasospasm subsides.

In this paper, the authors analysed 120 cases submitted to surgical treatment within 1 week of SAH comparing them with cases operated on later than 1 week. They discuss the indications for operation on ruptured aneurysms in the acute stage and possibility of prevention of vasospasm by early operation on aneurysms.

Clinical Material and Method

During last 10 years (January, 1970 to June, 1980), a total of 529 cases with ruptured aneurysms underwent direct operations using microsurgical technique at the University of Tokyo Hospital and its two affiliated hospitals. One of the authors took part in all of these operations. Of these 529 cases, 120 cases were operated on within one week of the SAH. These cases were submitted to operation immediately after admission or on the following day, and their Grade at operation was, in most cases, the same as that on admission. The clinical grade in this evaluation is that of Hunt (5) and adjustment of grade proposed in his original classification, however, has been made only in the presence of cerebral vasospasm on pre-operative angiograms, but not in light of hypertension or other coexistent systemic diseases.

In the early operation on ruptured aneurysms, the steps carried out are as follows: In the case of an aneurysm of the anterior circle of Willis, a little larger craniotomy is used compared with the usual small one after Yasargil (pterional approach). After opening the dura a silicone-rubber tube is inserted into the lateral ventricle and CSF is aspirated to the amount of 50 to 80 ml in order to obtain a slack brain. By this procedure, we can get a space large enough to approach the ruptured aneurysm in all cases. This tube is usually used as a ventricular drain postoperatively in order to control intracranial pressure (ICP). Operations are usually performed under normotension and normothermia and temporary clips are used for less than 10 minutes when the aneurysm shows rupture or leakage due to bleeding. In the 120 cases operated on within one week of the SAH, clipping of the ruptured aneurysm was feasible in all cases. After clipping the neck of the aneurysm, as much as possible of the subarachnoid clot is removed by suction and irrigation with saline (18). In the case of aneurysms of the anterior circle of Willis, the chiasmatic and interpeduncular cisterns and the Sylvian fissure of the operated side are opened in order to remove the clots. Before closure of the dura, 2% of Papaverin Hydrochloride is topically applied to the parent artery and main branches of the cerebral arteries. This drug can easily relieve any traumatic vasospasm induced by the early operation on the aneurysm.

For operations in the acute stage, we have routinely set up three kinds of drainage systems (16). The above-mentioned ventricular drain is placed for as long as two weeks for control of ICP postoperatively. A cisternal and an epidural drainage system is used for removal of blood from the basal cisterns for about 3 to 7 days after operation and from the epidural space of the operated area for a short time, respectively.

Results

The operative mortality (the deaths of patients occurring after operation and while still in hospital) of microsurgery performed within the first week of SAH was 12.5%, whereas that of operations done later than the first week was as low as 3.9%, the total operative mortality in 529 cases being 5.8%. Therefore, the operative mortality after the first week was about one-third of that within the first week. This difference was most marked in the internal carotid-posterior communicating aneurysms and the anterior communicating aneurysms (20.7% and 2.9% in the former and 8.6% and 5.1% in the latter).

Furthermore, in Table 1 the follow-up results of cases operated on within one week of SAH were detailed and compared with cases operated on later. The first week is divided into two periods, from day 0 (the day of aneurysmal rupture) to day 2 (48 hours after SAH) and from day 3 to day 7. Patients in Grade 1–2 showed excellent results regardless of timing of operation: in cases operated on within one week of the SAH, operative mortality was only 1.4% and the working rate in the follow-up (cases back to their previous occupations) was 93.2%. In contrast, follow-up results of cases in Grade 3 were varied. The working rate of cases operated on between day 3 and day 7 was statistically low as compared to cases operated on earlier or later than this period. This difference is chiefly due to development of postoperative vasospasm as mentioned above. Patients in Grade 4 within one week of the SAH usually show grave neurological symptoms pre-operatively caused by intracerebral haematoma or severe SAH and accordingly operative results were not good. All five cases with intracerebral haematoma as illustrated in Fig. 1 showed smooth postoperative courses and residual neurological deficits attributable to the haematoma determined the final outcome of patients. In contrast, three patients with severe SAH (Fig. 1) or intraventricular haematoma showed a deterioration of neurological state postoperatively due to development of vasospasm and died or became vegetative. In severe SAH, washout of cisternal blood-clots by early operation was incomplete and could not prevent development of severe vasospasms. Three out of 4 cases in Grade 4 submitted to operation between day 3 and day 7 were able to return to their previous occupations. These three cases showed pre-operatively a local type of vasospasm (16) which was not aggravated postoperatively. When cases in Grade 1 to 3 are surveyed, follow-up results of cases operated on within one week of the SAH are as good as those of cases submitted to operation later, except cases in Grade 3 operated upon between day 3 and day 7 as seen in the lowest row (N.B.) in Table 1.

Table 2 shows the relationship between the timing of operation and results in the two age groups, below and above 60 years of age. In cases operated on within 3 days and later than the 2nd week after SAH, the working rate was statistically higher among the younger patients. These results seem to derive from the fact that older patients could not easily recover from grave conditions caused by post- or preoperative vasospasm, intracerebral haematomas and other problems.

In Table 3, causes of mortality and morbidity in cases which could not return to useful social lives are shown. In cases undergoing operation on the aneurysm less than one week after SAH, intracerebral haematoma and postoperative vasospasm were the main causes of their mortality and morbidity. In the second week, intraoperative troubles such as premature rupture of aneurysms or clipping of vital arteries prevented patients

Table 1. Microsurgery of ruptured aneurysms. Timing, grade at operation and follow-up results (529 cases)

| | 1st week after SAH | | | | | | | | | | 2nd week after SAH | | | | | Later than 2nd week | | | | |
| | Day 0–2 | | | | | Day 3–7 | | | | | | | | | | | | | | |
Grade	Cases	Op. mt.	Wor-king	Caring for self	BD	Cases	Op. mt.	Wor-king	Caring for self	BD	Cases	Op. mt.	Wor-king	Caring for self	BD	Cases	Op. mt.	Wor-king	Caring for self	BD
I	3	0	3	0	0	5	0	5	0	0	17	0	15	2	0	267	5	236	16	10
II	30	1	27	2	0	35	0	33	1	1	19	0	18	0	1	28	3	23	0	2
III	13	0	11 a	2	0	14	5	5 a,b	3	1	26	1	24 b	1	0	25	1	16	1	7
IV	9	2	3	2	2	4	1	3	0	0	13	2	8	1	2	13	3	4	3	3
V	4	3	0	0	1	3	3	0	0	0	1	1	0	0	0	0	0	0	0	0
Total 59		6	44	6	3	61	9	46	4	2	76	4	65	4	3	333	12	279	20	22
		10.1%	74.6%	10.2%	5.1%		14.8%	75.4%	6.6%	3.3%		5.3%	85.5%	5.3%	3.9%		3.6%	83.8%	6.0%	6.6%

N.B.

	Cases	Op. mt.	Wor-king	Caring for self	BD	Cases	Op. mt.	Wor-king	Caring for self	BD	Cases	Op. mt.	Wor-king	Caring for self	BD	Cases	Op. mt.	Wor-king	Caring for self	BD
Grade I–III	46	1	41	4	0	54	5	43	4	2	62	1	57	4	0	320	9	275	17	19
Cases	(2.2%)		(89.1%)			(9.3%)		(79.6%)			(1.6%)		(91.9%)			(2.8%)		(85.9%)		

Op.mt.= operative mortality; BD= bed-ridden (20 cases) and died of other diseases after discharge (10 cases)

a p < 0.05. b p < 0.01

427

Table 2 Grade I–IV cases of ruptured aneurysm. Age, timing of microsurgery and results

Age	Timing of operation		Cases	Op. mt.	Working	Caring for self	BD
59 years	1st week	Day 0–2	39	0	35 [a](89.7%)	3(7.7%)	1(2.6%)
		Day 3–7	48	4(8.3%)	38 (79.2%)	4(8.3%)	2(4.2%)
	2nd week after SAH		57	2(3.4%)	52 (88.1%)	3(5.1%)	2(3.4%)
	Later than 2nd week		274	7(2.6%)	236 [a](86.1%)	14(5.1%)	17(6.2%)
	Subtotal		420	13(3.1%)	361 (86.0%)	24(5.7%)	22(5.2%)
60 years	1st week	Day 0–2	16	2(18.8%)	9 [a](56.3%)	3(18.8%)	1(6.3%)
		Day 3–7	10	2(20.0%)	8 (80.0%)	0	0
	2nd week after SAH		16	1(6.3%)	13 (81.3%)	1(6.3%)	1(6.3%)
	Later than 2nd week		59	5(8.5%)	43 [a](72.9%)	6(10.2%)	5(8.5%)
	Subtotal		101	11(10.9%)	73 (72.3%)	10(9.9%)	7(6.4%)
Grand Total			521	24(4.6%)	434 (83.3%)	34(6.5%)	29(5.6%)

Op.mt.= operative mortality; BD= bed-ridden (19 cases) and died of other diseases after discharge (10 cases)

[a] p < 0.01

Table 3. Causes of mortality and morbidity in those cases which could not return to social lives

	Cases	Intra-cerebral haematoma	Pre-op. and postop. vasospasm	Fixed deficit	Intraoperative troubles			Postop. compli-cations	Other disease	Others
					Rupture of aneurysm	Clipping of vital artery	Others			
1st week										
Day 0–2	15	5	9	0	1	0	0	0	0	0
Day 3–7	15	2	9	0	3	0	0	0	0	1
Subtotal	30	7(23.3%)	18(60.0%)	0	4(13.3%)	0	0	0	0	1
2nd week	10	0	3(30.0%)	2	2	2	1	0	0	0
Later than 2nd week	54	1	16(29.6%)	11(20.3%)	5(9.3%)	3	6	6(11.1%)	5(9.3%)	1
Total	94	8(8.5%)	37(39.4%)	13(13.8%)	11(11.7%)	5(5.3%)	7(7.4%)	6(6.4%)	5(5.3%)	2(2.1%)

50.0% 25.9% 24.5%

Table 4. Intra-operative and postoperative complications (in 120 cases)

1. Intra-operative rupture of aneurysms	
Massive bleeding	6(5.0%)
Leakage	23(19.2%)
2. Postoperative complications	
Vasospasm	43(38.1%) [a]
NPH	29(24.2%)
hyponatraemia (Na⟨130meq)	39(32.5%)
GI bleeding	5(4.8%)

[a] 7 cases with pre-operative vasospasm were excluded

from resuming normal lives. Meanwhile, regarding cases operated on later than the second week after SAH, pre-operative vasospasm, fixed neurological deficits, intra-operative troubles and postoperative complications such as meningitis, electrolyte inbalance and so on, are roughly equal and patients were not able to return to their normal lives.

Intra-operative and postoperative complications in cases operated on less than one week after SAH are listed in Table 4. Intraoperative rupture of aneurysms usually occurred during dissection of an aneurysmal neck or application of clips to the neck of the aneurysm. However, in one case with anterior communicating aneurysms submitted to operation in Grade 2 on day 1, massive bleeding from the aneurysm occurred when the frontal lobe was slightly elevated by a spatula and the patient finally died. Five out of six cases showing massive bleeding were fatal. But, there were no deaths in 23 cases showing leakage from an aneurysm, which was easily controlled by surgicel or temporary clips. Postoperative vasospasm developed in 38.1% of patients. The incidence of vasospasm in relation to clinical grade occurred as follows: Grade 1, 0%: Grade 2, 32.3%: Grade 3, 58.3%: Grade 4, 40%. Hyponatraemia (Na ⟨ 130mEq) mainly due to SIADH (syndrome of inappropriate secretion of antidiuretic hormone) usually occurred in association with postoperative vasospasm. Normal pressure hydrocephalus (NPH) developed in 24.2% of cases around the fourth week after SAH (19).

The purpose of early operation on ruptured aneurysms is to prevent not only rebleeding of aneurysms but also the development of vasospasm. As we already reported, if early operation on ruptured aneurysms within three days of the SAH can sufficiently wash out the cisternal clots surrounding the cerebral arteries, postoperative vasospasm will not develop or if present will be mild (17). Incidence of postoperative vasospasm in cases operated on within the first 3 days and that of pre-operative vasospasm which occurred in the natural course of SAH in cases remaining through the 2nd week after SAH are compared. Postoperative vasospasm developed in 35.8% of patients excluding three patients in Grade 5 and two cases with pre-operative vasospasm showing rebleeding. This 35.8% incidence of postoperative vasospasm is a little lower than that of pre-operative vasospasm (45.0%—54 in 120 cases), but there is no statistical difference between them. Furthermore, even if only severe vasospasm which produces death or permanent neurological deficits is considered, it is not yet possible to say that postoperative vasospasm (17.0%) has a lower incidence than pre-operative vasospasm (20.3%).

Discussion

Our early operation on ruptured cerebral aneurysms which has been performed is based upon four important points: namely, *(1)* ventricular tap and aspiration of CSF to obtain a slack brain immediately after dural opening, *(2)* illumination and magnification by surgical microscope, *(3)* washout of blood-clots surrounding the cerebral arteries after clipping of aneurysms, and *(4)* three kinds of drainages in the postoperative period. In all 120 cases operated on within one week of the SAH, clipping of the aneurysmal neck was completed. Sixty-eight patients (93%) out of 73 cases submitted to operation on aneurysms in Grade 1 or 2 returned to normal lives and there was only one death (1.4%) and four poor results (6.8%). Regarding 27 cases in Grade 3, sixteen (59%) returned to useful lives and five (18.5%) died: among 13 cases operated on within 3 days of bleeding, eleven (84.6%) returned to their previous work: whereas only five out of 14 cases operated on between day 3 and day 7 returned to their previous work, and the remaining nine cases showed poor results or died due to development of severe postoperative vasospasm. In patients in Grade 4, six (46%) of 13 cases were able to return to work and the prognosis of these patients was determined by the pre-operative neurological conditions due to intracerebral haematoma or postoperative vasospasm. In total, excluding seven cases in pre-operative Grade 5, we were able to return ninety (79.6%) out of 113 cases to their normal lives, with an operative mortality of 8%, by early operation on ruptured aneurysms within one week of the SAH.

Around the 1950's and 1960's, direct attack on ruptured aneurysms in the acute stage had been considered very dangerous. The reasons were increased ICP caused by presence of blood in the subarachnoid space or clots in the brain substance and the intense vasoconstriction supposed to be nearly always present shortly after SAH (9). Moreover, it was shown that if there was no selection of the better patients for operation, the patients' chances of recovery were as good with or without operation, except those cases with a large intracerebral haematoma in this acute stage (8). Therefore, the methods of treatment of ruptured cerebral aneurysms in those days, for the most part, had been directed at the prevention of recurrent bleeding among 70% of patients who survived the initial haemorrhage and also the prevention of neurological disability caused by repeated bleeding (12). These principles for the treatment of ruptured aneurysms seem to prevail even now in most clinics in the world. However, increased ICP is not an annoying condition because it can be controlled easily by a ventricular tap as mentioned above. Vasoconstriction or vasospasm is recently recognized as a phenomenon not present immediately after bleeding of aneurysms and early operations, particularly in the first three days after SAH, are not affected by vasospasm.

As for the timing of operation on ruptured aneurysms, many authors propose various optimal times for operation. Pool (11) recommended from the 7th day to the 9th day inclusive as an ideal time after SAH and mentioned that too early an operation (within six days) resulted in a forbiddingly high mortality [14 deaths (43%) in 32 cases with anterior communicating aneurysm], while this optimal time from the 7th to the 9th day inclusive resulted in a 17% mortality rate for the operation. Rowe (15) proposed 10 to 14 days after SAH and emphasized that this practice might reduce the operative mortality and the death of patients from rebleeding during the second and third week. Drake (2) also recommends that an operation should be performed later than one week after SAH. There is a great danger of producing postoperative vasospasm, and the mortality in drowsy patients (in Grade 3) operated on in less than 7 days was 35%; after a week it was only 17%; similarly, in Grade 1 and 2, mortality was 3% after one week as compared to 12.5% under 7 days. It was suggested, on the other hand, that patients in Grade 1 or 2 should be operated on as soon as possible (1, 4). We have shown here that the final outcome of patients operated on within one week of the SAH, particularly within three days, is as good as that of operations carried out later than one week. A few authors evaluated the timing of operation in relation to the onset of vasospasm. Our ten years experience of the treatment of ruptured aneurysms in the acute stage has shown that the most important factor that exerts a crucial influence upon the prognosis, is the development of vasospasm in the course of treatment (16). When vasospasm occurs postoperatively, patients usually show a deterioration in their neurological state and often a fatal outcome. In contrast, the prognosis of patients is only determined by pre-operative states if vasospasm does not develop. Secondly, vasospasm after aneurysmal rupture is never seen until a few days after SAH, as already reported (16). Therefore, timing of operation for ruptured aneurysms should be divided into two periods, namely, during the first three days when vasospasm is never seen and between day 3 and day 7 when vasospasm is inclined to develop, or is already in its initial stage (incipient vasospasm which does not yet produce neurological symptoms) and will be aggravated by any operative intervention.

Our division of the first week after SAH into two periods is also associated with possibility of preventing vasospasm by operation within 3 days and washout of the cisternal clots which are now regarded as the most important factor producing the vasospasmodic substances. As mentioned before, the results obtained so far, do not show that postoperative vasospasm was definitely prevented, although vasospasm developing after operations within three days was mild, if present. On the other hand, correlation between development of postoperative vasospasm and subarachnoid clots was examined by computerized tomography (CT) and angiography carried out pre- and postoperatively, in regard to the 42 cases submitted to operation within five days of the SAH (Table 5). Bloodclots in the subarachnoid space were washed out during the operation and by cisternal drainage postoperatively. Postoperative CT, however, still showed the presence of high density areas (clots) in 21 cases and of these cases, eleven developed postoperative vasospasm and six showed slight narrowing of the arteries surrounded by clots. In contrast, of the 21 cases in which pre- and/or postoperative CT did not show a high density area in the cisterns, only three showed postoperative vasospasm (one case) or slight narrowing of the cerebral arteries (two cases). It can be said that these results sugest the possibility of prevention of vasospasm when early operation could wash out the subarachnoid clots completely. Johnson, et al. (6), advocated an early operation to remove the subarachnoid clot that might maintain vasospasm, and Pool (10) also recommended early operation to prevent vasospasm. Drake (3) commenting on early operation stated that aggressive conservative measures such as Amicar, blood pressure reduction and partial carotid clamping for carotid aneurysms should lower rebleeding to less than 10% and death even more in the first week or two. In view of this early operation would be best justified if it càn be shown to prevent, by the toilet of the subarachnoid spaces, the development of vasospasm and the wondered how complete this toilet can be through an ordinary craniotomy if the clot is spread diffusely. Up to now, it has not always been

Table 5. Subarachnoid blood clots on CT and development of vasospasm

	Pre-op. CT	Postop. CT	Vasospasm (+) Slight narrowing (−)		
		(+) 21	11	6	4
Blood Clots	(+) 36	(−) 11	1	1	9
	(−) 6	(−) 10	0	1	9

(In 42 cases submitted to operation within five days of the SAH)

feasible to prevent postoperative vasospasm by early operation and this is mainly due to technical limitations, whereby it is difficult to remove the clots from the Sylvian fissure on the other side and from the posterior part of the Sylvian fissure of the operated side, when the blood clots occupy all the cisterns as shown in Fig. 1.

Antifibrinolytic treatment does not always guarantee the stopping of rebleeding of cerebral aneurysms (14). Quite a few patients show vasospasm during this treatment and cannot then be submitted to operation (13). This study has reinforced our inclination toward early operation on ruptured aneurysms, but the experience of ten and a half years urges us make some change in the policy of treatment of ruptured aneurysms in the acute stage. New principles, particularly in the treatment of ruptured aneurysms within one week of the SAH, are as follows:

1. For cases in Grade 1 or 2, microsurgery can be safely indicated.
2. During the first three days (day 1, 2 and 3), cases in Grade 3 can be submitted to clipping of the aneurysmal neck and removal of the subarachnoid clots. In cases in Grade 4 with intracerebral haematoma as shown in Fig. 1, operation is also indicated and the prognosis will depend upon the site of the haematoma. However, for patients in Grade 4 in whom there are severe neurological conditions due to diffuse and extensive cisternal clots or ventricular rupture, operation should be postponed until they show an improvement in their disturbance of consciousness. Cases in Grade 3 or 4 and aged over 60 years should also be treated conservatively.
3. During day 3 to 7 after SAH, no cases in Grade 3 and 4 can be safely submitted to operation except those cases with intracerebral haematoma or a local type of vasospasm.

Conclusion

During the last ten and a half years, 120 cases with ruptured aneurysms were operated on within one week of SAH and altogether, excluding seven cases in pre-operative Grade 5, 90 (79.6%) could return to their normal lives, with an operative mortality of 8%. Pre-operative Grade and the timing of operation determined the final outcome of these patients: particularly cases in Grade 4 operated on within three days of the SAH, and cases in Grade 3 or 4 operated on between day 3 and day 7 showed poor operative results because of the development of postoperative vasospasm or the presence of intracerebral haematoma. Up to now, it has been difficult to prevent development of vasospasm by washout of the cisternal clots when most cisterns were diffusely occupied by blood-clots.

References

1. Dinning, T.A.R.: Timing of surgery for leaking cerebral aneurysm: clinical, radiological and radio-isotopic considerations. Proc. Aust. Assoc. Neurol. *9*, 219–226 (1973)
2. Drake, C.G.: Discussion of Hunt, W.E., Hess, R.M.: Surgical risk as related to time of intervention in the repair of intracranial aneurysms. J. Neurosurg. *28*, 14–20 (1968)
3. Drake, C.G.: Postoperative arterial spasm. In: Cerebral arterial spasm. Wilkins, R.H. (ed), pp. 435–437. Baltimore: Williams & Wilkins 1980
4. Hunt, W.E., Kosnik, E.J.: Timing and perioperative care in intracranial aneurysm surgery. Clin. Neurosurg. *21*, 79–89 (1974)
5. Hunt, W.E.: Grading of risk in intracranial aneurysms. In: Recent progress in neurological surgery. Sano, K., Ishii, S., Le Vay, D. (eds.), pp. 169–175. Amsterdam: Excerpta Medica 1974
6. Johnson, R.J., Potter, J.M., Reid, R.C.: Arterial spasm in subarachnoid haemorrhage: mechanical considerations. J. Neurol. Neurosurg. Psychiatry *21*, 68 (1958)
7. Locksley, H.B.: Report on the cooperative study of intracranial aneurysms and subarachnoid hemorrhage. Section V, Part II. Natural history of subarachnoid hemorrhage, intracranial aneurysms and arteriovenous malformation: Bases on 6368 cases in cooperative study. J. Neurosurg. *25*, 321–368 (1966)
8. McKissock, W., Paine, K.W.E., Walsh, L.S.: An analysis of the results of treatment of ruptured intracranial aneurysms. J. Neurosurg. *17*, 762–776 (1960)
9. Norlen, G., Olivecrona, H.: The treatment of aneurysms of the circle of Willis. J. Neurosurg. *10*, 404–415 (1953)
10. Pool, J.L.: Early treatment of ruptured intracranial aneurysms of the circle of Willis with special clip technique. Bull. NY. Acad. Med. *35*, 357–369 (1959)
11. Pool, J.L.: Timing and techniques in the intracranial surgery of ruptured aneurysms of the anterior communicating artery. J. Neurosurg. *19*, 378–388 (1962)
12. Poppen, J.L., Fager, C.A.: Intracranial aneurysms. Results of surgical-treatment. J. Neurosurg. *17*, 283–296 (1960)
13. Post, K.D., Flamm, E.S., Goodgold, A., Ransohoff, J.: Ruptured intracranial aneurysms. Case morbidity and mortality. J. Neurosurg. *46*, 290–295 (1977)
14. Rossum, J.V., Wintzen, A.R., Endtz, L.J., Schoen, J.H.R., Jonge, H.D.: Effect of tranexamic acid on rebleeding after subarachnoid hemorrhage: A double-blind controlled clinical trial. Ann. Neurol. *2*, 238–242 (1977)
15. Rowe, S.N., Grunnagle, J.F., Susen, A.F., Davis, J.S.: Results of direct attack on intracranial aneurysm. J. Neurosurg. *12*, 475–486 (1955)
16. Saito, I., Ueda, Y., Sano, K.: Significance of vasospasm in the treatment of ruptured intracranial aneurysm. J. Neurosurg. *47*, 412–429 (1977)
17. Sano, K., Saito, I.: Timing and indication of surgery for ruptured intracranial aneurysms with regard to cerebral vasospasm. Acta Neurochir. *41*, 49–60 (1978)
18. Sano, K., Saito, I.: Early operation and washout of blood clots for prevention of cerebral vasospasm. In: Cerebral arterial spasm. Wilins, R.H. (ed.), pp. 510–513. Baltimore: Williams & Wilkins 1980
19. Shigeno, I., Aritake, K., Saito, I., Sano, K.: Hydrocephalus following early operation on ruptured cerebral aneurysms: Significance of long-term monitoring of intracranial pressure. In: Intracranial pressure IV. Shulman, K., Marmarou, A., Miller, J.D., Becker, D.P., Hockwald, G.M., Brock,.M. (eds.), pp. 235–240. Berlin, Heidelberg, New York: Springer 1980

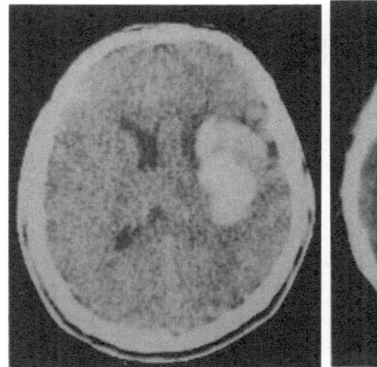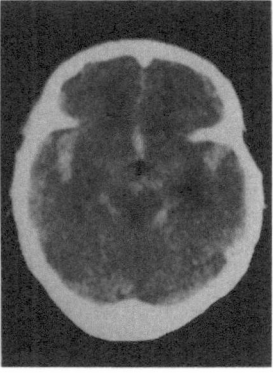

Fig. 1. CT scans of cases with ruptured aneurysms in the acute stage. Cases with intracerebral haematoma like the left picture usually show a smooth postoperative course and residual neurological deficits attributable to the haematoma determine the prognosis of patients. In contrast, cases with severe SAH occupying diffusely almost all cisterns as illustrated in the right picture develop vasospasm postoperatively and show poor results, because early operations cannot completely wash out the blood-clots and cannot always prevent the development of vasospasm

Direct Operation on Intracranial Aneurysms Within 48 Hours of Subarachnoid Haemorrhage—Correlation Between CT Findings and Vasospasm

H. Higuchi, Y. Nagamine, and H. Satoh

Introduction

CT findings from 137 cases of ruptured intracranial aneurysm, admitted to our department between 1977 to 1980, were graded from I to V. Comparisons were then made of the morbidity and mortality rates due to vasospasms between the 56 cases operated on within 48 hours of the onset of haemorrhage and the 52 cases operated on three or more days afterwards. It was found that early operations performed within 48 hours were remarkably successful in preventing cerebral vasospasm. The mortality rate for these early operations was 7.1%, compared to that of 17.4% for patients who waited longer for operations.

Clinical Materials

Between 1977 and 1980, a total of 137 cases of ruptured intracranial aneurysm were admitted to the Iwate Central Hospital. Operations were performed within 48 hours in 56 cases (Group A), and after three or more days in 52 cases (Group B). The remaining 29 died before operations could be performed.

Table 1 shows the sites of the aneurysms in these cases. In Group A the mortality rate was 7.1% (4/56 cases) and the morbidity rate was 10.7% (6/56 cases). The corresponding figures obtained for Group B were 0% (0/52 cases) and 50% (26/52 cases), respectively.

Among the 29 fatal cases not operated on, six patients died from recurrence of the bleeding while waiting for operation and five from vasospasm. Combining these cases, the mortality rate for those waiting for operations was 17.4% (11/63 cases). The remaining 18 of these 29 fatal cases were found to have massive intracerebral or intraventricular haematomas and would have been Grade IV or V according to Hunt and Kosnik's (4) criteria. All of these cases were inoperable and death occurred quickly.

CT findings on subarachnoid haemorrhage obtained within 48 hours of its onset were graded from I to V as follows according to the extent and density of the high density area;

Grade I   : No abnormality in CT findings.
Grade II   : High density area only in the cistern in which the ruptured intracranial aneurysm exists (Fig. 1).

Modern Neurosurgery 1. Edited by M. Brock
© Springer-Verlag Berlin · Heidelberg 1982

Table 1. Distribution of ruptured cerebral aneurysms

Group	ICA	MCA	ACOA	ACA	V–BA	Total	Mortality rate
(A) Within 48 hours	22	18	15	1		56	7.1%
(death)	(1)	(2)	(1)			(4)	
(B) After 48 hours	17	12	17	2	4	52	17.4%
Non- operative deaths — rebleeding	2		1		3	6	
Non- operative deaths — vasospasm	1		4			5	
Non- operative deaths — ICH or IVH	4	5	7	2		18	
Total	46	35	44	5	7	137	

Grade III : High density areas also in cisterns other than that in which the ruptured intracranial aneurysms exists (Fig. 2).

Grade IV : Symmetrical extremely high density areas in all cisterns (Fig. 3).

Grade V : CT findings also suggest the presence of massive intracranial or intraventricular haematomas (Fig. 4).

Comparisons were then made of morbidity and mortality due to cerebral vasospasms between Group A and Group B.

Results (Table 2)

There were 11 Grade I cases in Group A in which vasospasm did not occur. Two of the 12 cases in Group B developed pre-operative symptomatic vasospasm associated with neurological deficits such as hemiplegia.

Among the Grade II cases, postoperative symptomatic vasospasm occurred in two of the 20 cases in Group A and pre-operative symptomatic vasospasm in five of the 17 cases in Group B.

With Grade III cases, two of the nine cases in Group A showed postoperative symptomatic vasospasms, while pre-operative symptomatic vasospasms were seen in nine of the 13 cases in Group B.

In cases in which the CT findings were Grade IV, hemiplegia continued in two due to postoperative vasospasm and death occurred in four of the 12 cases in Group A. In Group B severe pre-operative vasospasm developed, leaving neurological deficits in all ten cases.

There were four Grade V cases in Group A and none in Group B. In these cases the patients lives were saved.

Table 2. Correlation between CT findings and surgical results

Group	CT grading					Total	Morbidity	Mortality	Total mortality
	I	II	III	IV	V				
	11	20	9	12	4	56			
(A) Within 48 hours		(2)ᵃ	(2)ᵃ	(2)ᵃ		(6)ᵃ	6/56	4/56	
				(4)ᵇ		(4)ᵇ	(10.7%)	(7.1%)	33/137
(B) After 48 hours	12	17	13	10		52	26/52		(24.0%)
	(2)ᵃ	(5)ᵃ	(9)ᵃ	(10)ᵃ		(26)ᵃ	(50%)		
								11/63	
(C) Non-operative deaths — rebleeding		1	1	4		6		(17.4%)	
vasospasm				(5)ᵇ		(5)ᵇ			
ICH or IVH					18	18			

ᵃ Neurological deficits due to vasospasm

ᵇ Deaths due to vasospasm

Discussion

The main objective of surgical treatment for ruptured intracranial aneurysm is to prevent recurrence of the rupture. Therefore, ideally, radical treatment should be performed as early as possible. However, since the results of early operation are clearly poorer than those performed more than two weeks after the onset of haemorrhage, not a few surgeons insist that operations should not be performed in the early stages, especially during the first week (1–3, 6, 9, 11).

On the other hand there are surgeons who make it a rule to perform early operations, namely within the first week because of the frequent recurrence of haemorrhage while waiting for operations (5, 7, 8).

Moreover, there are even some surgeons who perform the operations as early as possible, within 48 hours, aiming to prevent the recurrence of haemorrhage and vasospasms (10).

As a result of the introduction of CT, it has become possible to find out the extent and degree of subarachnoid haemorrhage in the early stages of the intracranial rupture of an aneurysm. It was found that an early operation performed within 48 hours of the rupture is useful in preventing not only recurrence of haemorrhage but also cerebral vasospasm through the removal of the subarachnoid clot at an early stage.

In our series, operations were delayed until the third day after the rupture or later in cases of vertebrobasilar aneurysms, geriatric cases over 65 years old, cases which would have been graded IV or V in terms of Hunt and Kosnik's criteria and cases with serious combined disturbances in other areas. However, even in these cases radical operations were performed as early as possible between the 3rd and 14th days if some improvement had been seen in the physical state and consciousness of the patients.

When operations were performed within 48 hours, a clearly more preventive effect against cerebral vasospasm was observed than with Grade I, II and III cases operated on on the third day or afterwards. With respect to Grade IV cases, death from post-operative vasospasms occurred in four of the 12 cases. All these four cases would have been classified as Grade II or III according to Hunt and Kosnik's criteria.

Based on the results of radical treatment performed within 48 hours, grading based on CT findings are more useful in predicting postoperative intracranial vasospasms than Hunt and Kosnik's gradings.

Among cases classified as Grade IV from the CT findings, 15 patients waited for operations. In five of these cases death occurred because of pre-operative vasospasm, and in the remaining ten cases operations were performed, but serious neurological deficits remained because of the pre-operative vasospasm. Among other cases waiting for operations six patients died without being operated on because of the recurrence of haemorrhage. When these six cases are included, the mortality rate for cases waiting for operations becomes 17.4%; inferior to that when operations were performed within 48 hours. Eighteen of the 22 cases classified as Grade V from the findings would have been classified as Grade IV or V according to Hunt-Kosnik's criteria. These patients died without operations being performed. In the remaining four cases, which would have been Grade III according to Hunt-Kosnik's criteria, the patients' lives were saved because of the operations being performed within 48 hours.

Conclusion

Our study shows that cerebral vasospasm can be prevented in many cases by surgically removing the blood clot in the subarachnoid space within 48 hours of the SAH.

References

1. Bohm, E., Hugosson, R.: Results of surgical treatment of 200 consecutive cerebral arterial aneurysms. Acta Neurol. Scandinav. 46, 43–52 (1970)
2. Crowell, R.M., Zeravas, N.T.: The management of intracranial aneurysm. Medical Clinics of North America 63, 695–713 (1979)
3. Drake, C.G.: Intracranial aneurysms. Proc. Roy. Soc. Med. 64, 477–481 (1971)
4. Hunt, W.E., Kosnik, E.J.: Timing and preoperative care in intracranial aneurysm surgery. Clin. Neurosurg. 21, 79–89 (1974)
5. Krayenbuhl, H.A., Yasargil, M.G., Flamm, E.S., Tew, J.M.: Microsurgical treatment of intracranial saccular aneurysms. J. Neurosurg. 37, 678–686 (1972)
6. Norlén, G., Olivecrona, H.: The treatment of aneurysms of the circle of Willis. J. Neurosurg. 10, 404–415 (1953)
7. Nornes, H., Wikeby, P.: Results of microsurgical management of intracranial aneurysms. J. Neurosurg. 51, 608–614 (1979)
8. Pool, J.L., Potts, D.G.: Aneurysms and arteriovenous anomalies of the brain, pp. 188–189. New York: Harper & Row 1965
9. Ransohoff, J., Goodgold, A., Benjamin, M.: Preoperative management of patients with ruptured intracranial aneurysms. J. Neurosurg. 36, 525–530 (1972)
10. Suzuki, J., Yoshimoto, T., Onuma, T.: Early operations for ruptured intracranial aneurysm – Study of 31 cases operated on within the first four days after ruptured aneurysm. Neurol. Med. Chir. (Tokyo) (Part 1), 83–89 (1978)
11. Uttley, D.: Subarachnoid haemorrhage, Br. J. Hosp. Med. 19, 138–154 (1978)

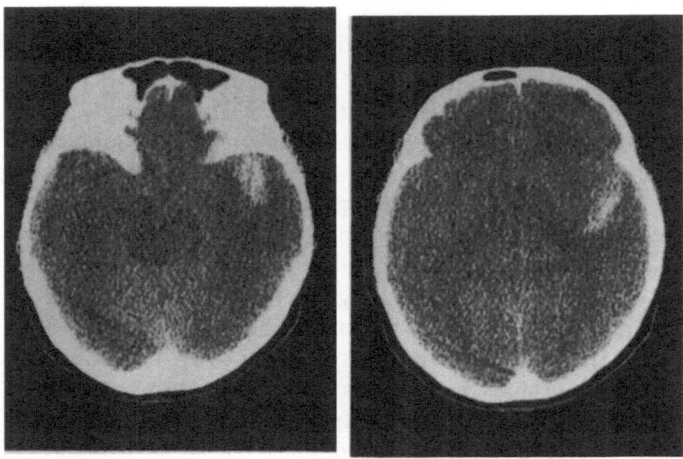

Fig. 1. *Grade II:* CT scan shows high density areas only in the cistern in which the ruptured intracranial aneurysm exists

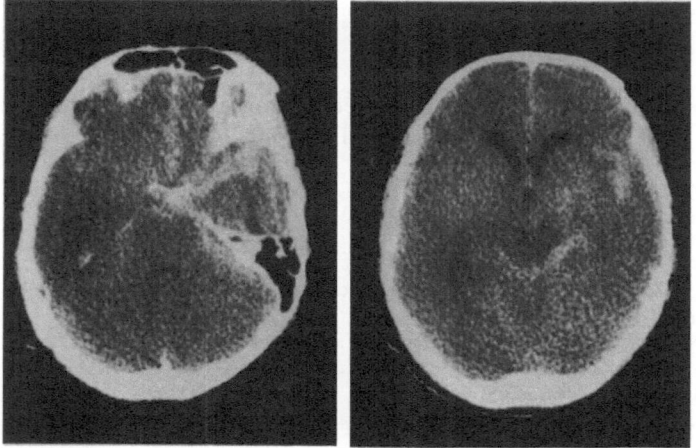

Fig. 2. *Grade III:* CT scan shows high density areas also in cisterns other than that in which the ruptured intracranial aneurysms exists

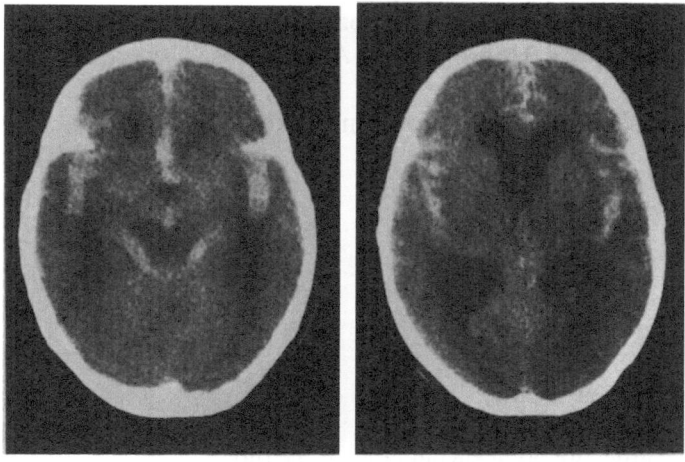

Fig. 3. *Grade IV:* CT scan shows symmetrical extremely high density areas in all cisterns

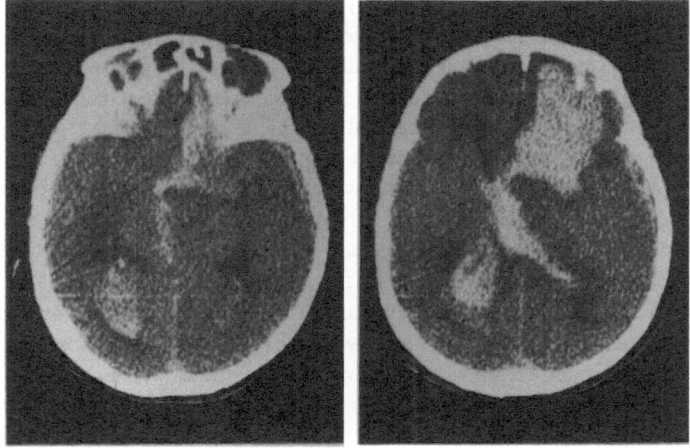

Fig. 4. *Grade V:* CT scan shows the presence of massive intracerebral or intraventricular haematomas

Transpetrosal Combined Supratentorial and Infratentorial Approach for Midline Vertebro-Basilar Aneurysms

K. Hashi, K. Nin, and K. Shimotake

Introduction

Difficulties are often encountered in the surgical approach to vertebrobasilar aneurysms situated in the midline at the level of the middle third of the clivus. The subtemporal transtentorial approach reported by Drake (2) gives inadequate room for manipulation of the lower side of the aneurysm neck, particularly when the aneurysm is large in size and fills the depths of the narrow operative field. A conventional lateral suboccipital approach has a similar limitation for the upper side of the aneurysm neck. The transoral clival approach has the serious drawback of a high risk of postoperative infection.

A combined supratentorial and infratentorial approach as described by Kasdon and Stein (4) allows wider exposure along the whole length of the clivus, but the division of the sigmoid sinus is not always without risk.

This paper presents an alternative method of exposure, by which the sigmoid sinus is preserved and a better view along the course of the vertebro-basilar trunk can be obtained. The approach consists of a combined subtemporal and lateral suboccipital craniotomy, removal of the bone at the postero-superior aspect of the petrous pyramid, and dural opening over the temporal lobe being extended inferiorly along the anterior border of the sigmoid sinus by division of the superior petrosal sinus and tentorium.

The technical details are described by the operation performed for a case with a midline situated right vertebral artery aneurysm (case 3).

Surgical Technique

The patient was placed in the head-up lateral position with the head flexed and tilted laterally so as to bring the sagittal plane of the head parallel to the horizontal plane. A hook-shaped scalp incision was made starting from a point 5 cm above the external auditory meatus extending down to a point 1 cm below and posterior to the tip of the mastoid process (Fig. 1A). The scalp flap was reflected. A small temporal bone flap and lateral suboccipital craniectomy were made. The bone over the transverse sinus was removed and both craniotomies were combined. The bone over the sigmoid sinus and posterior half of the mastoid process was carefully shaved off using an air drill, until the sigmoid sinus was fully exposed. Then, the petrous bone of the floor of the middle fossa and the portion anterior to the sigmoid sinus were drilled off to expose

 Modern Neurosurgery 1. Edited by M. Brock

the terminal portion of the superior petrosal sinus and a narrow dural strip of approximately 1 cm in width along the anterior border of the sigmoid sinus. In order to avoid possible damage of the semicircular canals situated in the petrous pyramid, the removal of the bone in the supero-posterior aspect of the petrous pyramid was confined to the thin layer necessary to expose a small area sufficient for dural incision (Fig. 1B).

The microscope was then used and the dura over the temporal lobe was opened. A vertical dural incision was extended inferiorly along the anterior border of the sigmoid sinus by division of the superior petrosal sinus at its junction with the sigmoid sinus. The tentorium was divided parallel to the petrous ridge up to the hiatus. The divided flaps were tugged and sutured to the surrounding tissues to facilitate the exposure (Fig. 1C).

The temporal lobe was retracted upward and the cerebellar hemisphere backward together with the mobilized sigmoid sinus. The lateral aspect of the brain stem was easily seen through the 5th and 7th and 8th cranial nerves. By changing the angle of the microscope, it was possible to see the third nerve superiorly, the twelfth nerve inferiorly and the whole length of the basilar artery by gentle retraction over the pons (Fig. 1D). The right vertebral artery and the aneurysm was found medial to the vagus group and handled easily through the space between the 7th and 8th nerves and the vagus group. The aneurysm, however, appeared unruptured and fusiform, although evidence of subarachnoid haemorrhage (SAH) was apparent in the cistern. A clip was applied to the part where the aneurysmal wall was thin and the whole aneurysm was coated with plastic adhesive (Biobond).

The dural opening was closed using a patch of lyophilized dura (Lyodura). The temporal bone flap was replaced and the space behind the petrous pyramid was packed with a piece of muscle.

Case Reports

Three cases operated on by this approach will be presented.

Case 1 (I.H.). A 62-year-old right-handed woman had sudden occipital headache followed by vomiting several times in the evening on January 25, 1978. Next morning lumbar puncture revealed SAH and a large aneurysm in the vertebrobasilar system was found by angiography in a neigbouring hospital (Fig. 2). On admission in the afternoon of the same day she was slightly obtunded but responded correctly to simple commands. She had marked stiff neck and headache with a blood pressure of 134/62 mm Hg. There was a positive Babinski sign on the left side. At 5 p.m. operation was begun with the approach described above, after placing a ventricular drain in the left frontal horn. The craniotomies were larger in this case compared to the one described earlier and the wedge-shaped removal of the posterior aspect of the petrous pyramid was deeper to the level of the internal auditory meatus. Another dural opening was made in the suboccipital region behind the sigmoid sinus in order to obtain an easy access to the proximal part of the vertebral arteries. Subarachnoid clot was removed. An aneurysm which was adherent to the clivus and the base of the brain stem was found between the level of the fifth nerve and the vagus group. The seventh and eighth nerves and anterior inferior cerebellar artery were stretched outward and adhered to the wall of the aneurysm. It was found that both the vertebral arteries were directly connected to the lower pole of the aneurysm, and that the basilar artery came from the right side of its upper pole. The aneurysm was separated from the brain stem and coated with plastic adhesive except for the part near the upper pole where a leak was encountered during the procedure and was controlled by gentle compression with gelatin cottonoid soaked with plastic adhesive. Postoperatively, she had sixth and seventh nerve weakness, which cleared up within a week, and nystagmus with difficulty of hearing on the left side. Ventriculo-peritoneal shunt was performed on February 9. When she was discharged on March 14, 1978, the left-sided hearing loss by 67.5 dB was her sole abnormality. This was still present at follow-up on July, 1981 when she was working well as a restaurant keeper.

Case 2 (T.T.). A 46-year-old right-handed woman was admitted to our hospital on April 3, 1978 for investigation of the cause of SAH which had occurred on January 20, 1975. There were no neurological abnormalities. Angiography demonstrated a right vertebral aneurysm pointing medially with irregularities on the wall of its parent artery (Fig. 3). We decided to use the combined approach because of the possibility of a partially thrombosed large aneurysm in which a trapping procedure would be necessary during the operation. On April 28, 1978 the operation was performed. The aneurysm was large and fusiform in shape, situated medial to the vagus group. Although the distal part of the right vertebral artery was identified, its junction to the aneurysm and the medial border of the aneurysm could not be seen. Clipping of the right vertebral artery distal to the origin of the posterior inferior cerebellar artery was then performed. Postoperatively, 7th, 9th and 12th nerve weaknesses on the right side and occasional dizziness developed, but these cleared up by the time of her discharge on May 20, 1978, She was well at follow-up in April, 1981.

Case 3 (I.S.). A 61-year-old right-handed man had severe headache and vomiting on May 15, 1978, Lumbar puncture revealed SAH, and a right vertebral aneurysm, situated in the midline, was found (Fig. 4). He was transferred to our clinic on May 26, when his state of consciousness was clear, and there was a stiff neck, and retinal haemorrhages on both sides. Operation was performed on May 26, 1978 using the combined approach because of the midline position of the aneurysm. The procedure was described in detail above. Postoperatively, he was without neurological deficits. Two weeks later the angiographic study was repeated, because the vertebral aneurysm was found unruptured. This revealed another aneurysm on the basilar artery an its junction with the left posterior cerebral artery. This was subsequently operated on on June 14, 1978 by the pterional approach. He was well until July 18, 1978, when a sudden abdominal pain and ileus developed. Thrombosis of the mesenteric artery was confirmed by emergency laparotomy. He died on July 21.

Discussion

A combined supra- and infratentorial approach for midline vertebro-basilar aneurysm was described by Kasdon and Stein (4): the advantage is to secure a wider exposure for both the distal and proximal part of the vertebro-basilar system simultaneously. The division of the sigmoid sinus, which is a serious drawback of the approach of Kasdon et al. and may limit the side of operation only to a non-dominant venous return, can be avoided with our technique as described above. In addition, the access created anterior to the sigmoid sinus provides a more lateral angle to look through, minimizing the retraction of the cerebellum and brain stem for exposure of the basilar artery.

The prototype of this approach was designed for the removal of a large acoustic neurinoma (5) or clivus meningioma (3). In these lesions the vestibular function has usually been disturbed already, so that any additional damage caused by destruction of the semicircular canals by the removal of the petrous pyramid would hardly cause any symptoms. In cases with an aneurysm, destruction of the semicircular canals may result in temporary dysequilibrium lasting for several weeks. In Case 1 and 2, where the bone removal was to the depth of the internal auditory meatus, nystagmus and dysequilibrium developed postoperatively, although the possibility of a direct injury of the 8th nerve intracranially in Case 1 or the effect of vertebral artery ligation in Case 2 could not be ruled out. This complication can be avoided by restricting the bone removal in the postero-superor part of the petrous pyramid to a small portion only to make dural incision possible in the space anterior to the sigmoid sinus. Because this, in turn, may restrict the lateral angle of the operative field, the decision as to how much bone should be removed would be dependent upon the position and size of the aneurysm.

Retrospectively, midline vertebral aneurysms such as Case 2 and 3 could have been operated via a conventional lateral suboccipital approach. However, the easy access to both distal and proximal parts of the parent vertebral artery obtained with this approach was an advantage over the standard method.

For an aneurysm at the vertebro-basilar junction or for low-lying basilar aneurysms only this combined approach could provide adequate access, and it should be the method of choice, particularly when the aneurysm was of large size such as Case 1 in this report.

Conclusion

The technique of a combined supra- and infratentorial approach for the midline vertebro-basilar aneurysm is described. In this approach the patency of the sigmoid sinus can be preserved. It permits a wide exposure through the whole length of the basilar trunk and both vertebral arteries at the same time, and provides satisfactory access for safer manipulation of the aneurysm in this particular region. The results of three cases were presented.

References

1. Chou, S.N., Ortiz-Suarez, H.J.: Surgical treatment of aneurysms of the vertebrobasilar system. J. Neurosurg. *41*, 671–680 (1974)
2. Drake, C.G.: Treatment of aneurysms of the posterior cranial fossa. Prog. Neurol. Surg. *9*, 122–294 (1978)
3. Hakuba, A., Nishimura, S., Tanaka, K., Kishi, H., Nakamura, T.: Clivus meningioma: six cases of total removal. Neurol. Med. Chir. (Tokyo) *17*, 63–77 (1977)
4. Kasdon, D.L., Stein, B.M.: Combined supratentorial and infratentorial exposure for low-lying basilar aneurysms. Neurosurgery *4*, 422–426 (1979)
5. King, T.T.: Combined translabyrinthine-transtentorial approach to acoustic nerve tumours. Proc. Roy. Soc. Med. *63*, 30–32 (1970)

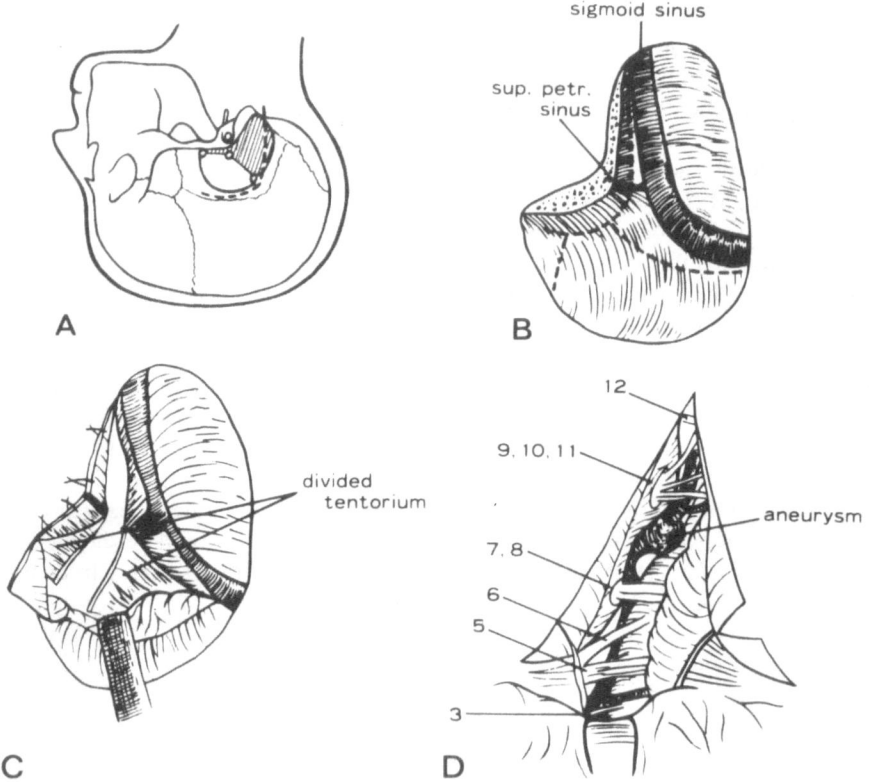

Fig. 1. A Scalp incision and craniotomy. Shaded portion shows the area of bone removed. **B** Dural incision. **C** Dural openings and division of the tentorium. The temporal lobe is retracted upward. **D** Microscopic view of the combined approach. The cranial nerves are marked with numerals. This drawing shows a reconstructed picture from the views which can be obtained by changing the angle of the microscope

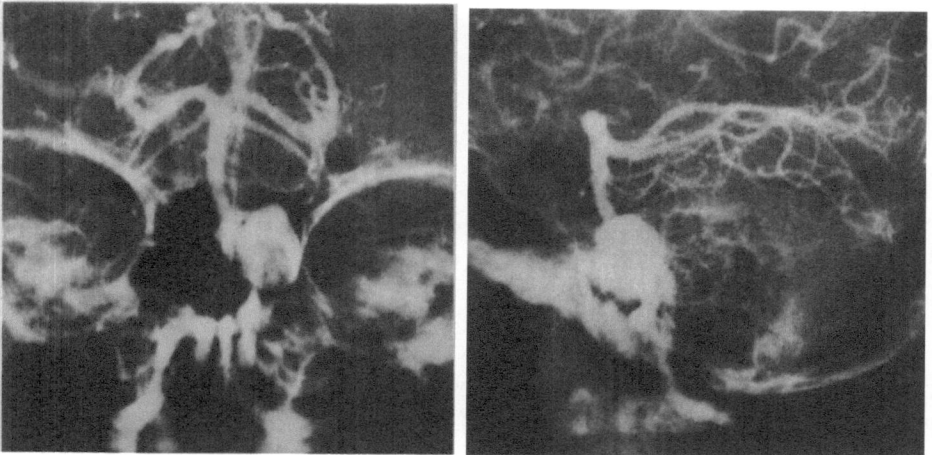

Fig. 2. Case 1. *Left:* antero-posterior (AP) view of vertebral arteriogram showing a large aneurysm at the vertebro-basilar junction. *Right:* lateral view

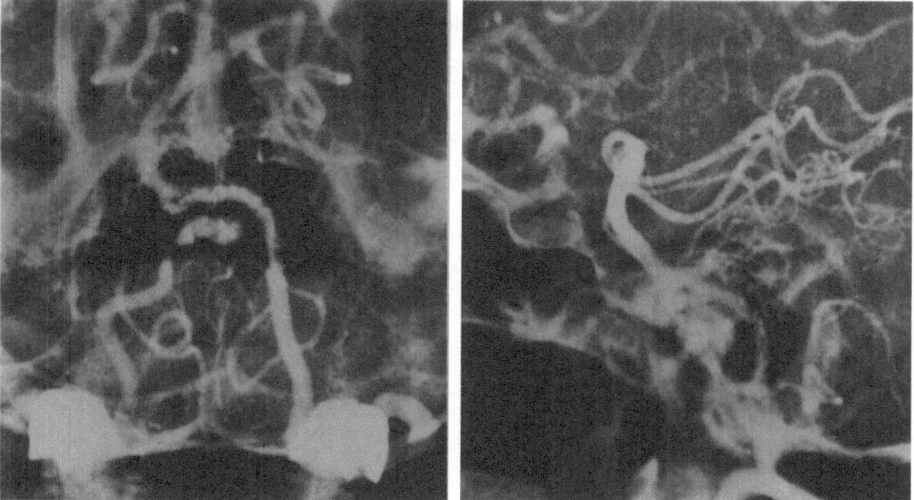

Fig. 3. Case 2. *Left:* AP view of a vertebral arteriogram showing an aneurysm pointing medially from the right vertebral artery. Parent arteries show irregularities of the wall indicating the presence of a thrombosed part in the aneurysm. *Right:* lateral view. The aneurysm is situated at the lower third of the clivus

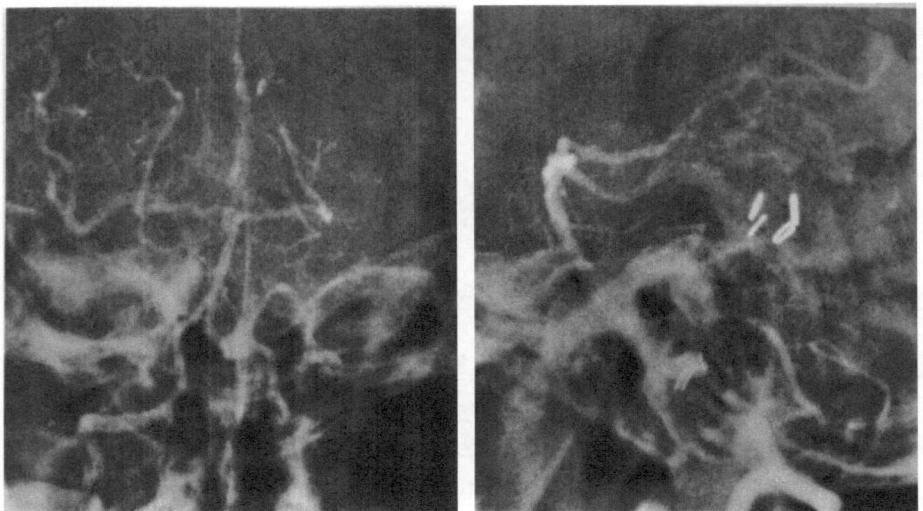

Fig. 4. Case 3. *Left:* AP view of bilateral vertebral arteriogram showing an aneurysm on the left vertebral artery. There is another aneurysm, faintly opacified in this film, on the basilar artery at its junction with the posterior cerebral artery. This aneurysm was confirmed afterwards to have been responsible for his SAH. *Right:* postoperative lateral view. A clip shows the position of the aneurysm

Long-Term Follow-Up of Deep Brain Stimulation for Relief of Chronic Pain in the Human

D.E. Richardson

Introduction

Stimulation techniques for the control of chronic pain have been used on our service since 1973, when Dr. Akil and I developed techniques for stimulating the periaqueductal and periventricular grey area. The technique is based on the demonstration by Reynolds (7) and by Mayer et al. (6), that stimulation of the periaqueductal grey in the rat produced diffuse and marked analgesia. Further investigation by Liebeskind et al. (5), also demonstrated the efficacy of periaqueductal stimulation for pain relief, with little or no side effects. After demonstrating, in acute operations, that stimulation of this area of the brain produced good analgesia and little or no side effects in the human (8, 9), we have done chronic implantation of cerebral electrodes in seventy-five patients for the relief of chronic pain. This is a brief review of the long-term results of deep brain stimulation for the relief of chronic intractable pain, and can be compared with the follow-up previously published on our first thirty patients (10).

Methods and Material

Questionnaires were sent to all patients operated on since 1973, on our service at Tulane Medical Centre and in the Pain Rehabilitation Unit at Hotel Dieu Hospital in New Orleans. Patients who did not respond to the questionnaire were contacted on the telephone by an unbiased technician and the questionnaire was filled out as directed by the patient. A summary of this material was then used to analyse the results in these 75 patients operated on between 1973 and 1981.

Results

Questionnaires were returned by, or telephone contact was established with, 57 patients; 7 patients could not be located and 12 patients had died — one of these during the period of acquisition of material for the study — resulting in 57 patients with adequate follow-up for analysis.

Diagnostic indications for a pain-relieving procedure are presented in Table 1. This reveals that a large majority (33 patients) were operated on for failure to recover from

Table 1. Indication for electrode implantation (Richardson, 1981)

Failed back syndrome	33
Cancer pain	9
Central pain	
Brain	7
Cord	8
Nerve injury	7
Phantom limb	4
Anaesthesia dolorosa	3
Miscellaneous	4
Total	75

spinal operations primarily directed toward the relief of herniated lumbar disc. Central nervous system injury in either the brain, spinal cord or peripheral nerves provided another 23 patients for operation. Deafferentation pain syndromes, such as phantom limb and anesthesia dolorosa, accounted for 7 patients.

Continued use of the brain stimulation device was presumed to be an indication of success, i.e. significant relief of pain. Therefore the number of patients still using the device is considered to be the number of patients with continued good results. This number is not further broken down because of the difficulty in ascertaining the degree of pain relief on written or telephone contact with the patient, without being able to examine the patient for more precise evaluation. Of the 57 patients available for adequate follow-up, 34 patients were still using the stimulator, giving a continued significant relief rate of about 60% of the patients over the period of the follow-up. This is presented in Table 2.

Patients who are not using their stimulator at this time are presented in Table 3. In five patients, the reasons for discontinuation include equipment failure, such as failure of the wiring system, electrode, or receiving device. They also include loss of pain relief for various reasons which could not be determined on the type of follow-up utilized for this study, and obvious cases of psychiatric failures of relief which should, under the present protocol of the Pain Rehabilitation Unit, have excluded many of this group of patients from consideration for operation.

Two patients had infections of late onset; one elderly patient had erosion of the electrode-retaining plug through the scalp, resulting in secondary infection requiring removal of the system. The second, a law enforcement officer, was struck on the side of the head, resulting in exposure of the wiring and secondary infection requiring removal.

Only one patient described side effects from stimualtion that would preclude his use of the stimulator even though it gave good pain relief. He suffered such acute and severe depression after stimulation that he elected to discontinue its use, despite the fact that it gave adequate pain relief for many hours following brief periods of stimulation.

Table 2. Results in all patients operated (Richardson, 1981)

Using stimulator	34 (60%)
Not using stimulator	23 (40%)
Dead	11
No follow-up	7
Total	75

Table 3. Reason for discontinuing stimulation (Richardson, 1981)

	Not using stimulator
Equipment failure	5
No pain relief	11
Psychiatric problems	5
Infection	2
Side effects	1
Dead	12
No follow-up	7
Total	43

We were surprised to find that twelve of our patients had expired since the time of surgery, although nine of these deaths were not unexpected, as the patients were operated on for relief of cancer pain.

A breakdown of the results of operations from 1973 to 1980, which is based on the percentage of good results per year, is presented in Fig. 1. This indicates that prolonged good results have been obtained from the early patients operated on, even though they represent a smaller number of patients. Significant improvement in results starting in 1978 is evident in this follow-up. While this may be attributed to the shorter period of follow-up, it is more likely related to the opening of our multidisciplinary Pain Rehabilitation Unit in the spring of 1978. All patients now have extensive psychological testing, psychiatric interviews, behavioural modification, and physical rehabilitation prior to consideration for operative pain relief.

One of the best results we obtained was our first patient, who was operated on in the spring of 1973. He continues to use his stimulator and functions quite adequately, and is at present managing his own electrical contracting company. However, he has required replacement of his electrode, and later the receiver and extension.

Discussion

An attempt has been made to obtain a follow-up on all patients who had deep brain electrodes placed over the past eight years to relieve chronic intractable pain. Although for many patients we could not obtain specific details of their problems following electrode implantation, several factors become relatively obvious. The use of deep brain stimulation for cancer pain has proven impractical, since most of these patients die relatively soon afer the procedure. We have now elected almost exclusively to use destructive procedures for cancer pain.

The screening process now used for evaluation of candidates for pain procedures is designed to rule out patients with emotional lability and psychogenic pain, and those patients whom we would not expect to get adequate pain relief from deep brain stimulation. This has significantly reduced the failure rate of the procedure. It is my impression that the number (five) of patients that we have characterized as psychiatric problems is probably low, and that most of the patients who have had no pain relief from stimulation probably could be lumped with those five. As our expertise in selecting patients for pain procedures improves, our failure rate should gradually be reduced.

It has been quite surprising that many patients who have experienced a decrease in pain relief after a successful period of stimulation do not return for a re-evaluation in an attempt to correct the cause for their loss of adequate pain control. This may indicate, of course, that a significant number of these patients has a need to continue their pain and suffering and they make very little attempt to continue their stimulation-induced pain relief even though they have classified it as adequate prior to failure of the system, for whatever reason.

The follow-up confirms the fact that deep brain stimulation can be effective in relieving pain over a long period and that the mechanical equipment failure problems resulting in failure of the stimulation system have been relatively rare. The analgesia produced by periventricular and periaqueductal stimulation is associated with the release of endogenous enkephalin and β-endorphin (3, 4) in the human and is blocked by naloxone in both animals and the human (2, 9). It is dependent on the raphe serotonin system. Our present concept is that at least two neurotransmitters are involved in this technique (1, 2). This has produced some concern that tolerance would develop with time and prolonged stimulation. However, only four patients in this series reported needing treatment for tolerance. All four recovered analgesic stimulation with the administration of L-tryptophan and tricyclic antidepressants to enhance serotonin production. Usually two to four weeks of treatment allowed recovery of pain control.

The over-all success rate continues to be 60% for long-term stimulation, despite our attempts to select our patients carefully and to provide variousforms of support for emotional factors in their illness.

Summary

Since 1973, deep brain stimulating electrodes have been placed in seventy-five patients for relief of chronic intractable pain. Long-term follow-up reveals that 60% of the patients have significant pain relief and that in 40% of those patients available for follow-up tich technique had failed for various reasons. Only five patients have had significant equipment failure resulting in loss of pain control and only two patients have had late onset infections. Most failures seem to have resulted from poor patient selction or a loss of the patient's desire to maintain adequate pain control.

References

1. Akil, H., Liebeskind, J.C.: Monoaminergic mechanisms of stimulation-produced analgesia. Brain Research *94*, 279–296 (1975)
2. Akil, H., Mayer, D.J., Liebeskind, J.C.: Antagonism of stimulation-produced analgesia by Naloxone, a narcotic antagonist. Science *191*, 961–962 (1976)
3. Akil, H., Richardson, D.E., Hughes, J. et al.: Elevation of levels of enkephalin-like material in the ventricular CSF of pain patients upon analgesic focal stimulation. Science *201*, 463–465 (1978)
4. Akil, H., Richardson, D.E., Barcus, J.D.: Appearance of β-endorphin-like immunoreactivity in human ventricular CSF upon analgesic electrical stimulation. Proc. Nat. Acad. Sci. USA Vol. *75*, No. 10, Oct. 1978
5. Liebeskind, J.C., Mayer, D.J., Akil, H.: Central mechanism of pain inhibition: studies of analgesia from focal brain stimulation. In: Advances in Neurology IV: Pain. Bonica, J.J. (ed.), pp. 261–168, New York: Raven Press 1974
6. Mayer, D.J., Wolfle, T.L., Akil, H., Carder, B., Liebeskind, J.C.: Analgesia from electrical stimulation in the brainstem of the cat. Science *174*, 1351–1354 (1971)
7. Reynolds, D.V.: Surgery in the rat during electrical analgesia induced by focal brain stimulation. Science *164*, 444–445 (1969)
8. Richardson, D.E., Akil, H.: Pain reduction by electrical brain stimulation in man. Part I: Acute administration in periaqueductal and periventricular sites. J. Neurosurg. *47*, 178–183 (1977)
9. Richardson, D.E., Akil, H.: Pain reduction by electrical brain stimulation in man. Part II: Chronic self-administration in the periventricular grey matter. J. Neurosurg. *47*, 184–194 (1977)
10. Richardson, D.E., Akil, H.: Long-term results of periventricular grey self-stimulation. Neurosurgery *1*, 199–202 (1977)

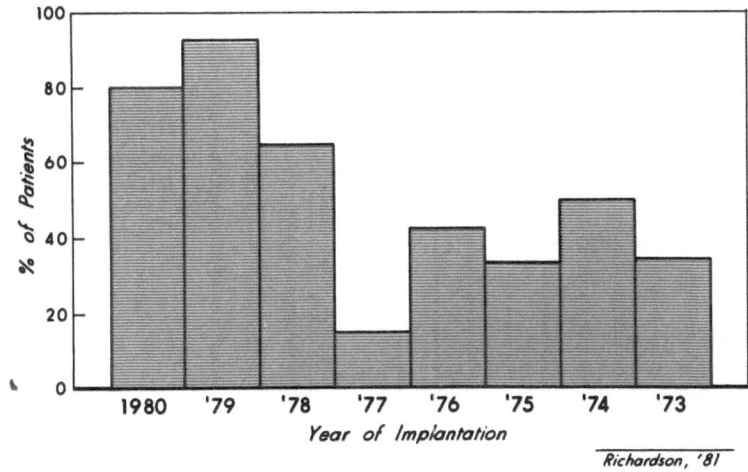

Fig. 1. Results by duration of implantation by year (percentage of patients currently using stimulator)

Results in 60 Cases of Deep Brain Stimulation for Chronic Intractable Pain

R. Plotkin

Abstract

Sixty cases have had deep brain stimulators implanted in the past 3 1/2 years. Forty-six cases have had PVG stimulation for peripheral pain, two PVG implants for central pain, and 12 have had specific sensory nucleus stimulation for central pain. Of the PVG cases, 80% have total pain relief or only slight residual pain, and 20% have failed. Those that have failed were probably poor candidates who should not have been selected. Of the specific sensory nucleus stimulation cases, only 33% are satisfied with their results and 50% have totally failed. Two cases had early complications (intraventricular haemorrhage) and four had late complications (sepsis and electrode drift).

The cases recorded here are the first 60 consecutive patients at this centre to have deep brain electrodes implanted to control chronic intractable pain. The programme was commenced after reports of this method by Adams et al. (1, 2), Hosobuchi et al. (8–11) Richardson et al. (17, 18), and many others (3–7, 13–16) appeared in the literature.

Material and Methods

Initially, patients were selected on clinical grounds, namely a history of chronic pain with clear organic cause. After 26 operations had been performed, morphine saturation testing using Hosobuchi's method (personal communication) was introduced, and all patients considered for deep brain stimulation were submitted to this test. When central pain was considered likely, the morphine saturation was followed after several days by a pentothal test.

Morphine Saturation Test

Through a fast running intravenous line, 1.5 mg morphine are given every 60 seconds until 30 mgs have been injected. The patient's pain level on a scale of 10 is charted each minute. If there is residual pain after this, a further 20 minutes is allowed to ensure complete saturation of morphine binding sites. Naloxone (0.8 mg) is then administered intravenously and the charting of pain levels continues for a further 20 minutes. Non-organic pain is indicated by total pain relief a few seconds

Modern Neurosurgery 1. Edited by M. Brock
© Springer-Verlag Berlin · Heidelberg 1982

after administration of 1.5 or 3.0 mg morphine, or a bizarre response. Gradually diminishing pain with naloxone reversal indicates peripheral pain of organic origin, and an anticipated good result with deep brain stimulation. No response to morphine suggests central pain. These patients are then subjected to a pentothal test. No analgesics are permitted for 12 hours prior to either test. Where hysteria is strongly suspected, normal saline is given in the same manner initially as part of the test, the patient being unaware of which substances are being injected at any particular moment (the author's modification).

Pentothal Test

25 mgs Pentothal is adminstered intravenously each minute until the patient is on the point of unconsciousness, at which time pain, if central, should entirely disappear. This test is carried out by an anaesthetist with full facilities for assisted respiration if required. (Tasker, R.R. reported by Hosobuchi, personal communication.)

The electrodes used were manufactured by Medtronic Inc., introduced in the alert state with a Leksell stereotaxic apparatus. Analgesics were witheld for 18 hours prior to operation. Patients were tested on the operating table to exclude placements where stimulation would produce undesirable side effects. All patients were tested via the external leads for at least one week, chronic implantation being undertaken only if an adequate response was obtained. An hourly pain chart was maintained during the test period with details of the stimulation given.

All cases had prophylactic antibiotics. Disulfiram 400 mg and amitriptyline 100 mg daily was administered for the first two weeks to those patients with periventricular grey implants, commencing on the day of electrode implantation. Thereafter the disulfiram was reduced to 200 mg daily (12), and the amitriptyline dosage adjusted according to the frequency of stimulation.

Forty-eight cases had electrodes introduced into the periventricular grey (PVG) 2 mm lateral to the edge of the third ventricle at the level of the posterior commissure. In two of these patients the pain was considered to be central in origin because of its nature and the response to the pentothal test. The types of pain treated and the number of cases are shown in Table 1.

Twelve patients had electrodes introduced into the specific sensory nucleus (VPL or VPM), all for apparent deafferentation pain. These cases are shown in Table 2.

The longest follow-up in this series is 42 months, and the shortest 6 months.

All patients had the best response when stimulated at 80 Herz, at an amplitude below discomfort. Stimulation time is half an hour.

Results

Of the 48 cases with PVG implants, 38 are pain-free or with only a small residuum of pain not requiring analgesics. Ten patients are failures in that either stimulation never relieved their pain, or pain was only controlled for a variable period. Nearly all patients who were initially relieved of their pain but subsequently failed, failed after approximately one year, only one at four months, and one at eighteen months. Seven of these failures were from the 26 cases selected without morphine saturation. Four of these were subsequently submitted to this test, and all gave hysterical reactions. Therefore three of the failures were positive to morphine saturation.

Table 1. Causes of pain and results in 48 cases of PVG stimulation

	Cases	Successes	Failures
Failed low back syndrome	35	28	7
Carcinoma lung	2	2	–
Cervical spondylosis	1	1	–
Sciatic nerve entrapment	2	1	1
Non-united fracture femur	1	1	–
Paraparesis	1	1	–
Tetraparesis	1	1	–
Diffuse disc disease	2	2	–
Stump pain	2	1	1
Osteoporosis	1	–	1
Total	48	38	10

Table 2. Causes of pain and results in 12 cases of specific sensory nucleus stimulation

	Cases	Pain free	Residual pain	Failures
Anaesthesia dolorosa, face	5	3	1	1
Thalamic facial pain	1	–	–	1
Phantom limb	2	1	1	–
Atypical facial pain	1	–	–	1
Paraplegia	1	–	–	1
Paraparesis	1	–	–	1
Brachial plexus avulsion	1	–	–	1
Total	12	4	2	6

The largest group of patients, 35, were the so-called "failed low back syndrome". Thirty-two of these cases had proven extradural fibrosis and/or arachnoiditis, and each had had an average of four low back operations.

The results in the other cases are shown in Table 1, each group being too small to allow individual conclusions, but having failures in three out of thirteen cases.

The number of cases receiving specific sensory nucleus stimulation for central pain is too small to permit any meaningful analysis, but failure of 50% has been found. The group that seem to do best with deafferentation pain are those with anaesthesia dolorosa of the face.

There were six cases with complications in this series. Two patients had intraventricular haemorrhage, presenting in the operating theatre in one, and several hours later in the other. Both were treated conservatively, recovered fully, and continue to derive benefit from stimulation. Two patients developed scalp sepsis, one three months after operation caused by a wig abrading the skin overlying the protuberance of the connecting plug. This was cleared with conservative management, and the patient — the first in the series — still remains pain-free. However, patients are no longer permitted to wear wigs after this procedure. The second case of sepsis presented one year after implant, the patient stating that her scalp was scratched by the hairdresser. Although the sepsis was confined to the scalp, it proved impossible to clear and eventually the apparatus was removed and reimplanted on the other side six months later. She, too, remains pain free on stimulation.

Two cases of electrode drift occurred, one 12 months and one 17 months after implantation. Both cases were successfully stimulating a specific sensory nucleus for central pain. Both were replaced from a different angle of approach and both continued to receive relief from stimulation, but one, a patient with a phantom foot, developed severe paraesthesiae of the contralateral limbs and trunk, with and without stimulation. He eventually requested removal of the apparatus, but his paraesthesiae have remained.

Discussion

At the third European Workshop on Electrical Neurostimulation in 1979 (19), delegates concluded that PVG stimulation for peripheral pain was no longer experimental and could be accepted as a routine legitimate procedure. However, the results of specific sensory nucleus stimulation for central pain could not yet be so considered. The results in this series confirm this decision. It is clear that the results of stimulation for central pain in this group of patients are not good, in contrast to those obtained for peripheral pain.

The failures in this group, in a high percentage of cases, are due to poor selection of cases, in that it can be exceedingly difficult to eliminate pain of non-organic origin. The overwhelming number of patients with "failed low-back syndrome" is a reflection of the incidence of this problem in cases presenting for treatment, but the combination of multiple low back operations, consequent arachnoiditis, and chronic pain does not necessarily mean that the pain is organic in origin. This is shown by the failed cases selected before morphine saturation and subsequently tested and found to have a hysterical response. Since the introduction of morphine saturation, many failed-low backs have been rejected as candidates for deep brain stimulation and referred for psychotherapy.

An 80% success rate for controlling chronic pain after three years compares very favourably with the three year follow-up of other procedures such as cordotomy and thalamotomy. So far there is no clinical evidence of harmful effects of intermittent stimulation over a period such as this.

Initially patients require stimulation several times in 24 hours, but the intervals increase during the first weeks so that many patients settle into a pattern of requiring to stimulate only once in 5 or 6 days, some very much more infrequently. In 14 of the

48 cases there seems to be a definite relationship between the daily dosage of amitriptyline and the pain-free period, the lower doses requiring more frequent stimulation.

One patient in this group developed tolerance, despite daily intake of disulfiram. Stimulation was stopped for two weeks during which he took 4g L-tryptophan daily, after which stimulation was again found to be effective, and continues to be so after six months on a maintainance dose of 2g L-tryptophan daily.

Conclusion

Periventricular grey stimulation for peripheral pain appears to be a good procedure in suitably selected cases, with so far no apparent ill effects from the intermittent stimulation. The main problem lies in selection of cases. The treatment of central pain by specific sensory nucleus stimulation has not produced satisfactory results in this series.

References

1. Adams, J.E., Hosobuchi, Y.: Session in deep brain stimulation. Technique and technical problems. Neurosurgery *1*, 196–199 (1977)
2. Adams, J.E., Hosobuchi, Y., Fields, H.L.: Stimulation of internal capsule for relief of chronic pain. Neurosurgery *41*, 740–744 (1974)
3. Boethuis, J., Carlsson, A.M., Meyerson, B.A.: Alleviation of malignant pain by electrical stimulation in the periventricular-periaqueductal region. Pain relief as related to stimulation sites. Second World Congress on Pain, IASP. Pain Abstr. *1*, 307 (1978)
4. Cosyns, P.: Management of severe chronic pain in humans by electrical central grey stimulation. Second World Congress on Pain, IASP. Pain Abstr. *1*, 76 (1978)
5. Crue, B.L., Felsööry, A.: Analgesia from percutaneous periaqueductal gray electrical stimulation in the human. Second World Congress on Pain. IASP. Pain Abstr. *1*, 308 (1978)
6. Fields, H., Adams, J.E.: Pain after cortical injury relieved by electrical stimulation of the internal capsule. Pain *79*, 169– 178 (1974)
7. Gybels, J.: Electrical stimulation of the central gray for pain relief in humans. A critical review. Second World Congress on Pain, IASP. Pain Abstr. *1*, 170 (1978)
8. Hosobuchi, Y.: Central grey stimulation for pain suppression in humans. Second World congress on Pain, IASP. Pain Abstr. *1*, 169 (1978)
9. Hosobuchi, Y., Adams, J.E., Fields, H.L.: Chronic thalamic and internal capsule stimulation for the control of anaesthesia dolorosa and dysesthesia of thalamic syndrome. International Symposium on Pain. In: Advances in neurology 4, Bonica, J.J. (ed.), pp. 785–787. New York: Raven Press 1974
10. Hosobuchi, Y., Adams, J.E., Linchitz, R.: Pain relief by electrical stimulation in the central gray matter and its removal by naloxone. Science *197*, 183–197 (1977)
11. Hosobuchi, Y., Adams, J.E., Rutkin, B.: Chronic thalamic stimulation for the control of facial anesthesia dolorosa. Arch. Neurol. *29*, 158–161 (1973)
12. Hosobuchi, Y., Wemmer, J.: Disulfiram inhibition of development of tolerance to analgesia induced by central gray stimulation in humans. Eur. J. Pharmacol. *43*, 383–387 (1977)
13. Mazars, G.J.: Intermittent stimulation of nucleus ventralis posterolateralis for intractable pain. Surg. Neurol. *4*, 93–95 (1975)
14. Nashold, B.S., Jr., Wilson, W.P.: Central pain observations in man with chronic implanted electrodes in the midbrain tegmentum. Confin. Neurol. *27*, 30–44 (1966)
15. Ray, C.D., Nida, G.A., Pelletier, G.J., Burton, C.V.: Control of severe, chronic pain by depth brain stimulator implantation: Aspects of anatomy behaviour evaluation and rehabilitation in 20 cases. Second World Congress on Pain, IASP. Pain Abstt., *1*, 307 (1978)

16. Richardson, D.E.: Brain stimulation for pain control. I.E.E.E. Trans. Biomed. Eng. B.M.E. *23,* 304–306 (1976)
17. Richardson, D.E., Akil, H.: Pain reduction by electrical brain stimulation in man. Part 1, Acute administration in periaqueductal and periventricular sites. J. Neurosurg. *47,* 178–183 (1977)
18. Richardson, D.E., and Akil, H.: Pain reduction by electrical brain stimulation in man. Part 11, Chronic self administration in the periventricular gray matter. J. Neurosurg. *47,* 184–194 (1977)
19. Unrecorded discussion, 3rd European Workshop on Electrical Neurostimulation. Megeve, March 30–31, 1979

Control of Pain in Brachial Plexus Avulsion, Spinal Paraplegia and Herpes Using DREZ Lesions

B.S. Nashold, R.H. Ostdahl, and E. Bullitt

Historical

In 1824, Rolando described a large area of grey matter in the dorsal spinal cord and named it the *substantia gelatinosa*. This grey matter of the dorsal horn is now known as the dorsal root entry zone (DREZ).

Anatomy and Functional Organization of the DREZ

Anatomically the dorsal root entry zone (DREZ) can be divided into six laminae, as proposed by the neuroanatomist Rexed (4). These anatomical divisions also have functional characteristics. Rexed (4) designated six laminae with lamina I made up of dense dentritic fibres running horizontally along the longitudinal aspect of the cord. The substantia gelatinosa is probably represented by laminae II and III which receives a very substantial efferent-afferent input. The neurons in this region develop prolonged discharge after stimulation which suggests that this area could be the origin of the intractable pain syndromes which are relieved after lesions of the dorsal root entry zone. Pharmacological studies reveal a number of chemical agents. There are synaptic excitatory transmitters such as glutamic acid, substance P, as well as enkephalins, neurotensin, cholecystokinin, neurophysin, oxytocin and glucagon, but the role of these agents in the genesis of pain is unknown.

Clinical

Fifty-four patients with intractable central pain syndromes due to spinal injury (*17*), brachial plexus avulsion (*27*), post-herpetic pain (*8*) and a peripheral nerve lesion (*2*) have been treated by this new technique of multiple focal coagulations of the dorsal root entry zone. Twenty-six patients sustained complete avulsion of the brachial plexus due to direct trauma, one patient had an incomplete avulsion and one patient suffered an avulsion of the pelvic plexus from the conus medullaris as the result of a traumatic leg amputation. Seventeen patients suffered traumatic paraplegia and seven patients suffered from herpetic infection and post-herpetic pain involving the arm and/or thoracic region. Two patients sustained multiple traumas to the ulnar nerve at the elbow

Modern Neurosurgery 1. Edited by M. Brock

resulting in a long term chronic pain syndrome. One patient included in the brachial plexus group sustained a gunshot wound of the cervical spine with partial tetraparesis and intractable pain in the distribution of the C6 nerve root.

Surgical Technique of DREZ Coagulation

The DREZ coagulations are made along the intermediolateral sulcus of the dorsal surface of the spinal cord (Fig. 1). In the patients with brachial plexus avulsion, the dorsal roots and, often, the ventral roots are absent, but the sulcus can be easily identified by magnification. At the present time we are using a standard percutaneous cordotomy type electrode with an exposed tip of 3 mm (Radionics). The dura over the involved area of the spinal cord must be opened cautiously, especially in patients with brachial plexus avulsion and spinal injury because of extensive arachnoiditis. These adhesions are carefully divided until the scar tissue around the spinal cord is freed. This is especially important in the paraplegic patient where there can be tethering of the spinal cord, usually on the inner surface of the dorsal dura. We have found several paraplegic patients in whom traction on the tethered cord has activated their central pain. In some patients, there appears to be hypervascularization on the dorsal surface of the cord involving the injured segment and this seems most noticeable in the paraplegic.

In one paraplegic patient with a T 4 thoracic transection, a large cyst extended above the site of the trauma into the cervical area, producing arm pain. Evacuation of the cyst relieved the pain for two years, but it then recurred without cyst formation, and the pain was only later relieved by DREZ lesions. Patients with herpes and ulnar neuropathy have normal cord morphology with intact dorsal roots, so that the identification of the lesion site becomes easier for the surgeon. The lesion electrode is introduced into the intermediolateral sulcus for a distance of 2–3 mm at an angle of 25° in the medial direction. The RF coagulation is then made (Radionics), and in our initial report in 1979 (2) we had used a current of 70 ma for 15 sec. for each separate coagulation, with a distance of 2–3 mm between each coagulation site. We now recommend in all cases 30–40 ma coagulation ofr 10 to 15 sec. and believe that this has reduced the post-operative complications. We may make as many as 15 to 20 lesions, especially in a patient with brachial plexus avulsion. In the paraplegics, the coagulation is bilateral, beginning at the level of the trauma and extending cephalad over at least two to three root segments. Where the dorsal roots are intact, such as in the patients with herpes or cancer, the site for the placement of the lesion can easily be determined because the rootlets are well defined in the dorsal intermediolateral column. In these patients, the selection of the dorsal roots to be treated by coagulation is determined clinically by the distribution of the pain over the extremity and in the case of cutaneous herpetic eruption, the dermatome involved is a good guide. There are often small arteries running in the dorsal sulcus of normal and injured cord, and these may be coagulated during the lesion without any serious consequence. The larger dorsal arteries must be preserved. The use of pre-operative and intra-operative steroids is routine. After the lesion, the spinal cord shows no visual evidence of change except at the individual lesion site.

Results

Brachial Plexus (27 patients). There was no surgical mortality in any of the groups. A 70% pain relief occurred in the patient with brachial plexus avulsion with the longest follow-up five years (2). One patient with an isolated injury to C 6 as the result of a gunshot wound to the spine was relieved after DREZ lesions of the C 6 rootlets and upper filaments of the C 7 root. The immediate postoperative morbidity included ipsilateral clumsiness and proprioceptive defects of the ipsilateral leg in 52% of the patients. Postoperative sensory changes such as hypo-aesthesia to pin-prick over the chest area, occurred in 28% of patients, but resolved in a short time.

Paraplegia (17 patients). Pain relief occurred in 50% of these patients, however, the follow-up time is shorter with the longest being three years (3). One patient had a transient loss of reflex bladder function, a second man lost his ability to walk, although he was completely wheelchair bound pre-operatively. One patient with arm pain associated with a cervical syrinx and pain, temporarily, lost finger mobility. Several recent patients with partial motor control in one leg have maintained this function postoperatively.

Herpes (8 patients). Excellent pain relief occurred in 4/8 patients with herpes, 2/8 poor relief and 1/8 failure. Two of these suffered from extensive involvement of the arm, shoulder and chest while the third had localized thoracic pain. Two patients, one with arm pain and another with arm and shoulder and chest pain, were partially relieved, while two with isolated thoracic pain were not helped. The follow-up averages six months in this group of patients with one patient with an excellent result now relieved for one year.

Peripheral Nerve Injury (2 patients). Two patients suffered pain in the ulnar distribution due to trauma and multiple surgical operations. Complete relief of pain with DREZ lesions of C 7, C 8 and T 1. Follow-up nine months.

References

1. Nashold, B.S., Urban, B., Zorub, D.S.: Phantom pain relief by focal destruction of substantia gelatinosa of Rolando. In: Advances in pain research and therapy, Vol. 1. Bonica, Albe-Fessard (eds.), pp. 959–963. New York: Raven Press 1976
2. Nashold, B.S., Ostdahl, R.: Dorsal root entry zone lesions for pain relief. J. Neurosurg. *51*, 59–69 (1979)
3. Nashold, B.S., Bullitt, E.: Dorsal root entry zone lesions to control central pain in paraplegics. J. Neurosurg. (in press)
4. Rexed, B.: A cytoarchitectonic atlas of the spinal cord in the cat. J. Comp. Neurol. *100*, 297–380 (1954)

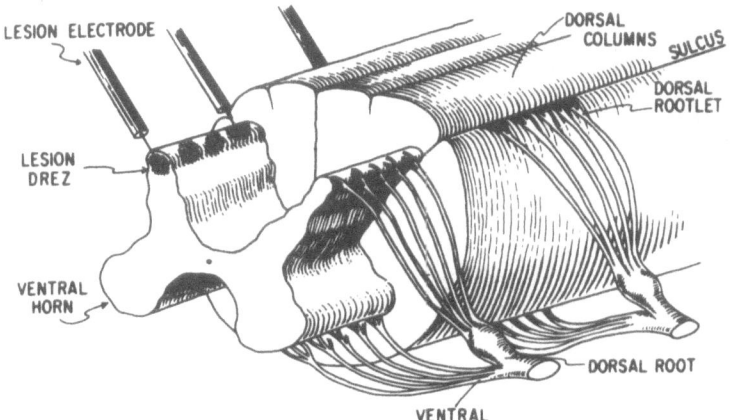

Fig. 1. Schematic drawing demonstrating the spinal cord and dorsal root entry zone (DREZ) (Permission of J. Neurosurg.)

CSF Endorphins Level in Patients with Cancer Pain Treated by Cervical Percutaneous Cordotomy

G. Salar, I. Job, M. Trabucchi, A. Bosio, and S. Mingrino

Introduction

Since 1975 various Authors (3, 5, 7, 13) have pointed out a clear correlation between endogenous polypeptides — endorphins and enkephalins — and pain mechanisms.

Terenius (14) found CSF endorphins level significantly lower in patients with chronic organic pain and much higher in patients with psychiatric disorders. He explains this finding by suggesting that the organic pain induces a general depression on the endorphinergic system followed by hypersensitivity to other painful stimuli. An alternative interpretation is that the low endorphins level in pain patients is caused by the increased consumption of the endorphinergic system which inhibits nociception. This system, chronically stimulated in subjects with persistent pain, could be saturated and unable to defend the patient from other nociceptive impulses.

It is already well known that stimulation of such descending pathways with pain inhibitory function, both at periaqueductal level (1, 4) or by percutaneous (12) or transcutaneous (6) electrostimulation, provokes analgesia or hypoalgesia and increases CSF endorphins level. This behaviour could signify an activation of the endorphinergic system, according to Terenius' hypothesis (14), with transient increase of CSF endorphin levels.

At this point, the main problem is: if electrotherapy definitely produces pain reduction by increasing CSF endorphins level, are the other pharmacologic or surgical procedures able to stimulate the endorphinergic system? In particular, if the afferent nociceptive pathway is interrupted by surgical procedures such as cervical percutaneous cordotomy in patients with chronic pain, do the CSF endorphins level remain unchanged — i.e. low with respect to normal subjects — or increase?

For this purpose we studied CSF levels of β-endorphins in a group of ten patients with chronic cancer pain before and after cervical percutaneous radiofrequency cordotomy.

Material and Methods

We examined ten patients, admitted during the first months of 1980 to the Institute of Neurosurgery of the University of Padua for lung cancer pain; seven of them had typical Pancoast syndrome and three showed multiple lesions in the bones.

All the patients were male, mean age 46. The youngest was 36, the oldest 57 years old.

Pain symptoms had been present from 7 to 2 months before, mean 3 months. During this period all our patients underwent several pharmacological treatments, in particular, all of them received morphine during the last three weeks before operation in doses ranging from 30 mg to 60 mg/die.

The surgical indication arose from the low analgesic effect of the drugs, the relatively young age of the patients, their good general condition and the unilateral localization of pain. Before treatment each patient underwent lumbar puncture to obtain 4 ml of CSF. At that time each subject had severe pain and did not receive any drugs in the preceding six hours. Immediately after the lumbar puncture the patients were operated on, and a cervical percutaneous radiofrequency cordotomy was done at C1–C2 level, following the usual standardized technique (9).

A further CSF sample was then obtained 24–36 hours after the surgical procedure. During this period none of the patients received drugs, particularly morphine.

The CSF samples obtained always had normal cytochemical findings. In a second group of ten patients (six males and four females) with no pain problem similar CSF samples were obtained from lumbar puncture performed for diagnostic procedures. Their mean age was 42, the oldest was 58, the youngest 31 years old. Even in this group the CSF cytochemical findings were completely normal.

The technique for the evaluation of CSF endorphin content has been that described by Rossier et al. (10), with minor modifications. The extraction of the endorphin fraction consisted in heating for ten minutes at 100°C, followed by lyophilization and a five-fold concentration. We used a radioimmunoassay (RIA), which is highly specific for Leu^{14} – His^{27} segment of β-endorphin. Since β-endorphin is the C-terminal 31 amino-acid fragment of β-lipotropin (β-LPH) this RIA detects both β-endorphin and β-LPH content in every sample. However using column chromatography the two molecules were separated, obtaining the CSF values of β-endorphin.

Results

The mean CSF endorphins levels in patients without pain problems is pg/ml 336.45– s.d. 60.47.

Table 1 indicates our group of patients with corresponding CSF endorphins levels before and after percutaneous cervical cordotomy and the clinical results 24–36 hours after the surgical treatment. The pain disappeared completely after operation in six patients, two had a marked reduction. In the last two cases the pain was slightly reduced but was tolerable without analgesic drugs.

Comparing the mean CSF endorphins levels before operation in our group of pain patients (pg/ml 278.2 –s.d. 51.72) with those obtained from the control group (pg/ml 336.45 –s.d. 60.47), the first appears lower; this mean variation is statistically significant (t: 2,32). Moreover the mean pre-operative CSF levels in the group with pain symptoms seem relatively lower with respect to those obtained in the same patients after the surgical treatment (pg/ml 315.4 –s.d. 86.48); this mean variation is not statistically significant (t: 1.53).

Table 1. The CSF endorphins levels are expressed in pg/ml. In the clinical results (+++) represents complete relief of pain, (++) marked reduction and (+) slight reduction of pain. The mean variation of CSF endorphins levels before and after cordotomy (278.2–s.d. 51,72 and 315.4–s.d. 86.48; t: 1,53) is not significant. Considering only cases with (+++) (Patients No. 1, 2, 3, 4, 5 and 6) the mean variation of CSF endorphins levels before and after cordotomy (274.5–s.d. 68.04 and 330.7 –s.d. 110.51; t: 1,43) is also not significant

No. of patient	CSF β-endorphins levels Precordotomy	Postcordotomy	Clinical results
1	305	523	+++
2	208	304	+++
3	395	360	+++
4	229	240	+++
5	270	345	+++
6	240	212	+++
7	285	315	++
8	270	245	++
9	305	318	+
10	275	292	+
Mean	278.2	315.4	
	–s.d. 51,72	–s.d. 86,48	

Considering only the six cases with good surgical results four of them had CSF endorphins level higher than before operation, but in two cases it was lower; the mean preoperative CSF levels of the six cases (pg/ml 274.5 –s.d. 68,04) is lower with respect to those obtained in the same patients after cordotomy (pg/ml 330.7 –s.d. 110.51); this mean variation is not statistically significant (t: 1,43).

The other four cases with marked or slight reduction of pain showed no significant variation of CSF endorphins level after the surgical treatment.

Discussion and Conclusion

The first important point which emerges from our data is that the mean CSF endorphins levels in subjects with chronic pain is significantly lower than those obtained from the control group without pain problems. This seems to confirm the hypothesis of Terenius (14) and Almay et al. (2), that chronic patients have a reduced endorphinergic activity.

The second point concerns the comparison between CSF endorphins levels before and after percutaneous cervical cordotomy: the postoperative values appear higher in the majority of cases, but the mean variation has no statistical significance. The interpretation of these findings is difficult because of the scanty experience; it seems that the endorphinergic system does not change in the same way in all cases after the surgical interruption of the painful sensation.

No final evidence about a correlation between reduction of pain and increased availability of morphine-like polypeptides can be obtained from our data. This is different from the recent reports of Hosobuchi et al. (4), Akil et al. (1), Sjolund et al. (12), von Knorring et al. (6) and Salar et al. (11), who found statistically significant variations of CSF endorphins levels during central or peripheral electrostimulation. It seems that these techniques can mobilize a large part of the endorphinic reserve in patients with or without pain problems, even if for a short time, inducing analgesia or hypoalgesia.

The limits of the present work may be summarized in the following points:

1. Postoperative evaluation has been carried out 24—36 hours after operation, and this might be too short a period to restore the normal level of endorphins, eventually worn by chronic pain.

2. All our patients made prolonged use of morphinic drugs before they were operated on. The chronic use of these drugs might have markedly altered the mechanisms of endorphin-mediated pain by a feedback mechanism, with reduction of these substances (8). For this reason the CSF samples obtained 6 hours after stopping the drugs (first lumbar puncture, before operation) and 30—42 hours later (second lumbar puncture, after operation) could be not sufficiently representative.

It would be interesting, therefore, to check the changes in endorphins levels after a longer interval, when the clinical results and the endorphinergic system are reasonably stabilized, in particular in the absence of pain and without any administration of drugs.

References

1. Akil, H., Richardson, D.E., Hughes, J., Barchas, J.D.: Enkephalin-like material elevated in ventricular cerebrospinal of pain patients after analgesic focal stimulation. Science 201, 463—465 (1978)

2. Almay, B.G.L., Johansson, F., v. Knorring, L., Terenius, L., Wahlstrom, A.: Endorphins in chronic pain. Difference in CSF endorphin levels between organic and psychogenic syndromes. Pain 5, 153—162 (1978)

3. Goldstein, A.: Opioid peptides (endorphins) in pituitary and brain. Science 193, 1081—1086 (1976)

4. Hosobuchi, Y., Rossier, J., Bloom, F.E., Guillemin, R.: Stimulation of human periaqueductal gray for pain relief increase immunoreactive-β-endorphin in ventricular fluid. Science 203, 279—281 (1979)

5. Hughes, J.: Isolation of an endogenous compound from the brain with pharmacological properties similar to morphine. Brain Res. 61, 417—422 (1975)

6. v. Knorring, L., Almay, B.G.L., Johansson, F.: Pain perception and endorphin levels in cerebrospinal fluid. Pain 5, 359—365 (1978)

7. Kosterlitz, N.W., Hughes, J.: Some throughts on the signification of enkephalins, the endogenous ligand. Life Science 17, 91—96 (1975)

8. Malfroy, B., Swerts, J.P., Guyon, A., Roques, B.P., Schwartz, J.C.: High-affinity enkephalin- degrading peptidase in brain is increased after morphine. Nature 276, 523—526 (1978)

9. Rosomoff, H.L.: Percutaneous radiofrequency cervical cordotomy technique. J. Neurosurg. 23, 639—644 (1965)

10. Rossier, J., Bayon, A., Vargo, T.M., Ling, N., Guillemin, R., Bloom, F.: Radioimmunoassay of brain peptides: evaluation of a methodology for the assay of β-endorphin and enkephalin. Life Sci. 21, 847—852 (1977)

11. Salar, G., Job, I., Mingrino, S., Bosio, A., Trabucchi, M.: Effect of transcutaneous electrotherapy on CSF β-endorphin content in patients without pain problems. Pain 10, 169—172 (1981)

12. Sjolund, B., Terenius, L., Eriksson, M.: Increased CSF levels of endorphins after electro-acupuncture. Acta Physiol. Scand. *100*, 382–384 (1977)
13. Snyder, S.M., Simantov, R.: The opiate receptor and opioid peptides. J. Neurochemistry *28*, 13–20 (1977)
14. Terenius, L.: The endorphins in endogenous antinociception. In: Advances in biochemical psychopharmacology: the endorphins, Vol. 1. Costa, E., Trabucchi, M. (eds.), pp. 321–332. New York: Raven Press 1978

Technique and Results of 800 Percutaneous Radiofrequency Thermocoagulations for Trigeminal Neuralgia

G.R. Nugent

In the early 1930's Kirschner popularized the electrocoagulation of the Gasserian ganglion for the treatment of trigeminal neuralgia. He used a very imaginative stereotaxic device which facilitated penetration of the foramen ovale and a large series of patients was treated with this technique (2). In the early 1970's Sweet introduced a refinement of this technique utilizing radiofrequency current which brought about a measure of control to the technique not possible with the electrocoagulation of Kirschner (4). The technique of Sweet is widely used in this country as well as other parts of the world.

We have altered the technique of Sweet in three ways. Most important of these is the use of a much smaller cordotomy-type electrode which permits the creation of the lesion while the patient is fully awake. This permits monitoring of the patient while the lesion is being made and thus permits control over the extent and location of the lesion and markedly reduces the incidence of corneal anaesthesia. To identify the AP and lateral coordinates of the target site, 54 cadaver skulls with a lead marker in Meckel's cave were placed in the Todd-Wells stereotaxic frame. The radiographic landmarks thus obtained have been previously reported and greatly facilitate penetration of the foramen ovale (3). Ordinarily, penetration of the foramen ovale is the easiest part of the entire procedure. Far more important and very often more difficult is the creation of an accurate and satisfactory lesion once the foramen has been penetrated.

Advantages

This technique is ordinarily carried out with little morbidity. It is therefore well tolerated by the elderly and the stay in hospital is brief. Our patients are treated in the morning and leave the hospital after lunch. There is no risk of facial paralysis.

Disadvantages

Theoretically the ideal way to treat trigeminal neuralgia is to stop the pain without creating numbness in the face. The vascular decompression procedure popularized by Dr. Jannetta may meet this theoretical ideal (1). A disadvantage of this radiofrequency procedure, therefore, is that cure is obtained at the expense of creating numbness in the face. Ordinarily this is no problem and most patients are happy to have the numb face to be rid of the severe pain. A problem, however, is that a small percentage of patients will develop annoying paraesthesias and dysaesthesias in the face. In our series this is 5%. There is a spectrum of this disorder running from most minimal and insignificant to anaesthesia dolorosa at the other end of the scale. Although it is true that the more dense the sensory deficit, the more sure the cure, it is also true that the more dense the sensory deficit the higher the incidence of these annoying sensations in the face associated with sensory deprivation. It is our aim therefore in this procedure, to create the most minimal sensory deficit consistent with lasting relief of the pain. This does mean that there will be a higher recurrence rate than otherwise (23% in our series) but this is such a simple and benign procedure that it can easily be repeated should the pain recur.

Anaesthetic Technique

No premedication is used but on arrival in the treatment room 2.5–5 mg (1–2ml) of Droperidol or, diazepam 3 to 5 mg is given I.V. In addition they receive 0.1 mg (2ml) of Fentanyl intravenously. Additional Fentanyl may be necessary in some cases. 1% plain lidocaine is used in the cheek. Penetration of the foramen ovale is usually the most painful part of the procedure and when the needle is aligned outside the foramen ovale, the patient is given between 30 to 50 mg of methohexital (Brevital). When asleep, the needle is passed through the foramen ovale.

Penetration of the Foramen Ovale

Various techniques have been recommended but we prefer the technique based upon our identification of the target site in cadaver skulls (3). To start the procedure a finger is placed in the mouth and an 18 gauge thin walled lumbar puncture needle measuring 10 cm in length is passed through the cheek approximately 2.5 cm lateral to the corner of the mouth. If a deviation from this landmark is to occur at this point it should be in the direction of a more inferior localization rather than superior. The needle is aimed at the pupil in the AP dimension and at a point on the zygoma approximately 2.5 cm anterior to the auditory meatus laterally. It is then brought to the base of the skull. The finger remains in the mouth throughout this part. We then use an image intensifier to obtain a lateral projection. The target site in this projection is the vertex of the angle produced by the shadow of the clivus and the petrous ridge (Fig. 1). The needle should be oriented so it is directed at this point. In the antero-posterior projection the target site is approximately 9 mm medial to the lateral wall of the internal auditory meatus as visualized on the AP projection which is made shooting down the orbito-meatal line (Fig. 2). This projection permits visualization of the internal auditory meati through the orbits. When the needle is oriented in these two projections, the methohexital is given and usually the needle is passed through the foramen without difficulty.

The Electrode

We use a 0.016 inch diameter cordotomy type electrode with a 3 mm exposed tip in preference to the much larger 19 gauge 5 or 7.5 mm temperature monitoring electrode which was introduced by Sweet (Fig. 3). We feel that the smaller electrode, which can be angled, permits the lesion to be made while the patient is awake and, therefore, allows more control over the extent and location of the lesion. Temperature monitoring is not possible with this smaller electrode but temperature monitoring is not necessary. More important than temperature monitoring is careful patient monitoring which is possible when the patient is awake. The temperature monitoring electrode is so large that it is impossible to avoid burning the Gasserian ganglion which is exceedingly painful. It is a fact that a heat lesion of the Gasserian ganglion or of the divisions distal to the ganglion is extremely painful but a heat lesion proximal to the ganglion in the retrogasserian rootlets is ordinarily well tolerated by the patient. If severe pain is produced while the radiofrequency generator is turned on it is because the electrode is in the ganglion or distal to it or is up against the pain sensitive dura which surrounds the nerve. The hub of the lumbar puncture needle acts as the indifferent or ground electrode.

Sometimes when using this small electrode, boiling may occur before the procedure has been completed. Once this occurs the current falls off and a larger lesion cannot be made with the electrode at that location. It will then have to be shifted to a slightly different position. One must remember that once the electrode is shifted the current has to be turned down to the original setting and the whole process started all over again.

Results

Table 1. Results of 800 procedures on 643 patients

	No.	%
Recurrence requiring a second procedure (10 of these were performed elsewhere)	146	23
Moderate paraesthesiae & dysaesthesiae	70	9
Annoying paraesthesiae & dysaesthesiae (44% rated the treatment Good to Excellent)	41	5
Anaesthesia Dolorosa	6	1
Loss of corneal reflex	25	3
Loss of corneal reflex in last 600 cases	13	2
Corneal reflex diminished	65	8
Neurolytic keratitis	5	1
Blind	0	
Motor root impaired	198	25

Average length of follow-up: 4.7 years

Discussion

Once the needle has penetrated the retrogasserian rootlets there should be a free flow of cerebral spinal fluid from the needle. At this point the localization depends upon three things: the depth of penetration, the response to stimualtion and the radiographic localization. The deeper the penetration the more likely the first division will be treated (Fig. 4), but it must be remembered that the gasserian ganglion and retrogasserian rootlets lie on a plane running from supero-medial to infero-lateral.

Unquestionably the single most important observation leading to the correct localization of the electrode is a low voltage response to stimulation. When the electrode tip lies within the retrogasserian rootlets the awake patient will experience electrical like tingling and paraesthesiae in the face at 60 Hz and 0.1 volt or less. When this is the case, and at the same time the radiographic landmarks are correct, the surgeon can usually be confident that he is going to be able to proceed with a satisfactory lesion without trouble. By rotating the angled electrode within the lumbar puncture needle it is possible to alter the location and response to stimulation without moving the entire assembly in or out. This facilitates the proper location of the needle in the rootlets to be treated. Ordinarily, when the needle is properly located radiographs will demonstrate it lying just below the petrous ridge, as seen on the AP projection and at or just posterior to the shadow of the clivus on the lateral view. If the tip of the electrode should project above the petrous ridge on the AP projection care must be taken to avoid unwanted involvement of the first division.

It is most important to appreciate that at times the retrogasserian rootlets can be almost destroyed by heat with no discomfort or awareness on the part of the conscious patient or the physician, that this is occuring. This seems to be particularly true for the first division fibres. Therefore, constant monitoring, along with numerous small incremental lesions in the conscious patient are important to avoid the creation of too much sensory deficit. During the creation of the lesion the patient may be aware of a burning sensation in the face in the area of the lesion. If the second division is being treated, this may creep up to involve the anterior temporal region lateral to the eye. If it then spreads into the globe or supraorbital area the first division is becomming involved. It is important when treating this area to constantly monitor the eyelash reflex. With the eyes closed the eyelashes are lightly stroked with a piece of twisted facial tissue and the direct and consensual blink response observed. When this starts to diminish the first division is becomming involved.

Sometimes a flush is noted in the face in the area in which the lesion is being made. This is a helpful guide to the location of the lesion.

In general the AP projection has proved to be far more useful for localizing the electrode than the lateral projection. There is extreme variability on the lateral view with some third division lesions being made with the electrode posterior the the clivus and first division lesions sometimes occurring with the electrode anterior to the clivus.

The end point is a judgment decision and it is our aim to create dense hypalgesia in the region of the trigeminal neuralgia pain but not analgesia. It is usually possible to treat trigeminal neuralgia triggering from the first division by creating moderate sensory deficit in the first division but with sparing of the corneal reflex. We were able to treat first division pain and spare the corneal reflex in 92% of patients.

If a motor response is produced during stimulation, the electrode is too medial in position.

Another reason for having the patient awake during the creation of the lesion is that occasionally the response to stimulation may indicate that the electrode tip is in one location but the lesion occurs in another.

It is important to appreciate that pain spreading from the second division up into the first division requires treatment of the second division only. It is only necessary to treat the first division when the patient's pain is triggered by touching the first division.

We usually make our first lesion at somewhere between 10–12 volts and 60 to 70 milliamps with a 15 to 20 second lesion. It no sensory deficit is created, a 40 second lesion is made, and if there is still no numbness in the face the current is increased and another 15 to 20 second lesion made. This process is continued until the endpoint is reached.

The best lesions are often made in the presence of a free flow of cerebro-spinal fluid, at a low voltage threshold of stimulation, and with surprisingly little discomfort in the face during the making of the lesion.

Complications

If the above described radiographic landmarks are not observed during the insertion of the needle the carotid artery can be punctured. When this occurs the needle is almost invariably too medial and too inferior in its location. Should this occur it is not necessary to abandon the procedure. Merely relocate the needle in the proper position and proceed with the treatment.

Corneal anaesthesia is usually unassociated with complications but neurolytic keratitis may occur, and meticulous eye care is necessary to prevent impairment of vision. No patients in our series have lost their vision though neurolytic keratitis occurred in five patients.

We had two patients with transient diplopia. One due to a fourth and the other to a sixth nerve palsy. A higher incidence of this has been reported by others.

Carotid cavernous sinus fistulas have been reported but when small and consisting of only a subjective and objective bruit, they may heal spontaneously. We had two such patients.

Meningitis has been reported by others but has never occurred in our series.

Conclusion

We present a technique of treating trigeminal neuralgia with radiofrequency current and outline our method of penetrating the foramen ovale, along with our use of a much smaller cordotomy-type electrode. With this smaller 3 mm electrode it is possible to thermocoagulate the retrogasserian rootlets where pain is minimal. The patient can, therefore, be awake throughout the lesion so that the extent and location of the sensory deficit can be carefully monitored. This permits a low incidence of: corneal anaesthesia, annoying paraesthesiae and dysaesthesiae, sensory deficit in unwanted areas and other complications.

References

1. Jannetta, P.J.: Observations on the etiology of trigeminal neuralgia, hemifacial spasm, acoustic nerve dysfunction, and glossopharyngeal neuralgia: Definitive microsurgical treatment and results in 117 patients. Neurochirurgia. *20*, 145–154 (1977)
2. Kirschner, M.: Zur Behandlung der Trigeminus Neuralgie. Med. Wochenschr. *89*, 235–239 (1942)
3. Nugent, G.R., Berry, B.: Trigeminal neuralgia treated by differential percutaneous radiofrequency coagulation of the Gasserian ganglion. J. Neurosurg. *40*, 517–523 (1974)
4. Sweet, W.H., Wepsic, S.G.: Controlled thermocoagulations of trigeminal ganglion and results for differential destruction of pain fibers. J. Neurosurg. *39*, 143–156 (1974)

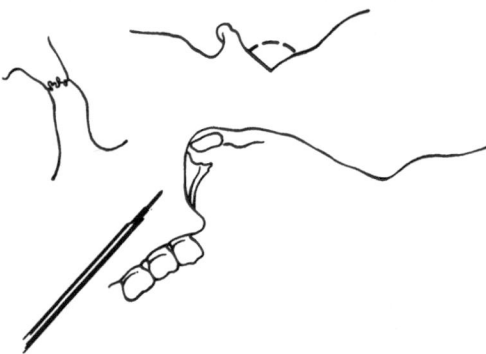

Fig. 1. Radiographic studies on cadaver skulls identified the lateral target site at the vertex of the angle produced by the clivus and petrous ridge. (Reproduced with permission from J. Neurosurg. 40:518, 1974)

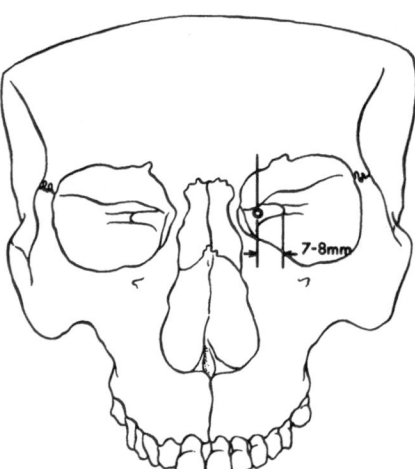

Fig. 2. The antero-posterior target is, considering radiographic magnification, approximately 9 mm directly medial to the lateral wall of the internal auditory meatus (Reproduced with permission from J. Neurosurg. 40:518, 1974)

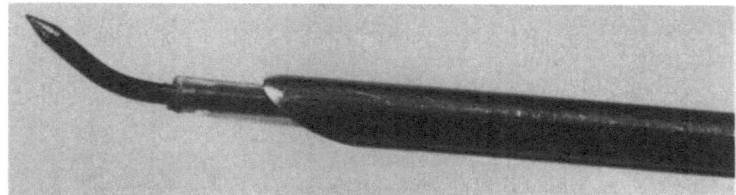

Fig. 3. The active element of the cordotomy-type electrode measures 0.406 mm by 3 mm and is angled to permit greater flexibility and control over the lesion

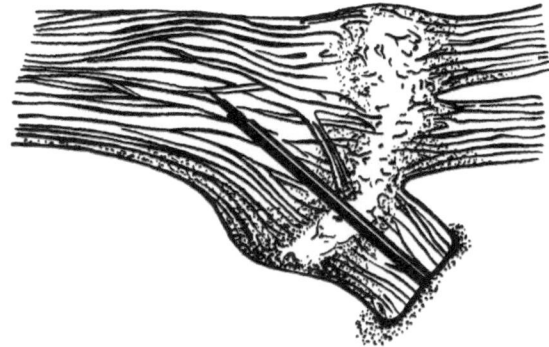

Fig. 4. The active component of the electrode lies behind the Gasserian ganglion within the rootlets bathed in cerebrospinal fluid. A second division lesion would be made at this location

Subject Index

Surgery of
Cervical Myelopathy
Infantile Hydrocephalus:
Long-Term Results

Editors: W. Grote, M. Brock, H. E. Clar,
M. Klinger, H. E. Nau

1980. 178 figures in 215 separate illustrations,
138 tables. XVII, 456 pages
(Advances in Neurosurgery, Volume 8)
ISBN 3-540-09949-2
Distribution rights for Japan:
Nankodo Co. Ltd., Tokyo

Contents:
Cervical Myelopathy. – Hydrocephalus in
Childhood. – Free Topics. – Subject Index.

Brain Abscess and
Meningitis Subarachnoid
Hemorrhage:
Timing Problems

Editors: W. Schiefer, M. Klinger, M. Brock

1981. 219 figures, 134 tables. XIX, 519 pages
(Advances in Neurosurgery, Volume 9)
ISBN 3-540-10539-5

Distribution rights for Japan:
Nankodo Co. Ltd., Tokyo

Contents:
Brain Abscess and Meningitis. – Subara-
chnoid Hemorrhage: Timing Problems. –
Free Topics. – Subject Index.

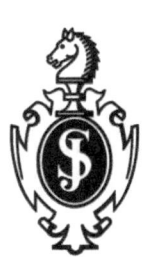

Springer-Verlag
Berlin
Heidelberg
New York

The Cranial Nerves

Anatomy · Pathology · Pathophysiology · Diagnosis · Treatment

Editors: M. Samii, P. J. Jannetta

1981. 410 figures. XVII, 664 pages
ISBN 3-540-10620-0

Contents:
History of Cranial Nerves Surgery. – Introductory Lecture. – Topographical Anatomy of the Cranial Nerves. – Cranial Nerve Injury. Structural and Pathophysiological Considerations and a Classification of Nerve Injury. – Experimental Studies on Neural Regeneration. – Olfactory Nerve (First Cranial Nerve). – Optic Nerve (Second Cranial Nerve). – Oculomotor, Trochlear and Abducens Nerves. – Trigeminal Nerve (Fifth Cranial Nerve). – Facial and Vestibulo-Cochlear Nerves (Seventh and Eight Cranial Nerves). – Clinical Aspects of Facial Nerve. – Cochleo-Vestibular Nerve. – Caudial Cranial Nerves.

This is the first book to present an interdisciplinary review of all aspects of the cranial nerves: anatomy, pathology, physiology, radiology and all relevant surgical disciplines. Outstanding scientists and pineers in their fields report their newest research and experience. In doing this they provide diverse views of diagnosis and treatment in respect of the individual cranical nerves and compare various techniques. This book is particularly concerned with the possibilities that now exist for interdisciplinary microsurgical treatment to conserve function by curing pathologic processes, and for reconstructive surgery.

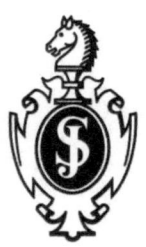

Springer-Verlag
Berlin
Heidelberg
New York